Computational Bioengineering

Computational Bioengineering

edited by
Guigen Zhang
Clemson University
South Carolina, USA

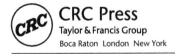
CRC Press
Taylor & Francis Group
Boca Raton London New York

CRC Press is an imprint of the
Taylor & Francis Group, an **informa** business

CRC Press
Taylor & Francis Group
6000 Broken Sound Parkway NW, Suite 300
Boca Raton, FL 33487-2742

First issued in paperback 2017

© 2015 by Taylor & Francis Group, LLC
CRC Press is an imprint of Taylor & Francis Group, an Informa business

No claim to original U.S. Government works

ISBN-13: 978-1-4665-1755-4 (hbk)
ISBN-13: 978-1-138-85020-0 (pbk)

Contents

Preface

This book is prepared with an intent to serve as a stepping stone toward establishing computational bioengineering as an area of study. Bioengineering, or biomedical engineering, is a field in which biomedical problems are solved based on myriad laws of physics and thermodynamics, as well as biology. Over the past decades, advances in bioengineering have contributed to numerous innovations and developments of medical devices, sensors, implants, prostheses, and so on, and they have resulted in significant improvement in our quality of life. However, one of the major challenges facing the field of bioengineering is its reliance on the knowledge and investigative approaches developed with reductive approaches originated in many traditional disciplines.

Computational bioengineering can take advantage of the latest computational capabilities to deal with biomedical problems using an integrative approach. Although computer modeling has been used to tackle bioengineering problems for decades, the types of problems tackled are mainly of hard and soft tissue mechanics and fluid mechanics. As a field of study, computational bioengineering should address not only problems of a mechanical nature but also electrical, electrostatic, electrochemical, chemical, biochemical, thermal, and electromagnetic problems, among others, either individually or combined, under the governing laws of physics, thermodynamics, and biology.

It is believed that a systematic study of computational bioengineering will not only help address many critical challenges facing bioengineering but also set a new direction for advancing the field. In the long run, this book is expected to foster integrative problem-solving mentality in engineering students and practitioners for the generation of new and novel solutions to future biomedical problems.

Each chapter in the book begins with a brief review of the advances in computational efforts in the selected topic area and ends with case studies with detailed technical information. The brief reviews are intended to provide a relevant overview of the selected topic area for readers, and the case studies aim to demonstrate the power of computational modeling in offering predictive capabilities to assess new surgical concepts and medical devices and postoperative surgical outcomes. In addition, this book aims to illustrate the expanded capabilities of computational bioengineering through discussions of a variety of bioengineering problems, ranging from orthopedic joint prostheses, bone remodeling, fixation devices, degeneration of load-bearing soft connective tissues and intervertebral discs, blood flow in the cardiovascular system, and treatment of heart valve disease, to cancer metastases and photodynamic cancer therapy. It also addresses crucial issues relevant to surface phenomena at cellular, protein–material, and solid–liquid levels. This book also discusses the interplay of the complex physics governing the operations of nanopore biosensors and explores the use of dielectrophoresis for the alignment and patterning of particles and cells. Finally, unlike modeling conventional engineering systems, modeling biological organs and constructs requires patient-specific models to capture the actual geometry and structure of the organs and constructs. These models are often obtained from volumetric images. Thus, issues in an image-based bioengineering modeling technique are discussed in this book as well.

MATLAB® is a registered trademark of The MathWorks, Inc. For product information, please contact:

The MathWorks, Inc.
3 Apple Hill Drive
Natick, MA 01760-2098 USA
Tel: 508 647 7000
Fax: 508-647-7001
E-mail: info@mathworks.com
Web: www.mathworks.com

Editor

Guigen Zhang, PhD, is a professor of bioengineering and of electrical and computer engineering at Clemson University. He is the executive director of the Institute for Biological Interfaces of Engineering, a research and education/training institute designated by the South Carolina Commission on Higher Education. Prof. Zhang is also a fellow of the American Institute for Medical and Biological Engineering (AIMBE). He has published extensively in the areas of biomechanics, biomaterials, and biosensors, and he holds numerous patents in nanotechnology-enhanced structures and biosensors.

Dr. Zhang has benefited tremendously from today's powerful computational modeling and simulation capabilities in his efforts to invent for a better tomorrow. In fact, several of his patents would not be possible without computer-aided investigations. Thus, he is very passionate about introducing engineering students and even practicing engineers to the skills of computational modeling. In his view, all engineers and researchers of today should be proficient in using computational tools to perform analysis, to design and invent, and to be able to tinker further along in a lab, a shop, or a garage. This is crucial to innovation by unleashing the hidden treasures of science, for computational modeling allows one to tackle real-world problems from a multidisciplinary perspective.

Contributors

Narayana R. Aluru
University of Illinois at
    Urbana-Champaign
Champaign, Illinois

Mark A. Baldwin
University of Denver
Denver, Colorado

Samuel Bearden
Clemson University
Clemson, South Carolina

Jozef Brcka
Tokyo Electron U.S. Holdings, Inc.
Austin, Texas

Pascal R. Buenzli
Monash University
Melbourne, Australia

Sarah E. Cisewski
Clemson University
Clemson, South Carolina

Chadd W. Clary
University of Denver
Denver, Colorado

Jacques Faguet
Tokyo Electron U.S. Holdings, Inc.
Austin, Texas

Guang Feng
Huazhong University of Science and
    Technology
Wuhan, China

Clare K. Fitzpatrick
University of Denver
Denver, Colorado

Mark A. Haidekker
University of Georgia
Athens, Georgia

Melinda Harman
Clemson University
Clemson, South Carolina

Johnie Hodge
Clemson University
Clemson, South Carolina

Chenyue W. Hu
Rice University
Houston, Texas

Guoqing Hu
Chinese Academy of Sciences
Beijing, China

Michele M. Kim
University of Pennsylvania
Philadelphia, Pennsylvania

Svetlana V. Komarova
McGill University
Montreal, Quebec, Canada

Ethan Kung
Clemson University
Clemson, South Carolina

Robert A. Latour
Clemson University
Clemson, South Carolina

Peter J. Laz
University of Denver
Denver, Colorado

Xianfeng Li
Clemson University
Clemson, South Carolina

Baochang Liu
University of Pennsylvania
Philadelphia, Pennsylvania

Adrienne M. Madison
University of Georgia
Athens, Georgia

Lorin P. Maletsky
University of Kansas
Lawrence, Kansas

Alison L. Marsden
University of California San Diego
La Jolla, California

Vandana Pandian
Clemson University
Clemson, South Carolina

Peter Pivonka
University of Melbourne
Melbourne, Australia

Christian M. Puttlitz
Colorado State University
Fort Collins, Colorado

Shizhi Qian
Old Dominion University
Norfolk, Virginia

Rui Qiao
Virginia Tech
Blacksburg, Virginia

Amina A. Qutub
Rice University
Houston, Texas

Sharan Ramaswamy
Florida International University
Miami, Florida

Rahul Rekhi
Rice University
Houston, Texas

Paul J. Rullkoetter
University of Denver
Denver, Colorado

David T. Ryan
Rice University
Houston, Texas

Marc D. Ryser
Duke University
Durham, North Carolina

Manuel Salinas
Florida International University
Miami, Florida

Snehal S. Shetye
Colorado State University
Fort Collins, Colorado

Kevin L. Troyer
Colorado State University
Fort Collins, Colorado

Yongren Wu
Clemson University
Clemson, South Carolina

Hai Yao
Clemson University
Clemson, South Carolina

Li-Hsien Yeh
National Yunlin University of Science and
    Technology
Douliu, Taiwan

Becky Zaunbrecher
Rice University
Houston, Texas

Guigen Zhang
Clemson University
Clemson, South Carolina

Yu Zhao
Clemson University
Clemson, South Carolina

Timothy C. Zhu
University of Pennsylvania
Philadelphia, Pennsylvania

1

An Integrative Way of Solving Bioengineering Problems

Guigen Zhang

CONTENTS

ABSTRACT The importance of establishing computational bioengineering as an area of study is argued here. It is believed that a systematic study of computational bioengineering will not only help address many critical challenges facing bioengineering and biomedical engineering but also set a new direction for advancing the field. As a stepping stone, this book is expected to foster integrative learning and thinking in students and practitioners for the generation of new options and novel solutions to solve bioengineering problems in academic research and industrial research and development activities. A brief summary of all the bioengineering problems discussed in this book is given to guide the readers.

1.1 The Need for a Transition from Reductive to Integrative Ways of Problem Solving

To facilitate learning, impart skills, and encourage specialized practices, the engineering field has witnessed, over the past centuries, subdivisions of the field into many specialized areas such as mechanical, agricultural, materials, civil, electrical, chemical, industrial, computer, biomedical, environmental, and so on. The benefit of such a compartmentalized division of disciplines is that in each discipline, certain selected or specialized knowledge, ways of thinking, procedures, and practices can be emphasized and imparted to students. This practice has been proven useful in the past as engineers played many crucial roles in bringing on the industrial as well as the digital revolutions. But time has changed and we live in a different world now. We can no longer afford to ignore the complex and interwoven issues as we used to do in our drive to seek simplicity. And yet, evidence is emerging that traditional compartmentalized disciplinary approaches are becoming insufficient for dealing with the unknowns and uncertainties of the real-world problems because our desire for simplicity has also led us to ignore opportunities to discover novel solutions to our problems. The design and production of tomorrow's systems and products will require an integrative approach rather than a reductive approach.

As argued by Roger Martin [1], integrative learning and thinking requires one to actively seek less obvious but potentially relevant factors, embrace the mess that is inherent with the inclusive approach, welcome complexity, consider multidirectional and nonlinear relationships, see the system of the problem, hold all relevant pieces of information suspended in mind at once, and reason how one decision might affect another.

Converting from a reductive way of learning and thinking to an integrative way of learning and thinking requires one to go beyond his or her comfort zone and break the barriers set forth by the traditional disciplinary boundaries. To begin, one might wander into other disciplinary fields to learn a thing or two or even steal some ideas per James March's suggestion [2]. Thus, examining problems using an integrative approach based on multidisciplinary principles may help us solve real-world problems, which never present themselves as subproblems in traditional discipline categories.

1.2 Computational Bioengineering as an Area of Study

Bioengineering, or biomedical engineering, is a field in which biomedical problems are solved based on myriad laws of physics and thermodynamics, as well as biology. Over the past decades, advances in bioengineering have contributed to numerous innovations and developments of medical devices, sensors, implants, prostheses, and so on, and they have resulted in significant improvement in our quality of life. However, one of the major challenges facing the field of bioengineering is its reliance on the knowledge and investigative approaches developed through the reductive method in the traditional compartmentalized disciplines.

Computational bioengineering takes advantage of the latest computational capabilities to deal with biomedical problems using an integrative approach. Although computer modeling has been used to tackle bioengineering problems for decades, the types of problems tackled are mainly of hard and soft tissue mechanics and vascular fluid mechanics. As a field of study, computational bioengineering should address problems of not only a mechanical nature but also electrical, electrostatic, electrochemical, chemical, biochemical, thermal, and electromagnetic problems, among others, either individually or combined, under the governing laws of physics, thermodynamics, and biology. This book illustrates these expanded capabilities of computational bioengineering through discussions of a variety of bioengineering problems, ranging from orthopedic joint prostheses, bone remodeling, fixation devices, degeneration of load-bearing soft connective tissues and intervertebral discs (IVDs), blood flow in the cardiovascular system and treatment of heart valve disease, to cancer metastases and photodynamic cancer therapy. In addition to these complex bioengineering problems, it also addresses crucial issues relevant to the underlying science and physics of bioengineering at a cellular level, and at protein–material as well as solid–liquid interfaces. Examples of some of these issues include cell phenotyping, protein–surface interaction, and the structure and effect of an electrical double layer. These issues are relevant to the design and development of engineering tissue constructs and biomaterials as well as to the elucidation of metal–fluid interaction that is crucial to the process of corrosion of metallic implants. To give a whole-picture view, this book also discusses the use of computational models to investigate the interplay of the complex physics governing the operations of a new generation of biosensors (specifically nanopore biosensors) and to explore the use of dielectrophoresis (DEP) for the alignment and patterning of particles and cells. Nanopore biosensors are regarded as a promising platform for single molecular detection and DNA sequencing, important to early-stage disease screening and diagnosis. Rapid patterning of cells and tissue constructs is also a key to the advance of tissue engineering and regenerative medicine. Finally, unlike modeling conventional engineering systems, modeling biological organs and constructs requires patient-specific models to capture the actual geometry and structure of the organs and constructs. These models are often obtained from volumetric images. Thus, issues in an image-based bioengineering modeling technique are discussed in this book as well.

In most deterministic problems, the physical phenomena encountered can be described by partial differential equations (PDEs) because these phenomena follow the laws of thermodynamics in terms of mass, momentum, and energy conservation. Solutions to these PDEs under certain initial and boundary conditions can shed in-depth and systemic insights into the underlying mechanisms governing these physical phenomena. Hence, solving a problem governed by multidisciplinary principles is to solve a set of coupled PDEs simultaneously. Doing so can provide valuable information toward the analysis of real-world problems as well as the design of engineering solutions to address the real-world problems. Solving coupled PDEs analytically for complex problems, however, is very difficult and sometimes impossible. But the explosion in computational powers and capabilities has made solving coupled multiple PDEs not only possible but also relatively easier to implement. For probabilistic problems, computational approaches based on molecular dynamics and Monte Carlo methods are becoming the norm in finding solutions.

In view of the great contributions computer modeling has made to the emerging fields like nanotechnology and synthetic biology in the past decades, it is believed that a systematic study of computational bioengineering will not only help address many critical challenges facing bioengineering but also set a new direction for advancing the field. This book is intended to serve as a stepping stone to the establishment of a field of study in computational bioengineering. In the long run, in addition to introducing the readers to the power of integrative computational approaches to advancing the field of bioengineering, this book is expected to foster integrative learning and thinking in engineering students for the generation of new options and novel solutions and to stimulate a sense of limitless possibility in bioengineering research and industrial research and development activities. As a reference book, this book also aims to demonstrate the value and power of computational modeling in offering predictive capabilities to assess new surgical concepts and medical devices and postoperative surgical outcomes and at the same time provide some relevant information for readers who want to follow up with the latest research developments in bioengineering and biomedical engineering using a computational approach.

1.3 A Summary of the Issues and Problems Discussed in This Book

1.3.1 Selected Problems Related to the Musculoskeletal System

Although joint replacement is a common treatment for arthritis, a significant number of total joint (hip and knee) replacement patients remain dissatisfied with the outcome of their procedure. To change this, premarketing assessment tools capable of predicting performance outcomes of joint prostheses, especially in younger and physically active patients, are needed. Chapter 2 explores a novel computational framework that combines both experimental and computational approaches, describing subject-specific deterministic and probabilistic modeling techniques suitable for generating functional performance assessments of joint prostheses.

Human bones constantly remodel over one's lifetime. When there is an imbalance between bone resorption and bone formation within basic multicellular units (BMUs), bone disorders such as osteoporosis and osteopetrosis can develop. While coupling between osteoclasts and osteoblasts is known to occur, the mechanisms of action for the involved molecules between spatially segregated populations of osteoclasts and osteoblasts within BMUs are by no means clear. Chapter 3 uses computational models to examine the functionalities of BMUs and their roles in bone remodeling.

External fixation is useful for the treatment of unstable fractures, limb lengthening, and congenital and pathological orthopedic deformities. The functionality of an external fixation device relies mainly on the use of tensioned wires to support bone fragments. One major problem with these wires is their yielding. Once the wires yield, the fracture healing process will be compromised. Chapter 4 provides an in-depth look at the cause of the nonlinear behavior observed in these tensioned wires and discusses how material yielding can be minimized to enhance the functionality of such a fixation device.

Soft tissue instability can cause or accelerate joint tissue degeneration, especially in situations during accidental fall, high-speed sports, or traumatic events. Understanding the viscoelastic mechanical behavior of connective tissues is a crucial first step in developing treatment modalities for joint instability. To address the limitations in current soft tissue viscoelastic characterization paradigms, enhance our ability to predict the functional role of soft connective tissues in whole joint mechanics, and develop future treatment options, Chapter 5 presents computational models for investigating the nonlinear viscoelastic behavior of load-bearing soft tissues based on a constitutive formulation along with a corresponding experimental characterization technique.

Back pain is a major public health problem, and more than 70% of all people will have back pain at some time in their life. Back pain is strongly associated with the degeneration of IVDs, which in the long run can lead to spinal stenosis. To help elucidate the etiology of human disc degeneration and develop strategies for restoring tissue function or retarding further disc degeneration, Chapter 6 presents a three-dimensional computational model to analyze the mechanical, chemical, and electrical signals within the IVD during axial unconfined compression and physiological loading conditions. By considering the human IVD as an inhomogeneous composite consisting of a charged elastic solid, water, ions (Na^+ and Cl^-), and nutrient solute (oxygen, glucose, and lactate), and by accounting for the effects of the endplate calcification and cell injection, this model sheds many valuable insights into the interplay among fluid pressurization, effective solid stress, charge density, and some new understanding toward disc biomechanics, pathology of IVD degeneration, and possible cell-based therapies for lower back pain.

1.3.2 Selected Problems Related to the Circulatory System

Simulations of blood flow in the cardiovascular system offer investigative and predictive capabilities to augment current clinical tools. With image-based patient-specific three-dimensional anatomical models coupled with associated hemodynamic and electro-dynamic behavior of the circulatory system, Chapter 7 shows that relevant physiological parameters such as wall shear stress and particle residence times can be estimated and correlated with clinical data for treatment planning and device evaluation. Chapter 8 presents, in addition to a brief overview of the structure of the human heart valves, their disease states and treatment options, and the use of computational fluid dynamics to elucidate the complex hemodynamics in the vicinity of the heart valve and the time-varying stresses on the leaflets. These computational results will surely provide valuable information in treating heart valve disease as well as surgical planning and preoperative, postoperative, and temporal, longitudinal functional assessment.

1.3.3 Selected Problems in Cancer Development and Treatment

Most cancer types develop the ability to metastasize, which is regarded as the most common cause of death among cancer patients. There is an immense clinical interest and societal value to understand the underlying biological mechanisms and develop preventive and therapeutic measures. Chapter 9 presents the important challenges in taking on the development of in silico tools for the study of cancer and cancer metastases and provides an overview of the existing deterministic and stochastic modeling approaches along with their potentials and limitations. Moreover, photodynamic therapy is an emerging cancer treatment modality that uses visible light to activate photosensitizers to generate cytotoxic oxygen radicals to kill cancer cells. Chapter 10 provides an in-depth review of the most important photochemical-based computational models dealing with the transport of light, photosensitizer drug and oxygen through vasculature in human tissues, and the interactions among them.

1.3.4 Other Bioengineering Problems

In addition to addressing problems directly related to the hard and soft tissues of the human musculoskeletal system, the flow dynamics and valves of the circulatory system, and cancer development and treatment, this book also addresses bioengineering issues such as cell phenotyping, protein–surface interaction, electrical double layer at a solid–liquid interface, biosensors, rapid alignment and patterning of particles and cells, and so on.

1.3.4.1 Cell Phenotyping

Advances in computational cell phenotyping are enabling scientists to characterize and transform biological systems in various laboratory, industrial plant, and clinical settings with impressive quantitative precision. This has resulted in transforming how biological research is conducted and how the results are interpreted in both basic research and translational stages. Chapter 11 explores ways computational cell phenotyping is being employed in research laboratories, industrial plants, and health care clinics, and highlights both the problems a computational phenotyping approach can solve and new challenges it may introduce.

1.3.4.2 Protein–Surface Interaction

In designing and developing a new biomaterial, it is of great value if the host reaction of the developed biomaterial is predictable. Protein–surface interaction is believed to be the most crucial event in affecting host reactions. Chapter 12 reviews various computational methods used for the simulation of protein–surface interaction. Among these methods, molecular simulations based on empirical force fields are used extensively in modeling protein–surface adsorption. When the complexity of the molecular systems becomes substantial, additional advanced sampling methods and coarse graining techniques are required to increase the efficiency of the simulation. All these relevant issues are discussed in Chapter 12.

1.3.4.3 The Electrical Double Layer at a Solid–Liquid Interface

At a solid–liquid interface, the ubiquitous electrical double layer plays an important role in affecting how the solid will interact with the surrounding liquid environment. Chapter 13 summarizes some key features of an electrical double layer structure based on theoretical and computational studies. An in-depth understanding of the structure is important to many bioengineering problems including the ion transport through charged channels of biological membranes, colloid stability on the surface of a biomaterial, electrochemical processes (e.g., corrosion) of a metallic implant, and electrokinetic phenomena within a biosensor channel, to name just a few.

1.3.4.4 Nanopore Biosensors

Development of biosensors is another active area of bioengineering. Among a few novel designs, nanopore devices are regarded as one promising platform for future biosensors. In particular, solid-state nanopores of different designs can be fabricated to suit various needs. However, the inherent complexity in understanding the operations of a nanopore device calls for computational modeling to deal with many interrelated physics including the effect of the electrical double layer, electrostatics in the presence of various materials with different work functions, mass transport through a nanopore in the presence of a complex electrical field, and concentration gradient. Chapter 14 discusses the interplay of all these factors and summarizes them in a case study of modeling a nanopore consisting of a single-walled carbon nanotube. In a more specific application, Chapter 15 describes the computational modeling of a nanopore-based DNA sequencing technique, in which DNA nanoparticles are electrophoretically driven through a single nanopore and the DNA sequence is determined on the basis of the change in the recorded ionic current flowing through the nanopore. Three types of nanopores, namely, ungated solid-state nanopore, gated solid-state nanopore by field effect transistor, and soft nanopore comprising functionalized polyelectrolyte brushes engrafted to the solid-state nanopore wall, are considered. This application sheds some new insights into the design and improvement of nanopore DNA sequencing technology via through-pore current measurements.

1.3.4.5 Rapid Alignment and Patterning of Particles and Cells

DEP has been widely used in micro- and nanofluidic systems for positioning, sorting, and separation of particles involved in medical diagnostics, drug discovery, cell therapeutics, and biosensor development. Chapter 16 uses a computational approach to reexamine the dielectrophoretic phenomenon and identifies some of the problems associated with evaluating the DEP forces experienced by particles and cells. It illustrates the consequences of ignoring some of the crucial factors in quantifying the DEP forces. To address some of the limitations in the current DEP theory, Chapter 16 also presents a new volumetric method for quantifying the DEP forces. To demonstrate the effectiveness of this mentod, this chapter provides case studies for investigating the alignment and movement of multiple particles under DEP along with experimental validation.

1.3.4.6 Issues in Image-Based Modeling for Bioengineering Problems

Modeling biological organs and constructs, unlike modeling mechanical systems, requires patient-specific models of organs. These patient-specific anatomic models are often obtained from volumetric images. Image-based modeling often deals with highly complex geometry, making the assignment of material properties to individual components from image information difficult. Chapter 17 discusses a four-step approach to address this problem. From geometry segmentation, meshing, simulation, to result analysis, it presents some important strategies to overcome some specific challenges of image-based computational modeling.

References

1. Martin R.L. 2009. *The Opposable Mind: How Successful Leaders Win through Integrative Thinking*. Harvard Business School Press, Boston.
2. Coutu D. 2006. Ideas as art: A conversation with James G. March. *The Harvard Business Review*, October, 83–89. Harvard Business School Press, Boston.

2

Toward Predicting the Performance of Joint Arthroplasty

Clare K. Fitzpatrick, Melinda Harman, Mark A. Baldwin, Chadd W. Clary,
Lorin P. Maletsky, Peter J. Laz, and Paul J. Rullkoetter

CONTENTS

ABSTRACT Joint arthroplasty is a common treatment for arthritis, involving the surgical implantation of prostheses to replace the bearing surfaces of diseased joints. While the clinical success of joint replacement is high, up to 25% of total knee replacement (TKR) patients remain dissatisfied with the outcome of their procedure. There is a recognized need for premarketing assessment tools capable of predicting performance outcomes of joint prostheses, in order to shorten development times, avoid disastrous prosthesis failures that threaten patient safety, and optimize design of components that are robust to patient and surgical variability. This chapter explores a novel computational framework that combines both experimental and computational approaches, describing subject-specific and probabilistic modeling techniques suitable for generating functional performance assessments of joint prostheses. Experimental and computational modeling approaches used in the past two decades are reviewed, including experimental kinematic and wear simulators, finite element models, lower limb musculoskeletal models, and deterministic and probabilistic techniques. The challenges of identifying and acquiring appropriate inputs for subject-specific computational models, experimentally verifying and validating model predictions, and incorporating population variability are discussed in detail. Throughout this chapter, the effectiveness of this modeling approach is documented through specific case studies of TKR prostheses, in which computational models are applied to questions of clinical and design importance.

2.1 Significance

The global burden of arthritis and other degenerative joint diseases, especially in aging populations, is widely recognized for its painful disability and associated socioeconomic costs [1,2]. The pain and severe joint destruction resulting from these diseases have a profoundly negative impact on a person's mobility and ability to maintain an active lifestyle. Joint arthroplasty, an orthopedic surgery involving implantation of medical devices that replace the bearing surfaces of the diseased joints, provides reliable pain relief and restoration of moderate function for arthritic patients. This is accomplished by replacing the bearing surfaces of the diseased joint with prosthetic components fabricated from metal alloys, ceramics, and ultrahigh molecular weight polyethylene. Total hip replacement (THR) and total knee replacement (TKR) are the most common joint arthroplasty procedures in the United States, affecting approximately 2 million Americans annually in 2006 [3]. Because of changing population demographics and increased demand from younger patients, annual utilization in the United States is projected to exceed 10 million by 2030, with considerably higher utilization of TKR than THR [3]. International utilization follows similar trends, with many countries reporting implantation rates exceeding 200 cases of joint arthroplasty for every 100,000 citizens [4,5].

Survivorship and functional outcomes after THR and TKR are typically very good, with joint arthroplasty registries in various countries reporting 90% to 95% survivorship of the prostheses at 10 years of in vivo function [6–9]. Unfortunately, a certain percentage of joint arthroplasties require revision surgery, with complete removal of the failed components (explants) and replacement with a new TKR prosthesis. Survivorship of these revised THR and TKR declines appreciably [6–9]. Prosthesis design plays a role in such failures, as most joint arthroplasty registries identify disparity among different prosthesis designs, with some THR and TKR prostheses having notably higher risks of revision than others [10–13].

The challenge of sustaining prosthesis longevity while meeting the higher demands of recreational and occupational activities among increasingly younger joint arthroplasty patients has led to the introduction of many new prosthesis designs and materials. Hundreds of different types of prostheses are currently available for joint arthroplasty, as prosthesis selection is considered a crucial aspect of the surgical decision-making process. However, long-term outcome studies do not provide real-time information useful for innovation and new prostheses are increasingly available through regulatory pathways that effectively bypass submission of extensive clinical data supporting prosthesis safety and effectiveness [14]. Alternative means of generating high-quality evidence demonstrating prosthesis safety and effectiveness are urgently needed to enhance regulatory and treatment pathways [15]. Specifically, premarketing assessment tools capable of predicting performance outcomes are highly desired, both to shorten development times of new concepts and to avoid disastrous prosthesis failures that threaten patient safety.

National health and regulatory agencies recognize the value of numerical models for enhancing the effectiveness of clinical studies and developing technology to augment subjective patient-specific assessments. For surgical treatments of musculoskeletal diseases such as osteoarthritis and rheumatoid arthritis, the translational pathway from basic discovery to therapeutic benefit involves developing novel surgical techniques, prosthesis designs, and bearing materials for joint arthroplasty [10,16,17]. The US Food and Drug Administration, in its acknowledgment to "stimulate innovation in clinical evaluations and personalized medicine to improve product development and patient outcomes," identifies two strategic areas with particular relevance to numerical modeling in medicine [18]. These include (1) continued refinement of computer modeling and simulation in clinical trial design to enhance the effectiveness of clinical studies and (2) promotion and development of scientific tools to better characterize and standardize measurements that rely on subjective readings. Others have further advocated that premarketing assessments proven to ensure device safety or reduce outcome variability be included as essential components of the regulatory pathway before larger multicenter clinical studies are initiated [10,15,19].

Novel computational frameworks are needed to fulfill a role in premarketing assessment of technologies in joint arthroplasty, providing for timely scientific evaluations related to prosthesis safety and effectiveness throughout its functional life cycle. Using a combined experimental and computational approach, it is possible to identify a translational pathway from bioengineering insight to therapeutic benefit. When successful and robust to patient variations, such premarketing assessment tools can aid innovation and inform the phased introduction of new technology in joint arthroplasty. For the remainder of this chapter, we will focus on TKR prostheses and review existing modeling approaches capable of quantifying and predicting their functional performance and generating evidence-based assessments. These models will describe subject-specific and probabilistic modeling techniques, which have proven suitable for identifying factors that can discriminate between poor and successful clinical outcomes in joint arthroplasty. The effectiveness of this approach in defining underlying mechanisms associated with functional performance and wear accumulation over the functional life cycle of TKR prostheses will be documented through detailed review of specific case studies.

2.2 Modeling Approaches

Computational models of TKR have evolved over the past 20 years from deterministic models of the tibiofemoral (TF) joint during fixtured testing to complete lower limb models that incorporate physiological soft-tissue representations; adaptive musculature and loading conditions at the hip, knee, and ankle joints; and simulation of activities of daily living (ADLs) [20]. Direct digitization of cadaver joints or segmentation of computed tomography (CT) and magnetic resonance (MR) images has made it possible to incorporate subject-specific representation of joint anatomy (bone, muscular attachments, soft tissues, etc.) into musculoskeletal models capable of calculating joint biomechanics [21–24]. Such modeling approaches have proven useful for reproducing in vivo kinematic and joint loading conditions, providing analytical tools that are complementary to in vitro simulations and other experimental testing, as well as in vivo clinical evaluations of prosthesis function in patients.

The predictive capability of these models is generally validated in combination with experimental studies. Direct modeling representations of experimental knee simulator kinematics have been validated against in vitro data generated by the mechanical simulators, with variations in complexity and functionality depending upon the use of static or dynamic loading conditions, inclusion of soft-tissue constraints, and inclusion of both the TF and patellofemoral (PF) joints in a full knee model [25–41]. Wear predictions from such models have been validated against tests from experimental wear simulators [42–46] and using in vivo kinematics and wear data acquired from patients [47].

Many of these previous approaches did not accommodate the significant variability in prosthesis alignment and loading conditions that exist in vivo for different prosthesis designs. For example, test standards for conducting knee joint wear simulation are typically performed using optimal component alignment and low-demand loading conditions representing a single ISO standard gait cycle [42,48,49] that do not sufficiently capture the lifetime function of TKR in active patients or generate wear patterns that agree with clinical retrievals [49,50]. Similarly, while some computational models using finite element (FE) analysis have addressed varied surgical alignment [51,52], they often report single deterministic results for simple loading conditions executed under optimal alignment [53,54]. Newer approaches capable of discriminating the performance of different TKR designs aim to accommodate variability that exists in TKR populations.

More recent computational models of TKR include complete lower limb models that incorporate physiological soft-tissue representations, adaptive musculature and hip and ankle loading conditions, and simulation of ADLs, which can be used to reproduce in vivo kinematic or joint loading conditions and account for uncertainty and subject-specific variability that is inherently present within the TKR population [25,55–59]. A key advantage of a multivariate computational approach, over in vivo or in vitro approaches, is that it can be utilized to describe interdependencies between model inputs and outputs over a broad range of clinically relevant conditions.

Generating model results that can be generalized to represent diverse conditions existing in entire populations of patients requires accounting for the uncertainty and variability that is inherently present within the TKR population [60]. Assessing sensitivity through deterministic parametric studies involves perturbing individual parameters or a matrix of parameters to determine which of the parameters has the most impact on the model outputs. Probabilistic analysis incorporated into the models accounts for the uncertainty and variability in model inputs, including aspects related to subject, surgical, and design parameter variability, and attempts to predict the likelihood of outputs [60,61]. Probabilistic methods, including Monte Carlo simulation and Latin Hypercube sampling techniques, can be implemented to investigate the influence of prosthesis design parameters (e.g., femoral sagittal plane radii, tibial insert conformity) and patient-specific factors (e.g., patient weight, gait pattern, muscle forces, ligament integrity) on the variability of TKR mechanics (wear, kinematics, contact mechanics) [57,60,62]. In these simulations, multiple parameters can be perturbed in a series of hundreds or thousands of separate simulations, in order to understand the influence of a single parameter on output metrics and interrelationships between difference parameters. Such statistical methods allow for a comprehensive understanding of TKR performance under the complex conditions that can exist during experimental and clinical performance assessments [46,55–58,63]. These research efforts constantly strive toward more physiological models and tools that can better predict and compare the performance of devices.

2.3 Acquiring Subject-Specific Metrics Suitable for Model Input

In order to design TKR prostheses that perform well throughout an entire patient population, it is necessary for tools to test the performance of new prostheses in situations representing the full scope of activities and loading conditions that are likely to occur in the lifetime of the device. Using subject-specific computational models that incorporate adequate patient information and are sensitive enough to appropriately differentiate between clinical conditions and outcomes, it is possible to define underlying mechanisms of functional outcomes in TKR patients. However, gathering subject-specific data suitable for modeling purposes can be challenging, requiring close cooperation between model developers, orthopedic surgeons and physical therapists, and laboratories capable of making precise measurements on relevant patient populations. In this manner, the substantial subject-specific variations in clinical outcomes, in knee mechanics and loading, and in the TKR surgical procedure can be captured.

Relevant inputs for subject-specific computational models of TKR patients often can be obtained from routine clinical assessments. Medical records contain pertinent information related to the functional history (e.g., patient demographics, reason for revision, prosthesis type, etc.), which can be used to identify representative TKRs that are characteristic of a given clinical outcome or failure mechanism (e.g., malalignment, patellar wear, polyethylene wear, instability, patellar complications, infection, etc.). Full-limb standing frontal and sagittal plane radiographs provide for assessment of prosthesis alignment relative to an anatomic axis (corresponding to axes defined by the midpoints of the femoral and tibial shafts) or relative to the limb's mechanical axis (a line connecting the center of the femoral head and the midpoints of the knee and ankle).

There are several options for gaining subject-specific joint and prosthesis anatomy. When available, CT and MR images provide for detailed three-dimensional (3D) information related to bone geometry, cartilage layers, soft-tissue structures, and prosthesis orientation. The Visible Human Project [64] consists of MR imaging, CT, and anatomical images useful for accurately representing bone and soft-tissue morphology in computational models, as well as estimating the origins and insertions of tendons and ligaments. In a similar manner, cadaver specimens can be imaged to gain morphological data and dissected for direct assessment of soft-tissue structures and their origins and insertions. Subject-specific TKR articular geometry can be obtained using geometric surface models of the implanted prosthesis design or by applying direct measurement and reverse engineering methods to acquire 3D surface models of explanted TKR prostheses.

More detailed laboratory assessments of subjects' motion and TKR function can include high-speed motion capture systems and biplane radiographic or fluoroscopic imaging systems to generate subject-specific kinetics and kinematics during dynamic activities [65–67]. In vivo loading conditions can be acquired through telemetric sensors embedded into the TKR bearing surfaces, providing a means for validating model estimates of muscle forces and associated articular contact forces during various activities [51,68].

In vivo studies involving the functional performance of TKR in patients have proven that evaluation of knee joint prostheses retrieved after in vivo service (explants) provides unique evidence related to the physiological environment in which the prostheses perform. The size and distribution of articular contact wear patterns on explants can address clinical issues associated with current surgical techniques and TKR performance during patient activities [69–72]. Consistent input data related to articular contact patterns can be acquired using stage II nondestructive analysis of the explants in accordance with international guidelines for standardized procurement and quantitative analysis of explanted devices [73,74]. Quantification of patient-specific articular contact patterns on TKR explants is possible using imaging and photogrammetric methods and damage classification protocols [50], which provide a mathematical representation of the TF articular contact relative to a defined prosthesis-based coordinate system [47,70,71,75]. Metrics generated from explants have proven useful for verifying outputs of experimental models through comparison with mechanical simulations of knee joint wear [50,76,77], as well as computational models of contact stress occurring at both the tibial [47,78,79] and patellar [80] articular surfaces.

2.4 Development, Validation, and Application of a Computational Knee Simulator

Evaluating the performance of an implanted device or the effect of surgical alignment on joint mechanics is of critical importance in determining the best component design or surgical technique for a patient. Clinical studies incorporate a host of unquantified sources of intersubject variation, including loading conditions (patient weight, limb alignment, gait pattern), ligament attachment sites and mechanical properties, and muscle efficiency. In the face of so much uncertainty, it is difficult to isolate the effect of a single parameter, such as implant design, on overall joint mechanics.

Experimental knee simulators provide a controlled and repeatable loading environment for comparative evaluation of component designs or surgical alignment under dynamic activities. Devices, or alignment conditions, can be implanted in the same cadaveric specimen, and directly compared under identical loading and soft-tissue conditions. However, the number of cadaveric simulations that may be performed is limited by the time and cost associated with each in vitro test; experiment simulators quickly become cost prohibitive as design-phase tools where tens or hundreds of component designs, sizes, and alignment conditions must be evaluated.

Computational models represent an efficient platform for performing component design evaluations under a variety of dynamic loading conditions that would otherwise be difficult and costly to accomplish experimentally. Experimental simulators and their computational counterparts are complementary tools; the experiments are required to validate the computational models, while the validated computational models can subsequently be utilized for early evaluation and ranking of component designs. In this section, we present a combined experimental and computational approach that was used to develop an FE counterpart to an experimental knee simulator. Once validated, the computational model was subsequently applied to address specific clinical issues by highlighting the work from Baldwin et al. [25], Fitzpatrick et al. [81], and Hoops et al. [82] on the development, validation, and application of a computational representation of an experimental knee simulator.

2.4.1 In Vitro Testing in an Experimental Knee Simulator

A variety of knee simulators, from quasi-static to fully dynamic, have been developed to answer clinical and design questions, evaluating kinematics, laxity, wear, ligament performance, and contact mechanics, and performing comparative analyses of TKR designs [48,49,83–88]. The Kansas knee simulator (KKS) is an electrohydraulic whole-joint mechanical knee simulator [89]. Five actuators at the hip, ankle, and quadriceps muscle are used to simulate a variety of dynamic activities, including a deep knee bend and a gait cycle, in cadaveric experiments. The five actuators of the experimental setup consist of a vertical load at the hip, medial–lateral (M–L) force at the ankle, vertical moment at the ankle, flexion moment at the ankle, and quadriceps excursion. Loading profiles are applied directly to the ankle and hip actuators, while quadriceps excursion is applied through feedback control to match a hip flexion profile (Figure 2.1).

A series of dynamic in vitro tests were conducted on three fresh-frozen cadaver knees implanted by a trained orthopedic surgeon with posterior-stabilized (PS) components. Each specimen was harvested from an intact leg by transecting tibial and femoral bones approximately 20 cm from the natural joint line, mounting the bones into aluminum fixtures and leaving the remaining tissues intact after TKR surgery. 3D kinematic data were collected using an Optotrak motion capture system (Northern Digital Inc., Waterloo, Canada). Each implanted knee specimen was subjected to a passive laxity envelope assessment by manually applying 5 Nm internal–external (I–E) and 10 Nm varus–valgus (V–V) torques in each direction to an instrumented prosthetic foot and recording resulting rotations at 30° intervals from 0° to 90° of femoral flexion. The magnitude of these torques was based on literature values [90–93] and provided sufficient rotation to characterize constraint without damaging the cadaveric specimen. After laxity assessments, cadaver specimens were placed in the KKS for whole-joint kinematic data collection. The proximal portions of the rectus femoris (RF) and vastus intermedius (VI) tendons were rigidly fixed to a linear actuator positioned to reproduce the original specimen quadriceps angle in the frontal plane.

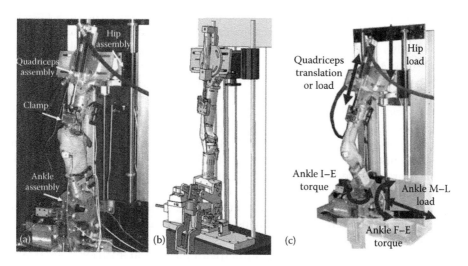

FIGURE 2.1
(a) Implanted cadaveric specimen in experimental KKS. (b) Computational representation of the KKS. (c) Loads applied to the simulator. (From Baldwin MA et al., *J Biomech*, 45:474–483, 2012.)

Simulated deep knee bend (up to 110° flexion) and gait activities were performed in the KKS using load-controlled actuators at a simulated hip and ankle, and a proportional–integral–derivative (PID)-controlled quadriceps actuator to apply the quadriceps excursion required to match a prescribed hip flexion profile. During each simulated dynamic activity, tibial, femoral, and patellar six-degree-of-freedom (6-DOF) motions were recorded along with position and load data from ankle, hip, and quadriceps actuators. Experimental kinematics were converted to relative joint motions (TF and PF) using digitized anatomic coordinate frames and a three-cylindrical open chain description of motion [94]. A hand-held digitization probe was used to record the position of the TKR components, bony surfaces, and ligament attachment sites relative to the local coordinate frames of their respective bones.

2.4.2 Development of a Computational Counterpart to the Experimental Simulator

A dynamic FE computational model of the experimental simulator was developed in Abaqus/Explicit (SIMULIA, Providence, Rhode Island) (Figure 2.1). Geometry of the KKS assembly was generated from computer-aided design (CAD) parts, with all mechanical joints and actuators present in the experimental setup represented. Specimen-specific tibial, femoral, and patellar bones were extracted from MR images via manual segmentation using ScanIP (Simpleware, Exeter, UK). Size-matched CAD PS components were aligned to the extracted bones using reference points digitized during the experiment. Similarly, each specimen-specific implanted knee model was aligned to initial positions within the KKS using digitized point data and recorded machine actuator positions. For all analyses, bones and femoral components were meshed with triangular shell elements, while polyethylene patellar and tibial components were represented by eight-noded hexahedral elements. To reduce computational cost, bones and implant components were considered rigid for all analyses, with a pressure–overclosure relationship, calibrated to match the contact behavior of fully deformable elastic–plastic polyethylene [33], used to define component contact. A coefficient of friction of 0.04 was applied at the articular surface interfaces [32,33].

TF soft tissues were represented by six capsular soft-tissue structures crossing the implanted TF joint, including the lateral collateral and popliteofibular ligaments (LCL and PFL, respectively), anterior lateral capsule (ALC), superficial medial collateral ligament (sMCL), and medial and lateral posterior capsule (Figure 2.2). These structures were chosen to provide adequate constraint to match the experimental laxity test data; specifically, the PFL and ALC were included to represent capsular contributions to I–E constraint not adequately provided by the sMCL and LCL alone. LCL and sMCL attachment sites were determined from dissection of the cadaveric specimens. Attachment sites of the PFL, ALC, and posterior capsular structures were difficult to identify from dissection or MR images; hence, attachments and dimensions were adopted from published literature [95–98].

Ligaments were represented as two-dimensional (2D) membranes embedded with fiber-reinforced tension-only nonlinear springs. Mechanical properties of the ligaments (initial stiffness, linear strain, attachment locations) were optimized using a simulated annealing optimization algorithm to match specimen-specific experimental laxity envelope results. Sixteen input parameters were included in the optimization: ALC and PFL initial strain and stiffness, localized LCL and sMCL strain (with individual anterior, medial, and posterior bundles), LCL and sMCL stiffness (applied to all bundles), and superior–inferior (S–I) and anterior–posterior (A–P) LCL and sMCL femoral attachment sites. Although the specimen-specific LCL and MCL tibial and femoral attachment sites were identified

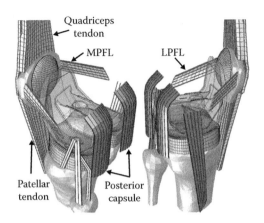

FIGURE 2.2
Soft tissues represented in the FE knee joint model. (From Baldwin MA et al., *J Biomech*, 45:474–483, 2012.)

through dissection, the fibers carrying load throughout the passive femoral flexion range were unknown and could exist anywhere within the attachment footprint. Since the model represents a subset of the actual ligament fibers, and mechanical characteristics of the ligaments were not available, both the A–P and S–I femoral attachment locations were included in the optimization. The optimization algorithm was applied to minimize differences between model-predicted and experimental I–E and V–V laxity responses at 0°, 30°, 60°, and 90° of femoral flexion. The optimized specimen-specific 2D TF ligament representations were incorporated into specimen-specific KKS computational models. The extensor mechanism and medial and lateral patellofemoral ligaments were represented by fiber-reinforced 3D structures using nonlinear tension-only springs embedded in a low-modulus, hyperelastic deformable hexahedral mesh. Stiffness of the patellar tendon, quadriceps tendon, and patellofemoral ligaments were established in separate uniaxial analyses to match literature values [99,100].

Hip and ankle actuator loads, measured from the experiment, were applied during deep knee bend and gait simulations. As per the experimental setup, PID control was integrated into the computational model to allow control of the quadriceps actuator in the same manner as the experiment. A sensor in the model was used to monitor hip flexion angle. At each increment in the analysis, the value of the sensor (instantaneous flexion angle) was passed to the PID controller (interface between the FE model and the PID controller was implemented through an Abaqus/Explicit user subroutine). In the controller, the instantaneous flexion angle was compared to the target hip flexion profile that the FE model is trying to match. The controller calculated the instantaneous quadriceps excursion required for the flexion angle to match its target profile. The output calculated by the controller is subsequently fed back and applied to the FE model.

2.4.3 Validation of the Computational Model with Experimental Data

Validation of the FE model was performed by comparing predicted TF and PF kinematics and KKS hip, ankle, and quadriceps actuator responses to experimental measurements at every 5° of femoral flexion during the deep knee bend activity and at every 5% of the gait cycle. Model-predicted and experimental root-mean-square (RMS) differences were averaged across all three specimens for each kinematic and mechanics output for each activity.

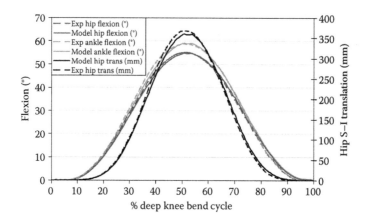

FIGURE 2.3
Comparison between experiment and PID-controlled hip flexion, ankle flexion, and hip translation during the simulated deep knee bend. (From Baldwin MA et al., *J Biomech*, 45:474–483, 2012.)

The 2D optimized TF ligament representations showed agreement with experimental laxity data and were acceptable for providing appropriate TF constraint; RMS I–E and V–V differences between model and experiment were 1.6° ± 0.5° and 0.7° ± 0.2°, respectively. With PID-controlled quadriceps actuation, model-predicted hip flexion angle matched the target experimental hip flexion profiles with an accuracy of less than 1°. Hip translation and ankle flexion also demonstrated excellent agreement between experiment and model (Figure 2.3). FE predictions for quadriceps load were a reasonable representation of the experimental loading. Trends and magnitude of both TF and PF kinematics showed good agreement between model predictions and experimental measurements. Deep knee bend TF flexion–extension had an average difference of 3.8° ± 1.9°, while I–E and V–V rotation differences were less than 1.3° ± 0.7°; A–P, S–I, and M–L TF translation differences were within 2.1 ± 1.2, 1.7 ± 1.2, and 0.9 ± 0.5 mm, respectively (Figure 2.4). Patellofemoral flexion, M–L tilt, and spin rotations in the deep knee bend activity produced average RMS differences of 2.7° ± 1.5°, 2.4° ± 1.2°, and 1.8° ± 1.1°, respectively, while local A–P, I–S, and M–L PF translations (with respect to the femur) differed by 2.2 ± 1.2, 3.6 ± 1.8, and 1.4 ± 0.8 mm, respectively. Similar accuracy was observed in both TF and PF kinematic predictions during gait simulations.

2.4.4 Application of Computational Models to Clinical Issues

Once confidence in model predictions has been established through experimental verification and validation, computational models may be applied to investigate a host of clinical and research questions. The FE model described above was utilized to investigate the issue of painful patellar crepitus in knee replacement patients. Painful patellar crepitus, a result of irritation of the quadriceps tendon in the suprapatellar region, is a potential complication in up to 14% of patients implanted with PS TKR components [101]. In some cases, tendon irritation leads to synovial overgrowth of a fibrous mass or nodule that can be trapped in the intercondylar box during active leg extension, limiting patellar excursion until the fibrosynovial hyperplasia escapes the intercondylar box, resulting in an audible patellar *clunk* sound and potentially patient discomfort [101–104]. The etiology of this inflammation has been attributed to factors that include prosthetic design, component

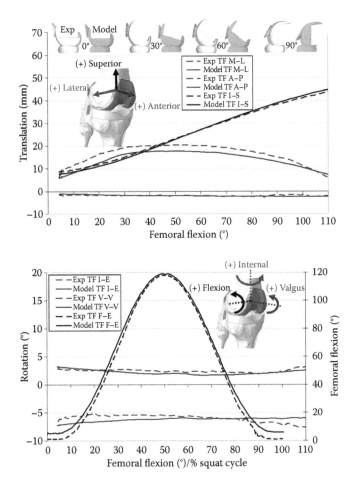

FIGURE 2.4
Comparison of experimental and model-predicted tibiofemoral translations and rotations during a simulated deep knee bend activity. (From Baldwin MA et al., *J Biomech*, 45:474–483, 2012.)

alignment, alteration of the joint line, patellar height, and patellar tracking [101,105–108]. Clinical observations have suggested that the quadriceps tendon may contact the anterior border of the femoral component intercondylar notch [102,104]; however, it is unclear what aspects of anatomic variation and component alignment increase the potential for tendon-to-notch contact and potentially lead to crepitation.

The computational KKS model is well suited for evaluating tendofemoral contact through the use of deformable, 3D representations of extensor mechanism structures articulating over a PS femoral component. Parameters hypothesized to affect patellar crepitus were selected from a clinical case–control study, comparing patients with a history of patellar crepitus to controls matched by sex, age, and body mass index [101]. Parameters of interest included the following: patellar tendon length, patellar component size, change in joint line, and femoral component flexion alignment. These parameters were perturbed in the computational model, with perturbation amounts based on standard deviations from data in the clinical study [101]. Patellar tendon length was modified by changing the tendon length in the computational model, resulting in patella alta or baja. The joint line was translated along the S–I direction by repositioning the femoral and tibial components relative to the patella, femur, tibia, and supporting ligamentous structures; both femoral and tibial components were shifted by the same amount in order to maintain consistent ligament balance at the start of the simulation. The full range of patellar component sizes was evaluated: 32, 35, 38, and 41 mm. Potential for crepitation was measured for each perturbed state as a function of tendofemoral contact over the deep knee bend cycle. Tendofemoral contact was defined by the cumulative region of tendon contact area on the femoral component over all flexion angles throughout the knee bend activity (Figure 2.5). Cumulative tendofemoral contact area near the intercondylar notch was defined by any contact within 2 mm.

The model was subsequently scaled to match patient-specific radiographic data and used to evaluate tendon articulation over the PS femoral component during the same simulated deep knee bend. The model was modified to match femoral and tibial dimensions in the sagittal and coronal planes, component sizes (tibial, femoral, and patellar), patellar height, medial/lateral patellar placement, medial/lateral patellar tilt, patellar tendon length, extensor mechanism attachment sites, femoral component flexion, anterior femoral offset, and posterior slope and offset of the tibial tray. Three matched crepitus–control patients [101] were selected to evaluate the tendofemoral contact differences between knees. Cumulative tendofemoral contact area within 2 mm of the intercondylar notch was calculated and compared for each patient-specific crepitus model and its matched control. In addition, for these patients, the minimum tendon-to-notch distance at 120° of flexion was also measured. Changes in joint line and femoral component flexion were also performed in the crepitus patient models in order to evaluate other potential surgical alignment options. The joint line was lowered by 3 and 6 mm. Separately, the femoral component was flexed by 2° and 4°. Finally, two combinations of femoral component flexion and decreased joint line were evaluated. The femoral component was flexed 2° while the joint line was lowered 3 mm, and the femoral component was flexed 4° while the joint line was lowered 6 mm.

Analysis of model perturbations showed that increasing patellar tendon length (alta), flexing the femoral component, and lowering the joint line improved tendofemoral contact by moving the contact away from the anterior edge of the notch and decreasing the cumulative contact area within 2 mm of the intercondylar notch. Conversely, decreasing the patellar tendon length (baja), extending the femoral component, and raising the joint line showed tendon contact on the femoral component closer to the notch and increased the contact area near the box (Figure 2.6). Perturbing the patellar tendon length by 6.5 mm (1 SD) and 13 mm (2 SD) showed the greatest effect on tendofemoral contact. Increasing patellar tendon length by 2 SD (positioning the patella in relative alta) held the tendon further away from the notch; the minimum distance between the anterior border of the intercondylar notch and the suprapatellar tendon increased by 1 mm compared with the original

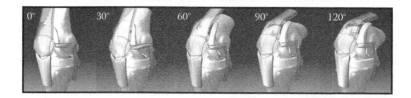

FIGURE 2.5
Contact between tendon and femoral component over the flexion cycle. (From Hoops HE et al., *J Orthop Res*, 30:1355–1361, 2012.)

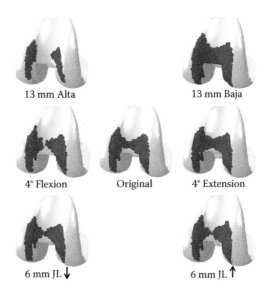

FIGURE 2.6
Composite tendofemoral contact patches from the originally aligned model (center) and changes owing to variation in patellar tendon length (alta and baja), flexion–extension alignment of the femoral component, and position of the joint line. (From Hoops HE et al., *J Orthop Res*, 30:1355–1361, 2012.)

alignment. Decreasing the patellar tendon length by 13 mm (2 SD) caused the quadriceps tendon to contact the anterior edge of the intercondylar notch and showed a large increase in contact area near the notch. In addition to the contact locations, the required quadriceps forces at deepest flexion in the model were approximately 13% higher with the 13 mm decreased (baja) position when compared with the increased (alta) position.

In the matched pair models, there were notable differences in tendofemoral contact locations between the crepitus patients and the matched controls. Contact patches of the crepitus patient models showed tendofemoral contact near the intercondylar notch, particularly along its anterior edge. The models of the matched controls show significantly less tendofemoral contact near this edge (Figure 2.7). The minimum tendon-to-notch distances from the three crepitus patient models were substantially less than the matched control models. Cumulative contact area within 2 mm of the notch was significantly greater in the crepitus models, compared to their matched controls. Perturbations testing possible alternate surgical alignments in the crepitus patient models showed improvements in tendofemoral contact conditions. Consistent with the perturbation analyses, flexing the femoral component to hide the notch and lowering the joint line held the tendon further from the notch and decreased the cumulative contact area. Combining these two surgical interventions produced the greatest improvement in tendofemoral contact.

2.4.5 Summary

Whole-joint mechanical simulators are useful design-phase tools capable of evaluating implant performance under simulated dynamic loading conditions and ligamentous constraint during in vitro testing, but are cost prohibitive for multiple evaluations. Computational models represent an effective platform for conducting parametric or probabilistic assessments of implant performance under a variety of loading and boundary

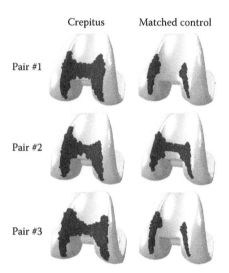

FIGURE 2.7
Composite tendofemoral contact patches from control-matched pairs, including both the crepitus and control knees. (From Hoops HE et al., *J Orthop Res*, 30:1355–1361, 2012.)

conditions, but they must be verified against experimental measurements to ensure accuracy of model predictions.

Incorporation of the PID controller into the FE model allows for evaluation of implant performance under a consistent set of kinematic conditions (specifically a controlled hip flexion profile) in the same manner as the experimental simulator. Different component geometries, surgical alignment, and anatomic variability affect the muscle force and excursion required to achieve a particular kinematic profile. The control system ensures that the flexion profile of the experimental simulator is accurately reflected in the computational setup, allowing the model to properly adapt to changes in implant design or alignment, as was implemented in the patellar crepitus study described above.

Computational models of in vivo situations are inherently difficult to validate because of substantial uncertainty; hence, in vitro models of dynamic activities are an intermediate step toward evaluation of components under in vivo conditions. Once the computational model had been appropriately validated, modifications, made with suitable acknowledgment and consideration of the conditions in which the model was initially validated, may be made to move toward component evaluation under more physiological conditions (multiple bundles of the quadriceps, relative hip–ankle A–P motion, etc.)—this concept is expanded upon in Section 2.5. This study represents a complete computational representation of the experimental KKS setup. The ability of the explicit FE model to predict kinematics will be valuable in providing implant designers with relevant information to reduce the design-phase timeline.

2.5 Toward Simulations Which Reproduce Conditions during ADLs

As described in Section 2.4, experimental simulators for knee replacement evaluation or in vitro testing provide valuable insight into the mechanics of the implanted joint.

Computational models complement these experimental tests, by facilitating tens or hundred of simulations in a cost- and time-efficient platform and allowing design-phase or parametric component or alignment evaluation. Computational representations of experimental simulators provide an efficient platform for evaluation of multiple component designs under consistent loading conditions, carrying out parametric analysis of surgical alignment, and assessment of design-phase changes to component geometry. In addition to tracking kinematics, outputs of interest may include joint forces, contact mechanics, muscle forces, polyethylene stresses, or bone strains, some of which are difficult or infeasible to obtain from the experiment. Most computational knee simulators are designed to create a specific kinematic profile or loading condition at the joint. However, changing the geometry of the TKR components, implant position, or limb alignment influences the forces, torques, and kinematics produced during the activity. A model that can adapt to changes in geometry and alignment to produce a consistent set of loading and boundary conditions provides a repeatable platform across which joint mechanics and muscle forces for different implant designs can be directly compared. Additionally, there are some limitations in the ability of an experimental simulator, and hence an exact computational representation, to recreate dynamic ADLs. In the KKS or an Oxford-type simulator, the relative A–P position of the hip and ankle is fixed; hence, relative hip–knee–ankle kinematics for activities requiring significant A–P motion, like a chair rise, cannot be exactly reproduced. In addition, muscles are represented with point-to-point *muscle* actuators, rather than physiological muscle paths, which influence the muscle force requirements during the activity. This study includes selected details from studies by Fitzpatrick et al. [55,56,81], which aims to develop computational cycles that better represent physiological joint loading during ADLs.

2.5.1 Incorporating Feedback Control of Joint Loads in Computational Simulations

Model development began with the computational representation of the KKS, as described in Section 2.4. In order to provide a platform for comparative evaluation of devices under consistent joint loading conditions, a controlled KKS model was developed. This model incorporated additional measures to control loading of the TF joint. Sensors, measuring all six load components on the tibial insert, were incorporated into the FE model. The PID control system, which initially just allowed control of flexion angle through the quadriceps actuator, was extended to allow simultaneous control of TF compressive joint force, A–P force, V–V and I–E moments, and hip flexion angle, through the vertical hip, flexion–extension ankle moment, M–L ankle force, vertical ankle moment, and quadriceps actuators, respectively (Figure 2.8). Instantaneous measurements from the joint load sensors were fed to a series of PID controllers, interfacing with the FE model through an Abaqus/Explicit user subroutine. On the basis of comparison between current sensor values (hip flexion angle, compressive joint force, A–P force, and V–V and I–E torques) and target profiles, a value for each actuator (quadriceps actuator, vertical hip load actuator, flexion–extension ankle torque, M–L ankle force actuator, and vertical I–E ankle torque, respectively) was applied in the FE model, with each actuator having an independent PID controller. Target TF joint loading profiles were adopted from published instrumented telemetric tibial tray data measuring all six load components of in vivo knee joint loading during a dynamic squat activity [109,110].

The controlled KKS model was able to match experimentally measured in vivo conditions. RMS differences between FE simulations and target profiles were 0.7°, 42 N, 0.4 Nm, and 0.2 Nm for knee flexion angle, compressive joint load, V–V torque, and I–E torque,

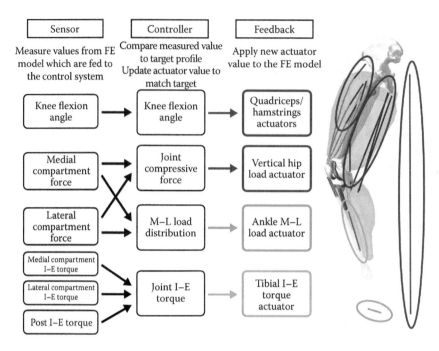

FIGURE 2.8
Schematic of implementation of the feedback control system to update actuators in the computational model to match specific loading conditions at the tibiofemoral joint. (From Fitzpatrick CK et al., *Comput Methods Biomech Biomed Engin*, 17:360–369, 2014.)

respectively, throughout a 90° deep knee bend activity (Figure 2.9). This model can be used for comparative evaluation of component designs under consistent joint loading conditions. In addition to development of cycles that reproduce physiological joint loads, loading profiles can be derived for use in the experimental simulator; the control system can be used to achieve a desired set of loading conditions, and the resulting actuator load profiles can be applied directly to the experimental simulator to induce the same loading conditions at the joint.

2.5.2 Enhanced Simulations to Better Reproduce ADLs

In order to better reproduce experimentally measured in vivo joint mechanics for complex activities, an enhanced simulator was developed, which extended the capabilities of the computational model beyond the experimental setup. To apply or measure I–E torque directly about the long axis of the tibia, an additional actuator was included in the model in order to better control I–E torque in deep flexion. To allow A–P motion of the hip, an actuator was created and used to prescribe relative hip–ankle A–P kinematics during simulation. The quadriceps muscle, which in the experimental simulator consisted of the RF and VI tendons together with a point-to-point line of action, was divided into four muscles (addition of vastus lateralis [VL] and vastus medialis [VM]) (Figure 2.10). Muscle lines of action for each muscle bundle were estimated from the Visible Human data set. Muscle geometry from cryosection data was reconstructed (ScanIP, Simpleware). The centroid of each muscle was estimated and used as the muscle path. The hamstrings muscle (semimembranosus, semitendinosus, long and short heads of

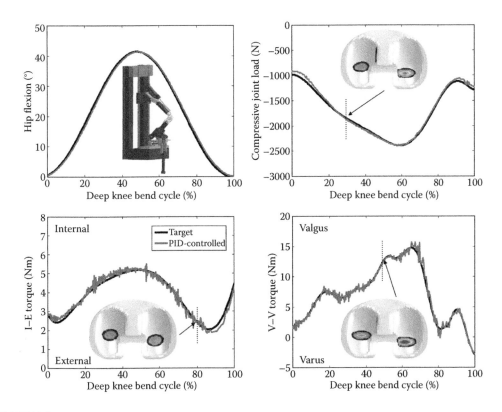

FIGURE 2.9
Accuracy of the control system in reproducing target tibiofemoral joint loading conditions in the controlled KKS model. (From Fitzpatrick CK et al., *Comput Methods Biomech Biomed Eng*, 17:360–369, 2014.)

the biceps femoris), which was not present in the experiment, was represented by four point-to-point actuators, with origins and insertion sites estimated from Visible Human data. Similar to quadriceps actuation, hamstrings actuation was controlled to match flexion angle. These measures allowed for a more physiological estimation of flexor/extensor muscle force required to perform a given activity. The overall quadriceps and hamstrings actuation calculated by the PID controller was distributed equally among the four bundles.

The enhanced simulator was evaluated during a chair rise simulation (tested with loading conditions from three different subjects), in addition to stance-phase gait and stepdown simulations (tested with loading conditions from a single subject). In the chair rise simulations, four actuators were simultaneously controlled through the PID system to match knee flexion angle, joint compressive force, M–L load distribution, and I–E torque to target profiles. Target profiles were taken from gait laboratory kinematics (flexion angle), in vivo telemetric data (compressive load, I–E torque), and a consistent M–L load distribution ratio (each of the three chair rise simulations was nominally assigned 50:50, 60:40, and 70:30 M–L target load split). In the stance-phase gait and stepdown simulations, five actuators were simultaneously controlled to match knee flexion angle, compressive joint load, M–L load distribution, I–E torque, and A–P force. RMS differences in knee flexion angle, compressive force, M–L and A–P load distribution, and I–E torque between the FE measurements and target profiles were compared throughout each cycle. Results from the

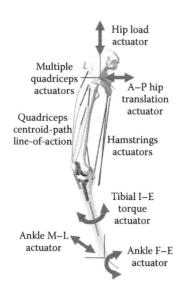

FIGURE 2.10
Actuators of the enhance simulator, with additional actuation (hip A–P and tibial I–E), hamstrings muscles, and physiological quadriceps muscle paths. (From Fitzpatrick CK et al., *Comput Methods Biomech Biomed Eng*, 17:360–369, 2014.)

simulations with four (chair rise) and five (stance-phase gait, stepdown) controlled actuators were compared to determine if increasing the level of control resulted in degradation in the accuracy of the control system.

The enhanced simulator model, with four actuators controlled, reproduced TF joint loading conditions with an RMS accuracy of less than 1.0°, 80 N, 2%, and 0.3 Nm for each of the three chair rise simulations (Figure 2.11). Control of a fifth actuator (controlling A–P force) during stance-phase gait and stepdown activities was implemented without any loss in accuracy of the control system; RMS differences of 0.5°, 65 N, 1.6%, 0.8 Nm, and 17 N for knee flexion angle, compressive joint load, M–L load split, I–E torque, and A–P force, respectively, were measured during the stance-phase gait simulation, and 0.8°, 65 N, 0.4%, 0.1 Nm, and 12 N for the stepdown activity (Figure 2.12).

2.5.3 Developing External Loading Conditions to Match Physiological Joint Loads

The methodology described in Sections 2.5.1 and 2.5.2 uses the control system to apply external loads at the hip, ankle, and muscle actuators to create a consistent set of loading conditions at the TF joint. This facilitates comparison of devices under consistent, physiological joint loading, and the resulting changes in kinematics and external loads can be compared. Oftentimes, however, it is desirable to evaluate the effect that a change in design or alignment would have on joint loads; a change in component design or alignment will likely affect both kinematics and forces at the joint. In order to be able to predict changes in both joint kinematics and forces, the methodology described in the previous sections' study may be applied initially to a baseline component or predicate device, and the resulting actuator load profiles applied by the FE model can be measured. Subsequently, these external actuator loading conditions can be applied directly in the FE model in order to perform a comparative analysis of implant geometry or alignment. In this manner, the

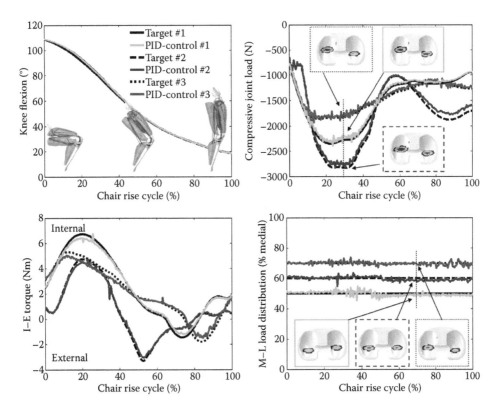

FIGURE 2.11
Comparison of target profiles with PID-controlled joint loads during a chair rise for three subjects in the enhanced simulator. (From Fitzpatrick CK et al., *Comput Methods Biomech Biomed Eng*, 17:360–369, 2014.)

model can simultaneously predict both kinematics and forces for a particular implant and compare these metrics between implant designs [55,56].

2.5.4 Summary

The controlled KKS model can be used for comparative evaluation of component designs under consistent joint loading conditions. In addition, loading profiles can be derived for use in the experimental simulator; the control system can be used to achieve a desired set of loading conditions, and the resulting actuator load profiles can be applied directly to the experimental simulator to induce the same loading conditions at the joint. The enhanced simulator representation described in Section 2.5.2 develops the computational model further than is currently feasible in the experimental setup. Relative hip–ankle A–P motion, inclusion of hamstrings, and more physiological muscle representations allow for improved modeling of ADLs; A–P motion facilitates modeling of activities such as a chair rise, hamstrings allow flexion activities such as gait to be modeled, and physiological moment arms of the quadriceps provide a more accurate estimate of the quadriceps muscle force required to perform an activity. These representations provide a suite of tools that can be used during design-phase evaluation of component geometries to assess performance under in vivo conditions.

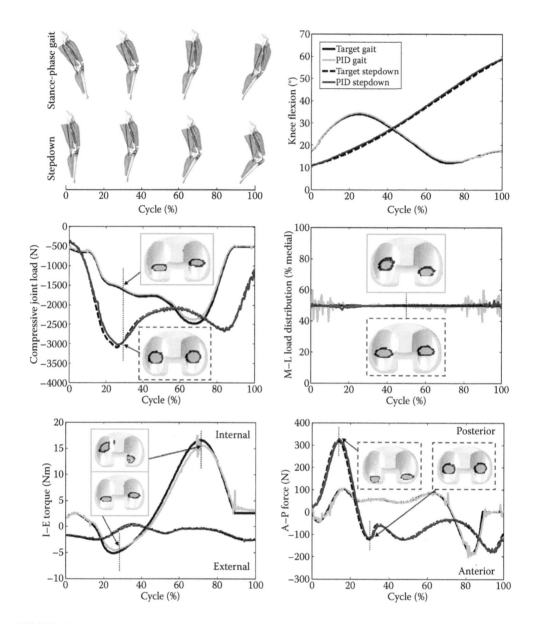

FIGURE 2.12

Comparison of target profiles with PID-controlled joint loads for a single subject in the enhanced simulator during stance-phase gait and stepdown cycles. (From Fitzpatrick CK et al., *Comput Methods Biomech Biomed Eng,* 17:360–369, 2014.)

Depending on the research question of interest, it may be advantageous to allow PID control of a subset of actuators (e.g., maintain control of the quadriceps actuator so that all devices are compared across the same flexion profile). Alternatively, M–L load distribution is affected by soft-tissue structures as well as component geometries. In order to evaluate the effect of weakening (or strengthening) medial ligaments or the medial muscle groups, an M–L force profile may be consistently applied across different implants rather

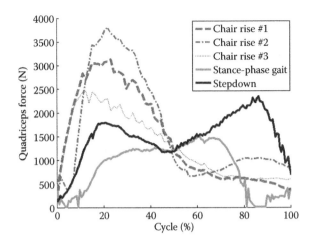

FIGURE 2.13
Quadriceps load during chair rise, stance-phase gait, and stepdown simulations. (From Fitzpatrick CK et al., *Comput Methods Biomech Biomed Eng*, 17:360–369, 2014.)

than controlled at the ankle, and the M–L load distribution may be measured under a variety of ligament or muscle conditions. The control system may also be used to evaluate quadriceps activation under different loading conditions. For instance, there was clear differentiation in the magnitude of quadriceps loading between the three chair rise simulations under different sets of loading conditions, as well as differences in loading pattern between ADLs (Figure 2.13). The flexibility of the control system allows the researcher to customize the FE environment to answer specific questions of interest. The platform described in this study is ideally suited to answer a wide variety of *effect of* research questions that will provide insight into the relationship between component geometry and patient and surgical variables.

2.6 Incorporating Variability into Computational Models

Uncertainty is inherently present in many aspects of biomechanics and orthopedics; factors such as patient geometry, kinematics and joint loading, and implant alignment are all variable in nature. Correspondingly, there is substantial variation in the outcome of TKR procedures within the patient population [111–116]. Patient-specific loads are imposed on the TKR components as a result of limb alignment, gait pattern, weight, muscle physiology, soft-tissue properties, and level of activity. Additional variability is introduced by the TKR procedure itself; components are available in a range of designs, and surgical technique and accuracy may vary from surgeon to surgeon. All of these factors contribute to variability in clinical outcome. Clinical studies and in vitro experiments, however, do not allow for adequate systematic investigation into the factors that influence TKR outcome. It is difficult to assess the individual contributions of these factors to overall variability in TKR mechanics, because of the limited number of trials that may be performed experimentally and sources of variation that cannot be quantified in vivo (muscle forces, ligament attachment sites, mechanical properties, etc.)—large-scale clinical studies are required to identify trends in TKR performance owing to subject-specific variation, rather than surgical technique or implant design.

Computational models, however, allow all sources of variation to be controlled or measured, so that relationships can be assessed in the absence of uncertainty. Prior computational studies have performed a variety of analyses to investigate factors that influence clinical outcomes. Several researchers have performed optimization or design-of-experiments style analysis of TKR design parameters, including sagittal and coronal plane radii and conformity, in order to evaluate the influence of design on implant constraint, flexion kinematics, contact locations, and wear [31,117–120]. Others have investigated the impact of variation in joint or muscle forces on mechanics of the knee [121,122]. A host of computational studies have evaluated the influence of various alignment parameters on TKR mechanics [123–128]. While several prior studies have considered multiple parameters, they have focused on a single source of variability (design, alignment, or loading) in isolation, without considering the relative contributions of each source of variability to the overall variation in TKR mechanics; for instance, designs are evaluated under a consistent set of loading conditions, or surgical alignment is evaluated for a single design. In reality, the patient population includes all of these parameters, which affect joint mechanics and should be accounted for in current computational models. This section describes work presented in Fitzpatrick et al. [55,56], which details a combined FE and probabilistic method in order to evaluate the relative contributions of implant design, surgical, and patient-specific variation to TF and PF joint mechanics during ADLs.

2.6.1 Development of an Efficient FE Model

Probabilistic analyses represent uncertain or variable parameters with a distribution in order to predict bounds of performance. Probabilistic methods typically require hundreds, if not thousands, of trials, to assess the contributions of each parameter and potential interaction effects between parameters. Hence, when applied in conjunction with FE models, the models must be sufficiently computationally efficient to perform the required number of probabilistic trials in a feasible timeframe. The lower limb model described in Sections 2.4 and 2.5 was modified to create a simplified knee joint model—this work required several thousand analyses; hence, a simplified model was necessary as computational efficiency was crucial. TF ligaments were represented by one-dimensional, nonlinear tension-only spring elements with reference strain and linear stiffness parameters adopted from prior work [25]. The quadriceps muscle, which was separated into RF plus VI (RF + VI), VL, and VM bundles, was represented by 2D fiber-reinforced membrane elements to allow for contact and wrapping in deep flexion, with line of action for each bundle based on cadaveric data [129]. Actuators in the model were used to apply loads and muscle forces to the knee. I–E and V–V torques were applied to the tibia, with the remaining tibial DOFs constrained. Quadriceps load was applied to the RF + VI, VL, and VM actuators; vertical load was applied at the hip; A–P force was applied to the femur, with femoral I–E rotation constrained, M–L translation free, and knee flexion determined by a combination of vertical hip and quadriceps load, creating a 6-DOF TF joint. Similarly, the patella was kinematically unconstrained in all 6-DOF, with constraint provided by the patellar tendon, patellofemoral ligaments, and quadriceps (Figure 2.14). Loads were applied to the model using the method described in Section 2.5.3, whereby the control system was initially implemented to create a specific loading condition at the joint and derive the corresponding external loading condition.

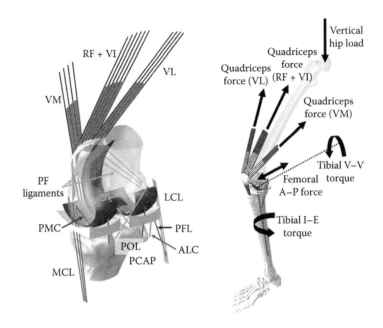

FIGURE 2.14
FE model of the knee joint including TF and PF ligaments, patella tendon, and quadriceps muscles (left); loading condition applied to the knee joint, including quadriceps force, vertical hip load, A–P force applied to the femur, and I–E and V–V torques applied to the tibia (right). (From Fitzpatrick CK et al., *J Biomech*, 45:2092–2102, 2012.)

2.6.2 Sources of Variability

Three sources of variability (implant design, surgical alignment, and patient-specific factors) were incorporated into the FE model. Implant design features were parameterized based on nine variables: femoral condyle distal, posterior, and coronal radii; tibial insert anterior, posterior, and coronal plane conformity; trochlear orientation and M–L position; and coronal plane curvature of the cam mechanism, with variability levels quantified from measurements of current TKR components (Figure 2.15). Values for each parameter were randomly generated assuming a uniform distribution. Custom-scripted software was developed to automatically generate surfaces of the femoral medial and lateral condyles,

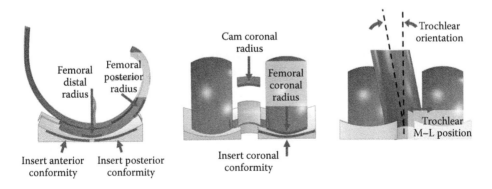

FIGURE 2.15
Design parameters perturbed in the probabilistic analysis. (From Fitzpatrick CK et al., *J Biomech*, 45:2092–2102, 2012.)

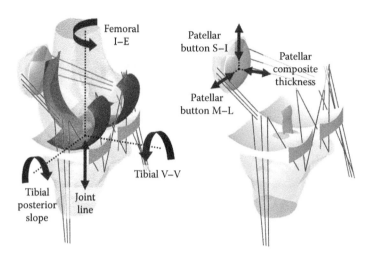

FIGURE 2.16
Surgical parameters perturbed in the probabilistic analysis. (From Fitzpatrick CK et al., *J Biomech*, 45:2092–2102, 2012.)

trochlear and cam geometries, and tibial insert medial and lateral condyles and post geometries, on the basis of the design parameters. A dome-shaped patellar button design was used in all analyses. Surgical variability was accounted for through seven alignment parameters: femoral I–E alignment, tibial insert coronal plane (V–V) alignment, tibial posterior slope, S–I joint line position, patellar composite thickness, and patellar button M–L and S–I position (Figure 2.16). Values for each parameter were randomly generated based on a normal distribution, with variability levels quantified from values reported from clinical studies or in prior computational work [35,57,111,130–136].

Patient-specific variability was accounted for by eight parameters: vertical hip load, femoral A–P force, tibial I–E and V–V torques, patella S–I position (alta–baja), patellar tendon M–L attachment on the tibial tubercle, and percentage of quadriceps load carried by the VM and VL bundles (Figure 2.17). Values for alta–baja, patellar tendon attachment, and quadriceps force distribution parameters were randomly generated based on a normal distribution, with variability levels determined based on clinical and cadaveric studies [111,129,137,138]. Variability in external loading profiles (vertical hip, femoral A–P force, tibial I–E and V–V loads) was derived from telemetric TKR patient data [109]. Compressive, A–P, I–E, and V–V loads at the TF joint were extracted for five patients during three dynamic activities—squat, stance-phase gait, and stepdown cycles. The PID control system was implemented for each of these five patients, and the corresponding external loading conditions were reported. Means and standard deviations of these external profiles, assuming a normal distribution, were used to define in vivo loading variability for each activity. Flexion profiles were adopted from video recordings of the patients during each activity [68]. Although there was some intersubject variation in flexion profiles, a single representative flexion profile was applied in the current analysis so that TKR mechanics could be directly compared as a function of flexion angle across probabilistic trials.

2.6.3 Integrating Probabilistic Methods with FE Simulations

Four separate Monte Carlo probabilistic simulations, with 250 trials each, were performed for each activity, investigating design, surgical, and patient-specific factors individually, in

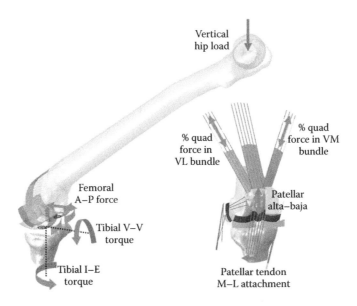

FIGURE 2.17
Subject-specific parameters perturbed in the probabilistic analysis. (From Fitzpatrick CK et al., *J Biomech*, 45:2092–2102, 2012.)

addition to all factors simultaneously. In the probabilistic analyses, the control system was implemented to control quadriceps actuation, ensuring that a consistent flexion profile was achieved across trials, allowing for evaluation of muscle force and quadriceps efficiency. Probabilistic bounds were calculated for TF and PF mechanics, including contact area, peak contact pressure, 6-DOF kinematics, joint loads, ligament forces, and quadriceps force for each of the four Monte Carlo simulations during each activity (squat, stance-phase gait, and stepdown). The relative contributions of each of the three sources of variability to the overall (combined) variability were calculated as a ratio of the area within the 5% and 95% probabilistic bounds for an individual source of variability to the area within the 5% and 95% probabilistic bounds for the combined analysis, identifying which source of variability contributed most to specific TKR mechanics (Figures 2.18 and 2.19). A ratio of 0 indicates that an individual source of variability has no effect on the output measure, while a ratio 1 indicates that the variation for an individual source of variability is equal to the variation for the combined analysis (i.e., contributes strongly to variation in the output measure). Sensitivity analysis, assessed through correlation coefficients between individual probabilistic parameters and output measures, was carried out to determine the most influential parameters for each source of variability.

Quantifying the relative contributions of design, surgical, and subject-specific variation to overall TKR variability, design factors were the primary contributors to condylar contact mechanics, patellar contact area was primarily determined by subject-specific factors, and post-cam contact mechanics were influenced by all sources of variation (Figure 2.18). The main contributors to TF I–E rotation, A–P translation, and V–V rotation were subject-specific, design, and surgical factors, respectively (Figure 2.19). PF kinematics were more influenced by subject-specific and surgical factors than the trochlear design parameters evaluated. TF joint loads were primarily influenced by subject-specific factors, as was normal PF force. TF ligament forces depended on surgical factors, while forces in the extensor mechanism were dependent on subject-specific factors.

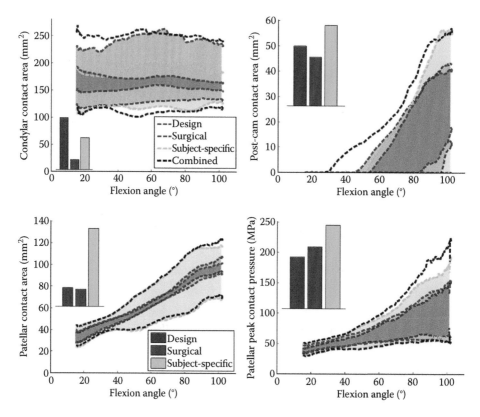

FIGURE 2.18

The 5% and 95% probabilistic bounds of contact mechanics for the squat simulation for all four probabilistic analyses. Insets show the relative contributions of each source of variability (design, surgical, and subject-specific) to the output measure. (From Fitzpatrick CK et al., *J Biomech*, 45:2092–2102, 2012.)

2.6.4 Summary

Frequently, in preclinical cadaveric or computational studies, devices are evaluated under a single set of boundary conditions [32,139,140]. Given the wide range in TKR mechanics attributed to subject-specific variation, additional analyses and experiments, under a range of loading conditions, are necessary to ensure robustness of a device and adequate performance throughout the entire population. Methods presented in this section can be applied to provide insight into which measures can be influenced through design and surgical decisions, and which measures are inherently dependent on variation in the patient population and should be considered in the robustness of implant design and surgical procedure. Given the large number of FE simulations (3000) that needed to be performed for the probabilistic analysis, a number of assumptions and simplifications were necessary to develop a model of sufficient computational efficiency. The model created a physiological loading condition at the knee joint, but not in a perfectly physiological fashion. The compressive load at the joint is primarily controlled by the vertical hip load, I–E and V–V moments are controlled by moments applied at the tibia, and the A–P force at the joint is controlled by an A–P force applied to the femur. Only the quadriceps muscle was included; hence, the net contribution from the rest of the muscles was incorporated, but

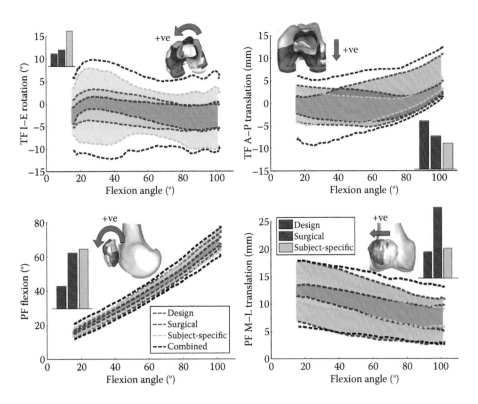

FIGURE 2.19
The 5% and 95% probabilistic bounds of tibiofemoral (top) and patellofemoral kinematics for the squat simulation for all four probabilistic analyses. Insets show the relative contributions of each source of variability (design, surgical, and subject-specific) to the output measure. (From Fitzpatrick CK et al., *J Biomech*, 45:2092–2102, 2012.)

no other individual muscles were represented. There are a variety of other parameters that could be evaluated using the current framework. For instance, the geometry of the trochlea and the patellar button (a dome-shaped design was used in the current analysis) was held constant, but trochlear and patellar geometry/conformity could also be included as probabilistic factors. Also, in the current study, the line of action of the quadriceps was consistent throughout all probabilistic trials. Preliminary evaluation of sensitivity to the quadriceps line of action indicated that there was a negligible effect on TF mechanics but may have a notable influence on PF mechanics, particularly patellar rotations, M–L translation, and PF contact forces. The results from the study are sensitive to the variability levels chosen for each parameter perturbed in the probabilistic analysis. Hence, care was taken to ensure that the variability levels selected were representative of current implant design measures, clinically reported surgical variation, and physiological loading and anatomic variability.

This type of analysis provides insight into interactions between implant design, surgical alignment, and inherently present subject-specific loading and anatomic variation and their respective influences on TKR mechanics. Understanding the relative contributions from multiple sources of variability will aid in clarifying the role of the designer, surgeon, and patient in contributing to and accommodating variation in TKR mechanics and patient outcomes.

2.7 Future Perspectives

Orthopedic surgery has long benefitted from computational and experimental models used to investigate important issues in prosthesis design and clinical performance. Considering the multifactorial etiology of joint replacement failure, computational frameworks are important tools in distinguishing among the many factors contributing to poor functional performance in TKR. Already, models proven capable of differentiating the complex interplay between variations in prosthesis alignment, prosthesis geometry, and patient loading and anatomy are helping to elucidate the underlying mechanisms of biomechanical function and wear. In this manner, models can be used to provide parameters suitable for targeting surgical instrumentation used for prosthesis alignment, identifying at-risk populations, and aiding treatment decisions before or during joint replacement surgery. Extending such computational frameworks to musculoskeletal disease before joint replacement has tremendous potential for aiding treatment decisions.

Continued refinement of existing computational platforms to improve analysis time will benefit more efficient probabilistic models. These efficient models are a compromise between fidelic representation of the in vivo situation and computational efficiency. Simplifying assumptions, for example, the number of muscles modeled and their line of action throughout various loaded activities, requires further validation with detailed experimental studies. More efficient models will provide prosthesis designers analytical tools for evaluating prosthesis designs over the kinematic, stability, and joint loading ranges encountered across the entire patient population. This will aid in design of prostheses that are robust to inherent variability in anatomy, surgical alignment, and patient function. Models that can elucidate interactions between subtle changes in prosthesis design and resulting joint mechanics or preoperatively identify patients at risk from clinical complications such as patellar crepitation or anterior knee pain have broad applications for implant designers and clinicians. When validated against defined in vivo conditions, which provide substantial population uncertainty, computational models have the potential to aid in optimizing component design on a population basis and help surgeons in determining alternative clinical pathways for patients at risk of poor clinical performance and mechanical function with current surgical conventions.

References

1. World Health Organization. The burden of musculoskeletal conditions at the start of the new millennium. Technical Report Series No. 919. Geneva: World Health Organization, 2003.
2. Vignon E, Valat JP, Rossignol M, Avouac B, Rozenberg S, Thoumie P, Avouac J, Nordin M, Hilliquin P. Osteoarthritis of the knee and hip and activity: A systematic international review and synthesis (OASIS). *Joint Bone Spine.* 73:442–455, 2006.
3. Kurtz SM, Lau E, Ong K, Zhao K, Kelly M, Bozic KJ. Future young patient demand for primary and revision joint replacement: National projections from 2010 to 2030. *Clin Orthop Relat Res.* 467:2606–2612, 2009.
4. Kurtz SM, Ong KL, Lau E, Widmer M, Maravic M, Gomez-Barrena E, de Pina M, Manno V, Torre M, Walter WL, de Steiger R, Geesink RGT, Peltola M, Roder C. International survey of primary and revision total knee replacement. *Int Orthop (SICOT).* 35:1783–1789, 2011.

5. Merx H, Dreinhofer K, Schrader P, Sturmer T, Puhl W, Gunther KP, Brenner H. International variation in hip replacement rates. *Ann Rheum Dis.* 62:222–226, 2003.

6. Australian Orthopaedic Association National Joint Replacement Registry. Annual Report. Adelaide: AOA, 2011. Available at http://www.aoa.org.au (accessed February 1, 2013).

7. National Joint Registry for England and Wales. 9th Annual Report. Hertfordshire, England: NJR Centre, 2012. Available at http://www.njrcentre.org.uk (accessed February 1, 2013).

8. Swedish Hip Arthroplasty Register: Annual Report 2011. Available at http://www.shpr.se (accessed February 1, 2013).

9. Swedish Knee Arthroplasty Register: Annual Report 2011. Available at http://www.knee.se (accessed February 1, 2013).

10. Carr AJ, Robertsson O, Graves S, Price AJ, Arden NK, Judge A, Beard DJ. Knee replacement. *Lancet.* 379:1331–1340, 2012.

11. Hardoon SL, Lewsey JD, Gregg PJ, Reeves BC, van der Meulen JHP. Continuous monitoring of the performance of hip prostheses. *J Bone Joint Surg.* 88B(6):716–720, 2006.

12. Jameson SS, Baker PN, Mason J, Porter ML, Deehan DJ, Reed MR. Independent predictors of revision following metal-on-metal hip resurfacing: A retrospective cohort study using National Joint Registry data. *J Bone Joint Surg Br.* 94(6):746–754, 2012.

13. Royal College of Surgeons of England. An investigation of the performance of the 3M Capital hip system. London: The Royal College of Surgeons of England, 2001. Available at http://www.rcseng.ac.uk (accessed December 1, 2014).

14. Mahomed NN, Syed K, Sledge CB, Brennan TA, Liang MH. Improving the postmarket surveillance of total joint arthroplasty devices. *Open Rheumatol J.* 2:7–12, 2008.

15. Challoner DR, Vodra WW. Medical devices and health: Creating a new regulatory framework for moderate-risk devices. *N Engl J Med.* 365(11):977–979, 2011.

16. Ulrich SD, Mont MA, Bonutti PM, Seyler TM, Marker DR, Jones LC. Scientific evidence supporting computer-assisted surgery and minimally invasive surgery for total knee arthroplasty. *Expert Rev Med Devices.* 4(4):497–505, 2007.

17. Sonntag R, Reinders J, Kretzer JP. What's next? Alternative materials for articulation in total joint replacement. *Acta Biomater.* 8(7):2434–2441, 2012.

18. US Food & Drug Administration. A strategic plan: August 2011, 1–36. Available at http://www.fda.gov/ScienceResearch/SpecialTopics/RegulatoryScience/ucm267719.htm (accessed February 1, 2013).

19. Nelissen RGHH, Pijls BG, Karrholm J, Malchau H, Nieuwenhuijse MJ, Valstar ER. RSA and registries: The quest for phased introduction of new implants. *J Bone Joint Surg.* 93(Suppl 3):62–65, 2011.

20. Mackerle J. Finite element modeling and simulations in orthopaedics. A bibliography 1998–2005. *Comput Methods Biomech Biomed Eng.* 9(3):149–199, 2006.

21. Damsgaard M, Rasmussen J, Christensen ST, Surma E, de Zee M. Analysis of musculoskeletal systems in the AnyBody modeling system. *Simul Model Pract Theory.* 14(8):1100–1111, 2006.

22. Delp SL, Kocmond JH, Stern SH. Tradeoffs between motion and stability in posterior substituting knee arthroplasty design. *J Biomech.* 28(10):1155–1166, 1995.

23. Pandy MG, Kotaro S, Seonfil K. A three-dimensional musculoskeletal model of the human knee joint. Part 1: Theoretical construction. *Comput Methods Biomech Biomed Eng.* 1(2):87–108, 1997.

24. Pandy MG, Sasaki K. A three-dimensional musculoskeletal model of the human knee joint. Part 2: Analysis of ligament function. *Comput Methods Biomech Biomed Eng.* 1(4):265–283, 1998.

25. Baldwin MA, Clary C, Fitzpatrick CK, Deacy JS, Maletsky LP, Rullkoetter PJ. Dynamic finite element knee simulation for evaluation of knee replacement mechanics. *J Biomech.* 45:474–483, 2012.

26. Baldwin MA, Clary C, Maletsky LP, Rullkoetter PJ. Verification of predicted specimen-specific natural and implanted patellofemoral kinematics during simulated deep knee bend. *J Biomech.* 42(14):2341–2348, 2009.

27. Barink M, van Kampen A, de Waal Malefijt M, Verdonschot N. A three-dimensional dynamic finite element model of the prosthetic knee joint: Simulation of joint laxity and kinematics. *Proc Inst Mech Eng H: J Eng Med.* 219(6):415–424, 2005.

28. Dhaher YY, Kahn LE. The effect of vastus medialis forces on patellofemoral contact: A model-based study. *J Biomech Eng.* 124(6):758–767, 2002.

29. D'Lima DD, Chen PC, Kester MA, Colwell CW, Jr. Impact of patellofemoral design on patel-lofemoral forces and polyethylene stresses. *J Bone Joint Surg.* 85-A(Suppl 4):85–93, 2003.

30. Elias JJ, Wilson DR, Adamson R, Cosgarea AJ. Evaluation of a computational model used to predict the patellofemoral contact pressure distribution. *J Biomech.* 37(3):295–302, 2004.

31. Fregly BJ, Marquez-Barrientos C, Banks SA, DesJardins JD. Increased conformity offers dimin-ishing returns for reducing total knee replacement wear. *J Biomech Eng.* 132:021007(1–7), 2010.

32. Godest AC, Beaugonin M, Haug E, Taylor M, Gregson PJ. Simulation of a knee joint replace-ment during a gait cycle using explicit finite element analysis. *J Biomech.* 35(2):267–275, 2002.

33. Halloran JP, Petrella AJ, Rullkoetter PJ. Explicit finite element modeling of total knee replace-ment mechanics. *J Biomech.* 38(2):323–331, 2005.

34. Halloran J, Clary C, Maletsky L, Taylor M, Petrella A, Rullkoetter P. Verification of predicted knee replacement kinematics during simulated gait in the Kansas knee simulator. *J Biomech Eng.* 132:081010, 2010.

35. Heegaard JH, Leyvraz PF, Hovey CB. A computer model to simulate patellar biomechanics following total knee replacement: The effects of femoral component alignment. *Clin Biomech.* 16(5):415–423, 2001.

36. Li G, Gil J, Kanamori A, Woo SLY. Validated three-dimensional computational model of a human knee joint. *J Biomech Eng, Trans ASME.* 121(6):657–662, 1999.

37. Pena E, Calvo B, Martinez MA, Doblare M. A three-dimensional finite element analysis of the combined behavior of ligaments and menisci in the healthy human knee joint. *J Biomech.* 39(9):1686–1701, 2006.

38. Perillo-Marcone A, Taylor M. Effect of varus/valgus malalignment on bone strains in the proxi-mal tibia after TKR: An explicit finite element study. *J Biomech Eng.* 129:1–11, 2007.

39. Powers CM, Chen YJ, Scher I, Lee TQ. The influence of patellofemoral joint contact geometry on the modeling of three dimensional patellofemoral joint forces. *J Biomech.* 39(15):2783–2791, 2006.

40. Shirazi-Adl A, Moglo KE. Effect of changes in cruciate ligaments pretensions on knee joint lax-ity and ligament forces. *Comput Methods Biomech Biomed Eng.* 8(1):17–24, 2005.

41. Zelle J, Van der Zanden AC, Malefijt MDW, Verdonschot N. Biomechanical analysis of posterior cruciate ligament retaining high-flexion total knee arthroplasty. *Clin Biomech.* 24:842–849, 2009.

42. Knight LA, Pal S, Coleman JC, Bronson F, Haider H, Levine DL, Taylor M, Rullkoetter PJ. Comparison of long-term numerical and experimental total knee replacement wear during simulated gait loading. *J Biomech.* 40(7):1550–1558, 2007.

43. Rawlinson JJ, Furman BD, Li S, Wright TM, Bartel DL. Retrieval, experimental, and computa-tional assessment of the performance of total knee replacements. *J Orthop Res.* 24(7):1384–1394, 2006.

44. Zhao D, Sakoda H, Sawyer WG, Banks SA, Fregly BJ. Predicting knee replacement damage in a simulator machine using a computational model with a consistent wear factor. *J Biomech Eng.* 130(1):011004(1–10), 2008.

45. Lanovaz JL, Ellis RE. Dynamic simulation of a displacement-controlled total knee replacement wear tester. *Proc Inst Mech Eng H.* 222(5):669–681, 2008.

46. Pal S, Haider H, Laz PJ, Knight LA, Rullkoetter PJ. Probabilistic finite element modeling of TKR wear. *Wear.* 264:701–707, 2008.

47. Fregly BJ, Sawyer WG, Harman MK, Banks SA. Computational wear prediction of a total knee replacement from in vivo kinematics. *J Biomech.* 38:305–314, 2005.

48. DesJardins JD, Walker PS, Haider H, Perry J. The use of a force-controlled dynamic knee simu-lator to quantify the mechanical performance of total knee replacement designs during func-tional activity. *J Biomech.* 33(10):1231–1242, 2000.

49. Sutton LG, Werner FW, Haider H, Hamblin T, Clabeaux JJ. In vitro response of the natural cadaver knee to the loading profiles specified in a standard for knee implant wear testing. *J Biomech.* 43:2203–2207, 2010.

50. Harman MK, DesJardins J, Benson L, Banks SA, LaBerge M, Hodge WA. Comparison of poly-ethylene tibial insert damage from in vivo function and in vitro wear simulation. *J Orthop Res.* 27(4):540–548, 2009.
51. D'Lima DD, Patil S, Steklov N, Colwell CW. The 2011 ABJS Nicolas Andry award: 'Lab'-in-a-knee: In vivo knee forces, kinematics, and contact analysis. *Clin Orthop Relat Res.* 469(10):2953–2970, 2011.
52. Piazza SJ, Delp SL, Stulberg SD, Stern SH. Posterior tilting of the tibial component decreases femoral rollback in posterior-substituting knee replacement: A computer simulation study. *J Orthop Res.* 16(2):264–270, 1998.
53. Buechel FF, Buechel FF, Pappas MJ, ALessio JD. Twenty-year evaluation of meniscal bearing and rotating platform knee replacements. *Clin Orthop Relat Res.* 388:41–50, 2001.
54. Delp SL, Loan JP. A graphics-based software system to develop and analyze models of musculoskeletal structures. *Comput Biol Med.* 25(1):21–34, 1995.
55. Fitzpatrick CK, Clary CW, Laz PJ, Rullkoetter PJ. Relative contributions of design, alignment and loading variability in knee replacement mechanics. *J Orthop Res.* 30:2015–2024, 2012.
56. Fitzpatrick CK, Clary CW, Rullkoetter PJ. The role of patient, surgical, and implant design variation in total knee performance. *J Biomech.* 45:2092–2102, 2012.
57. Fitzpatrick CK, Baldwin MA, Clary CW, Wright A, Laz PJ, Rullkoetter PJ. Identifying alignment parameters affecting implanted patellofemoral mechanics. *J Orthop Res.* 30(7):1167–1175, 2012.
58. Fitzpatrick CK, Rullkoetter PJ. Influence of patellofemoral articular geometry and material on mechanics of the unresurfaced patella. *J Biomech.* 45:1909–1915, 2012.
59. Fitzpatrick CK, Baldwin MA, Ali AA, Laz PJ, Rullkoetter PJ. Comparison of patellar bone strain in the natural and implanted knee during simulated deep flexion. *J Orthop Res.* 29:232–239, 2011.
60. Laz PJ, Browne M. A review of probabilistic analysis in orthopaedic biomechanics. *J Eng Med (Proc Inst Mech Eng: Part H).* 224:927–943, 2010.
61. Easley SK, Pal S, Tomaszewski PR, Petrella AJ, Rullkoetter PJ, Laz PJ. Finite element-based probabilistic analysis for orthopaedic applications. *Comput Methods Programs Biomed.* 85:32–40, 2007.
62. Fitzpatrick CK, Baldwin MA, Laz PJ, FitzPatrick DP, Lerner AL, Rullkoetter PJ. Development of a statistical shape model of the patellofemoral joint for investigating relationships between shape and function. *J Biomech.* 44(13):2446–2452, 2011.
63. Laz PJ, Saikat P, Fields A, Petrella AJ, Rullkoetter PJ. Effects of knee simulator loading and alignment variability on predicted implant mechanics: A probabilistic study. *J Orthop Res.* 24:2212–2221, 2006.
64. Visible Human Project. US National Library of Medicine, National Institutes of Health. Available at http://www.nlm.nih.gov/research/visible/visible_human.html (accessed December 1, 2014).
65. Banks SA, Hodge WA. 2003 Hap Paul Award Paper of the International Society for Technology in Arthroplasty. Design and activity dependence of kinematics in fixed and mobile-bearing knee arthroplasties. *J Arthroplasty.* 19(7):809–816, 2004.
66. Fregly BJ, Besier TF, Lloyd DG, Delp SL, Banks SA, Pandy MG, D'Lima DD. Grand challenge competition to predict in vivo knee loads. *J Orthop Res.* 30(4):503–513, 2012.
67. Papaioannou G, Nianios G, Mitrogiannis C, Fyhrie D, Tashman S, Yang KH. Patient-specific knee joint finite element model validation with high-accuracy kinematics from biplane dynamic Roentgen stereogrammetric analysis. *J Biomech.* 41(12):2633–2638, 2008.
68. Bergmann G. (ed). *Orthoload.* Charite—Universitaetsmedizin Berlin, 2008. Available at http://Orthoload.com (accessed July 1, 2011).
69. Banks SA, Harman MK, Hodge WA. Mechanism of anterior impingement damage in total knee arthroplasty. *J Bone Joint Surg.* 84-A(Suppl 2):37–42, 2002.
70. Harman MK, Banks SA, Hodge WA. Polyethylene damage and knee kinematics after total knee arthroplasty. *Clin Orthop Relat Res.* 392:383–393, 2001.
71. Harman MK, Banks SA, Hodge WA. Backside damage corresponding to articular damage in retrieved tibial polyethylene inserts. *Clin Orthop Relat Res.* 458:137–144, 2007.

72. Harman MK, Schmitt S, Rössing S, Banks SA, Scharf HP, Viceconti M, Hodge WA. Polyethylene damage patterns and deformation in unicondylar knee replacement corresponding to progressive changes in component alignment and fixation. *Clin Biomech.* 25(6):570–575, 2010.

73. International Organization for Standardization. Standard Number 12891-1: Implants for surgery—Retrieval and analysis of surgical implants: Part 1. Retrieval and handling. Geneva, Switzerland: International Organization for Standardization, 2011.

74. ASTM International. F561-05a: Standard practice for retrieval and analysis of medical devices and associated tissues and fluids. West Conshohocken, PA: ASTM International, 2005.

75. Teeter MG, Naudie DDR, McErlain DD, Brandt JM, Yuan X, MacDonald SJ, Holdsworth DW. In vitro quantification of wear in tibial inserts using microcomputed tomography. *Clin Orthop Relat Res.* 469:107–112, 2011.

76. Benson LC, DesJardins JD, Harman MK, LaBerge M. Effect of stair descent loading on ultra-high molecular weight polyethylene wear in a force-controlled knee simulator. *J Eng Med (Proc Inst Mech Eng: Part H).* 216:409–418, 2002.

77. Harman M, Affatato S, Spinelli M, Zavalloni M, Stea S, Toni A. Polyethylene insert damage in unicondylar knee replacement: A comparison of in vivo function and in vitro simulation. *J Eng Med (Proc Inst Mech Eng: Part H).* 224(7):823–830, 2010.

78. Harman MK, Banks SA, Fregly BJ, Sawyer WG, Hodge WA. Biomechanical mechanisms for damage: Retrieval analysis and computational wear predictions in total knee replacements. *J Mech Med Biol.* 5(3):469–475, 2005.

79. Morra EA, Harman MK, Greenwald AS. Computational models can predict polymer insert damage in total knee replacements. In *Insall & Scott Surgery of the Knee*, 4th edition, Scott WN (ed.), Vol. 1 (13):271–283. Philadelphia, PA: Elsevier Inc., 2005.

80. Fitzpatrick CK, Harman MK, Rullkoetter PJ. Comparison of mobile bearing patella wear patterns in computational and retrieval studies. Submitted to the 18th Congress of the European Society of Biomechanics, Lisbon, Portugal, 2012.

81. Fitzpatrick CK, Baldwin MA, Clary C, Maletsky LP, Rullkoetter P. Evaluating knee replacement mechanics during ADL with PID-controlled dynamic finite element analysis. *Comput Methods Biomech Biomed Eng.* 17:360–369, 2014.

82. Hoops HE, Johnson DR, Kim RH, Dennis DA, Baldwin MA, Fitzpatrick CK, Laz PJ, Rullkoetter PJ. Control-matched computational evaluation of tendo-femoral contact in patients with posterior-stabilized total knee arthroplasty. *J Orthop Res.* 30:1355–1361, 2012.

83. Matsuda S, Ishinishi T, White SE, Whiteside LA. Patellofemoral joint after total knee arthroplasty. *J Arthroplasty.* 12(7):790–797, 1997.

84. Powers CM, Lilley JC, Lee TQ. The effects of axial and multi-plane loading of the extensor mechanism on the patellofemoral joint. *Clin Biomech.* 13:616–624, 1998.

85. Li G, Rudy TW, Sakane M, Kanamori A, Ma CB, Woo SL-Y. The importance of quadriceps and hamstring muscle loading on knee kinematics and in-situ forces in the ACL. *J Biomech.* 32:395–400, 1999.

86. D'Lima DD, Poole C, Chadha H, Hermida JC, Mahar A, Colwell CW. Quadriceps moment arm and quadriceps forces after total knee arthroplasty. *Clin Orthop Relat Res.* 392:213–220, 2001.

87. Haider H, Walker PS. Measurements of constraint of total knee replacement. *J Biomech.* 38:341–348, 2005.

88. Becher C, Heyse TJ, Kron N, Ostermeier S, Hurschler C, Schofer MD, Fuchs-Winkelmann S, Tibesku CO. Posterior stabilized TKR reduce patellofemoral contact pressure compared with cruciate retaining TKA in vitro. *Knee Surg Sports Traumatol Arthrosc.* 17:1159–1165, 2009.

89. Maletsky LP, Hillberry BM. Simulating dynamic activities using a five-axis knee simulator. *J Biomech Eng.* 127(1):123–133, 2005.

90. Gollehon DL, Torzilli PA, Warren RF. The role of the posterolateral and cruciate ligaments in the stability of the human knee. A biomechanical study. *J Bone Joint Surg Am.* 69(2):233–242, 1987.

91. Markolf KL, Kochan A, Amstutz HC. Measurement of knee stiffness and laxity in patients with documented absence of the anterior cruciate ligament. *J Bone Joint Surg Am.* 66(2):242–252, 1984.

92. Markolf KL, Mensch JS, Amstutz HC. Stiffness and laxity of the knee—The contributions of the supporting structures. A quantitative in vitro study. *J Bone Joint Surg Am*. 58(5):583–594, 1976.

93. Seering WP, Piziali RL, Nagel DA, Schurman DJ. Function of the primary ligaments of the knee in varus-valgus and axial rotation. *J Biomech*. 13(9):785–794, 1980.

94. Grood ES, Suntay WJ. Joint coordinate system for the clinical description of three-dimensional motions: Application to the knee. *J Biomech Eng, Trans ASME*. 105(2):136–144, 1983.

95. LaPrade RF, Engebretsen AH, Ly TV, Johansen S, Wentorf FA, Engebretsen L. The anatomy of the medial part of the knee. *J Bone Joint Surg Am*. 89(9):2000–2010, 2007.

96. LaPrade RF, Ly TV, Wentorf FA, Engebretsen L. The posterolateral attachments of the knee: A qualitative and quantitative morphologic analysis of the fibular collateral ligament, popliteus tendon, popliteofibular ligament, and lateral gastrocnemius tendon. *Am J Sports Med*. 31(6):854–860, 2003.

97. Shahane SA, Ibbotson C, Strachan R, Bickerstaff DR. The popliteofibular ligament. An anatomical study of the posterolateral corner of the knee. *J Bone Joint Surg Br*. 81(4):636–642, 1999.

98. Shelburne KB, Torry MR, Pandy MG. Contributions of muscles, ligaments, and the ground-reaction force to tibiofemoral joint loading during normal gait. *J Orthop Res*. 24(10):1983–1990, 2006.

99. Atkinson P, Atkinson T, Huang C, Doane R. A comparison of the mechanical and dimensional properties of the human medial and lateral patellofemoral ligaments. 46th Annual Meeting of the Orthopaedic Research Society, 0776, 2000.

100. Stäubli HU, Schatzmann L, Brunner P, Rincón L, Nolte LP. Mechanical tensile properties of the quadriceps tendon and patellar ligament in young adults. *Am J Sports Med*. 27(1):27–34, 1999.

101. Dennis DA, Kim RH, Johnson DR, Springer BD, Fehring TK, Sharma A. Control matched evaluation of painful patellar crepitus after total knee arthroplasty. *Clin Orthop Relat Res*. 439:10–17, 2011.

102. Pollock DC, Ammeen DJ, Engh GA. Synovial entrapment: A complication of posterior stabilized total knee arthroplasty. *J Bone Joint Surg Am*. 84-A, 2174–2178, 2002.

103. Beight JL, Yao B, Hozack WJ, Hearn SL, Booth RE, Jr. The patellar *clunk* syndrome after posterior stabilized total knee arthroplasty. *Clin Orthop Relat Res*. 139–142, 1994.

104. Hozack WJ, Rothman RH, Booth RE, Jr., Balderston RA. The patellar clunk syndrome. A complication of posterior stabilized total knee arthroplasty. *Clin Orthop Relat Res*. 203–208, 1989.

105. Anderson JA, Baldini A, Sculco TP. Patellofemoral function after total knee arthroplasty: A comparison of 2 posterior-stabilized designs. *J Knee Surg*. 21:91–96, 2008.

106. Maloney WJ, Schmidt R, Sculco TP. Femoral component design and patellar clunk syndrome. *Clin Orthop Relat Res*. 199–202, 2003.

107. Ranawat AS, Ranawat CS, Slamin JE, Dennis DA. Patellar crepitation in the P.F.C. sigma total knee system. *Orthopedics*. 29:S68–S70, 2006.

108. Yau WP, Wong JW, Chiu KY, Ng TP, Tang WM. Patellar clunk syndrome after posterior stabilized total knee arthroplasty. *J Arthroplasty*. 18:1023–1028, 2003.

109. Kutzner I, Heinlein B, Graichen F, Bender A, Rohlmann A, Halder A, Beier A, Bergmann G. Loading of the knee joint during activities of daily living measured in vivo in five subjects. *J Biomech*. 43:2164–2173, 2010.

110. Heinlein B, Graichen F, Bender A, Rohlmann A, Bergmann G. Design, calibration and pre-clinical testing of an instrumented tibial tray. *J Biomech*. 40:S4–S10, 2007.

111. Dennis DA, Kim RH, Johnson DR, Springer BD, Fehring TK, Sharma A. Control-matched evaluation of painful patellar crepitus after total knee arthroplasty. *Clin Orthop Relat Res*. 469:10–17, 2010.

112. Harman MK, Banks SA, Kirschner S, Lützner J. Prosthesis alignment affects axial rotation motion after total knee replacement. A prospective study combining computed tomography and fluoroscopic evaluations. *BMC Musculoskel Dis*. 13(1):206, 2012.

113. Jenny JY, Miehlke RK, Giurea A. Learning curve in navigated total knee replacement. A multicentre study comparing experienced and beginner centres. *Knee*. 15:80–84, 2008.

114. Mahaluxmivala J, Bankes MJK, Nicolai P, Aldam CH, Allen PW. The effect of surgeon experience on component positioning in 673 press fit condylar posterior cruciate-sacrificing total knee arthroplasties. *J Arthroplasty.* 16:635–640, 2001.

115. Siston RA, Patel JJ, Goodman SB, Delp SL, Giori NJ. The variability of femoral rotational alignment in total knee arthroplasty. *J Bone Joint Surg Am.* 87:2276–2280, 2005.

116. Siston RA, Goodman SB, Patel JJ, Delp SL, Giori NJ. The high variability of tibial rotational alignment in total knee arthroplasty. *Clin Orthop Relat Res.* 452:65–69, 2006.

117. Willing R, Kim IY. Design optimization of a total knee replacement for improved constraint and flexion kinematics. *J Biomech.* 44:1014–1020, 2011.

118. Dargahi J, Najarian S, Amiri S. Optimization of the geometry of total knee implant in the sagittal plane using FEA. *Biomed Mater Eng.* 13:439–449, 2003.

119. Sathasivam S, Walker PS. The conflicting requirements of laxity and conformity in total knee replacement. *J Biomech.* 32:239–247, 1999.

120. Walker PS, Sathasivam S. Design forms of total knee replacement. *Proc Inst Mech Eng H.* 214(1):101–119, 2000.

121. Lin YC, Haftka RT, Queipo NV, Fregly BJ. Surrogate articular contact models for computationally efficient multibody dynamic simulations. *Med Eng Phys.* 32:584–594, 2010.

122. Imran A, Huss RA, Holstein H, O'Connor JJ. The variation in the orientations and moment arms of the knee extensor and flexor muscle tendons with increasing muscle force: A mathematical analysis. *Proc Inst Mech Eng H.* 214:277–286, 2000.

123. Strickland MA, Arsene CT, Pal S, Laz PJ, Taylor M. A multi-platform comparison of efficient probabilistic methods in the prediction of total knee replacement mechanics. *Comput Methods Biomech Biomed Eng.* 13:701–709, 2010.

124. Fitzpatrick CK, Baldwin MA, Rullkoetter PJ, Laz PJ. Combined probabilistic and principal component analysis approach for multivariate sensitivity evaluation and application to implanted patellofemoral mechanics. *J Biomech.* 44(1):13–21, 2011.

125. Yang NH, Canavan PK, Nayeb-Hashemi H. The effect of the frontal plane tibiofemoral angle and varus knee moment on the contact stress and strain at the knee cartilage. *J Appl Biomech.* 26:432–443, 2010.

126. Mihalko WM, Williams JL. Computer modeling to predict effects of implant malpositioning during TKA. *Orthopedics.* 33(10 Suppl):71–75, 2010.

127. D'Lima DD, Chen PC, Colwell CW. Polyethylene contact stresses, articular congruity, and knee alignment. *Clin Orthop Relat Res.* 392:232–238, 2001.

128. Lin YC, Haftka RT, Queipo NV, Fregly BJ. Two-dimensional surrogate contact modeling for computationally efficient dynamic simulation of total knee replacements. *J Biomech Eng.* 131:041010, 2009.

129. Farahmand F, Naghi Tahmasbi M, Amis A. The contribution of the medial retinaculum and quadriceps muscles to patellar lateral stability—An in-vitro study. *Knee.* 11:89–94, 2004.

130. Srivastava A, Lee GY, Steklov N, Colwell CW, Ezzet KA, D'Lima DD. Effect of tibial component varus on wear in total knee arthroplasty. *Knee.* 19:560–563, 2012.

131. Maestro A, Harwin SF, Sandoval MG, Vaquero DH, Murcia A. Influence of intramedullary versus extramedullary alignment guides on final total knee arthroplasty component position: A radiographic analysis. *J Arthroplasty.* 13:552–558, 1998.

132. Nagamine R, Miura H, Urabe K, Matsuda S, Hirata G, Moro-oka T, Kawano T, Iwamoto Y. A new concept for precise patella resection in total knee arthroplasty. *Am J Knee Surg.* 14:227–231, 2001.

133. Akagi M, Matsusue Y, Mata T, Asada Y, Horiguchi M, Iida H, Nakamura T. Effect of rotational alignment on patellar tracking in total knee arthroplasty. *Clin Orthop Relat Res.* 366:224–227, 1999.

134. Lee TQ, Budoff JE, Glaser FE. Patellar component positioning in total knee arthroplasty. *Clin Orthop Relat Res.* 366:274–281, 1999.

135. Anouchi YS, Whiteside LA, Kaiser AD, Milliano MT. The effects of axial rotational alignment of the femoral component on knee stability and patellar tracking in total knee arthroplasty demonstrated on autopsy specimens. *Clin Orthop Relat Res.* 287:170–177, 1993.

136. Gomes LS, Bechtold JE, Gustilo RB. Patellar prosthesis positioning in total knee arthroplasty. A roentgenographic study. *Clin Orthop Relat Res.* 236:72–81, 1988.
137. Bonnin MP, Saffarini M, Mercier PE, Laurent JR, Carrillon Y. Is the anterior tibial tuberosity a reliable rotational landmark for the tibial component in total knee arthroplasty? *J Arthroplasty.* 26:260–267, 2011.
138. Defrate LE, Nha KW, Papannagari R, Moses JM, Gill TJ, Li G. The biomechanical function of the patellar tendon during in-vivo weight-bearing flexion. *J Biomech.* 40:1716–1722, 2007.
139. Merican AM, Ghosh KM, Iranpour F, Deehan DJ, Amis AA. The effect of femoral component rotation on the kinematics of the tibiofemoral and patellofemoral joints after total knee arthroplasty. *Knee Surg Sports Traumatol Arthrosc.* 19:1479–1487, 2011.
140. Mizu-uchi H, Colwell CW, Jr., Matsuda S, Flores-Hernandez C, Iwamoto Y, D'Lima DD. Effect of total knee arthroplasty implant position on flexion angle before implant-bone impingement. *J Arthroplasty.* 26:721–727, 2011.

3

Mathematical Modelling of Basic Multicellular Units: The Functional Units of Bone Remodeling

Pascal R. Buenzli and Peter Pivonka

CONTENTS

ABSTRACT Bone remodeling denotes the continual renewal of the bone matrix over our lifetime. This renewal is operated by self-contained groups of bone-resorbing cells called osteoclasts and bone-forming cells called osteoblasts. These functional groups of cells ensure the tight coordination between bone resorption and bone formation required for skeletal maintenance and mineral homeostasis. Many bone disorders such as osteoporosis and osteopetrosis are associated with a deregulation of the balance between resorption and formation within basic multicellular units (BMUs). While usually recognized as the basic functional unit of bone remodeling, BMUs are still incompletely understood. Coupling between osteoclasts and osteoblasts is known to occur through several signaling molecules such as the receptor activator of nuclear factor kappa-B ligand (RANKL), osteoprotegerin (OPG), transforming growth factor beta (TGFβ), and parathyroid hormone (PTH). However, the mechanisms of action of these molecules between spatially segregated populations of osteoclasts and osteoblasts within BMUs are unclear. How a BMU initiates and progresses through bone and terminates and how these events translate to cell distribution and cellular interactions is also unclear. To shed light on the spatio-temporal dynamics of BMUs and the complex interactions of their constituents, several computational models describing BMU behavior have been developed in recent years. These modeling efforts have focused on different aspects of BMU regulation including (i) chemotactic effects of RANKL signaling in trabecular BMUs [1,2]; (ii) timing of RANKL and OPG signaling in trabecular BMUs [3]; (iii) cellular organization in cortical BMUs owing to biochemical pathways [4]; (iv) stages of the BMU's life, initiation, and progression stages—implications for tetracycline-based assessment of matrix apposition rates [5]; (v) formation of the resorption cavity and osteoclast resorption pattern [1,2]; (vi) refilling of the resorption cavity and osteoblast secretory activity [5,6]; (vii) repair of microdamage in the bone matrix and biomechanical steering of BMU progression [7]; and (viii) mechanical feedback in trabecular BMUs [8]. The objective of this book chapter is to give an overview of the state-of-the-art computational models of BMUs and their application to bone remodeling with a special emphasis on model developments from our own research.

3.1 Introduction

Human skeletal tissues undergo continuous renewal at rates ranging from 5% to 30% per year depending on the type of bones [9,10]. This renewal process is referred to as bone remodeling [9,10]. Bone remodeling occurs through a coordinated process of bone resorption and bone formation by specialized bone cells. These bone cells are organized into groups called basic multicellular units (BMUs) (see Figure 3.1). At the front of a BMU, osteoclasts (bone-resorbing cells) dissolve the bone matrix, creating a resorption cavity (cutting cone). Toward the rear of a BMU, osteoblasts (bone-forming cells) secrete osteoid, an organic matrix of collagen fibers gradually refilling the resorption cavity. This organic matrix becomes gradually mineralized to form new bone. The mineralization of osteoid is a process believed to be partly regulated by osteoblasts and osteocytes during the formation of osteocytes. Osteocytes are mechanosensing cells derived from osteoblasts that become trapped in the bone matrix during matrix deposition. The primary physiological functions of bone remodeling are believed to be (i) the repair of microdamage resulting from repeated mechanical loading and (ii) the regulation of calcium and phosphate homeostasis. Many bone disorders including osteoporosis and osteopetrosis have been associated with dysfunctional cell communication in remodeling.

The development of bone histomorphometry in the late 1950s led to the observation that bone renewal occurs in local *packets* of bone resorption and bone formation by different cell types, segregated spatially and temporally [11]. These packets of bone remodeling were termed *basic multicellular units* by Harold M. Frost, who first described them as the

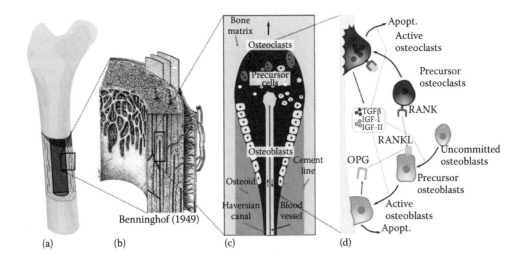

FIGURE 3.1
Bone tissue is renewed by BMUs. Osteoclasts and osteoblasts communicate with each other through several signaling molecules such as RANKL, OPG, and TGFβ. This couples bone formation to bone resorption in bone remodeling. Panels (a) through (d): from bone to tissue to BMUs to cells.

basic functional unit of bone remodeling [12]. There are approximately 1.7×10^6 BMUs in a normal adult skeleton [12–15]. In cortical bone, BMUs proceed through the bulk of the tissue, leaving new secondary osteons in their wake (Figure 3.1a through c). Osteons are cylindrical tissue structures approximately 100–200 μm in diameter and up to 10 mm in length; they are aligned with the main loading direction [16–18]. In trabecular bone, BMUs proceed along the surfaces of plates and struts, forming hemi-osteons, or trenches of new bone tissue approximately 60–70 μm deep [17]. Because trabecular bone remodeling operates on the bone surface, it can be associated with either negative bone balance (net bone loss) or positive bone balance (net bone gain). The situation in cortical bone depends on the mode of remodeling. Cortical remodeling either creates a new Haversian canal (*type I osteons*), which always implies net bone loss, or uses a preexisting Haversian canal (*type II osteons*) [15,19]. In the latter case, net bone gain may occur if the diameter of the Haversian canal is reduced by the passage of the BMU. The exact proportion of type I over type II osteons in cortical bone remodeling is still a subject of controversy: vascular channels increase with age [15] but age-related bone loss is attributed to increased pore area rather than increased pore density [20].

Dynamic histomorphometry techniques such as tetracycline labeling and radionuclide imaging have considerably helped in the elucidation of kinetic properties of matrix apposition and cell development within BMUs [21–23]. In the following, we describe the different phases of BMU remodeling starting with activation, followed by resorption, and by formation, the so-called ARF sequence. While trabecular bone exhibits the same sequence of surface activation, resorption, and formation, its three-dimensional (3D) organization is difficult to visualize from two-dimensional histological sections. Here, we will focus primarily on cortical BMUs.

The activation of BMU remodeling in a specific region of the bone surface starts with lining cells retracting from the bone surface [21]. Mononuclear preosteoclasts are then recruited to the uncovered bone matrix. Under preferable biochemical conditions (see below), the preosteoclasts nucleate to form multinucleated osteoclasts. An important component of cortical BMU initiation and progression is the generation of a blood vessel that provides stem cells and nutrients to the site of remodeling and enables the transport of minerals and waste products away from that site. In trabecular BMUs, recent experimental observations have confirmed the presence of a so-called canopy sealing off the region of bone undergoing remodeling from the marrow. In some cases, the canopy is seen to be perfused with blood vessels [24,25]. At the front of the BMU, in a region called the resorption zone (see Figure 3.1c and d), multinucleated osteoclasts attach to the bone surface and dissolve the bone matrix by secreting a mixture of hydrogen ions and proteases such as Cathepsin-K [26,27]. Hydrogen ions reduce the pH and dissolve the minerals into the microenvironment. Cathepsin-K is then able to break down the demineralized collagenous matrix. The average BMU progression speed is directly linked to the osteoclast resorption activity. The rate of progression of BMUs is estimated at 20–40 μm/day [28]. Toward the back of the BMU, in the so-called formation zone, active osteoblasts refill the cavity by laying down a collagen-rich substance known as osteoid (Figure 3.1c and d). Osteoid subsequently mineralizes over the following weeks to form new bone (see Refs. [9,21]). The region between the resorption zone and the formation zone, called the reversal zone, contains precursor cells of the osteoclast and osteoblast lineages [21]. In cortical bone, the blood vessel supplying the BMU with new precursor cells and nutrients grows at the same rate as the BMU progresses into the bone. The net effect of the passage of a cortical BMU at a specific location of bone is the local renewal of the bone matrix. In cortical bone, this leads to the formation of a so-called secondary osteon, which includes a Haversian canal. In trabecular bone, the completion of bone renewal by a BMU is seen as a new lamellar bone structural unit on the surface of the trabecular struts or plates.

Over the last several decades, bone biologists have identified a large number of biochemical and biomechanical regulatory factors secreted and received by the cells composing a BMU. These factors influence BMU behavior and the spatial and temporal organization of the cells within the BMU [29]. The formation of osteoclasts has been shown to rely crucially on macrophage colony-stimulating factor [30] and on the receptor activator of nuclear factor kappa-B (RANK) cell signaling pathway, which involves the receptor RANK, the ligand RANKL, and osteoprotegerin (OPG) [31–33]. RANKL activates the RANK receptor on precursor osteoclasts, which triggers their development and sustains their activity. The soluble molecule OPG is a decoy receptor of RANKL that can prevent RANKL from binding to RANK. Another important molecule mediating the communication between osteoblasts and osteoclasts is transforming growth factor beta (TGFβ). TGFβ is stored in high concentrations in the bone matrix. During matrix resorption by active osteoclasts, TGFβ is released into the bone microenvironment, where it exerts its action on several bone cells [34]. The existence of a mechanical regulation of bone remodeling has long been suspected. It is now well established that mechanical feedback is a key regulatory mechanism to maintain bone mass [35,36]. The commonly accepted view is that osteocytes act as mechanosensors that transduce local mechanical signals into biochemical signals through the production of nitric oxide, prostaglandin E_2, and sclerostin [37,38]. These biochemical signals are thought to regulate the initiation of bone remodeling processes and to help modulate the coupling between bone resorption and formation.

The above description of the cell types and biomechanical and biochemical factors involved in BMU regulation shows the complexity of the communication network of bone cells in a BMU (Figure 3.1d). In vitro and in vivo experiments generate ever-increasing amounts of information on different factors affecting BMU remodeling. A challenging problem is to integrate these experimental observations gained through different experimental conditions or models into an understanding of whole system behavior. To this end, several computational models describing BMU behavior have been developed in recent years.

This chapter is organized as follows: In Section 3.2, we first discuss the role of mathematical modeling in predicting bone remodeling and BMU regulation. Mathematical models focusing on different spatial and temporal scales are reviewed, such as the cellular, the tissue, and the organ scales. In Section 3.3, we present a continuous model of the spatio-temporal dynamics of a single cortical BMU based on partial differential equations (PDEs). In Section 3.4, we present a discrete model focusing on osteoclast resorption in cortical BMUs based on an agent-based modeling approach. Concluding remarks and an outlook are given in Section 3.5.

3.2 State of the Art of Mathematical Models of Bone Remodeling

Bone is a complex adaptive and self-repairing biological system owing to the multiple spatial and temporal scales involved in its modeling and remodeling. Only subsets of these scales are generally investigated experimentally depending on the biological questions tested. Indeed, this complexity is challenging to address using current experimental techniques. For example, how the underlying biochemical and biomechanical regulatory mechanisms lead to BMU initiation, to cell organization in BMUs, to the steering of progressing BMUs, and to the balanced bone resorption and formation is still unclear. Recent reviews have stressed the insights that mathematical modeling can bring to our understanding of the bone remodeling processes [39–41]. Mathematical and computational models are powerful tools to help us formalize conceptual models of BMU regulation. They enable simulation of complex biological mechanisms to test hypotheses *in silico*. Mathematical and computational models are particularly useful in the following situations: (i) when simultaneous multiple events make it difficult to predict intuitively the behavior of the system, (ii) when the time and length scales of various events under investigation are significantly different, and (iii) when the system exhibits nonlinear (nonobvious) behavior. In silico models can be regarded as an additional and complementary tool to the commonly employed in vitro and in vivo models. They can be used to test hypotheses that are difficult to address with current experimental techniques. They can help us interpret experimental data or help connect different types of data obtained by different experimental techniques.

Computational models of bone remodeling may be distinguished based on the particular regulatory mechanisms that are considered (e.g., purely biomechanical models, biochemical models, and coupled models) [39] or based on the particular scale that they have been applied to (e.g., cellular, tissue, and organ scale) [42]. In the following, we review some recently developed models of bone remodeling and of BMU regulation using the latter classification.

3.2.1 Cellular Scale Models

At the cellular scale, one is generally concerned with investigating the behavior of a single BMU. Mathematical models formulated on this scale describe the interactions of different cell types and biochemical and biomechanical regulatory mechanisms (Figure 3.1c and d). These models can be described using PDEs or agent-based approaches.

Ryser and Komarova developed a mathematical model of a single trabecular BMU describing the evolution in time and space of the concentrations of RANKL and OPG, the evolution of osteoclast and osteoblast numbers, and the evolution of bone mass [1,2]. These authors assume that (i) osteocytes surrounding a microfracture produce RANKL; (ii) osteoclasts are attracted to regions of high RANKL content; (iii) OPG and RANKL are produced by osteoblasts and diffuse through bone; (iv) RANKL is eliminated when binding to OPG or RANK. This set of assumptions in effect models a biochemical coupling between osteoblasts and osteoclasts. The evolution of the BMU arising from this model is studied numerically. The model recapitulates the spatio-temporal dynamics believed to occur in vivo in a cross section of bone: in response to a gradient of RANKL, osteoclasts move as a well-confined cutting cone. The coupling of osteoclasts to osteoblasts then recruits osteoblasts in sufficient numbers to refill the resorbed surfaces. The RANKL concentration is highest at the microfracture in front of the BMU, whereas the OPG concentration peaks at the back of the BMU, resulting in the formation of a RANKL/OPG gradient. In the model, this gradient strongly affects the rate of BMU progression and the size of the BMU. An interesting aspect of this model is to propose a mechanism for the termination of the BMU. If the diffusion of OPG is fast enough, OPG may gradually diffuse from the back of the BMU toward the front, where it may inhibit the availability of free RANKL. This may inhibit osteoclastogenesis sufficiently to eventually depopulate the BMU from all its cells. Thus, the spatial organization of a BMU provides important constraints on the roles of RANKL and OPG as well as possibly other regulators in determining the outcome of remodeling in the BMU.

Ji et al. have proposed a model of the trabecular bone remodeling cycle based on a predator–prey model [8]. The model simulates a remodeling event occurring at a fixed position in bone, integrating bone removal by osteoclasts and formation by osteoblasts. The model is developed to construct the variation in bone thickness at a particular point during the remodeling event. This is compared with observations derived from standard bone histomorphometric analyses. The analogy of a local bone remodeling event with a predator–prey system is based on the fact that during remodeling, the population of osteoblasts (predators) closely follows the population of osteoclasts (preys) with a small temporal delay. Furthermore, the remodeling rate of the bone surface can be represented by the periodicity of the solution of the predator–prey system; that is, bursts of osteoclasts followed by osteoblasts occur at periodic intervals. A feedback mechanism in the bone formation activity is included to co-regulate bone thickness. An interesting aspect of this model is that the number of parameters of the model is fairly small. This enables the authors to calibrate the model against experimental data recorded for normal (healthy) bone remodeling. Two sample pathological conditions, hypothyroidism and primary hyperparathyroidism, are also examined.

3.2.2 Tissue-Scale Models of BMU Regulation

At the tissue scale ($\sim 2 \times 2 \times 2$ mm^3), one is concerned with investigating the behavior of an ensemble of BMUs and its effect on the bone tissue structure including the mechanical properties. At this scale, two different types of modeling approaches can be distinguished.

The first type of models uses spatial averaging over a so-called representative volume element (RVE) of the tissue. Only temporal changes of biochemical and biomechanical quantities such as average cell densities, average concentration of regulatory factors, and bone volume in the RVE can be investigated. The advantage is that these models are usually described by ordinary differential equations (ODEs), which are simpler to study mathematically and numerically than PDEs or discrete models. Models neglecting mechanical effects (such as, e.g., osteocyte feedback) are commonly referred to as cell-population models. Commonly employed temporal models in bone remodeling applications are based on the models of Komarova et al., Lemaire et al., or Pivonka et al. [43–45]. In the model of Komarova et al., biochemical signaling between active osteoclasts and osteoblasts has been lumped into exponential parameters. In the models of Lemaire et al. and Pivonka et al., biochemical regulatory factors such as TGFβ, RANK, RANKL, and OPG have been included explicitly. In recent model developments, the mechanical features of bone have also been taken into account using a so-called micromechanical model of bone stiffness [46,47]. These coupled biochemical–biomechanical models are very powerful to investigate different aspects of biochemical and biomechanical regulation on bone remodeling and changes in mechanical properties of bone tissue. One advantage of these models is that they can be readily applied to the whole organ scale. On the other hand, no spatial information on the RVE scale is provided.

The second type of modeling approach fully takes into account the microstructure of bone. Hence, the distribution of stresses and strains in individual regions of bone such as in individual trabecular struts (and plates) can be estimated using finite element analysis (FEA). BMU remodeling in these models is taken into account in different ways. While some groups use a cellular Potts model to describe interactions of the bone matrix with osteoblasts and osteoclasts [7,48], others use so-called Wolff-type rules that essentially add bone in areas where mechanical loading is larger than normal and remove bone in areas where mechanical loading is lower than normal [49–56]. Due to very small fractions of bone removed in a single remodeling event compared to the tissue scale, the spatial discretization needs to be of the size of the resorption volume. Most commonly cubical elements of micron size are chosen and the respective finite element model has been commonly referred to as the microFE model. The initiation of new BMUs has been assumed random [51,57,58] or targeted using a damage criterion [59]. The advantage of such models is that the tissue spatial resolution is preserved. Their disadvantage is that they are computationally very intensive. Particularly, 3D models require supercomputing facilities. Mostly, the biomechanical aspects of bone are emphasized in these models. The regulation of the BMUs on the cellular and molecular level is usually not considered with as much detail as in the models mentioned in Section 3.2.1.

The model of van Oers, Ruimerman, and coworkers is particularly interesting [7,48]. This model proposes a unified theory for osteonal and hemi-osteonal remodeling by BMUs in which osteoclasts and osteoblasts are coupled entirely through local mechanical stimuli generated around evolving resorption cavities. The model is particularly suited to address the question of how mechanical forces guide bone cells and BMUs during remodeling. The hypothesis implemented in this microFE model is that strain-induced osteocyte signals inhibit osteoclast activity and stimulate osteoblast activity. While the structural model dealing with the mechanical aspects of bone is a classical microFE model calculating local stresses, the remodeling algorithm uses a cell simulation model based on a cellular Potts model. The simulation results of van Oers et al. capture some key features of BMU-based remodeling, such as (i) an effective coupling between resorption and formation in response to changing strains around the resorption sites (this effective coupling describes both cortical BMU tunneling through bone and trabecular BMU trenching on the bone surface), (ii) alignment of osteons in cortical bone and alignment of trabecular struts in trabecular bone with the main loading axis, and (iii) BMU initiation and BMU steering near regions of damaged bone (e.g., owing to osteocyte death).

3.2.3 Organ-Scale Models

Organ-scale models of bones (e.g., whole femur bone) primarily focus on the effect of changes in mechanical loading on adaptation of the bone microstructure. This type of models is generally based on the theory of (poro)elasticity and uses FEA to compute mechanical quantities such as stress, strain, strain energy density (SED), and so on. A Wolff-type adaptation algorithm is used to model a modeling or remodeling response: bone is gained in regions of high mechanical loading and lost in regions of low mechanical loading. The bone structure evolves to a state in which similar mechanical conditions are attained (in the form of stress, strain, SED, etc.) across different regions. Wolff-type phenomenological approaches of bone adaptation are useful in addressing questions related to structural biomechanics. We refer the reader to excellent recent reviews on these types of models [41,42,47,60].

3.3 Modeling the Spatio-Temporal Structure of Cell Distribution in BMUs

Bone resorption and formation in a BMU are strongly regulated by biochemical cell coupling. Biochemical coupling between cells involves several signaling molecules binding to specific cell receptors. Receptor–ligand bindings trigger intracellular signaling pathways inducing a cell response, such as an up- or down-regulation of the expression of a protein, chemotaxis, differentiation, proliferation, or apoptosis (see Figure 3.2). Intracellular pathways are often complex and may involve several dozens of molecules. They enable an understanding of the behavior and organization of a single cell. To understand the behavior and organization of a single BMU, we focus here on the intercellular communications at are play in the BMU. Intracellular pathways will be modeled phenomenologically, by specifying directly the strength of the cell response to a ligand (output) as a function of the fraction of cell receptors bound to the ligand (input).

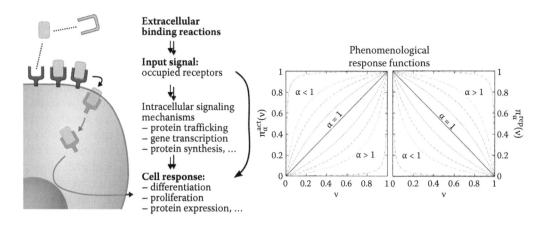

FIGURE 3.2

Intracellular pathways are modeled implicitly through phenomenological response functions $\pi_\alpha^{\text{act}}(v), \pi_\alpha^{\text{rep}}(v)$ integrating complex intracellular pathways. The response functions $\pi_\alpha^{\text{act}}(v), \pi_\alpha^{\text{rep}}(v)$ determine the strength of the cell response as a function of the fraction of occupied receptors v.

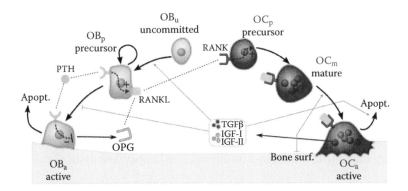

FIGURE 3.3
Biochemical intercellular communication between osteoclasts and osteoblasts of different maturity in the model of cell development in a single BMU.

In bones, the formation and activity of osteoclasts require RANKL, which is expressed on preosteoblasts (see Figure 3.3). Bone matrix resorption releases TGFβ in active form into the microenvironment, which helps promote the commitment of mesenchymal stem cells to the osteoblast lineage. This closes a positive feedback loop in which the creation of osteoblasts and the creation and activity of osteoclasts are self-reinforcing. In bone remodeling, this is a good thing: the more resorption there is, the more formation there will be. However, without control, this feedback loop would quickly lead to ever-increasing osteoblasts and osteoclasts. The control of this feedback loop in bone remodeling occurs in at least two ways: (i) TGFβ inhibits the differentiation of osteoclasts, and (ii) active or mature osteoblasts reduce their production of RANKL and increase their production of OPG. OPG binds RANKL, preventing its subsequent binding to RANK and thus preventing osteoclastogenesis.

The above controlled feedback loop of bone cell coupling leading to an overall biochemical regulation of bone remodeling was implemented at the tissue scale in the form of rate equations by several teams [43,44,61]. When supplemented with basic transport properties of osteoclasts and osteoblasts, the above mechanisms can be shown to be also responsible for the emergence and stability of the spatial organization of cells within a single BMU [4]. To do so, the rate equations in ODEs must be extended into PDEs.

3.3.1 Description of the Model

The creation and elimination of cells, cell migration, receptor–ligand binding reactions, and protein diffusion are all phenomena that modify locally the quantity of the concerned compounds. Such phenomena are described in general by the material balance equation of each cell type or molecule. In the material balance equation, source and sink terms account for nonconservative modifications of the local densities (as attributed to, e.g., cell differentiation, cell apoptosis, receptor–ligand binding reactions, protein expression by cells, and microenvironmental protein degradation). Transport terms account for conservative modifications of the local densities (as attributed to, e.g., cell migration, chemotaxis, and protein diffusion) [4].

The core assumptions of the spatio-temporal model of cell development in a single BMU that we propose are summarized below with the network of biochemical regulations illustrated in Figure 3.3. These assumptions are implemented as source/sink terms or transport terms in the material balance equation. The model considers a single spatial dimension, the BMU's longitudinal axis x.

3.3.1.1 Osteoclasts

Three stages of osteoclast development are considered: preosteoclasts (OC_p), mature osteoclasts (OC_m), and active osteoclasts (OC_a) (Figure 3.3). In bone remodeling, preosteoclasts are mononucleated cells while mature and active osteoclasts are multinucleated cells formed by fusion of preosteoclasts. In the model presented below, OC_m and OC_a are assumed to denote single nuclei incorporated in a multinucleated entity. We assume the following:

- OC_ps are distributed around the tip of a blood vessel growing at a rate commensurate with the BMU progression (20–40 µm/day) [9,15,21,62], taken to be $v_{BMU} = 30$ µm/day.
- OC_ps differentiate into mature osteoclast nuclei OC_ms at a rate $\mathcal{D}_{OC_p}$ accelerated by activation of the receptor RANK by the ligand RANKL [27,63].
- OC_m nuclei migrate toward the front of the BMU with a velocity $v_{OC_m} > v_{BMU}$. Once at the bone surface, they join an actively resorbing multinucleated osteoclast, hence, becoming OC_as [62].
- OC_as progress forward along the x axis owing to bone resorption, at a rate $v_{OC_m} = v_{BMU} = 30$ µm/day [9,15,21].
- OC_as undergo apoptosis at a rate $\mathcal{A}_{OC_a}$ accelerated by TGFβ [23,44].

Osteoclast development in the model can therefore be summed up schematically as the following sequence:

$$OC_p \xrightarrow{\text{RANKL+}} OC_m \xrightarrow{\text{bone surface+}} OC_a \xrightarrow{\text{TGFβ+}} \varnothing. \tag{3.1}$$

The continual supply of OC_ps from the blood vessel is assumed unbounded and not rate limiting. OC_p is taken as a given density distribution along the BMU peaked around the tip of the growing blood vessel:

$$OC_p(x,t) = OC_p(x - v_{BMU}t) = OC_p^0 \exp\left\{ -\frac{1}{2}\left(\frac{x - x_{bv}^0 - v_{BMU}t}{L_{rev}} \right)^2 \right\}. \tag{3.2}$$

The material balance equations for OC_m and OC_a corresponding to this sequence are as follows:

$$\frac{\partial}{\partial t}OC_m = \mathcal{D}_{OC_p}(RANKL)OC_p - \mathcal{D}_{OC_m}(R)OC_m - \frac{\partial}{\partial x}J_{OC_m} \tag{3.3}$$

$$\frac{\partial}{\partial t}OC_a = \mathcal{D}_{OC_m}(R)OC_m - \mathcal{A}_{OC_a}(TGFβ)OC_a - \frac{\partial}{\partial x}J_{OC_a}, \tag{3.4}$$

where R denotes the radius of the cavity and

$$J_{OC_m} = OC_m v_{OC_m} \tag{3.5}$$

$$J_{OC_a} = OC_a v_{OC_a} \tag{3.6}$$

are the fluxes of OC_m and OC_a, $\mathcal{D}_{OC_p}(\text{RANKL})$ is the RANKL-dependent differentiation rate of OC_ps, and $\mathcal{A}_{OC_a}(\text{TGF}\beta)$ is the TGFβ-dependent apoptosis rate of OC_as. As in Ref. [44], the up-regulation and down-regulation of cellular responses by a ligand are assumed proportional to the fraction of occupied receptors. The consideration of mass action kinetics for the receptor–ligand binding reactions shows that the fraction of receptors on a cell bound to the ligand L is given by $\dfrac{L/k}{1+L/k}$ [64], where k is the dissociation constant of the binding reaction. We therefore modulate the cellular responses by (dimensionless) *activator* and *repressor* functions of the ligand concentration as follows:

$$\mathcal{D}_{OC_p}(\text{RANKL}) = D_{OC_p} \pi_{\text{act}} \left(\frac{\text{RANKL}}{k_{OC_p}^{\text{RANKL}}} \right) \tag{3.7}$$

$$\mathcal{A}_{OC_a}(\text{TGF}\beta) = A_{OC_a} \pi_{\text{act}} \left(\frac{\text{TGF}\beta}{k_{OC_a}^{\text{TGF}\beta}} \right) \tag{3.8}$$

$$\mathcal{D}_{OC_p}(\text{RANKL}) = D_{OC_p} \pi_{\text{act}} \left(\frac{\text{RANKL}}{k_{OC_p}^{\text{RANKL}}} \right) \tag{3.9}$$

$$\mathcal{A}_{OC_a}(\text{TGF}\beta) = A_{OC_a} \pi_{\text{act}} \left(\frac{\text{TGF}\beta}{k_{OC_a}^{\text{TGF}\beta}} \right), \tag{3.10}$$

where

$$\pi_{\text{act}}(x) = \frac{x}{1+x}, \quad \pi_{\text{rep}}(x) = 1 - \pi_{\text{act}}(x) = \frac{1}{1+x}. \tag{3.11}$$

To model the transition from OC_m to OC_a at the bone surface of the genuinely 3D BMU cavity in this one-dimensional setup, we assume that $\mathcal{D}_{OC_m}(R)$ is proportional to the fraction of bone matrix seen in a cylindrical cross section of the BMU of radius R_c (cement line radius):

$$\mathcal{D}_{OC_m}(R) = D_{OC_m} \left(1 - \frac{R^2}{R_c^2} \right). \tag{3.12}$$

$\mathcal{D}_{OC_m}(R)$ interpolates between the maximum value D_{OC_m} at the tip of the BMU ($R = 0$) and the value 0 in the reversal zone ($R = R_c$).

3.3.1.2 Osteoblasts

Three stages of osteoblast development are considered: uncommitted osteoblast progenitors (such as mesenchymal stem cells) (OB_u), preosteoblasts (OB_p), and active osteoblasts (OB_a) (Figure 3.3). The fate of active osteoblasts is either to be buried in osteoid and become osteocytes during BMU refilling, to undergo apoptosis (e.g., via anoikis) if in surplus to perform the refilling, or to become bone lining cells covering the surface of the new Haversian canal at the end of refilling [9]. In the model presented below, all three alternatives are modeled by a single elimination rate from the active cell pool. We assume the following:

- OB_us are distributed around the tip of the blood vessel growing along x at 30 μm/day, similarly to OC_ps [9,21,22,62].
- OB_us differentiate into OB_ps at a rate $\mathcal{D}_{OB_u}$ accelerated by TGFβ [21,65–67].
- OB_ps differentiate into OB_as at a rate $\mathcal{D}_{OB_p}$ inhibited by TGFβ [4,44].
- OB_as are eliminated from the active cell pool at a rate A_{OB_a}.
- OB_ps and OB_as are stationary with respect to bone: $v_{OB_a} = v_{OB_p} = 0$ [9,21,68,69].

Osteoblast development in the model can therefore be summed up schematically as the following sequence:

$$OB_u \xrightarrow{\text{TGFβ+}} OB_p \xrightarrow{\text{TGFβ−}} OB_a \rightarrow \varnothing. \tag{3.13}$$

The material balance equations for OC_m and OC_a corresponding to this sequence are as follows:

$$\frac{\partial}{\partial t} OB_p = \mathcal{D}_{OB_u}(TGFβ)OB_u - \mathcal{D}_{OB_p}(TGFβ)OB_p \tag{3.14}$$

$$\frac{\partial}{\partial t} OB_a = \mathcal{D}_{OB_p}(TGFβ)OB_p - A_{OB_a}OB_a, \tag{3.15}$$

where $\mathcal{D}_{OB_u}(TGFβ)$ and $\mathcal{D}_{OB_p}(TGFβ)$ are the TGFβ-dependent differentiation of OB_us and OB_ps, respectively, given by

$$\mathcal{D}_{OB_u}(TGFβ) = D_{OB_u} \pi_{act}\left(\frac{TGFβ}{k_{OB_u}^{TGFβ}}\right) \tag{3.16}$$

$$\mathcal{D}_{OB_p}(TGFβ) = D_{OB_p} \pi_{rep}\left(\frac{TGFβ}{k_{OB_p}^{TGFβ}}\right). \tag{3.17}$$

Similarly to OC_p, the unbounded and non-rate-limiting supply of OB_us from the blood vessel is modeled as a peaked distribution around the tip of the growing blood vessel:

$$OB_u(x,t) = OB_u(x - v_{BMU}t) = OB_u^0 \exp\left\{-\frac{1}{2}\left(\frac{x - x_{bv}^0 - v_{BMU}t}{L_{rev}}\right)^2\right\}. \tag{3.18}$$

3.3.1.3 Signaling Molecules and Binding Reactions

The biochemical coupling between osteoclasts and osteoblasts is mediated in the model by RANKL and TGFβ, as in Refs. [4,44] (TGFβ may also represent other regulatory factors stored in the bone matrix, such as insulin-like growth factors, (Figure 3.3). RANKL is influenced by OPG and parathyroid hormone (PTH). RANKL, OPG, and TGFβ are driven by cellular actions (Figure 3.3):

- RANKL is expressed on the membrane of OB_ps; OPG is expressed by OB_as; RANK is expressed on OC_ps [4,70,71].
- RANKL binds both RANK and the decoy receptor OPG competitively (RANK signaling on OC_p is thereby diminished in the presence of OPG) [27,63].
- PTH promotes the expression of RANKL and inhibits the expression of OPG [72]. Here, a constant level of systemic PTH is assumed, uniformly distributed along the BMU [4].
- TGFβ is stored in the bone matrix at a constant concentration $TGFβ_{bone}$; it is released in the microenvironment in proportion to bone resorption by OC_as [27,66,67].
- All of the signaling molecules RANKL, OPG, and TGFβ undergo microenvironmental degradation at a constant rate. A constant number of RANK per OC_p is assumed.

Binding reactions between receptors and ligands are considered through mass action kinetics with reaction rates proportional to population sizes. Transport properties of RANK and RANKL are bound to transport properties of the osteoclasts and osteoblasts that express these molecules on their membrane. Not much is known of the transport properties of the other signaling molecules within BMUs. However, they do not need to be accounted for under the adiabatic hypothesis presented below, under which binding reaction rates dominate transport phenomena.

3.3.1.4 Adiabatic Approximation

Because of the separation of time scales between the fast reaction rates of ligands binding to their receptors on cells, and comparatively slow cell responses, a considerable simplification of the mass action kinetic equations considered for the competitive bindings between RANK, RANKL, and OPG can be performed. This simplification is based on the fact that cell population dynamics vary slowly in regard to receptor–ligand binding reaction rates and can be assumed constant in a first approximation when solving for the receptor and ligand concentration. This approximation is called adiabatic. We examine here the consequence of this separation of time scales in the presence of transport terms in a generic mass balance equation for the density n of a signaling molecule with source/sink terms $\sigma(x,t)$ and flux $J(x,t)$. Let r be the slowest reaction rate (e.g., in day^{-1}) to be found in σ. Dividing the mass balance equation by r, one has

$$\frac{1}{r}\frac{\partial}{\partial t}n(x,t) = \frac{1}{r}\sigma(x,t) - \frac{1}{r}\frac{\partial}{\partial x}J(x,t). \qquad (3.19)$$

If reaction binding dominates transport phenomena, $\left|\frac{1}{r}\frac{\partial}{\partial x}J\right| \ll 1$ and $r\sigma = O(1)$. Thus, changes in the local concentration of the free ligand occur on the short time scale r^{-1}, and only quasi–steady states of this signaling molecule need to be considered for the cellular dynamics, leading to

$$\sigma(x, t) \approx 0, \forall x, t. \tag{3.20}$$

This equation can then be solved for the quasi–steady-state value of the concentration of the signaling molecule as a function of the slowly varying cell densities:

$$L(x, t) = \text{function } (OB_p(x, t), OB_a(x, t), OC_m(x, t), OC_a(x, t)). \tag{3.21}$$

This simplification is exactly of the same form as in the temporal-only model of Ref. [44] (Equations 3.16 through 3.20). We assume here that it holds for RANKL, OPG, and PTH. With the production and elimination characteristics listed above, one obtains the following (see Refs. [4,44] for more details):

$$PTH(x,t) = \frac{\beta_{PTH}}{D_{PTH}}, \tag{3.22}$$

$$OPG(x,t) = \frac{\beta_{OB_a}^{OPG} OB_a \pi_{rep}\left(\dfrac{PTH}{k_{OB,rep}^{PTH}}\right)}{\beta_{OB_a}^{OPG} OB_a \pi_{rep}\left(\dfrac{PTH}{k_{OB,rep}^{PTH}}\right)\bigg/ OPG_{sat} + D_{OPG}}, \tag{3.23}$$

$$RANKL(x,t) = \frac{\beta_{RANKL}}{1 + k_{RANK}^{RANKL} RANK + k_{OPG}^{RANKL} OPG}\left\{ D_{RANKL} + \frac{\beta_{RANKL}}{N_{OB_p}^{RANKL} OB_p \pi_{act}\left(\dfrac{PTH}{k_{OB,act}^{PTH}}\right)}\right\}^{-1}, \tag{3.24}$$

$$RANK(x,t) = N_{OC_p}^{RANK} OC_p. \tag{3.25}$$

The production of TGFβ in the BMU cavity occurs during bone resorption by active osteoclasts and thus on a slower cellular time scale. TGFβ also acts differentially on osteoblasts of various maturity. It can be expected to be degraded by the BMU microenvironment at time scales matching the slower characteristic times of the cellular dynamics. The differential description of TGFβ is therefore kept:

$$\frac{\partial}{\partial t} TGF\beta(x,t) = TGF\beta_{bone} k_{res} OC_a - D_{TGF\beta} TGF\beta. \tag{3.26}$$

3.3.1.5 Boundary Conditions and Numerical Solution

The governing equations for cells and signaling molecules need to be supplemented with appropriate boundary conditions. These boundary conditions depend on how the equations are numerically resolved. Equations 3.3 and 3.4 are advection–reaction equations that require one boundary condition (first order in space). Advection–reaction equations are numerically unstable and often stabilized by adding a small diffusive term. This requires supplying two boundary conditions (second order in space). Because of the finite lifespan of all cells and signaling molecules in the model, boundary conditions have a limited influence on the density distributions along the BMU compared to the supply of precursor cells OB_u and OB_p. In fact, the boundary conditions influence the density distributions only in a limited region near the boundaries of the integration domain.

To model the progression of a BMU through bone during a long lifespan, it is worthwhile to solve the system of equations in a frame co-moving with the BMU. The position of the tip of the blood vessel is stationary in this co-moving frame. This enables restricting the spatial integration domain to a fixed region around the supply of precursor cells. The change of frame adds a convective term $u\dfrac{dn}{dx}$ to the material balance equation for n. Dirichlet boundary conditions (advection–reaction equation) or Dirichlet and Neumann boundary conditions (advection–diffusion–reaction equation) were specified in this co-moving frame at a fixed distance ahead of the tip of the blood vessel. This distance was chosen large enough (850 µm) to not interfere with the peaked distribution of precursor cells. The BMU cavity radius $R(x)$, which influences the activation of osteoclasts, was assumed to have a given shape with $R(x) = 0$ at a distance 350 µm ahead of the tip of the blood vessel. The system of PDEs was solved using Mathematica's PDE solver NDSolve with the method of lines [73].

3.3.2 Numerical Results and Discussion

3.3.2.1 BMU Initiation and Propagation

The precise physiological mechanisms leading to BMU initiation are still unclear. A combination of local signals from osteocytes or bone lining cells (e.g., in response to a local mechanical stimulus) attracts precursor cells near the bone interface. Bone lining cells detach from the bone interface to let osteoclasts start resorbing the bone matrix. In the model, we start with an initial condition consisting of the given peaked distributions of precursor cells (OB_u, OC_p) and a localized concentration of TGFβ around the tip of the blood vessel. No other cell types is present initially (Figure 3.4a). The controlled feedback loop between the different cell types involved in the BMU enables this initial condition to evolve into fully developed distributions of all cell types (Figure 3.4a through d). These structured cell distribution profiles propagate forward through bone similarly to a traveling wave, with active osteoclasts toward the front and active osteoblasts toward the rear of the BMU, corresponding to the cellular organization observed in BMUs in vivo (Figure 3.4d).

Each cell type reaches a stable spatial distribution at a different rate. Because of the longer lifespan of osteoblasts compared to osteoclasts, the cell distribution profile of active osteoblasts takes longer to evolve to a quasi–steady shape. The life history of a BMU is usually divided into three separate stages: initiation (resorption alone, early life), progression (resorption and formation, midlife), and termination (formation alone, late life) [15]. From the dynamics of cell development observed in our model, these stages can be decomposed further into several levels of quasi–steady states until the progression stage is fully developed. Indeed, while the population of certain cell types may have reached a quasi–steady state within the BMU, the population of other cell types may still be developing. Because of the longer lifespan of osteoblasts compared with osteoclasts, we observe that osteoclast densities reach a steady state earlier in the BMU's life than osteoblast densities. The sequence of cell types reaching a steady-state spatial distribution within the BMU is as follows: (1) precursor cells (OB_u, OC_p) (this is assumed to occur instantly), (2) mature and active osteoclasts (OC_m, OC_a), (3) preosteoblasts (OB_p), and (4) active osteoblasts. The appearance of the first active osteoblasts in the BMU (which denotes the transition from the

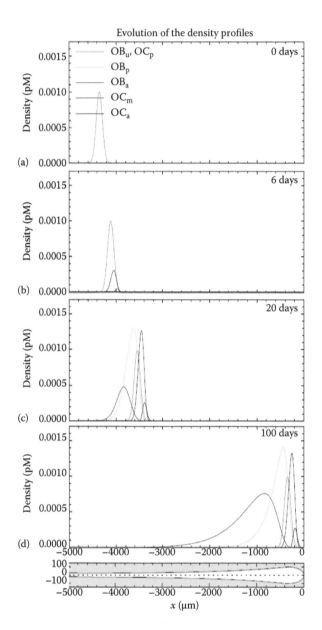

FIGURE 3.4

Density profiles within the BMU cavity at different time points: (a) initial state ($t = 0$ days); (b) early resorption phase with not fully developed OC_a profile ($t = 6$ days); (c) full resorption phase with only partially developed formation phase ($t = 20$ days); (d) fully developed cell profiles at steady state ($t = 100$ days).

initiation to the progression stage according to the usual picture) occurs between stages (1) and (2). In Figure 3.4c (at $t = 20$ days), the density of active osteoclasts (OC_as) and the front of the density of preosteoblasts (OB_p) have already reached a quasi–steady-state distribution, but not the density of OB_as near the back of the BMU. This state is situated between stages (3) and (4) above and corresponds to an early (still developing) progression stage. According to this picture of cell and BMU development, a significant portion of the BMU's lifespan of 6–12 months [21] could be spent in a developing stage (i.e., non–steady state) owing to the slow development of the osteoblast population. In fact, the stabilization of the spatial distribution profiles of cells occurs only once the BMU has traveled sufficiently far away from its point of origin (approximately 90 days).

3.3.2.2 Effect of Cell Transport Properties

Motile properties of osteoblasts and osteoclasts and the regulation of these properties within a BMU are not often mentioned in the literature [67,74,75]. However, these motile properties can influence dramatically the spatio-temporal coordination of the bone cells and thus the functional behavior of the BMU. In Figure 3.4, the wave-like propagation of the populations of OB_ps and OB_as is attributed to their creation upstream and elimination downstream: cells were assumed stationary with respect to bone. If individual OB_ps and OB_as are assumed to progress forward at the rate v_{BMU}, their distribution profile still progresses as a traveling wave. But cell segregation according to cell type in the BMU is lost in this situation. The simulation results corresponding to this situation are shown in Figure 3.5.

3.3.2.3 Effect of Swapping RANKL and OPG Expression

Osteoblasts of different maturity express RANKL or OPG with different strengths. Experimental findings suggest that less-mature osteoblasts express RANKL more than OPG. The functional importance of this differential expression pattern for the spatio-temporal coordination of bone cells in a BMU can be investigated with the model. The density profiles predicted by the model when RANKL is only expressed on OB_as and OPG is only expressed on OB_ps are shown in Figure 3.6. The lack of availability of RANKL near preosteoclasts owing to its expression on OB_as at the back of the BMU and its further screening by OPG expressed on OB_ps blunt the generation of osteoclasts. Very few active osteoclasts are therefore generated in this situation, leading to a dysfunctional BMU. These results provide a functional reason for the RANKL/OPG expression patterns observed experimentally.

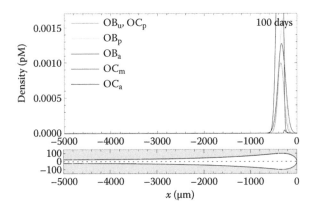

FIGURE 3.5
Density profiles within the BMU cavity when wrong fluxes are assigned; that is, $v_{OB_p} = v_{OB_a} = v_{OC_a} = v_{BMU}$.

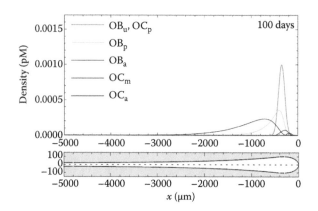

FIGURE 3.6
Density profiles within the BMU cavity when RANKL is expressed on active osteoblasts and OPG is expressed by preosteoblasts.

3.4 Investigation of Microscopic Resorption Behavior in Cortical BMUs

The one-dimensional PDE model presented in Section 3.3 is instructive as to how different cell types organize themselves along the longitudinal axis of the BMU because of cell coupling. In this section, we focus on a more detailed aspect of cortical BMU function: the resorption process by which osteoclasts open up the cutting cone at the front of the BMU. The resorption process determines the shape of the bone substrate on which new bone formation will occur. It determines the diameter and morphology of the secondary osteons created by the BMUs and their network.

Serial histological sectioning of bone in humans and other animals reveals that osteons are irregular cylindrical structures that vary in cross-sectional shape and anastomose extensively with one another, forming a complex network structure [76–79]. MicroCT imaging enables the direct visualization of resorption cavity shapes and of the network structure of Haversian canals in three spatial dimensions [80,81]. Resorption cavities are found to be varied and include unidirectional, bidirectional, and branched BMU morphologies (see Figure 3.7c and d).

On the other hand, experimental insights into the behavior of osteoclasts have been gained from in vivo and in vitro studies. In vivo autoradiographic studies have revealed that thymidine-labeled nuclei from osteoclast precursor cells fuse randomly with existing osteoclasts [21,23,82,83]. This fusion process leads to the continual renewal of the nuclei within the active osteoclasts at the front of BMUs, which is believed to account for an increase in the osteoclasts' lifespan or the persistence of their resorptive activity. In vitro cell cultures have shown that microscopic bone dissolution by active osteoclasts is achieved by the release of hydrogen ions and proteases into the *resorption pit* beneath the ruffled border of the osteoclast [84,85]. In vitro, osteoclasts resorb bone matrix for a period and then detach from the bone surface, before continuing resorption at a different site of the bone surface [84–86]. This behavior may enable further dissolution of the collagenous component of the bone matrix through exposure to several proteases (such as matrix metalloproteinases) secreted by other cells in the extracellular microenvironment [85,87]. It is unclear if this detachment–delay–reattachment behavior occurs in vivo as well [87].

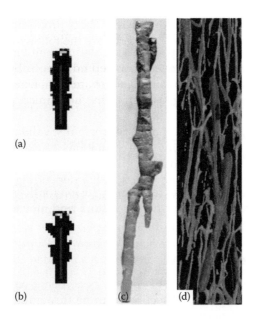

FIGURE 3.7
Resorption cavities obtained (a) without and (b) with an osteoclast lifespan increase through nuclei renewal by fusion. All the parameters of the simulations are identical in panels (a) and (b) except E^{fusion}. (c) Osteonal morphology in dogs. (Modified from Cohen, J. and W.H. Harris, *The Journal of Bone and Joint Surgery. American Volume*, 40:419–434, 1958.) (d) BMU resorption cavities and Haversian canal network in humans. (Modified from Cooper, D.M.L. et al., *The Anatomical Record Part A: Discoveries in Molecular, Cellular, and Evolutionary Biology*, 288A(7):806–816, 2006.)

Linking observations on osteoclast behaviors with observations on osteon morphologies is experimentally challenging and has not been done to date. However, insights into how osteoclast behaviors influence osteon morphologies can be gained through hypothesis testing from computational models. Below, we present a model of bone resorption by a population of osteoclasts [6] with the aim to investigate

   i. How the resorption cavity shape depends on the development and behaviour of osteoclasts

   ii. How osteoclasts move and fuse with each other within the resorption cavity

The second point is important to understand the life history of an osteoclast in BMUs. Where young and mature osteoclasts are likely to be found, for example, has important consequences for our understanding of cell regulation and cell communication (e.g., with osteoblasts) within the BMU [15,83,88–90].

The above points (i) and (ii) are best investigated utilizing a discrete modeling approach in which each osteoclast is followed individually. The cutting cone of a BMU consists of relatively few cells. There are approximately 10 active osteoclasts (each containing approximately 10 nuclei) at the front of a BMU [21,23]. Fluctuations in the number of cells or in their activity are visible as irregularities or roughness of the resorption cavity surface [76,81] (see Figure 3.7c and d). In a continuous model, cell densities represent local spatial averages. This prevents the investigation of individual cell movement patterns, cell fusion, and sequences of migration resorption of a single cell.

The assumptions of the discrete model of osteoclasts proposed are summarized below. The specific questions investigated by the model are the following:

i. Can the repeated sequences of resorption and migration observed in vitro be consistent with BMU cavity development and progression observed in vivo?

ii. Does bone dissolution necessitate exposure to the extracellular matrix for complete resorption?

iii. What are the specific influences of (a) total number of osteoclasts in the BMU and (b) osteoclast lifespan for the shape of the resorption cavity and progression rate of the BMU?

iv. What is the importance of nuclei renewal by fusion for the shape and progression of the resorption cavity and for the life history and movement pattern of osteoclasts within the BMU?

3.4.1 Description of the Model

We consider a two-dimensional slice of cortical bone being resorbed by osteoclasts, as would be seen in a thin longitudinal section running through the centerline of a cortical BMU (Figure 3.8). Each osteoclast is tracked individually, and the position and activity of the osteoclasts (resorbing or not) are updated at regular time intervals. This type of modeling approach is known as *agent-based modeling* and has been widely used in recent years for computational models of tumors and other biological systems [91–96]. The space is discretized into a square lattice with step size $\sigma = 40$ μm. Each lattice site is occupied by either (1) bone matrix, (2) one osteoclast (either migrating or active), (3) blood vessel components, or (4) connective tissue stroma (see Figure 3.8).

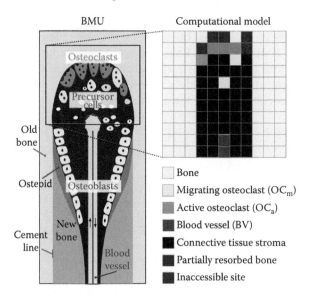

FIGURE 3.8
Schematic representation of a BMU and two-dimensional lattice corresponding to a longitudinal section of the BMU running through the centerline. Each lattice site of the model can be occupied by a single entity from the list at one time.

Osteoclast development and activity in the resorption cavity of the BMU are modeled by the following assumptions:

- Fully mature osteoclasts are generated at a rate η_{OC} (in day^{-1}) at a distance 160–240 μm (depending on site availability) ahead of the tip of a blood vessel (BV). The process of osteoclast maturation itself is not modeled explicitly, but assumed to take place over this distance [62]. The blood vessel grows vertically toward the front of the BMU at a maximum rate v_{BV} (in micrometers per day). This rate may be slowed down to ensure that a minimal vertical distance of 280 μm is kept between the tip and the bone surface.

- A mature osteoclast is in either of two states: *migrating* (not resorbing) or *active* (resorbing). We denote a migrating osteoclast by OC_m and an active osteoclast by OC_a. An osteoclast becomes active as soon as it reaches a bone surface. It remains active and immotile until all of its surrounding bone sites are resorbed, at which point it becomes a migrating osteoclast again.

- Dissolution of the bone matrix by an OC_a is represented by a kinetic dissolution law that gradually reduces the bone density $m(t)$ in time according to $\dfrac{dm}{dt} = -\gamma m$. Bone matrix at a lattice site that has been resorbed by more than 90% becomes a cavity site filled with connective tissue stroma. Such a site is deemed inaccessible to OC_ms for a period τ_{inhib} to allow for possible extracellular collagen digestion (blue state in Figure 3.8).

- The migration of OC_ms through the connective tissue stroma is modeled as a *biased random walk*. At each time increment, an OC_m chooses a lattice site i to migrate to with a probability P_i that depends on the presence of other components in the vicinity. The interaction of the OC_m with these components is described by *interaction energies* E_{ij}. The probability to migrate to site i is assumed to be

$$P_i \propto e^{-E_i/F_T}, \tag{3.27}$$

where $E_i = \sum_j E_{ij}$ is the total energy that the OC_m would have on site i. Depending on the constitution of the lattice sites j, E_{ij} is either: E_{ij}^{OC-OC}, the adhesion interaction energy with another osteoclast at j; $E_{ij}^{OC-BONE}$, the adhesion interaction energy with a bone site at j; or E_{ij}^{OC-BV}, the interaction energy with blood vessel components at j. Clearly from Equation 3.27, the OC_m migrates preferentially toward neighboring sites i of lowest energies E_i. Only adjacent or diagonal sites (Moore neighborhood) can be reached in a single time increment. The ranges of the interaction energies are limited to the Moore neighborhood:

$$E_{ij}^{OC-OC} = \begin{cases} E_{OC-OC}^{fusion}, & |i-j| = 0, \\ E_{OC-OC}, & |i-j| \le 1, \\ 0, & |i-j| > 1, \end{cases} \tag{3.28}$$

$$
E_{ij}^{\text{OC–BONE}} = \begin{cases} +\infty, & i \dashv j = 0, \\ E_{\text{OC–BONE}} < 0, & i \dashv j \leq 1, \\ 0 & i \dashv j > 1, \end{cases}
\tag{3.29}
$$

$$
E_{ij}^{\text{OC–BV}} = \begin{cases} +\infty, & |i - j| = 0, \\ 0 & |i - j| \geq 0, \end{cases}
\tag{3.30}
$$

where $|i - j|$ denotes the so-called *maximum norm* of the vector $i - j$ (i.e., the maximum of the absolute value of the vector's components).

- Osteoclasts that are newly generated are initially assigned a fixed lifespan τ_{OC}. To account for a lifespan-increasing nuclei renewal process in our simulations, a migrating OC_m can fuse with an existing OC_a or OC_m (with different probabilities, depending on the *fusion energies* $E_{\text{OC}_m\text{-OC}_a}^{\text{fusion}}$ and $E_{\text{OC}_m\text{-OC}_m}^{\text{fusion}}$, respectively). The lifespan of the osteoclast resulting from this fusion is increased by the remaining lifetime of the fusing OC_m.

- When the age of an osteoclast reaches its allotted lifespan (whether that lifespan has been increased by nuclei renewal or not), the cell is removed from the system.

The concept of *interaction energies* is a high-level simplification for complex molecular processes, but it allows to integrate the underlying biochemical signals and resultant cell properties into a single concept. The interaction energies are normalized by the so-called *metabolic energy* F_T in Refs. [97–99]. The metabolic energy F_T accounts for a background of metabolic fluctuations that give the OC_m more or less erratic motion. Metabolic fluctuations represent, for example, inhomogeneity in the connective tissue or fluctuations in signaling pathways or in biochemical reactions. If the metabolic energy is high ($F_T \gg |E_i|$), biases in the probabilities P_i are reduced, leading to more erratic OC_m migration. If the metabolic energy is low ($F_T \ll |E_i|$), biases in the probabilities P_i are accentuated, leading to more persistent OC_m migration toward the local minimum of energy. In Refs. [97–99], it is estimated that interaction energies are typically of the order $1F_T - 10F_T$. In the model, all energies are measured in units of the metabolic energy F_T and their physiological range is assumed to be within $0F_T - 10F_T$.

3.4.2 Numerical Results and Discussions

Numerical simulations of the model start from an initial lattice configuration consisting of a small circular cavity around the tip of the blood vessel. The system is evolved for 30 days with time increments of 0.1 days.* At each time increment, all osteoclasts are selected in random order and an update of their state and position is performed (asynchronous update). The dissolution of bone sites by the OC_as is performed in this selected order too. The possible growth of the blood vessel and the generation of new OC_ms are performed last.

---

* The time increment and lattice step determine the diffusion coefficient of the OC_m in a homogenous stromal tissue environment (i.e., unbiased random walk). With the value chosen and the Moore neighborhood, OC_ms have an effective diffusion coefficient $D_{\text{OC}_m} = \dfrac{\sigma^2}{3\Delta t} = 6.2 \times 10^{-10} \text{ cm}^2/\text{s}$ [6].

3.4.2.1 Sequences of Migration–Resorption and Extracellular Collagen Dissolution

For the simulations to create resorption cavities corresponding to observed osteon diameters of 200–350 µm progressing through bone at rates of 20–40 µm/day [15,21,35], small values of τ_{inhib} and of ν_{BV} values of 20–40 µm/day need to be chosen (see Figure 3.9). At such values of τ_{inhib}, osteoclasts are not observed to migrate away from a previous resorption site before starting to resorb again in the simulations. This suggests that the *detachment–delay–reattachment* behavior of an osteoclast described in vitro is unlikely to occur within a cortical BMU with significant migration before reattachment.

3.4.2.2 Influence of Number of Osteoclasts and Osteoclast Lifespan

If all the osteoclasts have the same lifespan, the total number of osteoclasts in the resorption cavity is given by

$$N_{OC} = \eta_{OC}\,\tau_{OC} \tag{3.31}$$

and the renewal rate of the osteoclast population is $1/\tau_{OC}$. Such a situation occurs in the simulations when preventing osteoclast lifespan increases through nuclei renewal by fusion $\left(E_{OC-OC}^{fusion} = \infty\right)$. This case is considered in Figure 3.10. Clearly, the total number of osteoclasts in the cavity strongly influences the width of the resorption cavity (i.e., the diameter of the osteon). The effect of population renewal rate (inverse of osteoclast lifespan) for identical osteoclast number is more subtle and seems to affect the roughness of the resorption cavity interface.

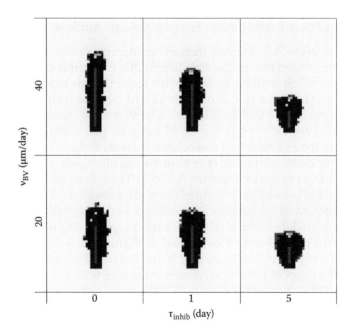

FIGURE 3.9
Resorption cavities obtained after 30 days for different values of the maximum rate of growth of the blood vessel and extracellular collagen digestion period τ_{inhib}. Each snapshot represents a 1600 µm × 2240 µm portion of the lattice.

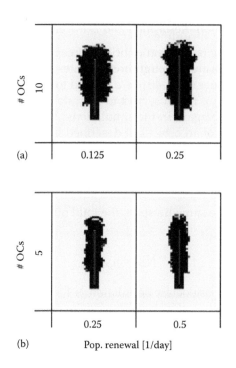

FIGURE 3.10
Influence of number of osteoclasts and osteoclast population renewal on the size and morphology of the resorption cavity: (a) large OC_a population; (b) lower OC_a population.

3.4.2.3 Influence of Osteoclast Lifespan Increase through Nuclei Renewal by Fusion

The mechanism of osteoclast lifespan increasing through nuclei renewal is conditional upon fusing of two osteoclasts. In the simulation, this is controlled in part by the fusion energy E_{OC-OC}^{fusion}. Depending on their position with respect to the blood vessel, which regularly produces new osteoclasts, not all osteoclasts will increase their lifespan. The effect of nuclei renewal by fusion is thereby different from increasing osteoclast lifespan globally on all osteoclasts (controlled by τ_{OC}). Figure 3.7 suggests that enabling a lifespan increase by fusion increases the propensity of osteoclasts to create *budding branches* from the main resorbing cavity. The osteonal structures in humans and other animals are known to branch and anastomose into a network structure [76–79,81]. These branches are not followed further in the simulations because branching of the central blood vessel is not modeled.

The trajectories followed by individual osteoclasts within a BMU in vivo are unknown [15,90]. Our discrete model of osteoclasts does not presuppose any preferential direction of motion except for the growth of the blood vessel. In Figure 3.11, we show the relative trajectories taken by all osteoclasts created during 30 days in our simulations. These trajectories are shown from the point of view of an observer moving with the tip of the blood vessel and thus represent the trajectories of the osteoclasts within the resorption cavity.

Our simulations suggest that during their lifespan, osteoclasts follow a path going from the tip of the blood vessel to the front of the BMU, and from there back down the sides of the cavity. This movement pattern is suggestive of the *treadmill* movement pattern hypothesized by Burger et al. [90]. Interestingly, enabling increases in osteoclast lifespan through nuclei renewal by fusion seems to accentuate this movement and to enable osteoclasts to progressively come further toward the back of the BMU.

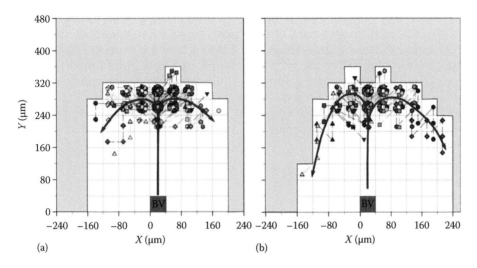

FIGURE 3.11
Relative trajectories of individual osteoclasts in a reference frame co-moving with the tip of the blood vessel. Each osteoclast is assigned a different symbol and is slightly offset within a lattice site so as to distinguish overlapping paths. (a) Without lifespan increase by fusion $\left(E_{\text{OC-OC}}^{\text{fusion}} = \infty\right)$. (b) With lifespan increase by fusion $\left(E_{\text{OC-OC}}^{\text{fusion}} < \infty\right)$.

3.5 Concluding Remarks and Future Outlook

The importance of developing comprehensive models of BMUs lies in the fact that bone remodeling is operated by these functional structures. Mathematical modeling can help link experimental observations made at a certain scale or on a particular system (e.g., in vitro observations of osteoclast behavior in response to a number of signaling molecules) and observations made at another scale or another system (e.g., in vivo histomorphometric measurements of osteon size or of matrix apposition rates). We exemplified this approach with two particular models recently developed by our group.

In the first model, a detailed account of cell–cell signaling through receptor–ligand binding reactions is implemented to account for biochemical coupling between osteoclasts and osteoblasts in a BMU. This biochemical coupling between the cells is seen to lead to the emergence of structured cell distributions progressing through bone as in a BMU. In the second model, osteoclasts are generated and followed through the simulation individually using a so-called agent-based modeling approach. This enables studying the specific influence of various aspects of osteoclast behavior (such as generation rate, lifespan increase through nuclei renewal by fusion, migration versus resorption sequences) on the size and morphology of a developing osteon.

Future advances of bioengineering and tissue engineering will heavily rely on how well experimental findings can be integrated into computational models. It is of paramount importance for these fields to be able to describe and predict the key behaviors of the biological systems considered. Computational modeling in tissue engineering, for instance, will be able to optimize tissue structures and composition without the need for extensive experimental search. In bone, degradable scaffolds are slowly remodeled into new bone by the coordinated action of osteoclasts and osteoblasts. Mathematical models of BMUs can help understand how fast or how likely bone integration may occur depending on the scaffold porosity, its microstructure, or biological compounds embedded into the scaffold or onto its surface. Undoubtedly, strong collaborations between experimental and theoretical groups are essential to develop such models and capture the most important biological and biomechanical features of the system. A prerequisite for such collaborations is the mutual understanding of research methodologies employed. We hope that this chapter will provide some inspiration on how theoretical tools such as mathematical modeling can be used in biomedical research in general and in tissue engineering and bone research in particular.

Acknowledgments

The work of the authors is supported by the Australian Research Council. A/Prof. Pivonka received Discovery Project funding (DP0988427), and Dr. Buenzli is the recipient of a Discovery Early Career Researcher Fellowship (DE130101191).

References

1. Ryser, M.D., N. Nigam, and S.V. Komarova, Mathematical modeling of spatio-temporal dynamics of a single bone multicellular unit. *Journal of Bone and Mineral Research*, 2009. **24**(5): pp. 860–870.
2. Ryser, M., S. Komarova, and N. Nigam, The cellular dynamics of bone remodeling: A mathematical model. *SIAM Journal on Applied Mathematics*, 2010. **70**(6): pp. 1899–1921.
3. Ryser, M.D., Y. Qu, and S.V. Komarova, Osteoprotegerin in bone metastases: Mathematical solution to the puzzle. *PLoS Computational Biology*, 2012. **8**(10): p. e1002703.
4. Buenzli, P.R., P. Pivonka, and D.W. Smith, Spatio-temporal structure of cell distribution in cortical bone multicellular units: A mathematical model. *Bone*, 2011. **48**(4): pp. 918–926.
5. Buenzli, P.R., P. Pivonka, and D.W. Smith, Bone refilling in bone multicellular units: Insights into tetracycline double labelling from a computational model. *arXiv*, 2012. **1208.6075**.
6. Buenzli, P.R. et al., Investigation of bone resorption within a cortical basic multicellular unit using a lattice-based computational model. *Bone*, 2012. **50**(1): pp. 378–389.
7. van Oers, R.F.M. et al., Simulations of trabecular remodeling and fatigue: Is remodeling helpful or harmful? *Bone*, 2011. **48**(5): pp. 1210–1215.
8. Ji, B. et al., A novel mathematical model of bone remodeling cycles for trabecular bone at the cellular level. *Biomechanics and Modeling in Mechanobiology*, 2012. **11**(7): pp. 973–982.
9. Martin, R.B., D.B. Burr, and N.A. Sharkey, *Skeletal Tissue Mechanics*. 1998, New York: Springer.
10. Currey, J.D., *Bones—Structure and Mechanics*. 2002, New Jersey: Princeton University Press.
11. Frost, H.M. and M.D. Springfield, Bone Remodeling Dynamics. 1963, Springfield, IL: Charles C. Thomas Company.
12. Frost, H.M., Bone remodeling dynamics, ed. M.D. Springfield. 1963, Illinois: Charles C. Thomas.
13. Webster, S.S.J., Integrated bone tissue physiology: Anatomy and physiology. In *Bone Mechanics Handbook*, 2nd ed., ed. S.C. Cowin. 2001, Boca Raton, FL: CRC Press.
14. Frost, H.M., The skeletal intermediary organization. *Metabolic Bone Disease and Related Research*, 1983. **4**(5): pp. 281–290.

15. Parfitt, A.M., The physiological and clinical significance of bone histomorphometric data. In *Bone Histomorphometry: Techniques and Interpretation*, ed. R.R. Recker. 1983, Boca Raton, FL: CRC Press. 143–223.

16. Lanyon, L.E., and S. Bourn, The influence of mechanical function on the development and remodeling of the tibia. An experimental study in sheep. *The Journal of Bone and Joint Surgery. American Volume*, 1979. **61**(2): pp. 263–273.

17. Smit, T.H., and E.H. Burger, Is BMU-coupling a strain-regulated phenomenon? A finite element analysis. *Journal of Bone and Mineral Research*, 2000. **15**(2): pp. 301–307.

18. Smit, T.H., E.H. Burger, and J.M. Huyghe, A case for strain-induced fluid flow as a regulator of BMU-coupling and osteonal alignment. *Journal of Bone and Mineral Research*, 2002. **17**(11): pp. 2021–2029.

19. Robling, A.G., and S.D. Stout, Morphology of the drifting osteon. *Cells Tissues Organs*, 1998. **164**: pp. 192–204.

20. Thomas, C.D.L., S.A. Feik, and J.G. Clement, Increase in pore area, and not pore density, is the main determinant in the development of porosity in human cortical bone. *Journal of Anatomy*, 2006. **209**: pp. 219–230.

21. Parfitt, A.M., Osteonal and hemi-osteonal remodeling: The spatial and temporal framework for signal traffic in adult human bone. *Journal of Cellular Biochemistry*, 1994. **55**: pp. 273–286.

22. Jaworski, Z.F.G., and C. Hooper, Study of cell kinetics within evolving secondary Haversian systems. *Journal of Anatomy*, 1980. **131**: pp. 91–102.

23. Jaworski, Z.F.G., B. Duck, and G. Sekaly, Kinetics of osteoclasts and their nuclei in evolving secondary Haversian systems. *Journal of Anatomy*, 1981. **133**: pp. 397–405.

24. Hauge, E.M. et al., Cancellous bone remodeling occurs in specialized compartments lined by cells expressing osteoblastic markers. *Journal of Bone and Mineral Research*, 2001. **16**(9): pp. 1575–1582.

25. Eriksen, E.F., G.Z. Eghbali-Fatourechi, and S. Khosla, Remodeling and vascular spaces in bone. *Journal of Bone and Mineral Research*, 2007. **22**(1): pp. 1–6.

26. Vaananen, H.K. et al., How do osteoclasts resorb bone? *Materials Science and Engineering: C*, 1998. **6**(4): pp. 205–209.

27. Roodman, G.D., Cell biology of the osteoclast. *Experimental Hematology*, 1999. **27**(8): pp. 1229–1241.

28. Jaworski, Z.F.G., and E. Lok, The rate of osteoclastic bone erosion in Haversian remodeling sites of adult dog's rib. *Calcified Tissue Research*, 1972. **10**(2): pp. 103–112.

29. Jilka, R.L., Biology of the basic multicellular unit and the pathophysiology of osteoporosis. *Medical and Pediatric Oncology*, 2003. **41**(3): pp. 182–185.

30. Wiktor-Jedrzejczak, W. et al., Total absence of colony-stimulating factor 1 in the macrophage-deficient osteopetrotic (op/op) mouse. *Proceedings of the National Academy of Sciences of the United States of America*, 1990. **87**(12): pp. 4828–4832.

31. Lacey, D.L. et al., Osteoprotegerin ligand is a cytokine that regulates osteoclast differentiation and activation. *Cell*, 1998. **93**(2): pp. 165–176.

32. Simonet, W.S. et al., Osteoprotegerin: A novel secreted protein involved in the regulation of bone density. *Cell*, 1997. **89**(2): pp. 309–319.

33. Yasuda, H. et al., Osteoclast differentiation factor is a ligand for osteoprotegerin/osteoclastogenesis-inhibitory factor and is identical to TRANCE/RANKL. *Proceedings of the National Academy of Sciences of the United States of America*, 1998. **95**(7): pp. 3597–3602.

34. Dallas, S.L. et al., Proteolysis of latent transforming growth factor-beta (TGF-beta)-binding protein-1 by osteoclasts. *Journal of Biological Chemistry*, 2002. **277**(24): pp. 21352–21360.

35. Robling, A.G., A.B. Castillo, and C. Turner, Biomechanical and molecular regulation of bone remodeling. *Annual Review of Biomedical Engineering*, 2006. **8**: pp. 455–498.

36. Robling, A.G. et al., Mechanical stimulation of bone *in vivo* reduces osteocyte expression of sost/sclerostin. *The Journal of Biological Chemistry*, 2008. **283**(9): pp. 5866–5875.

37. Bonewald, L.F., and M.L. Johnson, Osteocytes, mechanosensing and Wnt signaling. *Bone*, 2008. **42**(4): pp. 606–615.

38. Bonewald, L.F., The amazing osteocyte. *Journal of Bone and Mineral Research*, 2011. **26**(2): pp. 229–238.

39. Geris, L., J. Vander Sloten, and H. Van Oosterwyck, In silico biology of bone modelling and remodeling: Regeneration. *Philosophical Transactions of the Royal Society A: Mathematical, Physical and Engineering Sciences*, 2009. **367**(1895): pp. 2031–2053.
40. Pivonka, P., and S.V. Komarova, Mathematical modeling in bone biology: From intracellular signaling to tissue mechanics. *Bone*, 2010. **47**(2): pp. 181–189.
41. Trüssel, A., R. Müller, and D. Webster, Toward mechanical systems biology in bone. *Annals of Biomedical Engineering*, 2012. **40**(11): pp. 2475–2487.
42. Webster, D., and R. Müller, In silico models of bone remodeling from macro to nano—From organ to cell. *Wiley Interdisciplinary Reviews: Systems Biology and Medicine*, 2011. **3**(2): pp. 241–251.
43. Komarova, S.V. et al., Mathematical model predicts a critical role for osteoclast autocrine regulation in the control of bone remodeling. *Bone*, 2003. **33**(2): pp. 206–215.
44. Pivonka, P. et al., Model structure and control of bone remodeling: A theoretical study. *Bone*, 2008. **43**(2): pp. 249–263.
45. Pivonka, P. et al., Theoretical investigation of the role of the RANK-RANKL-OPG system in bone remodeling. *Journal of Theoretical Biology*, 2009. **262**(2): pp. 306–316.
46. Scheiner, S., P. Pivonka, and C. Hellmich, Coupling systems biology with multiscale mechanics, for computer simulations of bone remodeling. *Computer Methods in Applied Mechanics and Engineering*, 2013. **254**: pp. 181–196.
47. Pivonka, P. et al., The influence of bone surface availability in bone remodeling—A mathematical model including coupled geometrical and biomechanical regulations of bone cells. *Engineering Structures*, 2013. **47**: pp. 134–147.
48. van Oers, R.F.M. et al., A unified theory for osteonal and hemi-osteonal remodeling. *Bone*, 2008. **42**(2): pp. 250–259.
49. van der Linden, J.C., J.A.N. Verhaar, and H. Weinans, A three-dimensional simulation of age-related remodeling in trabecular bone. *Journal of Bone and Mineral Research*, 2001. **16**(4): pp. 688–696.
50. van der Linden, J.C. et al., A simulation model at trabecular level to predict effects of antiresorptive treatment after menopause. *Calcified Tissue International*, 2003. **73**(6): pp. 537–544.
51. Liu, X.S. et al., Dynamic simulation of three dimensional architectural and mechanical alterations in human trabecular bone during menopause. *Bone*, 2008. **43**(2): pp. 292–301.
52. Adachi, T. et al., Trabecular surface remodeling simulation for cancellous bone using microstructural voxel finite element models. *Journal of Biomechanical Engineering*, 2001. **123**(5): pp. 403–409.
53. Müller, R., Long-term prediction of three-dimensional bone architecture in simulations of pre-, peri- and post-menopausal microstructural bone remodeling. *Osteoporosis International*, 2005. **16**(2): pp. S25–S35.
54. Huiskes, H.W.J. et al., Effects of mechanical forces on maintenance and adaptation of form in trabecular bone. *Nature*, 2000. **405**(6787): pp. 704–706.
55. Mullender, M. et al., Effect of mechanical set point of bone cells on mechanical control of trabecular bone architecture. *Bone*, 1998. **22**(2): pp. 125–131.
56. Ruimerman, R. et al., A theoretical framework for strain-related trabecular bone maintenance and adaptation. *Journal of Biomechanics*, 2005. **38**(4): pp. 931–941.
57. Thomsen, J.S. et al., Stochastic simulation of vertebral trabecular bone remodeling. *Bone*, 1994. **15**(6): pp. 655–666.
58. Christen, P. et al., Bone morphology allows estimation of loading history in a murine model of bone adaptation. *Biomechanics and Modeling in Mechanobiology*, 2012. **11**(3–4): pp. 483–492.
59. Mc Donnell, P. et al., Simulation of vertebral trabecular bone loss using voxel finite element analysis. *Journal of Biomechanics*, 2009. **42**(16): pp. 2789–2796.
60. Pivonka, P., and C.R. Dunstan, Role of mathematical modeling in bone fracture healing. *BoneKEy*, 2012. **221**: pp. 1–10.
61. Lemaire, V. et al., Modeling the interactions between osteoblast and osteoclast activities in bone remodeling. *Journal of Theoretical Biology*, 2004. **229**(3): pp. 293–309.
62. Parfitt, A.M., Osteoclast precursors as leukocytes: Importance of the area code. *Bone*, 1998. **23**(6): pp. 491–494.

63. Martin, T.J., Paracrine regulation of osteoclast formation and activity: Milestones in discovery. *Journal of Musculoskeletal & Neuronal Interactions*, 2004. **4**(3): pp. 243–253.

64. Lauffenburger, D.A., and J.J. Linderman, *Receptors: Models for Binding, Trafficking, and Signalling*. 1996, Oxford: Oxford University Press.

65. Harada, S.-I., and G.A. Rodan, Control of osteoblast function and regulation of bone mass. *Nature*, 2003. **423**: pp. 349–355.

66. Iqbal, J., and M. Zaidi, Coupling bone degradation to formation. *Nature Medicine*, 2009. **15**(7): pp. 757–765.

67. Tang, Y. et al., TGF-β1–induced migration of bone mesenchymal stem cells couples bone resorption with formation. *Nature Medicine*, 2009. **15**(7): pp. 757–765.

68. Pazzaglia, U.E. et al., The shape modulation of osteoblast–osteocyte transformation and its correlation with the fibrillar organization in secondary osteons. *Cell and Tissue Research*, 2010. **340**(3): pp. 533–540.

69. Pazzaglia, U.E. et al., A model of osteoblast-osteocyte kinetics in the development of secondary osteons in rabbits. *Journal of Anatomy*, 2012. **220**(4): pp. 372–383.

70. Gori, F. et al., The expression of osteoprotegerin and RANK ligand and the support of osteoclast formation by stromal-osteoblast lineage cells is developmentally regulated. *Endocrinology*, 2000. **141**(12): pp. 4768–4776.

71. Thomas, G.P. et al., Changing RANKL OPG mRNA expression in differentiating murine primary ostoblasts. *Journal of Endocrinology*, 2001. **170**: pp. 451–460.

72. Ma, Y.L. et al., Catabolic effects of continuous human PTH (1–38) *in vivo* is associated with sustained stimulation of RANKL and inhibition of osteoprotegerin and gene-associated bone formation. *Endocrinology*, 2001. **142**(9): pp. 4047–4054.

73. Wolfram Research, Inc., Mathematica, Version 8.0, Champaign, IL: 2010.

74. Ishii, M. et al., Sphingosine-1-phosphate mobilizes osteoclast precursors and regulates bone homeostasis. *Nature*, 2009. **458**(7237): pp. 524–528.

75. Ishii, T. et al., Control of osteoclast precursor migration: A novel point of control for osteoclastogenesis and bone homeostasis. *IBMS BoneKEy*, 2010. **7**(8): pp. 279–286.

76. Cohen, J., and W.H. Harris, The three-dimensional anatomy of Haversian systems. *The Journal of Bone and Joint Surgery. American Volume*, 1958. **40**: pp. 419–434.

77. Tappen, N.C., Three-dimensional studies of resorption spaces and developing osteons. *The American Journal of Anatomy*, 1977. **149**: pp. 301–332.

78. Stout, S.D. et al., Computer assisted 3D reconstruction of serial sections of cortical bone to determine the 3D structure of osteons. *Calcified Tissue International*, 1999. **65**: pp. 280–284.

79. Moshin, S., D. Taylor, and L.C. Lee, Three-dimensional reconstruction of Haversian systems in ovine compact bone. *European Journal of Morphology*, 2002. **40**: pp. 309–315.

80. Britz, H.M. et al., The relation of femoral osteon geometry to age, sex, height and weight. *Bone*, 2009. **45**(1): pp. 77–83.

81. Cooper, D.M.L. et al., Three-dimensional microcomputed tomography imaging of basic multicellular unit-related resorption spaces in human cortical bone. *The Anatomical Record Part A: Discoveries in Molecular, Cellular, and Evolutionary Biology*, 2006. **288A**(7): pp. 806–816.

82. Miller, S.C., Osteoclast cell-surface specializations and nuclear kinetics during egg-laying in Japanese quail. *The American Journal of Anatomy*, 1981. **162**: pp. 35–43.

83. Parfitt, A.M. et al., A new model for the regulation of bone resorption with particular reference to the effects of bisphosphonates. *Journal of Bone and Mineral Research*, 1996. **11**: pp. 150–159.

84. Hall, B.K., Bone: The osteoclast. In *Bone*, Vol. 2, ed. B.K. Hall. 1991, Boca Raton, FL: CRC Press.

85. Väänänen, H., and H. Zhao, Osteoclast function: Biology and mechanisms. In *Principles of Bone Biology*, eds. J.P. Bilezikian, L.G. Raisz, and T.J. Martin. 2008, San Diego: Academic Press, pp. 193–209.

86. Martin, T.J., Some light shines on the resorption cavity. *BoneKEy-Osteovision*, 2002. doi:10.1138/2002025.

87. Everts, V. et al., The bone lining cell: Its role in cleaning Howship's lacunae and initiating bone formation. *Journal of Bone and Mineral Research*, 2002. **17**: pp. 77–90.

88. Bronkers, A.L.J.J. et al., DNA fragmentation during bone formation in neonatal rodents assessed by transferase-mediated end labeling. *Journal of Bone and Mineral Research*, 1996. **11**: pp. 1281–1291.

89. Boyce, B.F. et al., Apoptosis in bone cells. In *Principles of Bone Biology*, eds. J.P. Bilezikian, L.G. Raisz, and G.A. Rodan. 2002, San Diego: Academic Press, pp. 151–168.

90. Burger, E.H., J. Klein-Nulend, and T.H. Smit, Strain-derived canalicular fluid flow regulates osteoclast activity in a remodeling osteon—A proposal. *Journal of Biomechanics*, 2003. **36**(10): pp. 1453–1459.

91. Mansury, Y. et al., Emerging patterns in tumor systems: Simulating the dynamics of multicellular clusters with an agent-based spatial agglomeration model. *Journal of Theoretical Biology*, 2002. **219**: pp. 343–370.

92. Walker, D.C. et al., The epitheliome: Agent-based modelling of the social behaviour of cells. *Biosystems*, 2004. **76**(1–3): pp. 89–100.

93. Zhang, L. et al., Multiscale agent-based cancer modeling. *Journal of Mathematical Biology*, 2009. **58**: pp. 545–559.

94. Anderson, A.R.A. et al., Tumor morphology and phenotypic evolution driven by selective pressure from the microenvironment. *Cell*, 2006. **127**(5): pp. 905–915.

95. Gerlee, P., and A.R.A. Anderson, An evolutionary hybrid cellular automaton model of solid tumour growth. *Journal of Theoretical Biology*, 2007. **246**(4): pp. 583–603.

96. Jeon, J., V. Quaranta, and P.T. Cummings, An off-lattice hybrid discrete-continuum model of tumor growth and invasion. *Biophysical Journal*, 2010. **98**: pp. 37–47.

97. Beysens, D., G. Forgacs, and J.A. Glazier, Cell sorting is analogous to phase ordering in fluids. *Proceedings of the National Academy of Sciences of the United States of America*, 2000. **97**: pp. 9467–9471.

98. Drasdo, D., and S. Höhme, A single-cell-based model of tumor growth in vitro: Monolayers and spheroids. *Physical Biology*, 2005. **2**(3): pp. 133–147.

99. Block, M., E. Schöll, and D. Drasdo, Classifying the expansion kinetics and critical surface dynamics of growing cell populations. *Physical Review Letters*, 2007. **99**(24): p. 248101.

4

Effect of Nonlinearity in Tensioned Wires of an External Fixation Device

Guigen Zhang

CONTENTS

ABSTRACT External fixation is widely used in the treatment of unstable fractures, limb lengthening, and congenital and pathological orthopedic deformities because of its attractive features such as minimal invasiveness, maximum tailorability, and extreme versatility. These features are made possible by the use of tensioned wires to support bone fragments. These seemingly simple wires actually fulfill a very complex duty. One major problem with these wires is their yielding. Once the wires yield, the fracture healing process will be compromised. Thus, to maximize the benefit of these wires, it is necessary to know their fundamental characteristics. This chapter provides an in-depth look at the cause of the nonlinear behavior observed in these tensioned wires using a computational approach. It illustrates that the nonlinear behavior of the wires originates not only from the material hardening and yielding but also from the induced large deformation. Pretensioning the wires is beneficial for stiffening a fixation device but is disadvantageous to maintaining the wire elasticity. By limiting the level of the pre-tension, one can avoid the material nonlinearity, which is the main cause for material yielding, hence the loss of tension in the wires and the loss of functionality of the fixation device.

4.1 Introduction

External fixation devices are widely used for treating unstable bone fractures in order to prevent excessive shortening and angulations [1–6]. It is also popular in limb lengthening and correction of congenital and pathological orthopedic deformities [5,7,8]. Recently, external fixation has even found applications in engineered tissue repair [9] and veterinary medicine [10]. The main attractive features of these devices include minimal invasiveness, maximum tailorability, and extreme versatility for maintaining alignment and allowing desired movement simultaneously during fracture healing. It seems that these unique features were made possible by the use of tensioned fine wires for supporting bone fragments. Because the wires have small diameters, minimal invasion is required for the transfixation procedure. These wires offer surgeons the flexibility to adjust the wire tension in order to change the stiffness of the fixation for achieving desirable interfragmentary movement to promote proper bone healing [11–13].

The mechanical environment imposed on a fracture by an external fixator plays a significant role in influencing both the rate of fracture healing and the mode by which bone-healing union occurs [14,15]. The exact nature of the optimal mechanical environment for fracture healing still remains unknown. But in general, low levels of cyclic axial strain in the fracture gap promote fracture healing at an early stage, and high levels are beneficial at a later stage for the bone to regain the physiological rigor and strength. Gaining control of the interfragmentary motion requires an understanding of the various factors affecting the overall characteristics of a fixation device. Over the years, researchers have come to know that the wire tension, the number of wires, as well as the frame configuration, among others, are important factors influencing the overall performance of the fixation devices [6,16,17].

So far, much attention has been directed to searching for better configurations, instead of understanding the fundamental characteristics of the tensioned wires. Given the important role these wires play in a fixation device, the importance of knowing the fundamental mechanical and material characteristics of these tensioned wires has not been recognized. As many researchers observed, there is a nonlinear relationship between the applied load and wire transverse deflection [8,18], but the causes for the observed nonlinearity are by no means well understood.

Indeed, these seemingly simple wires actually fulfill a very complex duty, which makes it very difficult to predict their performances because a single stiffness value for predicting the deflection based on the load does not exist. Therefore, in such a situation, only reporting the stiffness value without giving the load information would be less helpful [18–20], thus making it very difficult, if not impossible, to control the interfragmentary motion. To make matters worse, issues such as material yielding, plastic deformation, and residual stresses will all come to play when dictating the performances of the tensioned wires and subsequently the fixation device [16].

Recently, the nonlinear behavior of these tension wires have been investigated thoroughly [21,22]. It was found that the observed nonlinearity can be geometrical and material. From an engineering standpoint, geometrical nonlinearity refers to the nonlinear behavior of a structure caused by the change in its geometrical configuration, and material nonlinearity is the result of material yielding. Geometrical nonlinearity is of elastic nature, and material nonlinearity is of plastic nature. With geometrical nonlinearity, the device will exhibit a nonlinear load–deflection relationship, but the deformation in its members will be within the elastic limit. In this case, the stresses and deformations in the device will disappear when the applied load is removed. Thus, geometrical nonlinearity has no adverse effect on the elastic behavior of a material or structure. With material nonlinearity, the device will endure elastic yielding (i.e., the material is partially yielded with reduced ability to resist further loading) and subsequently plastic yielding (i.e., the material is fully yielded with no ability to resist further loading). Once yielding occurs, residual stresses and permanent deformations will develop in the device, which in turn will lead to altered behavior for the device. Thus, it would be prudent to avoid material nonlinearity.

This chapter aims to provide an overview of the underlying mechanics, the cause for both the geometrical and material nonlinearity, the effect of wire tension, and how the material nonlinearity can be minimized in an external fixation device in order to stiffen the fixation device and retain the elastically predicted mechanical performance of the device.

4.2 Geometrical Nonlinearity and Plastic Failure of a Wire under Bending

Linear elastic analysis is only valid and useful for predicting mechanical behavior of a material or a structure undergoing a linear and elastic deformation. When the material/structure undergoes a deformation that is beyond linear and elastic, such an analysis will no longer be valid. In the following section, we will provide some distinctions between linear, elastic, nonlinear, and plastic relationship and behavior; discuss the origin of nonlinear elastic behavior; and determine the plastic limit of a material in resisting combined bending and tension.

4.2.1 Defining Linear, Nonlinear, Elastic, and Plastic Deformations

To begin, it would be helpful to define some relevant terms in order to help distinguish between linear elastic, nonlinear elastic, and nonlinear plastic deformations. The terms *linear* and *nonlinear* are geometrical terms often used to refer to the relationship between two variables such as in a load–displacement curve or a stress–strain curve. When these relationship curves are straight lines, we call them linear, and when they are curved lines, we call them nonlinear. On the other hand, the terms *elastic* and *plastic* refer to material or structural deformational behavior, specifically the ability to regain the original shape after the removal of a load. When a material/structure regains its original shape (all deformations vanish) after the removal of a load, we consider it deforming with elastic behavior, and when it does not regain its original shape, we call it deforming with plastic behavior. For plastic deformation, it can occur partially or fully. In partial plastic deformation, part of the deformation will vanish after unload, and in full plastic deformation, all deformation will remain after unload.

To put these terms in a practical sense, we often use them in combination to describe certain mechanical behavior. For example, a material/structure can exhibit elastic behavior with either linear or nonlinear relationship between load (or stress) and displacement (or strain). As illustrated in Figure 4.1a, linear elastic behavior is one in which the load–displacement curve is a straight line (linear) and the loading and unloading curves follow the same trace such that the displacement will vanish when the load is reduced to zero (elastic). Nonlinear elastic behavior (see Figure 4.1b) describes a curved load–displacement relationship (nonlinear) and the displacement will disappear when the load is decreased to zero (elastic). While these two cases show elastic behavior, the difference between linear and nonlinear elastic behavior is that the former occurs when the deformation is very small (often invisible) and the latter occurs when the deformation is slightly larger

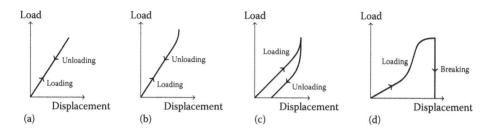

FIGURE 4.1

Load–displacement curves for four typical mechanical cases: (a) linear elastic behavior, (b) nonlinear elastic behavior, (c) partial plastic behavior, and (d) full plastic behavior.

(sometime visible; for instance, when one gently pinches an aluminum can and then lets go of it without causing any shape change). When plastic deformation occurs, the load–displacement curve will always be nonlinear. Figure 4.1c shows a partial plastic load–displacement curve in which part of the displacement will disappear and part will remain after unloading. The remaining displacement in the material or structure is often called residual deformation or permanent deformation. Here, we use the words *displacement* and *deformation* interchangeably. Figure 4.1d shows a case of full plastic load–displacement curve. In this case, the material is in a state of full plastic yielding and it eventually will break as the plastic deformation keeps increasing.

It is worth noting that these four types of load–displacement curves are not necessarily originated from four different materials. They may appear within a single material at different stages of loading. Figure 4.2a shows a load–displacement curve for a material undergoing linear elastic, nonlinear elastic, elastic yielding, and plastic yielding deformations. Here, the term *yielding* is used to refer to plastic deformation. Elastic yielding describes the same situation as partial plastic deformation in which the elastic part of the total deformation will vanish and the plastic part will remain after unloading, while plastic yielding means the same thing as full plastic deformation. Figure 4.2a shows that linear elastic behavior will occur when the induced displacement is extremely small. When the displacement increases slightly, the material may exhibit nonlinear but elastic behavior. This behavior is sometimes referred to as large-deformation nonlinearity, or geometrical nonlinearity. When the displacement increases further, the material will reach an elastic yielding zone in which it still exhibits elastic behavior but with reduced Young's modulus. As the displacement continues

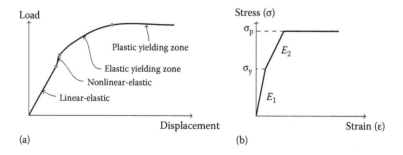

FIGURE 4.2

Four types of mechanical behavior seen in a single material or structure: (a) a load–displacement curve over a large displacement range and (b) its corresponding stress–strain curve.

to increase, the material will enter a plastic yielding zone in which the displacement or deformation will keep increasing without needing any increase in loading.

Figure 4.2b shows a stress–strain curve depicting the same deformational behavior as shown in Figure 4.2a. When the material behaves elastic (both linear and nonlinear), it has Young's modulus of E_1. When the stress in the material reaches its elastic yielding point (σ_y), it will exhibit reduced elastic behavior with Young's modulus of E_2, where $E_2 < E_1$. As the strain in the material further increases, the material will reach its plastic yielding point (σ_p) after which full plastic deformation will occur and the stress in the material will remain the same until the material breaks.

4.2.2 Geometric Nonlinearity in a Wire

To demonstrate the origin of geometrical nonlinearity, we will take a look at a wire subjected to a transverse load (P) at its mid-span with fixed constraints at its two ends as illustrated in Figure 4.3. For a thin wire with a very small cross-section area, under the given loading and constraint conditions, the wire can be assumed (in a simplified view) to deform into a triangle configuration. According to the free-body diagram shown in Figure 4.3, to remain in equilibrium, the wire tension (T) and the applied transverse load (P) should satisfy

$$P = 2T \cos\theta = 2T \frac{\delta}{\sqrt{\delta^2 + (L/2)^2}} \tag{4.1}$$

in which δ is the transverse deflection at the mid-span and L is the length of the wire. The induced tension in the wire can be determined as $F = AE\varepsilon$, where A is the wire cross-section area, E is the Young's modulus of the material the wire is made of, and ε is the mechanical strain in the wire, which can be calculated as

$$\varepsilon = \frac{\sqrt{\delta^2 + (L/2)^2} - L/2}{L/2}. \tag{4.2}$$

By substituting these relationships into Equation 4.1, we establish the following load–deflection relationship:

$$P = \frac{4EA}{L} \frac{\delta\left(\sqrt{4\delta^2 + L^2} - L\right)}{\sqrt{4\delta^2 + L^2}}. \tag{4.3}$$

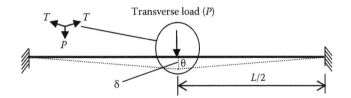

FIGURE 4.3
A wire with fixed constraints at two ends is subject to a transverse load and the wire is assumed to undergo a deformation in a triangle shape characterized by the wire's midpoint deflection (δ).

Clearly, Equation 4.3 describes a nonlinear relationship between the applied load (P) and the resulting deflection (δ). As long as the induced strain in the wire (see Equation 4.2) is small such that the wire exhibits elastic behavior, this type of nonlinearity will be of elastic nature as well. Therefore, this type of nonlinearity is often termed *geometrical nonlinearity*. It is worth noting that because a simplified wire deformation of a triangle configuration is assumed, this analysis only serves to illustrate the origin of the geometrical nonlinearity, and it should not be used to predict the wire performance discussed in this study owing to a much more complicated wire deformation.

4.2.3 Plastic Failure of a Wire under Combined Tension and Bending

As the applied transverse load increases, a further tension and bending moment will be generated in the wire. The combined tension (T) and bending moment (M) will cause the neutral axis (N.A.) for bending to shift to the compression side. Assuming that the wire possesses the stress–strain relationship shown in Figure 4.2b, the maximum tensile stress in the wire will first increase linearly with T and M (see Figure 4.4) until it reaches the elastic yielding point σ_y. After this point, the maximum stress will continue to increase as the strain in the material increases. Once the maximum stress reaches the plastic yielding point σ_p, plastic zones start to develop. While the maximum stress remains at the plastic yielding level, any further increases in loading (tension and bending) will be sustained by the expansion of the plastic zones until the wire goes fully plastic as depicted in Figure 4.5.

Once the wire reaches a fully plastic deformation, failure is assumed to occur. At the onset of such stress state, the wire is still in an equilibrium state. Thus, one has

$$\sum F = 0 : T = F_1 - F_2 = \sigma_p A_1 - \sigma_p A_2 \tag{4.4}$$

$$\sum M = 0 : M = F_1 y_1 + F_2 y_2 = \sigma_p A_1 y_1 + \sigma_p A_2 y_2. \tag{4.5}$$

Here, A_1 and A_2 are the areas of the tension and compression zones, respectively, y_1 and y_2 are the distances from the neutral axis (N.A.) to their respective centroids (C_1 and C_2 in Figure 4.5). In a polar coordinate system, one can express these values as $A_1 = r^2(\pi + 2\theta + \sin2\theta)/2$, $A_2 = r^2(\pi - 2\theta - \sin2\theta)/2$, $y_1 = c_1 + r\sin\theta$, and $y_2 = c_2 - r\sin\theta$, where

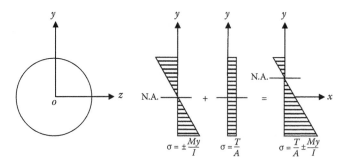

FIGURE 4.4
A wire with a circular cross-section area subjected to a combined tension and bending moment. The combined loading condition will cause the neutral axis (N.A.) of the wire to shift from its common location of $y = 0$ upward such that the cross section is under a higher tensile stress and a lower compressive stress.

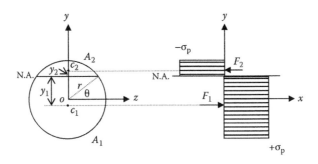

FIGURE 4.5
A circular wire is in a fully plastic deformation after the stresses in both tensile and compressive regions reach the plastic yielding point.

$c_1 = \dfrac{4r\cos^3\theta}{3(\pi + 2\theta + \sin 2\theta)}$, $c_2 = \dfrac{4r\cos^3\theta}{3(\pi - 2\theta - \sin 2\theta)}$, r is the radius of the wire, and θ defines the angular location of the neutral axis (N.A.). By substituting these values into Equations 4.4 and 4.5, we arrive at the following relationships:

$$T = r^2(2\theta + \sin 2\theta)\sigma_p \qquad (4.6)$$

$$M = \sigma_p\left[\frac{4r^3\cos^3\theta}{3} + r^3\sin\theta(2\theta + \sin 2\theta)\right] = \frac{4r^3\sigma_p}{3}\cos^3\theta + Tr\sin\theta. \qquad (4.7)$$

From Equation 4.6, we can determine the location of the neutral axis through $\theta_{N.A.}$ by the equation. Obviously, when there is no tension in the wire (i.e., $T = 0$), one has $\theta_{N.A.} = 0$; then, the neutral axis will overlap with the z-axis. For a given wire tension, $\theta_{N.A.}$ can be determined by solving $2\theta_{N.A.} + \sin\theta_{N.A.} = T/r^2\sigma_p$ using the Newton–Raphson method. Substituting the solved $\theta_{N.A.}$ into Equation 4.7, the limiting plastic bending moment (the moment that will cause a fully plastic deformation) in the presence of the wire tension can be found as

$$M_p = \frac{4r^3\sigma_p}{3}\cos^3\theta_{N.A.} + Tr\sin\theta_{N.A.}. \qquad (4.8)$$

This expression will be used to estimate the limiting plastic bending moment in the tensioned wires in the following sections.

4.3 A Tensioned Wire in a Fixation Device

4.3.1 Geometrical, Material, and Loading Considerations

We now discuss a detailed investigation of the fundamental characteristics of a tensioned wire in a fixation device by examining various factors including wire geometrical configuration, material nonlinearity, loading and unloading, levels of pre-tension, and full plastic deformation. To focus on the mechanical and material characteristics of the wires in an external Ilizarov ring frame (see Figure 4.6a), we isolate a single wire. To account for all possible factors including shearing, bending, torsion, axial displacement, and lateral movement, the single wire is analyzed as a three-dimensional (3D) beam structure. As illustrated Figure 4.6b, a stainless steel wire 150 mm in length and 1.8 mm in diameter is considered using the finite element analysis technique. To simulate the actual loading conditions, the left end of the wire is assigned a fixed boundary condition in which all six degrees of freedoms (DOFs) are restrained, and the right end is restrained in five DOFs except for the horizontal translation, for which an initial wire extension is applied to pre-tension the wire. A transverse load (P) is then applied at the midpoint of the wire.

To represent the actual stress–strain behavior of the stainless steel, the three-segment elastoplastic stress–strain diagram discussed early is used. As illustrated and listed with parametric values [23] in Table 4.1, the stress–strain curve has an initial linear elastic region with $E_1 = 193$ GPa. After reaching its elastic yield stress $\sigma_y = 520$ MPa, the material enters a strain-hardening region with reduced $E_2 = 96.5$ GPA. In this strain-hardening region, the stress continues to increase with the strain until it reaches the plastic yielding point $\sigma_p = 1300$ MPa, after which point the material will behave fully plastically. Poisson's ratio of $\nu = 0.3$ is used for the stainless steel. In this study, both elastic and plastic analyses are performed. For the elastic analyses, only the elastic material properties ($E_1 = 193$ GPa and $\nu = 0.3$) are used, and for the plastic analyses, all these material properties ($E_1 = 193$ GPa, $E_2 = 96.5$ GPA, $\sigma_y = 520$ MPa, $\sigma_p = 1300$ MPa, and $\nu = 0.3$) are used.

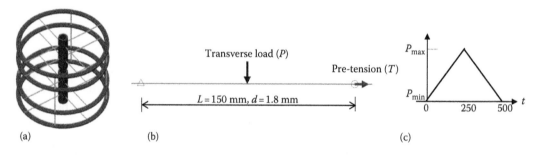

(a)   (b)   (c)

FIGURE 4.6
(a) A computer model of an Ilizarov ring frame fixation device, (b) a tensioned wire isolated from the frame along with the loading and boundary conditions, and (c) a triangle-shaped loading and unloading scheme for the transverse (or vertical) load.

TABLE 4.1

Material Properties of Stainless Steel along with Four Pre-Tension Cases for the Wire and Wires

		$E_1 = 193$ GPa, $E_2 = 96.5$ GPa, $\nu = 0.3$	
	Material Properties	$\sigma_y = 520$ MPa, $\sigma_p = 1300$ MPa	
	Transverse Loading	$P_{min} = 0$ N, $P_{max} = 250$ N	
		Initial Extension (mm)	**Pre-Tension (N)**
	Case 1	0	0/0[a]
	Case 2	0.1222	400/490[a]
	Case 3	0.2443	800/980[a]
	Case 4	0.3665	1200/1420[a]

Stress–strain diagram

[a] Calculated with the consideration of the embedment of part of the wire in the bone segment in the multiple-wire cases.

Table 4.1 also lists the four pre-tension cases analyzed in this study. In Case 1, no pre-tension is applied. In Case 2 through Case 4, an initial extension of 0.1222, 0.2443, and 0.3665 mm is applied to the wire, respectively. These values are chosen for generating a pre-tension of approximately 400, 800, and 1200 N in the wire, respectively. In actual simulation, the initial extension is applied first and held in position. Then, the transverse load (P) is applied to simulate a loading and unloading situation in a triangle shape (see Figure 4.6c) in 500 time steps, 250 time steps for loading, and 250 time steps for unloading with $P_{min} = 0$ N and $P_{max} = 250$ N.

In all the analyses, the resulting load–deflection curve is obtained first. After that, the tension and bending moment in the wire at locations close to the connectors are calculated at each time step. With the calculated wire tensions and bending moments, the upper limit for the plastic bending moment (the moment that will cause a fully plastic wire deformation) in the presence of wire tension is then determined.

4.3.2 Load–Deflection Curves

Figure 4.7 shows the load–deflection curves obtained for the four cases considered in both the elastic (dashed lines) and plastic (solid lines) situations. Obviously, these curves are of nonlinear relationships in all cases, indicating the nonlinear nature of the wire. The effect of pre-tension is apparent: increasing the pre-tension decreases the wire deflection at any given transverse load. Since all these curves are obtained under a load regime of loading and unloading, the loading curves in all the elastic cases (thin lines) overlap with the unloading curves, confirming the elastic behavior of the wire. At a lower load ($P < 100$ N), the level of pre-tension affects the stiffness (i.e., the slope of the curves) significantly, but at a higher load ($P > 150$ N), such effect seems not even distinguishable as indicated by the almost parallel tangents of these curves. This fact suggests that a single stiffness value is certainly insufficient to describe the wire performance. In all the elastic cases, the nonlinearity seen cannot come from material yielding because of the elastic nature of these analyses. Instead, it originates from the change in the wire geometrical configuration under the imposed loading and boundary conditions. With this kind of geometrical nonlinearity, the wire exhibits nonlinear load–deflection relationship, but the deflection-induced deformation in the wire will be within the material's elastic limit such that the deformation in the wire will disappear when the applied load is removed.

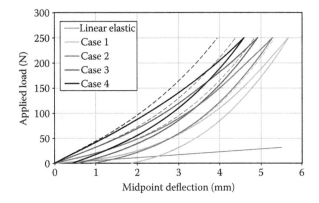

FIGURE 4.7
Load–deflection curves obtained from the nonlinear elastic (dashed lines) and nonlinear plastic (solid lines) analyses for the four pre-tension cases. The result from the linear elastic analysis is also shown as a reference.

The load–deflection curves from the plastic analyses (solid lines) are different: the loading curves (upper branches) do not overlap with the unloading ones (lower branches), indicating the existence of permanent deformation in the wire. In each pre-tension case, divergence between the plastic curve and the elastic curve confirms the existence of material yielding. This type of nonlinearity is known as the material nonlinearity, with which the wire will experience hardening and yielding. In a close inspection of the location of the diverging point, one can see that a higher pre-tension causes the wire to harden at a lower load, suggesting that a highly pre-tensioned wire will harden early.

From the loading–unloading curves for the plastic cases, it is also seen that after each loading cycle, certain wire deflection remains owing to the plastic deformation in the wire. The residual deflection in the wire varies with the level of pre-tension: the higher the pre-tension, the smaller the residual deformation. The residual deflection is found to be 1.861, 0.946, 0.589, and 0.437 mm for Case 1 through Case 4, respectively. This is so mainly because a highly tensioned wire will undergo less deformation and vice versa, and a wire experiencing a larger overall deformation will have a higher residual deformation.

To have a close look at the nonlinear elastic deformation, the result of a linear elastic study is also plotted as a reference (see Figure 4.7). This linear elastic result not only matches exactly the theoretical solution ($\delta = PL^3/192\ EI$) but also tangents the loading curve for the wire with no pre-tension at the onset of loading in both the nonlinear elastic and plastic cases. In other words, the wire with no pre-tension behaves linearly when the deflection is very small, and it gradually transitions into nonlinear behavior when its deflection becomes large. These phenomena are as expected.

As also seen in Figure 4.7, the early divergence between the linear elastic straight line and the loading curve for the wire with no pre-tension indicates that the valid range for the linear elastic analysis is very narrow. When the wire deflection goes beyond this small range, nonlinear load–deflection behavior emerges in all cases. Such nonlinearity, however, can be either elastic (or geometrical) or plastic (or material). If the load–deflection curve follows the thin lines, the nonlinearly is geometrical, and if it follows the thick lines, the nonlinearity is material. But in either case, the induced nonlinearity will cause the slope of these load–deflection curves (or stiffness) to increase; thus, it is beneficial in terms of stiffening the wire structure.

4.3.3 The Induced Tensions and Bending Moments in the Wire

Figure 4.8 shows that the wire tension increases from its respective pre-tension level as the transverse load increases in both the elastic (dashed lines) and plastic (solid lines) analyses. The amount of increase differs: the highest increase occurs in the wire with no pre-tension. An increase in wire tension of 1333, 1050, 796, and 531 N for Case 1 through Case 4, respectively, is found from the pre-tension level to the peak in the plastic cases. Because of the material yielding, after unloading, the wire tension drops below its pre-tension level in all cases except for Case 1 in which the wire tension drops to zero. The wire tension drops from 1200 to 753 N in Case 4, from 800 to 474 N in Case 3, and from 400 to 197 N in Case 2. Also, divergence of the plastic curves (solid lines) from the elastic curves (dashed lines) occurs at a lower load in the wire with a higher pre-tension, again confirming that a highly tensioned wire hardens early.

The four lower curves in Figure 4.9 show that the maximum bending moment in the wire also increases with the transverse load. At any given load, the bending moment generated in the wire with a lower pre-tension is higher than that with a higher pre-tension. This is attributed to the larger deflection induced in a less tensioned wire (see Figure 4.7). As shown in Figure 4.10, the induced bending moment has almost a single linear relationship

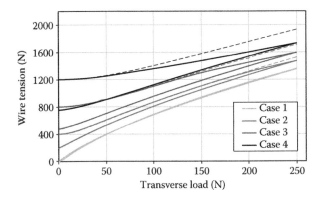

FIGURE 4.8
Variation of wire tension with the applied transverse load. Results from the four pre-tension cases in both the nonlinear elastic (dashed lines) and plastic (solid lines) are shown.

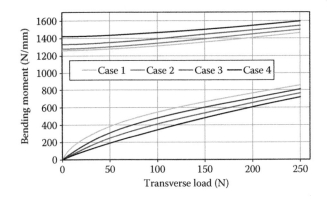

FIGURE 4.9
Variation of maximum bending moment (lower four curves) and limiting plastic moment in the wire (upper four curves) with the applied transverse load.

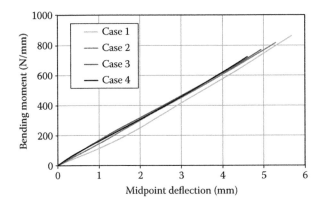

FIGURE 4.10
The bending moment generated in the wire varies with the midpoint transverse deflection in almost the same linear way regardless of the pre-tension level.

with the midpoint deflection regardless of its pre-tension level (note that the one with no pre-tension behaves slightly differently). This means that the more the wire deflects, the higher the induced bending moment. Because the wire with a lower pre-tension indeed deflects more, it thus generates higher bending moments. A highly tensioned wire will therefore generate less bending moment and bending stress in the wire.

4.3.4 Maximum Tensile Stress and Limiting Plastic Moment

Figure 4.11 shows the variation of the maximum tensile stress owing to the combined wire tension and bending moment. As the load increases, the maximum tensile stress increases in all cases until it reaches the full plastic yielding point (σ_p = 1300 MPa). The maximum tensile stress in a less tensioned wire increases in a much faster pace because of its large bending moment. The wire with no pre-tension deforms in full plastic behavior first. Thus, a less tensioned wire, though entering strain hardening later, develops a full plastic deformation earlier.

The variation of the limiting plastic moment (predicted by Equation 4.8) with the applied load is given in Figure 4.9 (the upper four curves). Interesting enough, the limiting plastic moment increases with the load in all cases. At any given load, the higher the pre-tension, the higher the limiting plastic moment. This fact suggests that the pre-tension in the wire actually pushes the limiting plastic moment high. Comparing to the actual bending moment generated in the wire (the lower four curves), these limits are much higher, thus indicating that full plastic bending failure of the wire is less likely to occur within the current loading range.

Taken together, the inevitable large deformation encountered in the wire will stiffen its load–deflection curve, and the addition of the wire pre-tension will make the curve even steeper. One major concern, however, is that the large deformation and the pre-tension will cause the wire to harden. Once the wire hardens, permanent deformations will develop. This will cause the wire tension to drop after each loading cycle, which may adversely affect the fracture healing process. To avoid material hardening or yielding, the deflection in the wire should be kept within the elastic–plastic diverging point. By so doing, one could reap two benefits: taking advantage of the geometrical nonlinearity to stiffen the wire structure and avoiding the material nonlinearity to minimize the plastic deformation in the wire.

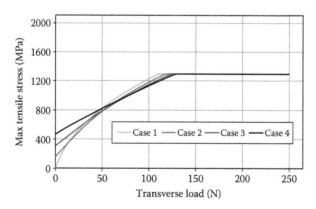

FIGURE 4.11
Variation of the maximum tensile stress owing to the combined wire tension and bending moment with the applied transverse load.

4.4 Multiple Tensioned Wires in a Fixation Device

4.4.1 Geometrical, Material, and Loading Considerations

Now we will discuss some nonlinear and large deformation analyses for the investigation of the mechanical characteristics of multiple tensioned wires supporting a bone segment. In Figure 4.12, a two-wire model and a four-wire model are shown. In the two-wire model, the two wires are cross-aligned at 90° and placed 4 mm apart vertically, and in the four-wire model, a second pair of wires, located 60 mm away vertically from the first pair, is used. The bone segment has a cylindrical shape with a length of 128 mm and a diameter of 38 mm, and the wires are round stainless steel with a span length of 152 mm and a diameter of 1.8 mm. For the bone segment, 3D brick elements are used, and for the wires, 3D beam elements are used in the models to account for their shearing, bending, torsion, axial displacements, and lateral movements. The wires are transfixed through the bone segment to mimic an actual situation. One end of the wires is fixed in all six DOFs, and the other end is restrained in five DOFs except for the axial translation. Initial extension is applied axially at these unfixed ends to pre-tension the wires. To load the bone segment supported by the transfixation wires, a vertical load (P) is applied to the bone segment at the top. For the material properties of the bone segment, isotropic elastic properties with E_{Bone} = 22 GPa and ν_{Bone} = 0.35 are used. For the material properties of stainless steel, the same elastoplastic stress–strain relationship shown in Table 4.1 is used.

To pre-tension the wires, initial extension at four different levels, as listed in Table 4.1, is applied. In each case, the initial extension is first applied and held in place, then the vertical load is linearly ramped up to its peak P_{max} = 250 N in 250 time steps and gradually ramped down in the same pace (for a total of 500 time steps; see Figure 4.6c).

4.4.2 Load–Deflection Curves for the Bone Segment

In all cases, the midpoint vertical deflection of the bone segment is first determined at each time step. Figure 4.13 shows the load–deflection curves obtained for the two-wire model. Here, results from both the elastic (dashed lines) and plastic (solid lines) analyses are shown. Clearly, all the curves for the four considered cases reflect nonlinear relationships. The effect of pre-tension on the load–deflection curve is significant. As the pre-tension

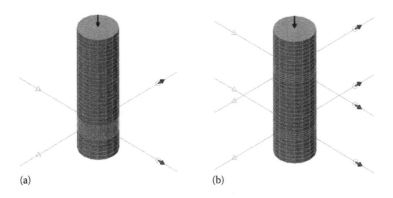

(a)   (b)

FIGURE 4.12
A bone segment transfixed by multiple wires: (a) a two-wire model and (b) a four-wire model.

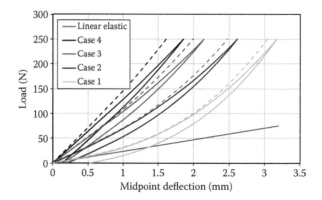

FIGURE 4.13
Load–deflection curves obtained for the two-wire model. The dashed lines are for the nonlinear elastic cases, and the solid lines are for the nonlinear plastic cases. The result of the linear elastic analysis is also shown as a reference.

increases (from Case 1 to Case 4 in both analyses), the steepness of the load–deflection curve increases. In other words, a higher pre-tension in the wires leads to a smaller deflection in the bone segment. Note that all these curves were obtained under a load regime of loading and unloading. Thus, the loading curve in each elastic case overlaps the unloading one, confirming the elastic behavior of the wires. In the plastic cases, however, the loading curves (upper branches) do not overlap their unloading counterparts (lower branches), indicating the existence of permanent deformation.

Noting the location of the diverging point between the elastic and plastic curves in each pre-tension case, one can see that a higher pre-tension will cause the wires to yield at a smaller load. Because of the high pre-tension in the wires in Case 4, the elastic and plastic curves diverge at the very beginning, indicating that the wires have already yielded even before the vertical load is applied.

As a reference, a linear elastic analysis for the two-wire model is performed and its result is plotted in Figure 4.13. The straight line of the linear elastic case tangents the upper branch (loading curve) of Case 1 in both the nonlinear elastic and plastic analyses at the onset of loading. This indicates that the wires with no pre-tension behave linearly when the deflection is very small, but they gradually transition into nonlinear behavior when the deflection becomes large. This phenomenon is as expected.

Figure 4.14 shows the load–deflection curves for the four-wire model. Again, results from both the elastic (dashed lines) and plastic (solid lines) analyses are given. As in the two-wire model, all curves show nonlinear relationships and the effect of pre-tension on the load–deflection curve is obvious. The load–deflection curve becomes steeper and straighter as the pre-tension increases. Although the elastic and plastic curves in Case 4 diverge at the beginning as in the two-wire model, divergence in the rest of the cases occurred at a much higher load (not even visible in Case 1).

4.4.3 The Induced Tensions in the Wires

Figure 4.15 shows that the wire tension increases as the load increases in both the two-wire model (solid lines) and the four-wire model (dashed lines). At the same level of pre-tension, more increase in wire tension is seen in the two-wire model than in the four-wire model. Because of the yielding in the wires, the wire tension drops below the pre-tension level

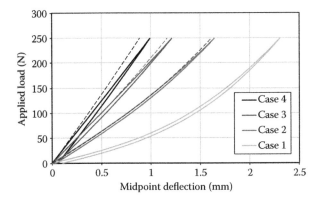

FIGURE 4.14
Load–deflection curves obtained for the four-wire model. The dashed lines are for the nonlinear elastic cases, and the solid lines are for the nonlinear plastic cases.

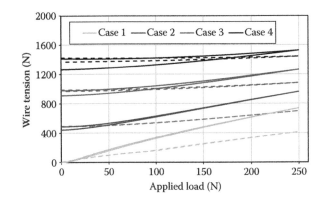

FIGURE 4.15
Variation of wire tension with the applied load for the two-wire (solid lines) and the four-wire (dashed lines) models.

after unloading in all pre-tension cases, but the drop is smaller in the four-wire model than in the two-wire model.

From the above results, one can see that increasing the pre-tension will reduce the wire deflection, or stiffen a fixation device. The drawback, however, is that a higher pre-tension will cause the wires to yield at a lower vertical load. Once the wires yield, the induced permanent deformations will cause the wire tension to drop after unloading, which may adversely affect the fracture healing process. Thus, pre-tensioning the wires is beneficial only when the applied pre-tension along with the service load (i.e., the vertical load in this study) does not cause the wires to yield. This requires that the stress generated in the wires must be kept below the elastic yielding stress of the stainless steel.

4.4.4 The Benefits and Limitations of Using More Wires

As seen in Section 4.4.3, adding two more wires has not only caused a significant decrease in the deflection of the bone segment under the same load but also slowed down the pace at which the wire tension increase with increasing load. These facts indicate that using more wires to support the bone segment will not only stiffen a fixation device but at the same time delay the onset of wire elastic yielding.

In Figures 4.13 and 4.14, one can see that a higher pre-tension causes the elastic–plastic divergence to occur at a lower vertical load, meaning that a smaller vertical load will be allowed without causing the wires to yield. In the two-wire model, this allowable load is 17.5 N for Case 3 and 49 N for Case 2, while in the four-wire model, it is 35 N for Case 3 and 98 N for Case 2. Since the vertical load is sustained by two wires in the two-wire model and by four wires in the four-wire model, the allowable load adjusted for a single wire is actually 8.75 N for Case 3 and 24.5 N for Case 2 in both models.

Recall that the higher the pre-tension, the stiffer the fixation device becomes. Thus, to maximize the stiffness of a fixation device, one could apply a high pre-tension to the wires. But doing so will reduce the allowable vertical load. With a small allowable load, more wires will be required to sustain the service load without causing any material nonlinearity. In view of the difficulty in dealing with a large number of wires during surgery, having a small allowable load is disadvantageous. Thus, when determining the level of wire pre-tension, it would be beneficial if the selected pre-tension could lead to a high stiffness in the wire structure without reducing the allowable load too much (so that the number of wires needed will be at minimum).

4.4.5 The Relationship between Allowable Load and Wire Pre-Tension

To help make the above arguments more clear, a range of pre-tension from 0 to 1100 N is applied to the wires, and the allowable load (adjusted for a single wire) is obtained when the maximum wire stress reaches 500 MPa (slightly below the elastic yielding stress of 520 MPa). At each pre-tension, two stiffness values are calculated: the first one is taken from the tangent of the load–deflection curve at the onset of loading, and the second one is taken at the level of the allowable load. These two values define the lower boundary (LB) and the upper boundary (UB) of the range in which the actual stiffness of the wire structure will vary.

Figure 4.16 shows the obtained results. The curve for the allowable load (refer to the left ordinate) increases slightly as the pre-tension increases from zero to approximately 200 N, where it reaches its maximum. After this point, the allowable load decreases as the

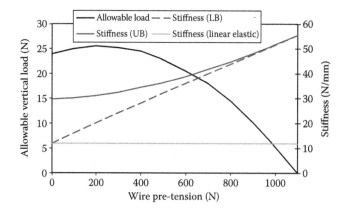

FIGURE 4.16
Variation of the allowable vertical load (refer to the left ordinate), and the upper and lower stiffness values (refer to the right ordinate) with the pre-tension.

pre-tension increases, and it drops to zero at 1100 N (this means that at this pre-tension, no additional vertical load can be applied without causing wire yielding). For the stiffness, both the UB and LB curves (refer to the right ordinate) go up as the pre-tension increases. The gap between the two curves is wider at a lower pre-tension than at a higher pre-tension, indicating that the higher the pre-tension, the less the actual stiffness varies. This fact agrees with that the load–deflection curve becomes steeper and straighter as the pre-tension increases (see Figures 4.13 and 4.14). The increasing trend in the stiffness (both UB and LB) suggests that it is possible to increase the wire stiffness several folds by pre-tensioning the wires without causing them to yield. One major advantage of avoiding wire yielding is that all the adverse consequences such as permanent deformation, residual stress, and reduction of wire tension will be eliminated, so that the wire structure will perform elastically with predictable repeatability. Taken together, since the allowable load and the stiffness change in opposite ways as the pre-tension increases, the region where the load and the stiffness curves cross (i.e., in between 620 and 650 N) can be considered as an optimal level for the pre-tension for avoiding material nonlinearity.

The graph in Figure 4.16 can also be used to estimate how many wires are needed and what stiffness can be derived for a fixation device. Here we present an example. If a pre-tension of 630 N is chosen, an allowable vertical load, 19 N, is determined from this graph. For an anticipated service load, say 225 N, 12 wires will be needed (225/19 = 11.84) for the fixation device. To further estimate the stiffness of this 12-wire fixation device, a stiffness value between 37 and 40 N/mm (adjusted for a single wire) is found from the graph. Multiplying this value by the number of wires determined earlier (i.e., 12), one estimates the stiffness to be within 444 and 480 N/mm. One precautionary note is that this example only serves to demonstrate that it is possible to predict the mechanical performance of a fixation device. Since this graph is obtained on the basis of the frame configuration considered in this study, any change in the frame configuration, in the angle between the two cross-aligned wires, or in the distance between the upper and lower wire pairs will affect the actual prediction.

4.5 Conclusions and Future Perspective

The nonlinear behavior of a tensioned wire originates not only from its material nonlinearity such as hardening and yielding but also from its geometrical nonlinearity caused by the large deformation experienced by the wires. Because of such nonlinear behavior, a single stiffness value is not sufficient to describe the wire performances. For better prediction of the performance of such an external fixation device, an entire load–deflection curve describing the load–deflection behavior of the wires is necessary.

Adding pre-tension to the wires will stiffen the wire structures, reduce the amount of wire deflection, generate less bending moment, delay the onset of the full plastic deformation, and elevate the limiting plastic moment. The drawback, however, is it will cause the wire to behave nonlinearly: geometrically, materially, or both. But this drawback can be overcome if the nonlinearity is limited to only geometrical. Thus, to enhance the wire performances, further efforts should be devoted to exploiting the geometrical nonlinearity and avoiding the material nonlinearity.

Pre-tensioning the wires in an external fixation device is beneficial for stiffening the device, but it is disadvantageous to maintaining the wire elasticity. By limiting the level of the pre-tension, it is possible to avoid the undesirable material nonlinearity. Doing so, one can stiffen the fixation device and at the same time retain predictable repeatability in its mechanical performance.

It is hoped that the computational modeling work presented above on elucidating the linear and nonlinear behavior of the tensioned wires in a fixation device will be subjected to more scrutiny and validation by practitioners and surgeons who use these devices. To maximize the benefits and minimize the drawbacks discussed in this chapter, it seems necessary to have a fully validated model for each design of such a fixation device so that the limits in pretension and in overall vertical load can be identified before the application of the device in order to avoid wire yielding and to retain desired elastic performance for an external fixation device.

References

1. Ilizarov, G.A., 1989. The tension–stress effect on the genesis and growth of tissues. Part I: The influence of stability of fixation and soft-tissue preservation. *Clin. Orthop. Relat. Res.*, 238, 249–281.
2. Ilizarov, G.A., 1989. The tension–stress effect on the genesis and growth of tissues. Part II: The influence of the rate and frequency of distraction. *Clin. Orthop. Relat. Res.*, 239, 263–285.
3. Brown, C., Henderson, S., Moore, S., 1996. Surgical treatment of patients with open tibial fractures. *AORN J.*, 63(5), 875–881, 885–896.
4. Goodship, A.E., Watkins, P.E., Rigby, H.S., Kenwright, J., 1993. The role of fixator frame stiffness in the control of fracture healing. An experimental study. *J. Biomech.*, 26, 1027–1035.
5. LaBianco, J., Vito, G.R., Kalish, S.R., 1996. Use of the Ilizarov external fixator in the treatment of lower extremity deformities. *J. Am. Pediatr. Med. Assoc.*, 86, 523–531.
6. Saleh, M., Royston, S., 1996. Management of nonunion of fractures by distraction with correction of angulation and shortening. *J. Bone Joint Surg.*, 78-B, 105–109.
7. Fleming, B., Paley, D., Kristiansen, T., Pope, M., 1989. A biomechanical analysis of the Ilizarov external fixator. *Clin. Orthop. Res.*, 241, 95–105.
8. Podolsky, A., Chao, E.Y.S., 1993. Mechanical performance of Ilizarov circular external fixators in comparison with other external fixators. *Clin. Orthop.*, 293, 61–70.
9. Itoh, S., Kikuchi, M., Takakuda, K., Nagaoka, K., Koyama, Y., Tanaka, J., Shinomiya, K., 2002. Implantation study of a novel hydroxyapatite/collagen (Hap/Col) composite into weight-bearing sites of dogs. *J. Biomed. Mater. Res. (Appl. Biomater.)*, 63(5), 507–515.
10. Radke, H., Dennis, N.A., Applewhite, A., Zhang, G., 2006. Biomechanical analysis of unilateral external skeletal fixators combined with IM-Pin and without IM-Pin using finite-element method. *Vet. Surg.*, 35, 15–23.
11. Caja, V.L., Kim, W., Larsson, S., Chao, E.Y.S., 1995. Comparison of the mechanical performance of three types of external fixators: Linear, circular and hybrid. *Clin. Biomech.*, 10, 401–406.
12. Saleh, M., 1998. The Sheffield hybrid fixator: Design considerations and clinical experience. *Orthop. Product News*, May/June, 33–35.
13. Yang, L., Nayagam, S., Saleh, M., 2003. Stiffness characteristics and inter-fragmentary displacements with different hybrid external fixators. *Clin. Biomech.*, 18(2), 166–172.
14. Aro, H.T., Chao, E.Y.S., 1993. Bone-healing patterns affected by loading, fracture fragment stability, fracture type and fracture site compression. *Clin. Orthop.*, 293, 8–17.
15. Chao, E.Y.S., Aro, H.T., Lewallen, D.G., Kelly, P.J., 1989. The effect of rigidity on fracture healing in external fixation. *Clin. Orthop.*, 241, 24–35.
16. Hillard, P.J., Harrison, A.J., Atkins, R.M., 1998. The yielding of tensioned fine wires in the Ilizarov frame. *Proc. Inst. Mech. Eng.*, 212(Part H), 37–47.

17. Matsuura, M., Lounici, S., Inoue, N., Walulik, S., Chao, E.Y., 2003. Assessment of external fixator reusability using load- and cycle-dependent tests. *Clin. Orthop. Relat. Res.*, 406, 275–281.
18. Watson, M.A., Mathias, K.J., Vulli, N.M., 2000. External ring fixators: An overview. *Proc. Inst. Mech. Eng.*, 214(Part H), 459–470.
19. Bronson, D.G., Samchukov, M.L., Birch, J.G., Browne, R.H., Ashman, R.B., 1998. Stability of external circular fixation: A multi-variable biomechanical analysis. *Clin. Biomech.*, 13, 441–448.
20. Windhagen, H., Glockner, R., Bail, H., Kolbeck, S., Raschke, M., 2002. Stiffness characteristics of composite hybrid external fixators. *Clin. Orthop.*, 405, 267–276.
21. Zhang, G., 2004. Geometric and material nonlinearity in tensioned wires of an external fixator. *Clin. Biomech.*, 19, 513–518.
22. Zhang, G., 2004. Avoiding the material nonlinearity in an external fixation device. *Clin. Biomech.*, 19, 746–750.
23. Beer, F.P., Johnson, E.R., Jr., DeWolf, J.T., Mazurek D., 2014. *Mechanics of Materials*, 7th Edition, McGraw-Hill, Columbus, OH.

5

Viscoelasticity of Load-Bearing Soft Tissues: Constitutive Formulation, Numerical Integration, and Computational Implementation

Christian M. Puttlitz, Snehal S. Shetye, and Kevin L. Troyer

CONTENTS

ABSTRACT Soft tissue instability can cause or accelerate joint tissue degeneration. This is especially relevant to dynamic loading during falls, sports, and trauma-related events. The associated degenerative sequelae can result in significant loss of function and general reduction in one's quality of life. Thus, understanding the dynamic viscoelastic mechanical behavior of the involved soft tissue structures is a crucial first step in developing treatment modalities for joint instability. Current soft tissue viscoelastic characterization paradigms utilize quasi-linear viscoelastic formulations that inherently do not allow for a single, inseparable elastic and viscous behavior description. Further, available nonlinear viscoelastic formulations lack a description of relaxation manifested during dynamic loading events. Consequently, finite element implementation of nonlinear soft tissue viscoelastic behavior has not been widespread. Thus, to address these shortcomings, the following work describes the development of a novel, nonlinear viscoelastic constitutive formulation and a corresponding experimental characterization technique that is computationally tractable and implementable in state-of-the-art finite element algorithms. Implementation of the important nonlinear viscoelastic behavior of orthopedic soft tissues into computational models will greatly accelerate our ability to understand the functional role of soft connective tissues in whole-joint mechanics and facilitate future treatment options.

5.1 Introduction

Orthopedic soft tissues play critical roles in the stability of the joints and load-bearing structures of the human body. Cartilage provides load-bearing structures the ability to articulate with minimal friction with efficient load-transfer capability. Tendons help muscles in actuation of motion and transmission of forces to joints. Ligaments are passive load-bearing structures that aid in joint stability. Thus, damage to these tissues can result in debilitation, loss of function, and decreased range of motion. Therefore, understanding their function and mechanical environment is paramount for designing effective treatments.

Many attempts have been put forth to describe the mechanical behavior of orthopedic soft tissues, which greatly deviate from classical isotropic linear mechanics. Accordingly, fully nonlinear, anisotropic, closed-form mathematical descriptions have been presented, including the application of hyperelastic constitutive formulae. These descriptions demonstrate large variations with regard to complexity and computational intensity. The latter concern is especially relevant because the goal of these formulae developments is eventually implementation into computational models, most commonly finite element models. Therefore, more recently, there has been a substantial amount of research that has attempted to balance predictive accuracy with computational tractability and expense.

Another confounding factor associated with modeling hydrated biological soft tissues is that they demonstrate a very high degree of time-dependent (i.e., viscoelastic) behavior. This aspect of soft tissue behavior is commonly disregarded or simplified because of the complexity of viscoelastic formulae and the associated difficulty in implementing these mathematical descriptors in computational models owing to numerical integration issues. Recently, our group has developed computational tractable formulae for implementing fully nonlinear viscoelasticity in a commercial finite element package for modeling ligaments and tendons.

5.1.1 Ligament and Tendon: Morphology and Function

Ligament and tendon are dense fibrous connective tissues with similar, primarily mechanical, functional roles that provide locomotion and stabilize the skeleton. Tendinous tissues transmit muscular contractions to bone and limbs in order to invoke locomotion and provide active joint stability (via the musculature). Ligamentous tissues span across a joint (connecting adjacent bones) in order to passively guide physiologic joint motion patterns and restrict potentially harmful movements. The gross (tissue-level) mechanical phenomena exhibited by these tissues are a result of their specific geometry and their biochemical and microstructural composition. However, it has been shown that all ligaments and tendons are highly viscoelastic and their normal physiologic function is highly dependent on this temporal mechanical behavior.

5.1.1.1 Tendon

Tendon is a natural fibrous composite material with a hierarchical structure. It is composed of collagen fibers (predominately type I) embedded in a highly hydrated PG matrix (ground substance). Collagen fibers dominate the solid-phase microstructure, constituting more than 85% of the tissue's dry weight [1]. The collagen structure exhibits its own hierarchical organization, and these collagen substructures are tightly packed and exhibit a high degree of anatomical alignment parallel to the longitudinal axis of the tendon. Intermolecular and intramolecular cross-links allow these tissues to achieve high mechanical integrity (high tensile stiffness and strength) [2,3]. Additionally, the collagen fibrils exhibit a wavy crimp pattern that is thought to play an important role in the tissue's mechanical behavior [4]. Although proteoglycans (PGs) constitute a relatively small portion of the total solid-phase tendinous microstructure (less than 2% of the total dry weight), these molecules are essential for maintaining tendon hydration (and therefore viscoelastic mechanical function) [2,5]. Water constitutes more than half (approximately 60%) of the total wet weight of tendon [6]. Cellular components (predominately fibroblasts) are sparsely embedded within the ground substance and are aligned in the direction of the fibrils [1]. These cells synthesize and secrete collagen fibers and extracellular matrix components [2,7,8]. Production of these extracellular components is regulated by mechanobiologic stimulation. Cellular nutrition is provided by diffusion or vascular supply [1,5].

5.1.1.2 Ligament

Although ligaments are biologically and morphologically similar to tendons, these tissues contain distinct differences that reflect upon their unique physiologic role. For example, ligaments must exhibit greater extensibility than tendons in order to facilitate joint motion [6]. Morphologically, this reduced stiffness is achieved via a reduced collagen fiber content (70% of the total dry weight) and a reduced degree of parallel collagen fiber arrangement as compared with tendons [1,6,9–11]. The increase in collagen fiber dispersion is a result of the different in vivo loading conditions experienced by these two tissue types. Whereas tendons predominately experience consistent uniaxial (longitudinal) forces, ligaments may be subjected to multiaxial loading patterns [6] (depending on their anatomical location) that require specific mechanical properties in the off-axis directions. For example, the cruciate and collateral knee ligaments exhibit a spatially varying anisotropic collagen fiber arrangement in order to withstand multidirectional loads [12,13]. Additionally, ligaments typically contain greater amounts of the structural protein elastin (typically 1% to 2% of the total dry weight) as compared with tendon [6]. In some specialized ligaments, such as the spinal ligamenta flava, elastin is the predominate fibrous component [14], which allows this tissue to undergo a greater amount of elastic deformation as compared with the other, predominately collagenous, spinal ligaments [15–17].

5.2 Mechanical Behavior of Orthopedic Connective Tissues

When considering the mechanical response of orthopedic connective tissues such as ligaments and tendons, it is important to study both the quasi-static and dynamic mechanical
response of these structures. During quasi-static loading, inertial considerations can be
largely neglected; however, inertial effects must be incorporated into investigations of tissue dynamic loading. For orthopedic tissues such as bone, where the correlation between
strength and the applied strain rate is relatively weak, quasi-static testing is usually sufficient to describe the material properties. However, this is not true for soft structures,
such as ligament and tendon, which require a more detailed examination of their time-
dependent properties.

5.2.1 Elastic Behavior

The quasi-static elastic behavior of ligament and tendon has been extensively studied.
These tissues experience nonlinear, finite deformations in vivo that cannot be described
by the infinitesimal strain theory (Hooke's law) of typical engineering materials [18]. When
these tissues are tensioned at a constant strain rate, they exhibit the nonlinear, hyperelastic force–displacement (or stress–strain, σ–ε) relationship shown in Figure 5.1 [19]. The
concave-up region from 0 to A is commonly referred to as the *toe region* of the curve. This
nonlinear region typically encompasses the physiologic range of the tissue; the relatively
linear region from A to B typically lies outside of this range [19]. The increased stiffness
(slope or $d\sigma/d\varepsilon$) in the A–B region serves as a protective mechanism for the tissue and its
associated joint by increasing the tissue's energy-absorbing capacity and restricting nonphysiologic joint motions. Following this linear region, a nonlinear subfailure region (from
B to C) is preceded by ultimate tissue failure at C.

Tendons and ligaments have unique load-deformation profiles that are specific to their
in vivo mechanical function. Tendons typically have a smaller toe region and a greater
stiffness and ultimate strength than ligaments. These properties maximize the efficiency
with which muscular contractions are transmitted to the bone and protect the tissue when
subjected to large musculoskeletal forces [1,6]. The high mechanical integrity (stiffness
and strength) of the tendon is derived from its relatively high proportion of longitudinally

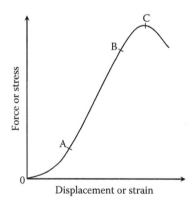

FIGURE 5.1
A typical force–displacement (or stress–strain) curve for dense connective tissue.

aligned collagen fibers [1]. Conversely, ligaments exhibit a longer toe region (i.e., they undergo a greater amount of deformation at a reduced stiffness) in order to facilitate joint movement [6]. This increased extensibility decreases the amount of muscular expenditure required to move the joint throughout physiologic motions [16].

The shape of the nonlinear loading curve is related to the tissue's microstructure, specifically collagen fiber recruitment and orientation. In the zero-force configuration, the collagen fibrils are crimped and offer negligible resistance to deformation. As a tensile load is applied to the tissue, these fibrils become successively straightened and recruited [20], resulting in the toe region of the loading curve. The linear region of the loading curve arises as more fibrils are recruited and become load-bearing [20]. By direct measurement of the collagen fiber spread of spinal ligaments during deformation (via x-ray diffraction techniques), Kirby et al. [11] and Hukins et al. [10] demonstrated an increase in fibril alignment toward the loading axis. As the fibers became more oriented with the loading axis, apparent stiffness of the tissue also increased.

5.2.2 Viscoelastic Behavior

While the elastic properties offer some insight into the functional mechanical role of tendons and ligaments, application of these static properties is severely restricted since these hydrated tissues are subjected to transient and dynamic deformations in vivo. As a result, these tissues exhibit a significant amount of viscoelastic, or time-dependent, behavior, such as creep, stress relaxation, hysteresis, and strain rate–dependent stiffness. Creep describes the continued increase in tissue strain over time when subjected to a constant stress. Stress relaxation describes the temporal stress decay within the tissue when it is subjected to a constant strain. The viscoelastic effects of hysteresis and strain rate–dependent stiffness arise during tissue loading and unloading. Hysteresis is defined as the energy lost during cyclic loading and is evidenced by energy dissipation (depicted as different loading and unloading profiles) on a stress–strain plot of a loading cycle. Finally, the effective stiffness of a viscoelastic material is dependent upon the rate to which the tissue is extended.

While it is widely accepted that the phenomenological viscoelastic behavior of soft connective tissues arises from its morphology, the specific microstructural mechanisms for this behavior are a subject of ongoing debate. Current theories speculate that the origin of tendon and ligament viscoelasticity arises from mechanisms acting on different length scales, including intermolecular viscoelasticity of the collagen fibrils, interactions between the solid-phase (collagen and PG) constituents, and movement of fluid through the tissue. Intermolecular viscoelastic effects within the collagen fibrils themselves have been reported via observation of changes in the periodic spacing between tropocollagen molecules in tendons subjected to creep experiments [21]. Additionally, development of theoretical constitutive models has led some to hypothesize that interactions between the glycosaminoglycan (GAG) and fibril constituents contribute to tissue-level viscoelasticity [22,23]. However, recent experimental work has demonstrated that GAG–fibril interactions do not significantly affect the viscoelastic behavior of the tissue [24]. Instead, the GAG constituents may contribute to tissue-level viscoelasticity by regulating fluid flow through the tissue. Similar to cartilage, the GAG constituents in ligament affect its transverse permeability in compression [25]. This compressive behavior may affect fluid flow through the matrix (inducing tissue-level viscoelasticity) during axial tensile loading because of the relatively large Poisson's ratio (lateral contraction) observed by these tissues [25–28]. Collectively, these previous experimental studies of molecular-level viscoelasticity and fiber-level fluid flow suggest that several mechanisms, at different length scales, are responsible for the gross viscoelastic behavior of the tissue.

As with the elastic mechanical behavior described above, the viscoelastic properties of tendon and ligament have important contributions to normal physiologic function by facilitating joint motion, minimizing muscular expenditure, and protecting the joint (and the tissue itself) during traumatic events. Both tendon and ligament exhibit strain rate–dependent stiffness [1], displaying a reduced stiffness at slow (physiologic) strain rates and a high stiffness at fast (traumatic) strain rates. For ligaments, reduced stiffness decreases the amount of muscular energy required to produce physiologic joint motions. At traumatic strain rates, the increased stiffness and ultimate load indicates an increased energy-absorbing capacity, improving the tissue's resistance to abnormal motions and mitigating ligamentous or joint injury. Similar strain rate–dependent behavior has been reported for muscle–tendon units [29], protecting these tissues from injury during fast loading rates. Additionally, tendon creep (lengthening under constant load) minimizes the rate of muscle fatigue during isometric contractions by allowing the muscle to shorten [1].

5.2.3 Viscoelastic Theory

Viscoelastic theory describes the time-dependent relationship between stress and strain for a solid material. Consequently, the current mechanical state of the material depends on previous loading events; that is, the mechanical behavior is dependent upon the loading history (history-dependent behavior). All biological tissues, especially soft tissues such as ligament and tendon, exhibit viscoelastic behavior. As detailed above, this time-dependent behavior is necessary to perform the important functional roles of the tissue. The following develops the mathematical formulae typically used to model viscoelastic phenomena in biological tissues.

5.2.3.1 Linear Viscoelasticity

Materials that exhibit time-dependent behavior such as stress relaxation and creep are typically referred to as viscoelastic materials. Consequently, different mechanical models have been developed to describe this behavior such as the Maxwell, Voigt, and Kelvin models. The Kelvin model, also referred to as the *standard linear solid* model, describes most accurately a linear viscoelastic material displaying relaxation and creep behavior and has been successfully used to describe materials such as rubber and typical engineering metals.

5.2.3.1.1 Transient Behavior

For typical engineering materials (e.g., steel, aluminum, titanium) at room temperature subjected to small strains, the one-dimensional stress response (σ) to an instantaneous application of strain (ε_0) is described by Hooke's law:

$$\sigma = E\varepsilon_0, \tag{5.1}$$

where E is the Young's modulus of the material that characterizes its resistance to deformation (stiffness). Similarly, the material's compliance (J) in response to an instantaneous stress application of σ_0 can be described by the inverse of Equation 5.1: $J = 1/E = \varepsilon/\sigma_0$. For a viscoelastic material, the intrinsic parameter relating stress and strain (analogous to E for elastic materials) depends on time, t. Thus, the time-dependent stress response to an instantaneous (transient) strain application of ε_0 is given by

$$\sigma(t) = E(t) \cdot \varepsilon_0, \tag{5.2}$$

where $E(t)$ is the *relaxation modulus* (or *relaxation function*) of the material that characterizes its stress decay (stress relaxation) over time. An analogous form of Equation 5.2 can be developed to describe the time-dependent strain in response to an instantaneous stress application of stress:

$$\varepsilon(t) = J(t) \cdot \sigma_0,\tag{5.3}$$

where $J(t)$ is the *creep compliance* of the material that characterizes its creep behavior. The mathematical form of the relaxation function is not arbitrary; thermodynamic restrictions require it to be a monotonically decreasing function [30,31]. A linear viscoelastic relaxation function that has been used among the biomechanics community is derived from the standard linear solid model [19]:

$$E(t) = E_\infty + E_0 e^{-t/\tau_r},\tag{5.4}$$

where E_∞ represents the (steady-state) elastic component of the mechanical behavior (as $t \to \infty$) and E_0 represents the strength of the viscous (time-dependent) relaxation component corresponding to the time constant τ_r.

5.2.3.1.2 Cyclic Behavior

If a linear viscoelastic material is subjected to harmonic oscillations, the strain will *lag* the stress because of internal material damping (Figure 5.2), which is a consequence of the viscous component of the material [31]. Thus, for a sinusoidal stress applied to a material at a specific frequency (v, expressed in units of hertz):

$$\sigma(t) = \sigma_0 \sin(2\pi v t).\tag{5.5}$$

The resulting out-of-phase strain is

$$\varepsilon(t) = \varepsilon_0 \sin(2\pi v t - \delta),\tag{5.6}$$

where δ represents the phase lag between stress and strain (Figure 5.2). The tangent of the phase lag, $\tan(\delta)$, is called the *loss tangent* and is a measure of a material's internal damping [31].

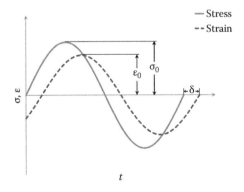

FIGURE 5.2
Cyclic behavior of a viscoelastic material. The strain lags the stress by a phase shift, δ.

As a consequence of the phase lag between stress and strain, the dynamic stiffness (E^*) of a material can be expressed as a complex number:

$$\frac{\sigma}{\varepsilon_0} = E^* = E' + iE'',$$
(5.7)

which has a magnitude of

$$|E^*| = \sqrt{(E')^2 + (E'')^2}.$$
(5.8)

The storage modulus (E') and the loss modulus (E'') in Equations 5.7 and 5.8 are defined as

$$E' = |E^*|\cos(\delta)$$
(5.9)

$$E'' = |E^*|\sin(\delta),$$
(5.10)

where E' represents the energy stored within the material and E'' represents the energy dissipated per cycle [32].

5.2.3.1.3 *Constitutive (Generalized) Behavior*

The equations developed above apply to very specific (transient and cyclical) loading histories. Since biological tissues are subjected to complex, arbitrary load applications *in vivo*, it is desirable to obtain general constitutive formulae to describe linear viscoelastic behavior. Such a mathematical form can be developed using the Boltzmann superposition principle, which postulates that the effect of a compound cause is a sum of the individual causes [31]. Utilizing a more rigorous mathematical approach [33], recall from above that for a single instantaneous input of strain:

$$\varepsilon(t) = \varepsilon_0 H(t),$$
(5.11)

where ε_0 is the input strain magnitude and $H(t)$ is the Heaviside step function defined as

$$H(t) = \begin{cases} 0 & \text{for} \quad t < 0 \\ \dfrac{1}{2} & \text{for} \quad t = 0 \\ 1 & \text{for} \quad t > 0. \end{cases}$$
(5.12)

The resulting stress output is $\sigma(t) = \varepsilon_0 E(t)$ for $t > 0$. A series of such step increases in strain can be used to describe any arbitrary strain input profile. Hence, for r discrete step increases in strain, Equation 5.11 can be recast as

$$\varepsilon(t) = \sum_{i=1}^{r} \Delta\varepsilon_i H(t - \tau_i),$$
(5.13)

where $\Delta\varepsilon_i$ is the change in strain magnitude for the ith step occurring at time τ_i and t is the current time. Utilizing the Boltzmann superposition principle, the resulting stress output (from Equation 5.2) is

$$\sigma(t) = \sum_{i=1}^{r} \Delta\varepsilon_i E(t - \tau_i) H(t - \tau_i). \tag{5.14}$$

As the number of strain steps increases to infinity, Equation 5.14 converges to the hereditary integral:

$$\sigma(t) = \int_0^t E(t - \tau) H(t - \tau)\, d\varepsilon(\tau), \tag{5.15}$$

where τ is a continuous time variable of integration representing the history effect [31,33]. In Equation 5.15, the term $H(t - \tau) = 1$ since $\tau > 0$ is imposed and falls within the bounds of integration [33]. Therefore, for a differentiable strain history, the final form of the constitutive relationship for a linear viscoelastic material can be cast as

$$\sigma(t) = \int_0^t E(t - \tau) \frac{d\varepsilon(\tau)}{d\tau}\, d\tau. \tag{5.16}$$

It can be shown that for a single instantaneous strain history of $\varepsilon(\tau) = \varepsilon_0 H(\tau)$, the transient stress response given by Equation 5.2 is recovered from Equation 5.16. Additionally, if a harmonic strain history $\varepsilon(\tau)$ is imposed, the stress given by Equation 5.16 can be represented as a complex number in the form of Equation 5.7 [31]. If the relaxation function given by Equation 5.4 is assumed and input into Equation 5.16, the complex moduli are determined by [31]

$$E'(\omega) = E_\infty + E_0 \frac{\omega^2 \tau_r^2}{1 + \omega^2 \tau_r^2} \tag{5.17}$$

$$E''(\omega) = E_0 \frac{\omega \tau_r}{1 + \omega \tau_r}, \tag{5.18}$$

where $\omega = 2\pi\nu$ (ν is the loading frequency as defined above).

Linear viscoelasticity assumes that both the elastic and the viscous components of the mechanical behavior are linear. Specifically, a material modeled utilizing linear viscoelasticity must satisfy two assumptions: (1) the relationship between stress and strain during stress relaxation experiments performed at different strain magnitudes (taken at isochrones) is linear (linear elastic behavior assumption), and (2) the relaxation modulus is independent of the applied strain level (linear viscous behavior assumption). Soft connective tissues that undergo finite deformations violate the assumptions of linear viscoelasticity. Therefore, more general, quasi-linear and fully nonlinear formulations have been developed to describe the nonlinear viscoelastic behavior of soft tissues.

5.2.3.2 Quasi-Linear Viscoelasticity

The quasi-linear viscoelastic (QLV) theory proposed by Fung [34] has been widely accepted as the gold standard to describe the time-dependent behavior of soft connective tissues [35–44]. This formulation incorporates the known nonlinear, hyperelastic behavior exhibited by soft connective tissues by generalizing the linear elastic behavior assumption of linear viscoelastic theory. Specifically, the strain- and time-dependent stress in response to an instantaneous (Heaviside) strain application is modeled as the separable convolution (*) of the hyperelastic $\sigma^e(\varepsilon)$ and viscous $G(t)$ components of the mechanical behavior:

$$\sigma(t, \varepsilon) = G(t)*\sigma^e(\varepsilon). \tag{5.19}$$

A restriction is imposed on the relaxation function $G(t)$ such that $G(0) = 1$. This normalized function is called the *reduced relaxation function*. For general strain histories, the QLV equation takes the following form [19]:

$$\sigma(t, \varepsilon) = \int_0^t G(t - \tau) \frac{\partial \sigma^e(\varepsilon)}{\partial \varepsilon} \frac{\partial \varepsilon(\tau)}{\partial \tau} d\tau. \tag{5.20}$$

Since $G(t)$ is independent of the applied strain magnitude, a fundamental assumption of QLV theory is linear viscous behavior.

5.2.3.3 Fully Nonlinear Viscoelasticity

Recent studies have conclusively demonstrated that both tendon [45] and ligament [46–50] exhibit fully nonlinear viscoelastic behavior (nonlinearity in both the elastic and the viscous aspects of the tissue's mechanical behavior) at strain magnitudes associated with physiologic joint motion. This nonlinear behavior cannot be accurately captured by Equation 5.20. Fully nonlinear viscoelastic formulations allow relaxation to occur as a function of the applied strain via a nonseparable formulation [31]:

$$\sigma[t, \varepsilon(t)] = \int_0^t E[\varepsilon(\tau), t - \tau] \frac{d\varepsilon(\tau)}{d\tau} d\tau, \tag{5.21}$$

where $E(\varepsilon, t)$ is the strain- and time-dependent relaxation modulus. The nonseparability condition in Equation 5.21 necessarily imposes the condition that $E(\varepsilon, t)$ simultaneously describes both elastic and viscous nonlinearities. Under a Heaviside strain application of ε_0, Equation 5.21 reduces to

$$\sigma[t, \varepsilon(t)] = E(\varepsilon, t) \cdot \varepsilon_0. \tag{5.22}$$

5.3 Numerical Implementation of Constitutive Viscoelastic Formulae

While the closed-form mathematical descriptions of QLV and fully nonlinear viscoelasticity presented above are well described, one needs to typically reformat these equations in order to implement them for numerical simulations. The QLV formulation can be recast as

$$\sigma(\varepsilon, t) = \int_0^t G(t - \tau) \frac{\partial \sigma^e(\varepsilon)}{\partial \varepsilon} \frac{\partial \varepsilon(\tau)}{\partial \tau} d\tau + \sigma_0, \tag{5.23}$$

where σ_0 represents the initial tissue pre-tension in the reference configuration. The reduced relaxation function can be approximated by the Prony series [37,48,51]

$$G(t) = G_\infty + \sum_{i=1}^4 G_i e^{-t/\tau_i} \tag{5.24}$$

subjected to the constraint

$$G_\infty + G_1 + G_2 + G_3 + G_4 = 1, \tag{5.25}$$

where G_∞ is the steady-state relaxation coefficient $\left[G_\infty = \lim_{t \to \infty} G(t)\right]$, and the G_i coefficients represent the relaxation strength corresponding to the τ_i time constants. This relaxation function is selected in this case because it is similar in form to the fully nonlinear relaxation modulus described in detail below. The Prony series representation (with fitted parameters G_∞, G_i, and τ_i) is known to yield nonunique solutions [19]. However, a unique solution can be achieved by fixing the τ_i time constants [52]. Additionally, previous work [48] has demonstrated that this Prony series representation is insensitive to initial guesses spanning five temporal decades (0.001 to 10). The shortest fixed time constant, $\tau_1 = 0.1$ s, is chosen to temporally coincide with typical experimental ramp times (<0.3 s). Succeeding time constants are incrementally increased by decadal values [37,48], ending at the decade value that corresponds with the length of the experiment: $\tau_2 = 1$ s, $\tau_3 = 10$ s, $\tau_4 = 100$ s. The instantaneous elastic stress, and its derivative, can be represented by the following nonlinear equations:

$$\sigma^e(\varepsilon) = A(e^{B\varepsilon} - 1) \tag{5.26}$$

$$\frac{\partial \sigma^e(\varepsilon)}{\partial \varepsilon} = ABe^{B\varepsilon}, \tag{5.27}$$

where A and B are the instantaneous elastic parameters [37,48,51].

If the applied strain ramp history is complex (not a pure linear ramp and constant hold), differentiation of the applied strain history $\varepsilon(\tau)$ complicates direct numerical integration of Equation 5.23. Therefore, in order to simplify the integration of Equation 5.23, the differential operator can be removed from the input strain history via integration by parts:

$$\sigma(\varepsilon, t) = ABe^{B\varepsilon}\left[-\int_0^t \frac{dG(t-\tau)}{d\tau}\varepsilon(\tau)d\tau + G(t-t)\varepsilon(t) - G(t-0)\varepsilon(0) \right] + \sigma_0$$

$$= ABe^{B\varepsilon}\left[-\int_0^t \frac{dG(t-\tau)}{d\tau}\varepsilon(\tau)d\tau + G(0)\varepsilon(t) \right] + \sigma_0.$$

(5.28)

Several finite ramp time correction methods have been developed for QLV formulations [36,53–55], with the method proposed by Abramowitch and Woo [55] being the most commonly adopted [44,48,56–60]. Limitations of the Abramowitch and Woo method include the assumption of QLV tissue behavior (linear viscous behavior) and the assumption of a pure linear strain ramp application, which require very long (nonphysiologic) ramp times. In order to elucidate errors associated with a pure linear strain assumption applied to an actual (nonlinear, fast-ramp) strain history, the fitted parameters obtained using the methodology of Abramowitch and Woo have been used to predict the full (ramp–relax) stress relaxation experiment, and the cyclic experiments, by numerically integrating Equation 5.28 with the actual strain history used as input.

For the fully nonlinear viscoelastic formulation, the constitutive equation can be recast as

$$\sigma[\varepsilon(t), t] = \int_0^t E[\varepsilon(\tau), t-\tau]\frac{d\varepsilon(\tau)}{d\tau}d\tau + \sigma_0. \tag{5.29}$$

The nonlinear (strain- and time-dependent) relaxation modulus can be approximated by the Prony series [61]:

$$E(\varepsilon, t) = E_\infty(\varepsilon) + \sum_{i=1}^4 E_i(\varepsilon)e^{-t/\tau_i}, \tag{5.30}$$

where $E_\infty(\varepsilon)$ represents the strain-dependent steady-state modulus $\left[E_\infty(\varepsilon) = \lim_{t\to\infty} E(\varepsilon, t)\right]$ and $E_i(\varepsilon)$ represents the strain-dependent moduli corresponding to the τ_i time constants. Analogous to Equation 5.28, Equation 5.29 can also be integrated by parts to simplify the numerical integration:

$$\sigma[\varepsilon(t), t] = -\int_0^t \frac{dE[\varepsilon(\tau), t-\tau]}{d\tau}\varepsilon(\tau)d\tau + E[\varepsilon(t), t-t]\varepsilon(t) - E[\varepsilon(0), t-0]\varepsilon(0)$$

$$= -\int_0^t \frac{dE[\varepsilon(\tau), t-\tau]}{d\tau}\varepsilon(\tau)d\tau + E[\varepsilon(t), 0]\varepsilon(t) + \sigma_0.$$

(5.31)

There are relatively few finite ramp time correction methods for fully nonlinear viscoelastic materials [62,63]. However, these previous attempts were developed specifically for the Schapery nonlinear viscoelastic material model, rather than the single integral formulation of the modified superposition method (i.e., Equation 5.29) [31,33], which has been recommended for modeling ligament viscoelasticity [64]. Instead of directly correcting for the finite ramp time, Equation 5.29 has traditionally been used with fast ramp times that approximate a true (Heaviside) step function, which has the following form:

$$\sigma[t, \varepsilon(t)] = E(\varepsilon, t) \cdot \varepsilon_0 + \sigma_0. \tag{5.32}$$

Data from the relaxation period of the experiment are then considered only after a specified amount of time in order to reduce the transient errors of the testing device. Multiples of the ramp time (t_0), such as $10t_0$ [31,46,47] and $2.5t_0$ [31,45,65], have been used or recommended for connective tissues. These methods negate important short-term relaxation information and may not be appropriate if the relative degree of short-term relaxation is substantial [66]. Since the short-term relaxation behavior plays an important role in the mechanical performance of soft tissues, the errors associated with the $10t_0$ and the $2.5t_0$ fitting methods are elucidated below by quantifying the ability of their fitted parameters to predict the full (ramp–relax) stress relaxation and cyclic experiments.

Relaxation during loading may play a vital role in soft tissue mechanics. For example, the spinal anterior longitudinal ligament exhibits a greater stiffness, ultimate load, and peak energy at faster loading rates than at slower ones [17,67,68]. This rate-dependent behavior facilitates and guides normal spinal motion patterns at slow loading rates but prevents excessive joint motion and tissue damage by absorbing additional energy during (fast loading rate) traumatic situations [69]. Unfortunately, this intrinsic relaxation mechanism during loading complicates the experimental viscoelastic characterization of these soft tissues.

From a modeling perspective, soft tissue viscoelasticity can be characterized via stress relaxation experiments to define the tissue's relaxation modulus. Theoretically, the relaxation modulus completely characterizes the temporal stress behavior of the tissue in response to an instantaneous (Heaviside or step) strain application. However, inertial limitations of physical testing devices prevent instantaneous strain applications, and very fast ramp times are intractable because of issues such as overshoot, vibration, and poorly approximated strain histories [35,44,55,65,66,70]. Empirical deviations from a true step strain application can cause significant errors in the determination of the tissue's relaxation modulus because of the intrinsic relaxation that occurred during the ramping (loading) period of the experiment.

Several methods have been developed to either correct for the finite ramp time of stress relaxation experiments or reduce the error associated with fast ramp times [31,36,45–47,53–55,62,63,65]. However, these methods either negate relaxation manifested during the short-term loading period or are restricted to very specific (linear) strain applications or viscoelastic formulations. The interrogation of errors associated with negating the important short-term relaxation behavior has been largely neglected in published studies. Additionally, for fast ramp times, which accurately represent in vivo loading conditions during the activities of daily living [65], the inertial effects of the testing device result in poor linear ramp approximations. Thus, a finite ramp time correction method that is restricted to a linear ramp assumption may introduce errors if physiologic loading rates are used for the experiment. Furthermore, multiple QLV [19,35,37,38,55] and fully nonlinear viscoelastic [45–47,64,65] formulations have been proposed to describe soft tissue viscoelasticity. Current finite ramp time correction methods are not transferrable between these various formulations. Therefore, there exists a significant need to develop a general method to characterize the viscoelastic behavior of these tissues that incorporates relaxation manifested during loading.

5.4 Comprehensive Viscoelastic Characterization Methodology

While the above numerical implementation techniques allow for computationally tractable formulations of the constitutive equations, these methods are reliant upon numerous material coefficients that differentiate the specific material behavior. Therefore, it is critical that the above techniques are paired with equally effective experimental and data fitting techniques in order to completely describe and model the material's mechanical behavior.

Recently, a finite ramp time correction method (hereafter referred to as the *comprehensive viscoelastic characterization* [CVC] method) that is generalizable to any viscoelastic formulation (QLV or fully nonlinear viscoelastic) and can accommodate an arbitrary strain history has been developed [52]. Thermodynamic limitations require the relaxation modulus to be a monotonically decreasing function [30,31]. Therefore, the CVC method was designed to fit only the decreasing (relaxation) period of the full experimental curve so that the fitted parameters are unconstrained. The relaxation manifested during loading is then incorporated by utilizing the following iterative algorithm:

a. *Fit the relaxation period of the experimental data, assuming a Heaviside strain application.* For the QLV formulation, an instantaneous strain application can be considered by assuming separability of the functions $\sigma^e(\varepsilon)$ and (t) [38,55]. Thus, Equation 5.26 is fitted to the ramping period ($0 < t < t_0$, where t_0 is defined by the maximum stress), and Equation 5.24, subjected to the constraint in Equation 5.25, is fitted to the normalized [$\sigma(t_0) = 1$] relaxation period ($t \geq t_0$) [38,55]. For the fully nonlinear formulation, a Heaviside step is assumed, and data in the relaxation period are fitted to Equation 5.32.

b. *Predict the full (ramp–relax) experiment by inputting the Heaviside assumption parameters obtained from step (a) into the integral form of the constitutive equation (Figure 5.3).* The integral formulations (Equation 5.28 for the QLV formulation, Equation 5.31 for the fully nonlinear formulation) are numerically integrated (the *quadgk* MATLAB® function can be used). The actual experimental strain history is included in this integration by use of a fitted cubic spline (this can be achieved using the *csaps* MATLAB function) to functionally describe $\varepsilon(\tau)$.

c. *Fit the relaxation period of the predicted curve obtained from step (b), assuming an instantaneous strain application (see step [a] for the analogous fitting procedure).*

d. *Calculate the difference {δ} between the fitted parameters for the experiment and the current prediction as*

$$\{\delta\} = \{\Theta\}_{exp} - \{\Theta\}_{pred'} \tag{5.33}$$

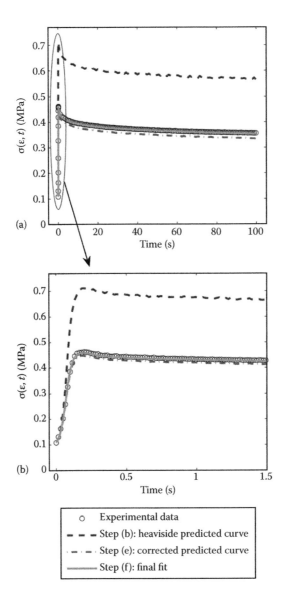

FIGURE 5.3
Depiction of the CVC method for a typical specimen for both (a) the long-term behavior and (b) the short-term behavior.

where $\{\Theta\}_{exp}$ is a vector containing the fitted parameters from step (a) and $\{\Theta\}_{pred}$ is a vector containing the fitted parameters determined form step (c). For the QLV fits: $\{\Theta\} = \{A, B, G_{\infty}, G_1, G_2, G_3, G_4\}$; for the fully nonlinear fits: $\{\Theta\} = \{E_{\infty}, E_1, E_2, E_3, E_4\}$.

e. *Define a new set of parameters $\{\Theta\}_{new}$ as input into the integral form of the constitutive equation and integrate to obtain a new predicted curve (Figure 5.3):*

$$\{\Theta\}_{new} = \{\Theta\}_{exp} + \{\delta\}. \tag{5.34}$$

f. *Iterate steps (c) through (e) until the following criterion (tolerance, TOL) is satisfied*:

$$|\max\{\delta\}| \le \text{TOL}. \tag{5.35}$$

By utilizing initial guesses within the range described above, and forcing the shape of the predicted curve to match the experimental curve (step [d]), the prescribed (relatively low; TOL = 10^{-6}) tolerance necessitates that the best set of (unique) coefficients has been obtained.

The predictive accuracy of the CVC method has been determined by applying this technique to experimentally derived stress relaxation and dynamic cyclic data on spinal ligaments [52]. Each ligament was tensioned to 5 N [57,65,71] and allowed to relax for 600 s. The resulting displacement was used as the reference configuration. Each ligament was then subjected to a cyclic (haversine) frequency sweep (0.001, 0.01, 0.1, and 1 Hz) at 10% and 15% peak-to-peak strain amplitudes. The slowest frequency (0.001 Hz) was performed as a preconditioning procedure. The remaining frequencies were chosen to observe the model's predictive accuracy with regard to varying physiologic loading rates, from quasi-static (0.01 Hz) to dynamic (1 Hz). Following this cyclic protocol, the reference configuration was redefined under 5 N of pre-tension, and the specimen was preconditioned (10% peak-to-peak strain amplitude, 1 Hz, 120 cycles) and subjected to stress relaxation experiments (ramp time: < 0.3 s, hold: 600 s, recover: 600 s [57,71] at 4%, 6%, 8%, 10%, 14%, 16%, 18%, 20%, and 25% engineering strain magnitudes). These strain magnitudes are well below the failure strains reported for these ligaments [72] and fall within the physiologic bounds predicted by computational and mathematical models [17,73]. The cross-sectional area of each ligament was measured using post hoc digital image capture [48].

Since the coefficient of determination (r^2 value) is a poor measure of goodness-of-fit for stress relaxation experiments owing to the disproportionately large amount of datum points in the long-term behavior [48], a weighted root-mean-squared error (RMSE) [66,74] was calculated in order to determine the probable error of the fitted stress relaxation curves:

$$\text{RMSE} = \sqrt{\frac{\sum_{k=1}^{n} \{w(t_k) \cdot [(\sigma_{\exp})_k - (\sigma_{\text{model}})_k]\}^2}{n}}, \tag{5.36}$$

where n is the number of datum points. The weighting function, $w(t_k)$, was defined as

$$w(t_k) = \frac{e^{-t_k/\tau_1} + e^{-t_k/\tau_2} + e^{-t_k/\tau_3} + e^{-t_k/\tau_4}}{4}, \tag{5.37}$$

where t_k is the kth time datum point and $(\sigma_{\exp})_k$ and $(\sigma_{\text{model}})_k$ are the kth experimental and model stress datum points, respectively. The RMSE was also calculated without the weighting function to quantify the error associated with the cyclic predictions. Additionally, the percent error between the kth datum points for the cyclic predictions were calculated as

$$\% \, \text{error} = \left| \frac{(\sigma_{\text{model}})_k - (\sigma_{\text{exp}})_k}{(\sigma_{\text{exp}})_k} \right| \cdot 100\%. \tag{5.38}$$

A significant amount of error was observed for the $10t_0$ and the $2.5t_0$ cyclic predictions (Figure 5.4). The CVC method, however, predicted the cyclic data extremely well, with percent errors and RMSE values that were an order of magnitude less than the experimental error (Table 5.1). The percent error and RMSE values for the CVC method predictions were also at least an order of magnitude less than the $10t_0$ and the $2.5t_0$ predicted curves (Table 5.1).

Since the CVC method is based on the shape of the relaxation curve, instead of the specific form of the constitutive equation, it can be applied to any viscoelastic formulation. Additionally, since the actual strain history is used as input for the integral form of the constitutive equation, no assumptions are made with regard to the applied strain history. Thus, this method is independent of the loading duration (i.e., can be applied to short or long ramp time experiments).

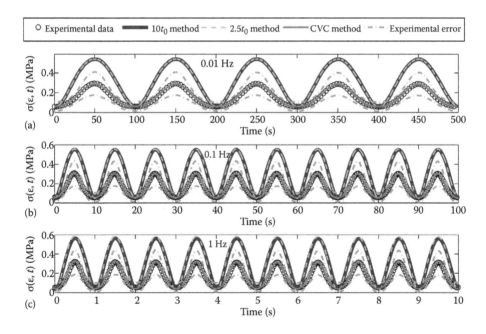

FIGURE 5.4

Comparison of the cyclic 10% strain amplitude predictions for the fully nonlinear viscoelastic fitting methods at the (a) 0.01 Hz, (b) 0.1 Hz, and (c) 1 Hz loading frequencies. The cyclic predictions for the 15% strain amplitude were similar. Experimental error was defined as one standard deviation from the experimental mean.

TABLE 5.1

Summary of the Error Calculations for the Fully Nonlinear Viscoelastic Cyclic Predictions at (a) the 10% and (b) the 15% Strain Amplitudes

	Percent Error (%)						RMSE (MPa)		
	0.01 Hz		0.1 Hz		1 Hz		0.01 Hz	0.1 Hz	1 Hz
(a) 10% Strain Amplitude									
CVC method	5.22	(5.18, 5.27)[a]	2.76	(2.67, 2.84)[a]	6.65	(6.17, 7.31)[a]	0.006	0.006	0.012
Experimental error	40.17	(40.14, 40.20)[b]	42.30	(42.22, 42.41)[b]	40.36	(40.03, 40.77)[b]	0.071	0.076	0.074
$10t_0$ method	105.96	(105.08, 106.72)[c]	104.10	(102.46, 105.71)[c]	103.68	(98.14, 109.39)[c]	0.188	0.188	0.188
$2.5f_0$ method	105.96	(105.17, 106.78)[c]	104.44	(102.82, 105.97)[c]	104.75	(99.69, 110.18)[c]	0.188	0.189	0.197
(b) 15% Strain Amplitude									
CVC method	6.48	(6.37, 6.58)[a]	6.16	(6.04, 6.28)[a]	6.06	(5.27, 9.18)[a]	0.019	0.025	0.032
Experimental error	44.93	(44.87, 44.98)[b]	43.96	(43.83, 44.09)[b]	44.34	(44.07, 44.58)[b]	0.121	0.125	0.126
$10t_0$ method	78.45	(77.37, 79.61)[c]	85.65	(83.70, 87.93)[c]	82.55	(75.48, 88.21)[c]	0.192	0.190	0.189
$2.5f_0$ method	78.29	(77.25, 79.51)[c]	86.83	(84.78, 89.02)[c]	92.92	(85.47, 99.95)[d]	0.193	0.193	0.203

Note: Superscript letters indicate statistical groupings within each strain amplitude and frequency; different letters indicate p < 0.008. The CVC method parameters predicted the cyclic data extremely well, exhibiting median percent error (95% lower confidence limit, 95% upper confidence limit) and RMSE values that were well within the bounds of experimental error (one standard deviation from the experimental mean) for both strain magnitudes and across all frequencies. Conversely, the parameters obtained from both of the $2.5f_0$ and the $10t_0$ fits poorly predicted the cyclic behavior. Statistical analyses were performed on the percent error by using a Kruskal–Wallis test within each strain amplitude and frequency grouping. Post hoc pairwise comparisons were performed by using a Wilcoxon rank-sum test with Bonferroni adjustment (statistical significance defined as p < 0.008).

5.5 Finite Element Implementation of Fully Nonlinear Viscoelasticity

The preceding theoretical, numerical, and material characterization modeling work is motivated by the final utility goal—implementation into finite element models in order to accurately describe the temporal behavior of orthopedic connective soft tissues.

In order to advance current FE modeling techniques to encompass fully nonlinear viscoelastic tissue response and accurately describe the physiologic static and dynamic loading scenarios, in the following we detail (1) nonlinear viscoelastic characterization of tendon experimental stress relaxation data, (2) an accurate nonlinear viscoelastic constitutive equation that accurately describes this experimental behavior and implementation of this relationship into FE algorithms, and (3) validation of this viscoelastic FE model by prediction of static and dynamic (cyclic) loading scenarios [75].

5.5.1 Experimental Data Acquisition

Ovine Achilles tendon ($n = 7$) were subjected to a series of physiologic [45] stress relaxation (randomized strain magnitudes: 1%, 2%, 3%, 4%, 5%, 6%, ramp rate: 10 mm/s, hold: 100 s, recover: 1000 s, data capture rate: 102.4 Hz) and dynamic (randomized strain amplitudes: 3% and 6%, frequencies: 1 and 10 Hz, data capture rate: 204.8 Hz) creep experiments. The cross-sectional area of each tendon was measured post hoc using an area micrometer technique [76–79].

5.5.2 Nonlinear Viscoelastic Formulations

The following two subsections describe both the analytical and FE nonlinear viscoelastic formulations. All fits and analytical predictions were performed with MATLAB (version 7.11; MathWorks, Inc., Natick, Massachusetts), and the FE simulations were performed using ABAQUS (version 6.9; Simulia, Providence, Rhode Island).

5.5.2.1 Analytical Formulation

Since tendon is a nonlinear viscoelastic material [45], the viscoelastic constitutive formulation given by Equation 5.29 was utilized for this study. The relaxation modulus was modeled using the five-term Prony series given by Equation 5.30 with fixed decadal time constants: $\tau_1 = 0.1$ s, $\tau_2 = 1$ s, $\tau_3 = 10$ s, $\tau_4 = 100$ s. Stress relaxation data at each strain magnitude were fitted to Equation 5.29 using two characterization techniques: (1) the CVC method described above, which incorporates viscoelastic effects during the loading event via an iterative algorithm [52], and (2) a previously described viscoelastic characterization technique [31,45,65] wherein strain is assumed to be applied instantly (i.e., a Heaviside step application; thereby neglecting relaxation experienced during loading) and data fitting begins after a multiple of 2.5 times the ramp time t_0 (referred to as the *2.5t₀ method*).

For each fitting method, the strain dependence of the moduli components were determined post hoc via a polynomial formulation [52,64,80–82]:

$$E(\varepsilon) = C_1\varepsilon + C_2\varepsilon^2, \tag{5.39}$$

where C_1 and C_2 were fit for each individual modulus component [$E_1(\varepsilon)$, $E_2(\varepsilon)$, $E_3(\varepsilon)$, $E_4(\varepsilon)$, $E_\infty(\varepsilon)$]. In order to examine differences between these two characterization techniques, the coefficients from each method (and strain level) were input into the analytical formulation (Equation 5.29) with the actual (ramp and relax) strain history to predict the experimental stress relaxation curve [52].

The relaxation period fits and the full predicted curves were compared via calculation of an exponentially weighted root-mean-squared error (wRMSE) (Equation 5.36) [52,74,82]. Statistical wRMSE comparisons were performed using the PROC MIXED procedure in SAS (SAS Institute, Inc., Cary, North Carolina; statistical significance: $p < 0.05$).

5.5.2.2 Finite Element Formulation

Consider a five-component mechanical model (Figure 5.5) composed of an elastic (steady-state) spring in parallel with four Maxwell components [61]. Under deformation, each component undergoes the same strain ε, whereas the total stress σ is a summation of the stress in each individual component (σ_∞ and σ_i) plus any initial pre-tension σ_0:

$$\sigma = \sigma_\infty + \sum_{i=1}^{4} \sigma_i + \sigma_0. \tag{5.40}$$

The steady-state stress σ_∞ component is given by the purely elastic relationship:

$$\sigma_\infty = E_\infty(\varepsilon) \cdot \varepsilon, \tag{5.41}$$

whereas the stress in each Maxwell component σ_i ($i = 1, 2, 3, 4$) is governed by the time-dependent differential equation [31]:

$$\dot{\sigma}_i + \frac{1}{\tau_i}\sigma_i = E_i(\varepsilon) \cdot \dot{\varepsilon}, \tag{5.42}$$

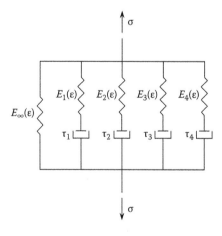

FIGURE 5.5
A five-component spring and dashpot nonlinear viscoelastic mechanical model. Nonlinearity of the spring constants $E_\infty(\varepsilon)$, $E_1(\varepsilon)$, $E_2(\varepsilon)$, $E_3(\varepsilon)$, and $E_4(\varepsilon)$ as modeled via a quadratic polynomial (Equation 5.38). The dashpots are characterized by their respective time constants τ_i ($i = 1, 2, 3, 4$).

where $[\dot{\ }]$ represents differentiation with respect to time and $E_\infty(\varepsilon)$, $E_i(\varepsilon)$, and τ_i are defined as the strain-dependent steady-state modulus $\left[E_\infty(\varepsilon) = \lim_{t\to\infty} E(\varepsilon, t) \right]$, and $E_i(\varepsilon)$ represents the strain-dependent moduli corresponding to the τ_i time constants. Equation 5.40 can be implemented numerically by use of the stable integration operator [83]:

$$\dot{f}_{t+\frac{1}{2}\Delta t} = \frac{\Delta f}{\Delta t}$$

$$f_{t+\frac{1}{2}\Delta t} = f^t + \frac{\Delta f}{\Delta t},$$

(5.43)

where f is an arbitrary function, f^t is its value at the current time, and Δf is the change in f over a time step Δt. Hence, by defining $\Delta f = f^t - f^{t-1}$, where f^{t-1} is the function value from the previous time step, the total stress at the current time (Equation 5.40) can be recast as

$$\sigma^t(\varepsilon^t, t) = E_\infty(\varepsilon^t) \cdot \varepsilon^t + \sum_{i=1}^{4} \frac{1}{1 + \dfrac{\Delta t}{\tau_i} + \dfrac{\Delta t}{2\tau_i}} \left[E_i(\varepsilon^t) \cdot \Delta\varepsilon + \left(1 + \frac{\Delta t}{2\tau_i} \right) \sigma_i^{t-1} \right] + \sigma_0,$$

(5.44)

where ε^t is the strain at the current time, $\Delta\varepsilon$ is the strain increment, and σ_i^{t-1} is the ith Maxwell component stress (Equation 5.42) from the previous time step.

In addition to the stress definition (Equation 5.44), the FE solution procedure also requires definition of a tangent stiffness. Utilizing the relations in Equations 5.40 through 5.43, the uniaxial tangent stiffness C^t can be cast as [83]

$$C^t = \frac{\partial \Delta\sigma}{\partial \Delta\varepsilon} = E_\infty(\varepsilon^t) + \sum_{i=1}^{4} \left[\frac{1}{1 + \dfrac{\Delta t}{2\tau_i}} \right] E_i(\varepsilon^t).$$

(5.45)

5.5.3 Finite Element Model

A single, two-node linear truss element (T3D2) was used to create a tension-only FE model of tendon in ABAQUS CAE. The inability to support bending/torsional moments makes this element ideal to represent long, slender structures supporting only axial loads [83], a typical geometry and mechanical behavior exhibited by tendon and several other connective tissues. A custom-written (FORTRAN) user-defined subroutine (UMAT) was developed to calculate the stress and tangent stiffness (Equations 5.44 and 5.45) using the coefficients obtained from either the CVC method or the $2.5t_0$ method. Gage length and cross-sectional area measurements obtained experimentally were used in the model geometry definitions.

In order to interrogate the predictive accuracy of the FE model and the two characterization methods, the FE models with material coefficients obtained from the each method were used to predict the average dynamic behavior via input of the average experimental cyclic displacement history. Accuracy of these predictions was evaluated with calculation of a nonweighted RMSE and the percent error [52,82]. For each strain amplitude, FE predictions for each characterization technique were compared with their corresponding analytical predictions (obtained via Equation 5.29) and with the experimental variability (defined as one positive standard deviation from the experimental mean).

5.5.3.1 Finite Element Model Predictions

Both characterization methods fit the stress relaxation period well (Figure 5.6). As compared with the CVC method, there was a significant increase in wRMSE or $2.5t_0$ method prediction of the entire (ramping and relaxation periods) curve (p < 0.001). The polynomial formulation (Equation 5.39) described the strain dependence of the moduli well ($r^2 \geq 0.89$). Comparison of the two fitting techniques indicated that there was no statistical difference between the $E_\infty(\varepsilon)$, $E_2(\varepsilon)$, $E_3(\varepsilon)$, $E_4(\varepsilon)$ moduli components (p ≥ 0.44). However, the $E_1(\varepsilon)$ modulus, corresponding to the 0.1 s time constant, was observed to be highly dependent on the fitting technique (p < 0.001).

The FE model predictions for each fitting method closely approximated the average cyclic analytical solution at both the 3% and the 6% (Figure 5.7) strain amplitudes. Data

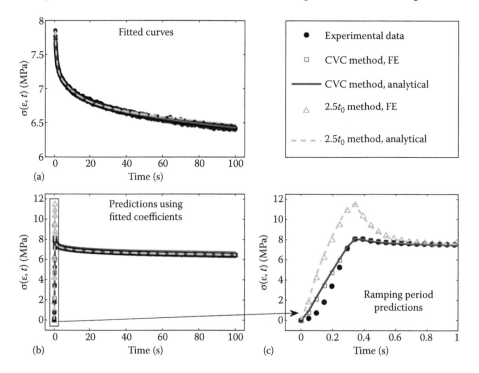

FIGURE 5.6
(a) A typical relaxation period curve fit (CVC method wRMSE = 2.62 kPa, $2.5t_0$ method wRMSE = 1.33 kPa); (b) the corresponding full (ramping and relaxation periods) analytical and FE curve predictions (CVC method wRMSE = 54.21 kPa, $2.5t_0$ method wRMSE = 182.51 kPa); and (c) the ramping period–only predictions. Since the inherent viscoelastic nonlinearity was determined post hoc, the CVC method predictions at individual strain magnitudes were not explicitly inclusive of the relaxation as a function of the applied strain. As a result, there was a minor disparity between the predicted stress relaxation behavior and the experimental ramping period (shown in [c]) that led to an increase in wRMSE with strain amplitude. The FE model closely approximated the analytical solution of both characterization methods.

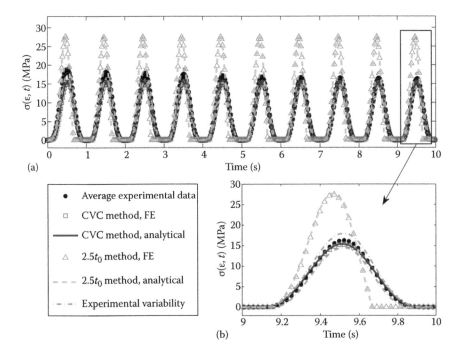

FIGURE 5.7
Average 6% strain amplitude cyclic behavior and the corresponding analytical and FE predictions from the two fitting techniques for (a) the full experiment and (b) the last full cycle. The $2.5t_0$ method predictions poorly approximated both the magnitude of the average experimental data and its phase. Conversely, the CVC method predictions were within the bounds of experimental variability and in-phase with the average experimental data.

taken from the last full cycle indicated that the material coefficients obtained using the CVC method (1) fell within the bounds of experimental variability, (2) closely approximated the average experimental peak stress (within the bounds of experimental variability), and (3) were in-phase with the average experimental data. Conversely, the coefficients obtained from the $2.5t_0$ method could not comprehensively capture these three criteria at either strain amplitude.

5.6 Future Directions

An important advantage of the proposed differential FE formulation (Equation 5.44) with regard to computational efficiency is that it requires storage of a single (axial) stress value from the previous step rather than the entire stress history (as necessitated by Equation 5.29). Even for FE models with relatively few elements, storage of the entire stress history at each integration point may be computationally expensive or intractable. Similar methods have been previously developed for an integral formulation, but its applicability has been restricted to QLV theory [84].

The constitutive formulae presented in this chapter are limited to uniaxial (one-dimensional) tensile deformations. Nevertheless, both the integral (Equation 5.29) and the differential (Equation 5.44) formulations may be generalized to multiaxial stress states [33], although tendon and ligament anisotropy is rarely considered in whole-joint simulations. Current whole-joint FE investigations, such as those of the cervical spine [85,86], the lumbar spine [87,88], the knee [89,90], the sacroiliac joint [91], and the pelvic joint [92], typically model these connective tissues as one-dimensional elastic spring or truss elements in order to reduce computational cost. Several tissue-level anisotropic phenomenological formulations have been suggested for modeling ligament viscoelasticity [32,84,93,94]. Nonetheless, most of these models are based on oversimplified QLV assumptions that cannot accurately capture nonlinear viscoelastic behavior [84,93,94]. However, a possible fully nonlinear viscoelastic formulation proposed by Rajagopal and Wineman [95] may offer the generality necessary to describe multidimensional soft tissue nonlinear viscoelasticity:

$$T = -p\mathbf{1} + F(t)\left\{ R[C(t),0] + \int_0^t \frac{\partial}{\partial(t-\tau)} R[C(\tau), t-\tau] \mathrm{d}\tau \right\} F^T(t), \qquad (5.46)$$

where T is the Cauchy stress tensor, $-p\mathbf{1}$ is the indeterminate stress (owing to the incompressibility constraint), $F(t)$ is the time-dependent deformation gradient, $C(\tau)$ is the right Cauchy–Green deformation tensor, and $R[C(\tau), t - \tau]$ is the tensorial relaxation modulus. Equation 5.46 is similar in form to the one-dimensional nonlinear superposition formulation utilized herein (Equation 5.29).

Implementation of Equation 5.46 is not straightforward. Several experimental and computational challenges exist, such as (1) the explicit definition of the form of the tensorial relaxation modulus R, (2) the protocol for conducting multiaxial nonlinear stress relaxation experiments (at multiple strain magnitudes) under controlled hydrothermal conditions, and (3) the complex (simultaneous) fitting of the multidimensional stress relaxation data to determine the material coefficients of R. It is likely that appropriate material symmetries (such as transverse isotropy) are requisite in order to reduce the number of tensorial components of Equation 5.46 and make the definition of R tractable [96]. Additionally, the form of R must satisfy previously established thermodynamic feasibility requirements [30,31]. It is postulated that fitting the multiaxial experimental data to Equation 5.46 may be carried out by developing an FE model of the experimental specimen (based on physical measurements) where the actual experimental forces or displacements can be used as the input FE boundary conditions. This FE model, which includes a custom user-defined material (UMAT) that implements Equation 5.46, can be used to create the predicted curves (step [b]) in the CVC algorithm. This protocol would be similar to a previous study that combined analytical and computational models to achieve the optimum coefficients for an anisotropic QLV model for brain stem [97].

Although several studies have demonstrated that the single integral nonlinear superposition model (Equation 5.29) can accurately capture the nonlinear viscoelastic effects of soft tissues subjected to temporally varying (stress relaxation and cyclic) loading conditions [45–49,52,64,98], recent evidence suggests that this formulation demonstrates reduced accuracy when describing other viscoelastic effects such as stress recovery [98] and creep. A single integral formulation developed by Schapery [99] may be more applicable to describe soft tissue recovery than Equation 5.29 [98]. In addition, multiple-integral nonlinear viscoelastic models, which contain more general nonlinear material definitions than the single integral models [31,33], may offer the ability to represent numerous soft tissue viscoelastic effects. To the best of this author's knowledge, there has been no effort to implement multiple integral formulations into soft tissue viscoelasticity.

As a final note, there are a number of relaxation moduli proposed to describe musculoskeletal soft tissue viscoelasticity, including Prony series (e.g., Equation 5.30) and power law formulations [45–47,64,65,81]. To date, there has been no general agreement in the literature over which specific form the relaxation modulus must take to describe soft tissue viscoelasticity.

References

1. S. R. Simon, and American Academy of Orthopaedic Surgeons, *Orthopaedic Basic Science* (American Academy of Orthopaedic Surgeons, Rosemont, IL, 1994).
2. J. A. Weiss, and J. C. Gardiner, *Critical Reviews in Biomedical Engineering* **29**, 303 (2001).
3. M. L. Tanzer, and J. H. Waite, *Collagen and Related Research* **2**, 177 (1982).
4. S. L. Y. Woo, G. A. Johnson, and B. A. Smith, *Journal of Biomechanical Engineering* **115**, 468 (1993).
5. W. R. Walsh, *Repair and Regeneration of Ligaments, Tendons, and Joint Capsule* (Humana Press, Totowa, NJ, 2006).
6. A. P. Rumian, A. L. Wallace, and H. L. Birch, *Journal of Orthopaedic Research* **25**, 458 (2007).
7. D. E. Birk, and R. L. Trelstad, *Journal of Cell Biology* **103**, 231 (1986).
8. B. R. Olsen, in *Cell Biology of Extracellular Matrix*, edited by E. D. Hay (Plenum, New York, 1991), p. 177.
9. C. B. Frank, *Journal of Musculoskeletal and Neuronal Interactions* **4**, 199 (2004).
10. D. W. Hukins, M. C. Kirby, T. A. Sikoryn, R. M. Aspden, and A. J. Cox, *Spine* **15**, 787 (1990).
11. M. C. Kirby, T. A. Sikoryn, D. W. L. Hukins, and R. M. Aspden, *Journal of Biomedical Engineering* **11**, 192 (1989).
12. A. A. Aims, in *Sciences Basic to Orthopaedics*, edited by S. Hughes, and I. D. McCarthy (Saunders, London, 1998), p. 232.
13. S. Arms, J. Boyle, R. Johnson, and M. Pope, *Journal of Biomechanics* **16**, 491 (1983).
14. A. L. Nachemson, and J. H. Evans, *Journal of Biomechanics* **1**, 211 (1968).
15. F. A. Pintar, N. Yoganandan, T. Myers, A. Elhagediab, and A. Sances, *Journal of Biomechanics* **25**, 1351 (1992).
16. M. M. Panjabi, V. K. Goel, and K. Takata, *Spine* **7**, 192 (1982).
17. P. C. Ivancic, M. P. Coe, A. B. Ndu, Y. Tominaga, E. J. Carlson, W. Rubin, F. H. Dipl-Ing, and M. M. Panjabi, *The Spine Journal* **7**, 659 (2007).
18. Y. C. Fung, *American Journal of Physiology* **213**, 1532 (1967).
19. Y. C. Fung, *Biomechanics: Mechanical Properties of Living Tissues* (Springer-Verlag, New York, 1993).
20. A. Viidik, *Anatomy and Embryology* **136**, 204 (1972).
21. E. Mosler, W. Folkhard, E. Knorzer, H. Nemetschekgansler, T. Nemetschek, and M. H. J. Koch, *Journal of Molecular Biology* **182**, 589 (1985).
22. P. Ciarletta, S. Micera, D. Accoto, and P. Dario, *Journal of Biomechanics* **39**, 2034 (2006).
23. R. Puxkandl, I. Zizak, O. Paris, J. Keckes, W. Tesch, S. Bernstorff, P. Purslow, and P. Fratzl, *Philosophical Transactions of the Royal Society of London Series B-Biological Sciences* **357**, 191 (2002).
24. T. J. Lujan, C. J. Underwood, N. T. Jacobs, and J. A. Weiss, *Journal of Applied Physiology* **106**, 423 (2009).
25. H. B. Henninger, C. J. Underwood, G. A. Ateshian, and J. A. Weiss, *Journal of Biomechanics* **43**, 2567 (2010).
26. J. Hewitt, F. Guilak, R. Glisson, and T. P. Vail, *Journal of Orthopaedic Research* **19**, 359 (2001).
27. H. A. Lynch, W. Johannessen, J. P. Wu, A. Jawa, and D. M. Elliott, *Journal of Biomechanical Engineering* **125**, 726 (2003).
28. L. H. Yin, and D. M. Elliott, *Journal of Biomechanics* **37**, 907 (2004).
29. D. C. Taylor, J. D. Dalton, A. V. Seaber, and W. E. Garrett, *American Journal of Sports Medicine* **18**, 300 (1990).

30. R. M. Christensen, *Transactions of the Society of Rheology* **16**, 603 (1972).
31. R. S. Lakes, *Viscoelastic Solids* (CRC Press, Boca Raton, FL, 1999).
32. J. S. Little, and P. S. Khalsa, *Journal of Biomechanical Engineering* **127**, 15 (2005).
33. W. N. Findley, J. S. Lai, and K. Onaran, *Creep and Relaxation of Nonlinear Viscoelastic Materials, with an Introduction to Linear Viscoelasticity* (Elsevier/North Holland, Amsterdam, 1976).
34. Y. C. Fung, in *Biomechanics: Its Foundations and Objectives*, edited by Y. C. Fung, N. Perrone, and M. Anliker (Prentice-Hall, Englewood Cliffs, NJ, 1972), p. 181.
35. J. R. Funk, G. W. Hall, J. R. Crandall, and W. D. Pilkey, *Journal of Biomechanical Engineering* **122**, 15 (2000).
36. M. K. Kwan, T. H. Lin, and S. L. Woo, *Journal of Biomechanics* **26**, 447 (1993).
37. S. R. Lucas, C. R. Bass, R. S. Salzar, M. L. Oyen, C. Planchak, A. Ziemba, B. S. Shender, and G. Paskoff, *Acta Biomaterialia* **4**, 117 (2008).
38. S. L. Woo, M. A. Gomez, and W. H. Akeson, *Journal of Biomechanical Engineering* **103**, 293 (1981).
39. S. L. Woo, B. R. Simon, S. C. Kuei, and W. H. Akeson, *Journal of Biomechanical Engineering* **102**, 85 (1980).
40. S. R. Toms, G. J. Dakin, J. E. Lemons, and A. W. Eberhardt, *Journal of Biomechanics* **35**, 1411 (2002).
41. D. M. Elliott, P. S. Robinson, J. A. Gimbel, J. J. Sarver, J. A. Abboud, R. V. Iozzo, and L. J. Soslowsky, *Annals of Biomedical Engineering* **31**, 599 (2003).
42. G. A. Johnson, D. M. Tramaglini, R. E. Levine, K. Ohno, N. Y. Choi, and S. L. Y. Woo, *Journal of Orthopaedic Research* **12**, 796 (1994).
43. J. C. Iatridis, L. A. Setton, M. Weidenbaum, and V. C. Mow, *Journal of Biomechanics* **30**, 1005 (1997).
44. S. D. Abramowitch, S. L. Y. Woo, T. D. Clineff, and R. E. Debski, *Annals of Biomedical Engineering* **32**, 329 (2004).
45. S. E. Duenwald, R. Vanderby, Jr., and R. S. Lakes, *Annals of Biomedical Engineering* **37**, 1131 (2009).
46. R. V. Hingorani, P. P. Provenzano, R. S. Lakes, A. Escarcega, and R. Vanderby, Jr., *Annals of Biomedical Engineering* **32**, 306 (2004).
47. P. Provenzano, R. Lakes, T. Keenan, and R. Vanderby, Jr., *Annals of Biomedical Engineering* **29**, 908 (2001).
48. K. L. Troyer, and C. M. Puttlitz, *Acta Biomaterialia* **7**, 700 (2011).
49. S. Ambrosetti-Giudici, P. Gedet, S. J. Ferguson, S. Chegini, and J. Burger, *Clinical Biomechanics* **25**, 97 (2010).
50. G. M. Thornton, A. Oliynyk, C. B. Frank, and N. G. Shrive, *Journal of Orthopaedic Research* **15**, 652 (1997).
51. S. R. Lucas, C. R. Bass, J. R. Crandall, R. W. Kent, F. H. Shen, and R. S. Salzar, *Biomechanics and Modeling in Mechanobiology* **8**, 487 (2009).
52. K. L. Troyer, D. J. Estep, and C. M. Puttlitz, *Acta Biomaterialia* **8**, 234 (2012).
53. B. S. Myers, J. H. McElhaney, and B. J. Doherty, *Journal of Biomechanics* **24**, 811 (1991).
54. I. Nigul, and U. Nigul, *Journal of Biomechanics* **20**, 343 (1987).
55. S. D. Abramowitch, and S. L. Woo, *Journal of Biomechanical Engineering* **126**, 92 (2004).
56. S. D. Abramowitch, X. Zhang, M. Curran, and R. Kilger, *Clinical Biomechanics* **25**, 325 (2010).
57. M. Kohandel, S. Sivaloganathan, and G. Tenti, *Mathematical and Computer Modelling* **47**, 266 (2008).
58. R. D. Mirani, J. Pratt, P. Iyer, and S. V. Madihally, *Biomaterials* **30**, 703 (2009).
59. S. L. Y. Woo, S. D. Abramowitch, R. Kilger, and R. Liang, *Journal of Biomechanics* **39**, 1 (2006).
60. F. Xu, K. Seffen, and T. J. Lu, Theoretical and experimental aspects of continuum mechanics, in *Proceedings of the 3rd IASME/WSEAS International Conference on Continuum Mechanics*, 14 (2008).
61. K. M. Pryse, A. Nekouzadeh, G. M. Genin, E. L. Elson, and G. I. Zahalak, *Annals of Biomedical Engineering* **31**, 1287 (2003).
62. L. O. Nordin, and J. Varna, *Mechanics of Time-Dependent Materials* **9**, 259 (2005).
63. J. Sorvari, M. Malinen, and J. Hamalainen, *International Journal of Non-Linear Mechanics* **41**, 1050 (2006).
64. P. P. Provenzano, R. S. Lakes, D. T. Corr, and R. Vanderby, Jr., *Biomechanics and Modeling in Mechanobiology* **1**, 45 (2002).
65. S. E. Duenwald, R. Vanderby, and R. S. Lakes, *Acta Mechanica* **205**, 23 (2009).

66. J. A. Gimbel, J. J. Sarver, and L. J. Soslowsky, *Journal of Biomechanical Engineering* **126**, 844 (2004).
67. P. Neumann, T. S. Keller, L. Ekstrom, and T. Hansson, *Spine (Phila Pa 1976)* **19**, 205 (1994).
68. N. Yoganandan, F. Pintar, J. Butler, J. Reinartz, A. Sances, Jr., and S. J. Larson, *Spine (Phila Pa 1976)* **14**, 1102 (1989).
69. A. A. White, and M. M. Panjabi, *Clinical Biomechanics of the Spine* (Lippincott, Philadelphia, 1990).
70. W. Yang, T. C. Fung, K. S. Chian, and C. K. Chong, *Journal of Biomechanical Engineering* **128**, 909 (2006).
71. S. Turner, in *The Physics of Glassy Polymers*, edited by R. N. Haward (Wiley, New York, 1973), p. 238.
72. C. R. Bass, S. R. Lucas, R. S. Salzar, M. L. Oyen, C. Planchak, B. S. Shender, and G. Paskoff, *Spine (Phila Pa 1976)* **32**, E7 (2007).
73. V. K. Goel, and J. D. Clausen, *Spine* **23**, 684 (1998).
74. L. Ott, and M. Longnecker, *An Introduction to Statistical Methods and Data Analysis* (Duxbury, Pacific Grove, CA, 2001).
75. K. L. Troyer, S. S. Shetye, and C. M. Puttlitz, *Journal of Biomechanical Engineering* **134** (2012).
76. D. L. Butler, E. S. Grood, F. R. Noyes, R. F. Zernicke, and K. Brackett, *Journal of Biomechanics* **17**, 579 (1984).
77. S. S. Shetye, K. Malhotra, S. D. Ryan, and C. M. Puttlitz, *American Journal of Veterinary Research* **70**, 1026 (2009).
78. M. J. Gibbons, D. L. Butler, E. S. Grood, D. I. Bylskiaustrow, M. S. Levy, and F. R. Noyes, *Journal of Orthopaedic Research* **9**, 209 (1991).
79. K. C. McGilvray, B. G. Santoni, A. S. Turner, S. Bogdansky, D. L. Wheeler, and C. M. Puttlitz, *Cell Tissue Bank* **12**, 89 (2011).
80. R. S. Lakes, and R. Vanderby, *Journal of Biomechanical Engineering* **121**, 612 (1999).
81. A. Oza, R. Vanderby, and R. S. Lakes, *Rheologica Acta* **42**, 557 (2003).
82. K. L. Troyer, and C. M. Puttlitz, *Journal of Biomechanics* **45**, 684 (2012).
83. ABAQUS, *Abaqus Analysis User's Manual (Version 6.9)* (Dassault Systèmes Simulia Corp., Providence, RI, 2009).
84. M. A. Puso, and J. A. Weiss, *Journal of Biomechanical Engineering* **120**, 62 (1998).
85. K. Brolin, and P. Halldin, *Spine* **29**, 376 (2004).
86. W. Womack, P. D. Leahy, V. V. Patel, and C. M. Puttlitz, *Spine (Phila Pa 1976)* **36**, E1126 (2011).
87. A. Rohlmann, N. K. Burra, T. Zander, and G. Bergmann, *European Spine Journal* **16**, 1223 (2007).
88. U. M. Ayturk, and C. M. Puttlitz, *Computer Methods in Biomechanics and Biomedical Engineering* **14**, 695 (2011).
89. J. Y. Bae, K. S. Park, J. K. Seon, D. S. Kwak, I. Jeon, and E. K. Song, *Medical and Biological Engineering and Computing* **50**, 53 (2012).
90. M. A. Baldwin, C. W. Clary, C. K. Fitzpatrick, J. S. Deacy, L. P. Maletsky, and P. J. Rullkoetter, *Journal of Biomechanics* **45**, 474 (2012).
91. P. H. Eichenseer, D. R. Sybert, and J. R. Cotton, *Spine* **36**, E1446 (2011).
92. A. T. M. Phillips, P. Pankaj, C. R. Howie, A. S. Usmani, and A. H. R. W. Simpson, *Medical Engineering and Physics* **29**, 739 (2007).
93. Z. A. Taylor, O. Comas, M. Cheng, J. Passenger, D. J. Hawkes, D. Atkinson, and S. Ourselin, *Medical Image Analysis* **13**, 234 (2009).
94. G. A. Johnson, G. A. Livesay, S. L. Y. Woo, and K. R. Rajagopal, *Journal of Biomechanical Engineering* **118**, 221 (1996).
95. K. R. Rajagopal, and A. S. Wineman, *Mathematics and Mechanics of Solids* **14**, 490 (2009).
96. J.-P. Boehler, *Applications of Tensor Functions in Solid Mechanics* (Springer-Verlag, Wien; New York, 1987).
97. X. G. Ning, Q. L. Zhu, Y. Lanir, and S. S. Margulies, *Journal of Biomechanical Engineering* **128**, 925 (2006).
98. S. E. Duenwald, R. Vanderby, and R. S. Lakes, *Biorheology* **47**, 1 (2010).
99. R. A. Schapery, *Polymer Engineering and Science* **9**, 295 (1969).

6

Physical Signals and Solute Transport in Human Intervertebral Disc: Multiphasic Mechano-Electrochemical Finite Element Analysis

Yongren Wu, Sarah E. Cisewski, and Hai Yao

CONTENTS

ABSTRACT A three-dimensional inhomogeneous finite element model for charged hydrated soft tissues containing charged/uncharged solutes was developed based on the triphasic theory. It was applied to analyze the mechanical, chemical, and electrical signals within the human intervertebral disc (IVD) during axial unconfined compression and physiological loading conditions. The human IVD was modeled as an inhomogeneous mixture consisting of a charged elastic solid, water, ions (Na^+ and Cl^-), and nutrient solute (oxygen, glucose, and lactate) phases. The effects of tissue properties and boundary conditions on the physical signals and the transport of fluid and solute were investigated. In addition, the effects of the endplate calcification and cell injection were simulated by a reduction of the tissue porosity and increasing the cell density. The numerical simulation showed that, during disc compression, the fluid pressurization and the effective (von Mises) solid stress were more pronounced in the annulus fibrosus (AF) region near the interface between the AF and nucleus pulposus (NP). The electrical signals were very sensitive to fixed charge density. Changes in material properties of the NP (water content, fixed charge density, and modulus) affected fluid pressure, electrical potential, effective stress, and solute transport in the disc. The physiological diurnal cyclic loading did not significantly change the nutrient environment in the human IVD during the day and night. Calcification of the cartilage endplate significantly reduced the nutrient levels in the human IVD. In cell-based therapies for IVD regeneration, excessive amounts of injected cells may cause further deterioration of the nutrient environment in the degenerated disc. This study is important for understanding the disc biomechanics and pathology of IVD degeneration and providing new insights into cell-based therapies for low back pain.

6.1 Introduction

Cartilaginous tissues, such as articular cartilage and the intervertebral disc (IVD), are avascular charged hydrated soft tissues [1–3]. The extracellular matrix (ECM) of cartilaginous tissues consists of a fibrous (collagen–proteoglycan [PG]) network, abundant interstitial water (~80%), and ions (mainly Na^+ and Cl^-) (Figure 6.1). The charged nature of the ECM derives from the charged groups (SO_3^- and COO^-) on the glycosaminoglycan (GAG) chains of PGs [1–5]. These charges are considered as *fixed* in the ECM and attract opposite ions (i.e., counter ions) in the interstitial fluid to maintain a tissue electroneutral state at a macroscopic level. Electrostatic interactions (at a microscopic level) between immobile, fixed charges (on the solid matrix) and mobile free ions (in the interstitial fluid) give rise to physicochemical and electrokinetic effects at a macroscopic level, such as Donnan osmotic pressure, swelling, streaming potential and current, negative osmosis, and electroosmosis effects [1–3]. The cell population in cartilaginous tissues is sparse and accounts for less than 10% of the tissue volume in adult articular cartilage and the IVD [6–8]. Because of the avascular nature of the tissue, the embedded cells survive on nutrient transport through the dense ECM by fluid flow (convection) and diffusion.

6.1.1 Physical Signals and Mechanobiology

The surrounding cell environment is complicated, including mechanical, chemical, and electrical signals. During the past two decades, increasing attention has been focused on

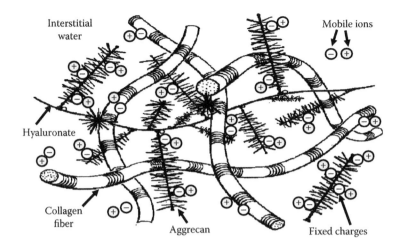

FIGURE 6.1
A schematic diagram of the structure of the charged hydrate ECM of cartilaginous tissues that consists of three major phases: a charged solid phase largely composed of collagen and PG aggregates, a fluid phase primarily composed of water with dissolved solutes, and an ion phase that is required to neutralize the charges fixed to the solid matrix.

the biological responses of cartilaginous tissues to mechanical forces and other physical stimuli to understand cellular mechanotransduction mechanisms. Figure 6.2 illustrates how the mechanical forces at the tissue level affect the physical signals at the cellular level. Thus, tissue remodeling (growth or degeneration) alters the physical signals through changes in the ECM material properties [9,10]. As pointed out by Grodzinsky et al. [11], "these physical stimuli and the resulting cellular responses should be studied at the molecular, cellular and tissue levels for fully understanding the feedback between applied macroscopic forces, ECM molecular structure, and the resulting macrocontinuum tissue material properties—a feedback process that is orchestrated by cells in vivo."

The quantitative determination of physical signals within the tissue is important for designing a strategy for either tissue regeneration (e.g., tissue engineering) or impeding tissue degeneration (e.g., osteoarthritis and disc degeneration). The physical signals are complex, composed of mechano-electrochemical events within the ECM (stress, strain, ion concentrations, fluid pressure, electrical potential, and flow of water, ions, and nutrient solutes). The physical signals may be quantified by appropriate, theoretical models with realistic material properties [12,13]. The development and assessment of these kinds of models will be described in this chapter.

6.1.2 Solute Transport and Nutrition

Transport of fluid and solutes through the matrix as well as other physical signals play a key role in tissue nutrition and tissue growth for avascular tissues. This is particularly important for the IVD because it is the largest avascular structure in the human body. The nutrients that disc cells require for maintaining disc health are supplied by blood vessels at the margins of the disc. Poor nutritional supply to the disc cells is believed to be one of the mechanisms for disc degeneration [14–18], which has been implicated as a possible primary etiological factor in the pathophysiology of low back pain [19–26].

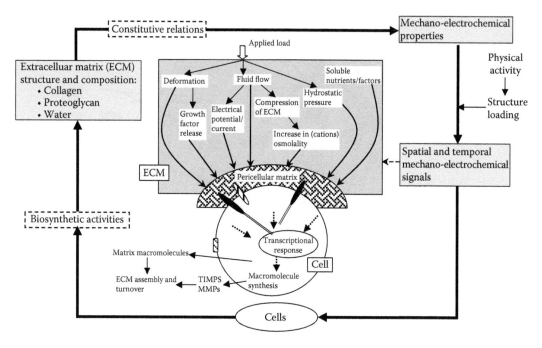

FIGURE 6.2
Illustration of the interrelationships between ECM composition and structure, mechano-electrochemical signals, and chondrocyte biosynthetic activities in cartilage. (Adapted from Mow, V.C. et al., *Osteoarthritis Cartilage* 7(1):41–58, 1999. With permission.)

Nutrition also plays an essential role in tissue engineering applications. During tissue growth in a bioreactor, the transport properties of the tissue or cell–matrix construct change, thus altering the transport rates of fluid and solutes within the tissue. As a result, constitutive relations for transport properties need to be developed in order to predict the changes in hydraulic permeability or solute diffusivity as the ECM composition changes. With these constitutive relations for transport properties, we would be able to quantitatively predict the physical signals (see Figure 6.2) and nutrient levels surrounding the cells during tissue growth or degeneration (e.g., osteoarthritis and disc degeneration).

6.2 General Background

This chapter focuses on the human IVD, which provides strength and flexibility to the spine. The broad, long-term research objectives are to (1) elucidate the etiology of disc degeneration, (2) develop strategies either for restoring tissue function or for retarding further disc degeneration, and (3) develop novel, less-invasive diagnostic tools for disc degeneration.

6.2.1 Composition, Structure, and Charged Nature of IVD

The IVD is composed of three major components: annulus fibrosus (AF), nucleus pulposus (NP), and cartilage endplate (CEP) (Figure 6.3a). The biochemical composition and

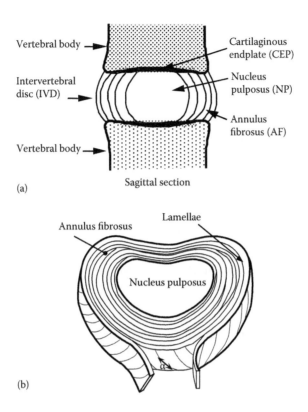

FIGURE 6.3
(a) Schematic view of a sagittal cross section of the motion segment composed of vertebral bodies and an IVD. (b) Schematic of the IVD's laminate structure of the AF. Part of the annulus is removed to show the lamina structure.

structure of each component are quite distinct [27,28], suggesting that each component may have a unique mechanical role. The NP is composed of randomly oriented collagen fibrils enmeshed in a mucoprotein gel. It is surrounded on its periphery by the AF, and superiorly and inferiorly by CEPs. For the nondegenerate lumbar spine, the AF is formed by a series of concentric encircling lamellae that are free from macroscopic ruptures. The lamellae consist of collagen fibers that run in the same direction within each lamella but opposite to those in adjacent lamellae, at approximately ±30° to the horizontal axis (Figure 6.3b) [29,30]. Because of this layered structure, the mechanical properties of the AF are anisotropic [31–34]. The CEP is a thin layer of hyaline cartilage surrounding the cranial and caudal surfaces of the central regions of the disc. The disc is composed mostly of water (65%–90% wet weight) with significant quantities of collagen (15%–65% dry weight), PG (10%–60% dry weight), and other matrix proteins (15%–45% dry weight) [20,35–40]. Differences in biochemical composition and structure distinguish the different regions of the disc. Significant variations in the composition of the disc from outer regions to inner regions have been reported, with water and PG contents being greatest in the NP and inner AF, while collagen content is greatest in the outer AF. Thus, from an engineer's point of view, the IVD can be well characterized as an inhomogeneous, anisotropic, multiphasic material.

The negatively charged nature of the IVD tissue arises from the carboxyl and sulfate groups of the GAGs in the disc, including chondroitin-6-sulfate, chondroitin-4-sulfate, keratan sulfate, biglycan, decorin, versican, and hyaluronan [20,27,28,36,41–47]. These GAGs will attach to a protein core to form an aggrecan molecule, which may further form large macromolecular aggregates with hyaluronan in the disc. The negative charges are considered as *fixed* in the ECM because aggrecans are entangled with the collagen network and restrained within the solid matrix. Electrostatic interactions between immobile, fixed charges (on the solid matrix) and mobile free ions (in the interstitial fluid) give rise to physicochemical and electrokinetic effects [38,48–61]. Thus, the transport of fluid and solutes in the IVD depends upon physicochemical factors, such as water content, fixed charge density (FCD), and the type and concentration of the bathing solutions [57,59,61–64]. In order to quantify the transport behavior of the human IVD, these physicochemical factors need to be included in the theoretical model.

6.2.2 Clinical Relevance and Significance

Back pain is a major public health problem in the United States [65], causing suffering and distress to patients and their families. More than 70% of all people have back pain at some time in their life, with an annual prevalence ranging from 15% to 45%. Back pain is the most frequent cause of activity limitation in people below 45 years of age and is a common reason for visiting a health care provider [22,23,65–67]. As a result, the diagnosis and treatment of back pain place an enormous economic burden on society. Back pain is strongly associated with the degeneration of IVDs [19–26,66,67]. Disc degeneration, although in many cases asymptomatic, may be associated with sciatica and disc herniation, or prolapse. It decreases IVD height and abnormally loads the surrounding muscles and ligaments, therefore altering the mechanics of the rest of the spinal column. In the long term, disc degeneration can lead to spinal stenosis, which is a major cause of pain and disability in the elderly.

Degeneration occurs in the IVD far earlier than in any other musculoskeletal tissues [68,69]. Approximately 20% of people in their teens have IVDs with mild signs of degeneration [69]. With disc degeneration, changes in disc morphology, biochemistry, function, and material properties occur. The most significant biochemical change seen in the degenerate disc is loss of PG [43]. The changes in collagen with disc degeneration are not as obvious as those associated with PGs [70]. The loss of PG is believed to be responsible for the decrease in osmotic pressure and tissue hydration [61], resulting in loss of load-support capability of the disc [71]. It also affects the movement of molecules into and out of the disc [7].

The disc is the largest avascular structure in the human body. The cells depend on blood vessels at the tissue margins to supply nutrients and remove metabolic waste [72–74]. The nutrients have to travel through the CEP layer to reach the disc ECM, which may be as far as 8 mm from the capillary bed in the surrounding vertebral bodies. One of the primary causes of disc degeneration is thought to be the failure of the nutrient supply to the disc cells [14–18]. It is believed that the endplate route is the main pathway for nutritional supply to the disc cells [75,76]. Because of aging and other pathological conditions, the CEP may calcify, which reduces PG and water content, thus changing the transport properties (e.g., hydraulic permeability and solute diffusivities) of the endplate [77,78]. Convection and diffusion through the calcified endplate is likely to be hindered, thus decreasing the nutritional supply to the disc [75,79]. Therefore, under physiological loading conditions, the calcification of the CEP may significantly affect the nutrient concentrations within the disc. However, to our knowledge, the effect of CEP calcification on nutrient transport (diffusion and convection) inside the human IVD has not been fully elucidated under physiological loading conditions (i.e., day–night cyclic loading).

Recently, the injection of IVD cells/stem cells into the NP region has been proposed for IVD regeneration in cell-based therapies for low back pain treatment [80–82]. The success of this therapeutic approach first depends on the viability after the injection. Usually, the nutrient transport in degenerated discs is hindered by the calcified endplate. The increased nutrient demand owing to the increase in cell density may further deteriorate the nutrient environment in the degenerate disc. Without restoring the nutrient environment, this procedure may accelerate the process of degeneration [81]. However, the impact of a cell injection coupled with already present degeneration on the nutrient environment of the disc has not been determined.

6.2.3 The Current State of Knowledge in the Field

The focus of this chapter is on the development of the mechano-electrochemical finite element model (FEM) as well as the recent advances involving the incorporation of strain-dependent constitutive relations of the transport properties (i.e., hydraulic permeability and solute diffusivity) for IVD tissues.

6.2.3.1 Continuum Porous Media Theory in Soft Tissue Mechanics

Significant progress in the macroscopic porous media theory has been made over the past decades (see review paper by de Boer [83]). Many studies concerning the fundamentals of the theory and development of mathematical models in the field of biomechanics have been published [12,49,50,56,58,83–90]. One of them is the biphasic theory for cartilage developed by Mow et al., which consider tissue as a mixture of water phase and solid phase [90]. This theory has been widely used for the investigation of biomechanical and fluid transport behaviors of hydrated soft tissues such as articular cartilage and hydrogels. It has also been extended to account for the viscoelastic solid and tension–compression nonlinearity behaviors of cartilaginous tissues [91–94].

In 1991, Lai et al. [58] developed a triphasic mechano-electrochemical theory for describing swelling and deformational behaviors of charged hydrated soft tissues based on a tertiary-mixture theory and the laws of thermodynamics [95,96]. This theory treats the fixed charges as being attached to the solid phase. This triphasic formulation represents the natural progression of constitutive modeling of charged hydrated soft tissues from the biphasic formulation [90]. In the triphasic theory, a charged hydrated tissue is modeled as a mixture consisting of three distinct phases (i.e., solid, water, and ion phases). The driving forces are the gradient of (electro)chemical potentials of each phase. This theory has been successfully used to study the swelling, negative osmosis and osmotic pressure, transport of fluid and ions, and electrokinetic phenomena in charged hydrated tissues [53,55,97–106]. Note that a similar theory was also developed by Huyghe and Janssen [87,88]. Microcontinuum models for charged hydrated soft tissues were also developed [84,86,107]. Contributions to the mechanical behavior of the fluid flow and electrokinetic coupling in bones have also been published [108–110].

In 1998, Gu et al. [56] extended the triphasic mixture theory to describe the swelling and passive transport of multi-electrolytes through charged hydrated soft tissues (such as cartilage and IVD tissues) and cell membranes. The general constitutive laws for an inhomogeneous, anisotropic solid phase, interstitial fluid phase, and an ion phase were also obtained. It was demonstrated that this theory could be used to predict not only the swelling behavior of charged tissues but also the electrical response of the cell under mechanical loading [98,111]. Thus, this comprehensive theory could provide a foundation for understanding mechanical and electrochemical behaviors of charged hydrated tissues. In this chapter, the triphasic mixture theory is used as a theoretical framework for the numerical simulation.

6.2.3.2 Numerical Analyses Using the Finite Element Method

Because of the unique composition and structure of the materials, the complexity of the mechano-electrochemical coupling phenomena as well as the difficulty in measuring the in vivo biomechanical response, transport of solutes, and cellular activities in the human IVD, numerical simulation using FEMs became an essential tool to help understand the biomechanical and nutrient environment in the IVD. Numerous works have been done to study the biomechanical behavior of spinal motion segments as well as isolated IVD samples [112–127]. Most FEM analyses for spinal motion segments were based on the model in which the NP was assumed to be an incompressible fluid and the AF was a linear or nonlinear, elastic or viscoelastic, and single-phase or composite material. Simon et al. and Laible et al. used the poroelastic (biphasic) theory for their finite element analysis of a spinal motion segment, which included fluid transport and swelling effects [116,122,123]. A two-dimensional (2D) poroelastic axisymmetric FEM was also presented by Whyne et al. recently [128]. The influence of load-induced fluid flow on solute transport within the IVD was investigated by Ferguson et al. using poroelastic FEM [129]. However, none of those models considered the charged nature of the IVD or coupled the solute transport with the fluid flow and thus lack the power to provide the comprehensive picture of the mechano-electrochemical environment within the disc under mechanical loading conditions.

The triphasic theory developed by Lai et al. provides a link between mechanical and electrochemical theories. However, because of the nonlinearity of the comprehensive, triphasic theory [56,58,87,88], it is almost impossible to find an analytic solution to most boundary-value problems. In order to investigate tissue behavior under various loading conditions, Sun et al. [105,130] and Yao and Gu [131] developed a triphasic finite element formulation. In this formulation, the solid displacement and (electro)chemical potentials of water and ions were chosen as the primary degrees of freedom. This finite element formulation has been used to investigate a one-dimensional stress relaxation problem [105,130] and a 2D dynamic unconfined compression problem [131]. A similar model, developed by Iatridis et al., was also applied to an IVD slice in a 2D plane stress problem [132].

In this chapter, three-dimensional (3D) mechano-electrochemical FEMs for IVD tissues were developed based on the specialized triphasic theory, which includes nutrient solute (uncharged) phases. These models were used to analyze the mechano-electrochemical signals and nutrient solute transport within the IVD tissue under various mechanical loading conditions. Effects of CEP calcification and the injection of IVD cells in cell-based therapy for IVD regeneration were also investigated.

6.2.3.3 Constitutive Modeling of Transport Properties in Fibrous Porous Media

Transport of water and solutes (including ions) in tissue is mainly governed by transport properties such as hydraulic permeability (or conductivity) and solute diffusivity [56,58]. Many constitutive models, based on the microcontinuum model, have been developed for predicting the hydraulic permeability of uncharged fibrous porous [133–138]. Models for charged fibrous porous media (such as cartilage ECM) were also developed by Eisenberg and Grodzinsky [86] and Chammas et al. [107] using a unit cell approach [135]. Note that for uncharged fibrous porous media, such as agarose gel, Eisenberg et al.'s models [86,107] for permeability are consistent with the model by Happel [135]. Recently, Gu and Yao developed a theoretical model based on experimental data that satisfactorily describe the constitutive relationship between intrinsic permeability and matrix composition in cartilaginous tissues [139,140].

Many constitutive models have also been developed for predicting solute diffusivity in fibrous porous media, including those based on steric effects [141,142], hydrodynamic effects (i.e., the effective medium/Brinkman model) [143,144], and the models based on both steric and hydrodynamic effects [145–147]. In the effective medium/Brinkman model, the structural information of the tissue is embedded in the Darcy permeability (κ). Experimental studies show that the major factors governing diffusion coefficients in cartilaginous tissues are solute size and pore size of tissue [148], which are related to tissue hydration and structure [7]. Recently, Yao and Gu developed a constitutive relation that is capable of satisfactorily describing the strain-dependent diffusion behavior of solutes in gels or biological soft tissues [149]. These unique constitutive relations of permeability and diffusivity developed by Yao and Gu were incorporated into the theoretical framework of finite element simulation described in this chapter.

6.3 A Specialized Triphasic Formulation for Charged Hydrated Soft Tissue

In models of the mechanical behavior of hydrated soft tissues, the most commonly used theory is that of mixtures (see the review in Section 6.2.3.1). The mixture theory views the tissue as a mixture of continuum materials. The mixture is regarded as a superposition of its constituents, each occupying the total mixture volume. The behavior of the mixture is the result of the behavior of the distinct constituents and the interaction between them. The theory of deforming porous media was originally developed by Biot [150]. Later, the modern mixture theory was derived from Biot's theory by Truesdell and Bowen [151].

The biphasic theory developed by Mow et al. [90], which considers the tissue as a mixture of solid and fluid phases, was the first mixture model for cartilage. This theory has been successfully employed to investigate biomechanical and fluid transport behaviors of hydrated soft tissues, such as articular cartilage and hydrogels. Further development by Lai et al. led to the triphasic mechano-electrochemical theory for describing swelling and deformational behaviors of charged hydrated soft tissues [58], which accounts for osmotic swelling by means of the third component (i.e., ion component). In this theory, a charged hydrated tissue is modeled as a mixture consisting of three distinct phases: (1) a charged solid phase (collagen–PG matrix), (2) a fluid phase (interstitial water), and (3) an ion phase with two species (cation and anion). This theory treats the fixed charges as being attached to the solid phase while all three phases are considered explicitly as integral parts of the tissue. The formulation of the triphasic theory is based on a tertiary-mixture theory and the laws of thermodynamics [95] and represents the natural progression of constitutive modeling of charged hydrated soft tissues from the biphasic formulation [90]. This theory has been successfully used to study the swelling, negative osmosis and osmotic pressure, transport of fluid and ions, and electrokinetic phenomena in charged hydrated tissues [53,55,97–106]. Furthermore, Gu et al. [56] extended the triphasic mixture theory to describe the swelling and passive transport of multi-electrolytes with polyvalence through charged hydrated soft tissues and cell membranes.

Nutrient transport plays a key role in maintaining tissue health for avascular tissues (e.g., IVD). The most basic nutrients, such as oxygen and glucose, are uncharged solutes contained in the interstitial fluid. In order to determine the nutrient level as well as physical signals within the cartilaginous tissues under different loading conditions, it is essential to have a theoretical model to take into consideration the uncharged solute. Therefore, a specialized triphasic model for charged hydrated soft tissues containing uncharged solutes was presented in this section.

6.3.1 Governing Equations

The formulation introduced in this section may be considered as a specific form of the more general triphasic theory under infinitesimal deformation [56,58]. The charged tissue is modeled as a mixture of four phases including the incompressible solid phase with fixed charges, interstitial water phase, ion phase with two monovalent species (e.g., Na^+ and Cl^-), and uncharged solute phase. In this formulation, the solid displacement and (electro) chemical potentials of water and ions were chosen as the basic continuous degrees of freedom [105]. This formulation has the advantage that jump conditions across the interface boundaries are satisfied automatically, which is convenient for the investigation of the mechano-electrochemical behavior of charged hydrated soft tissues with discontinuous material properties.

The balance of linear momentum for the mixture and the conservation of mass for each of the phases or species led to the following governing equations [56,58,105]:

$$\nabla \cdot \boldsymbol{\sigma} = 0, \tag{6.1}$$

$$\nabla \cdot (\mathbf{v}^s + \mathbf{J}^w) = 0, \tag{6.2}$$

$$\partial(\phi^w c^+)/\partial t + \nabla \cdot (\mathbf{J}^+ + \phi^w c^+ \mathbf{v}^s) = 0, \tag{6.3}$$

$$\partial(\phi^w c^-)/\partial t + \nabla \cdot (\mathbf{J}^- + \phi^w c^- \mathbf{v}^s) = 0, \tag{6.4}$$

$$\partial(\phi^w c^o)/\partial t + \nabla \cdot (\mathbf{J}^o + \phi^w c^o \mathbf{v}^s) = 0, \tag{6.5}$$

where ϕ^w is tissue porosity defined as a ratio of water volume to total tissue volume. The total stress tensor of the mixture $\boldsymbol{\sigma}$, the velocity of the solid phase $\mathbf{v}^s$, the fluxes relative to the solid phase $\mathbf{J}^\alpha$ (α = w, +, −, o), and concentrations (per unit water volume) c^α (α = +, −, o) were related to solid displacement $\mathbf{u}$, modified (electro)chemical potentials of water ε^w, cation ε^+, anion ε^-, and uncharged solute ε^o given by [105]

$$\mathbf{v}^s = \frac{\partial \mathbf{u}}{\partial t}, \tag{6.6}$$

$$\boldsymbol{\sigma} = -[RT\varepsilon^w + RT\phi(c^+ + c^- + c^o) - p_o] + (\lambda + B_w)\nabla \cdot \mathbf{u} + \mu[\nabla\mathbf{u} + (\nabla\mathbf{u})^T], \tag{6.7}$$

$$\mathbf{J}^w = -RTk\left(\nabla\varepsilon^w + \frac{c^+}{\varepsilon^+}\nabla\varepsilon^+ + \frac{c^-}{\varepsilon^-}\nabla\varepsilon^- + \frac{c^o}{\varepsilon^o}\nabla\varepsilon^o\right), \tag{6.8}$$

$$\mathbf{J}^+ = H^+ c^+ \mathbf{J}^w - \frac{\phi^w c^+ D^+}{\varepsilon^+} \nabla \varepsilon^+, \tag{6.9}$$

$$\mathbf{J}^- = H^- c^- \mathbf{J}^w - \frac{\phi^w c^- D^-}{\varepsilon^-} \nabla \varepsilon^-, \tag{6.10}$$

$$\mathbf{J}^o = H^o c^o \mathbf{J}^w - \frac{\phi^w c^o D^o}{\varepsilon^o} \nabla \varepsilon^o, \tag{6.11}$$

where R is the universal gas constant; T is the absolute temperature; ϕ is the osmotic coefficient; p_o is the prestress (see Equation 6.12); B_w is the interphase coupling coefficient; λ and μ are Lame coefficients of solid matrix; k is the intrinsic (i.e., closed-circuit) permeability; and D^+, D^-, and D^o are the intratissue diffusivities of cation, anion, and uncharged solute, respectively. The parameters H^α ($\alpha = +, -, o$) in Equations 6.9 through 6.11 are the convective coefficients since the convective velocity in a mixture is in general not equal to the water velocity. The value of the convective coefficients represents the hindrance factor of the solute for convection that incorporates hydrodynamic and steric interactions between solute and the matrix [152]. They are functions of the drag coefficients between a solute and other phases. Note that the mechanical interactions among solutes were assumed to be negligible.

The infinitesimal deformation assumption was considered when deriving Equations 6.6 and 6.7 [58,105]. The value of prestress (p_o) in Equation 6.7 depends on the choice of the reference configuration for strain. In this study, the free-swelling state of tissue equilibrated with the bathing (NaCl) solution of concentration c^* (no other uncharged solute) was chosen as the reference configuration for strain. Thus, the prestress (p_o) was given as

$$p_o = RT\left[\phi\left(c_o^+ + c_o^-\right) - 2\phi^* c^*\right] - B_w e_o, \tag{6.12}$$

where c_o^+ and c_o^- are the ion concentrations within the tissue at equilibrium (i.e., the initial ion concentrations) and e_o is the dilatation of tissue at equilibrium (relative to the hypertonic state). If one chooses the tissue configuration at the hypertonic state (load-free) as the reference configuration, then $p_o = 0$ and $e_o = 0$. In the following calculations, all strains were relative to the free-swelling state of tissue equilibrated with 0.15 M NaCl bathing solution [53].

In Equations 6.7 through 6.10, the modified (electro)chemical potentials (ε^w, ε^+, ε^-, ε^o) were related to fluid pressure (p), electrical potential (ψ), and solute concentrations (c^+, c^-, c^o) by [105]

$$\varepsilon^w = \frac{p}{RT} - \phi(c^+ + c^- + c^o) + \frac{B_w}{RT} e, \tag{6.13}$$

$$\varepsilon^+ = \gamma_+ c^+ \exp\left(\frac{F_c \psi}{RT}\right), \tag{6.14}$$

$$\varepsilon^- = \gamma_- c^- \exp\left(-\frac{F_c \psi}{RT}\right), \tag{6.15}$$

$$\varepsilon^o = \gamma_o c^o, \tag{6.16}$$

where e is the dilatation; F_c is the Faraday constant; and γ_+, γ_-, and γ_o are the activity coefficients of cation, anion, and uncharged solute, respectively. At equilibrium, the activity coefficient of the uncharged solute within the tissue (γ_o) was related to the partition coefficient (Φ) (i.e., the ratio of solute concentration in tissue to solute concentration in bathing solute at equilibrium) and the activity coefficient of the uncharged solute in bathing solution (γ_o^*) by

$$\gamma_o = \gamma_o^* / \Phi. \tag{6.17}$$

The ion concentrations were related to the value of the negative fixed charged density (c^F) through the electroneutrality condition in this model [58]:

$$c^+ = c^- + c^F, \tag{6.18}$$

where c^F is related to the tissue porosity, the reference FCD $\left(c_0^F\right)$ and reference porosity $\left(\phi_0^w\right)$ by

$$c^F = \frac{c_0^F(1-\phi^w)\phi_0^w}{(1-\phi_0^w)\phi^w}. \tag{6.19}$$

Since tissue porosity (ϕ^w) was related to tissue dilatation and the porosity at the reference configuration (i.e., at $e = 0$) [58]

$$\phi^w = \frac{\phi_0^w + e}{1+e}, \tag{6.20}$$

the FCD was strain dependent.

6.3.2 Boundary Conditions

To arrive at a unique solution, specific boundary conditions at the material surface are required. In this specialized triphasic formulation, the boundary conditions are the continuity of total stress and (electro)chemical potential for each component at the boundaries, or the solid displacement ($\mathbf{u}$) and the fluxes ($\mathbf{J}^\alpha$) of each component are continuous. It states that

$$\mathbf{u} = \mathbf{u}^*, \varepsilon^\alpha = \varepsilon^{\alpha*} \ (\alpha = w, +, -, o), \tag{6.21}$$

and

$$\boldsymbol{\sigma} \cdot \mathbf{n} = \mathbf{t}_{app}, \mathbf{J}^\alpha \cdot \mathbf{n} = \mathbf{J}^{\alpha*} \cdot \mathbf{n} \ (\alpha = w, +, -, o), \tag{6.22}$$

where $\mathbf{n}$ is the surface normal on the boundary, $\mathbf{t}_{app}$ is the traction, and * stands for the quantities in the bathing solution. Because of the continuity of the (electro)chemical potentials, the ion concentrations and fluid pressure are generally not continuous at the tissue–bath interface.

6.3.3 The Weak Formulation for the Finite Element Implementation

The mechanical, electrical, and chemical signals within the tissue under different loading conditions can be analyzed by solving Equations 6.1 through 6.5 with appropriate initial and boundary conditions using the finite element method. Using the standard Galerkin weight residual method [105], the finite element formulation was constructed. The weak formulation of the specialized triphasic theory (Equations 6.1 through 6.5) was given by

$$\int_\Omega \mathbf{w} \cdot \nabla \cdot \boldsymbol{\sigma} \, d\Omega = 0, \tag{6.23}$$

$$\int_\Omega w^{(1)} \left[\nabla \cdot (\mathbf{v}^s + \mathbf{J}^w) \right] d\Omega = 0, \tag{6.24}$$

$$\int_\Omega w^{(2)} \left[\partial(\phi^w c^+)/\partial t + \nabla \cdot (\mathbf{J}^+ + \phi^w c^+ \mathbf{v}^s) \right] d\Omega = 0, \tag{6.25}$$

$$\int_\Omega w^{(3)} \left[\partial(\phi^w c^-)/\partial t + \nabla \cdot (\mathbf{J}^- + \phi^w c^- \mathbf{v}^s) \right] d\Omega = 0, \tag{6.26}$$

$$\int_\Omega w^{(4)} \left[\partial(\phi^w c^\circ)/\partial t + \nabla \cdot (\mathbf{J}^\circ + \phi^w c^\circ \mathbf{v}^s) \right] d\Omega = 0, \tag{6.27}$$

where vector $\mathbf{w}$ and four scalar functions $w^{(1)}$, $w^{(2)}$, $w^{(3)}$, and $w^{(4)}$ are arbitrary admissible weighting functions for the five governing equations.

Applying the divergence theorem to Equations 6.23 through 6.27, one could obtain

$$\int_\Omega \mathrm{tr}[(\nabla \mathbf{w})^\mathsf{T} \cdot \boldsymbol{\sigma}] d\Omega = \int_{\Gamma_t} \mathbf{w} \cdot \mathbf{t}^* \, d\Gamma, \tag{6.28}$$

$$\int_\Omega w^{(1)} \nabla \cdot \mathbf{v}^s \, d\Omega + \int_\Omega \mathbf{J}^w \cdot \nabla w^{(1)} \, d\Omega = -\int_{\Gamma_{J^w}} w^{(1)} \mathbf{J}^{w*} \cdot \mathbf{n} \, d\Gamma, \tag{6.29}$$

$$\int_\Omega w^{(2)} \partial(\phi^w c^+)/\partial t \, d\Omega + \int_\Omega \mathbf{J}^+ \cdot \nabla w^{(2)} \, d\Omega + \int_\Omega w^{(2)} \nabla \cdot (\phi^w c^+ \mathbf{v}^s) d\Omega = -\int_{\Gamma_{J^+}} w^{(2)} \mathbf{J}^{+*} \cdot \mathbf{n} \, d\Gamma, \tag{6.30}$$

$$\int_\Omega w^{(3)} \partial(\phi^w c^-)/\partial t \, d\Omega + \int_\Omega \mathbf{J}^- \cdot \nabla w^{(3)} \, d\Omega + \int_\Omega w^{(3)} \nabla \cdot (\phi^w c^- \mathbf{v}^s) d\Omega = -\int_{\Gamma_{J^-}} w^{(3)} \mathbf{J}^{-*} \cdot \mathbf{n} \, d\Gamma, \tag{6.31}$$

$$\int_\Omega w^{(4)} \partial(\phi^w c^\circ)/\partial t \, d\Omega + \int_\Omega \mathbf{J}^\circ \cdot \nabla w^{(4)} \, d\Omega + \int_\Omega w^{(4)} \nabla \cdot (\phi^w c^\circ \mathbf{v}^s) d\Omega = -\int_{\Gamma_{J^\circ}} w^{(4)} \mathbf{J}^{\circ*} \cdot \mathbf{n} \, d\Gamma, \tag{6.32}$$

where $t^* = \sigma^* \cdot n$ is the traction on the boundary of the tissue and * stands for the quantities on the tissue boundary.

The spatial and temporal discretization of this weak formulation was followed by the procedure provided by Sun et al. [105]. The modified Newton–Raphson iterative procedure was employed to handle the nonlinear terms in the above set of equations. The resulting first-order ordinary differential equations with respect to time were solved using the implicit Euler backward scheme. The primary degrees of freedom, that is, the solid displacement u and the modified (electro)chemical potentials ε^α ($\alpha = w, +, -, o$) of water, cation, anion, and uncharged solute, were independently interpolated. Since the highest order of derivatives was the same for each degree of freedom, the same order shape functions were used. In this chapter, the weak formulation was solved using commercial finite element software COMSOL (COMSOL Inc., Burlington, Massachusetts).

6.4 Multiphasic FEMs of Human IVD

On the basis of the above weak formulation, a 3D multiphasic FEM of the human IVD was developed and applied to analyze the mechanical, chemical, and electrical signals within the human IVD under various mechanical loading conditions. Two simulation examples are presented here. The first example simulated the human IVD under an axial compression during stress relaxation. The effects of tissue properties and boundary conditions on the physical signals and the transport of fluid and solute were investigated. The numerical simulation showed that, during disc compression, the fluid pressurization and the effective (von Mises) solid stress were more pronounced in the AF region near the interface between AF and NP. In the NP, the distributions of the fluid pressure, effective stress, and electrical potential were more uniform than those in the AF. The electrical signals were very sensitive to FCD. Changes in material properties of the NP (water content, FCD, and modulus) affected fluid pressure, electrical potential, effective stress, and solute transport in the disc. This study is important for understanding disc biomechanics, nutrition, and mechanobiology.

This second example examined the effects of CEP calcification and the injection of IVD cells on the nutrition distributions inside the human IVD under physiological loading conditions using multiphasic finite element modeling. The simulation results showed that nutrient solute distribution inside the disc is maintained at a stable state during the day and night. Physiological diurnal cyclic loading does not change the nutrient environment in the human IVD. The CEP plays a significant role in the nutrient supply to human IVD. Calcification of the CEP significantly reduces the nutrient levels in human IVD. Therefore, in cell-based therapies for IVD regeneration, the increased nutrient demand as a result of cell injection needs to be addressed. Excessive numbers of injected cells may cause further deterioration of the nutrient environment in the degenerated disc. This study is important for understanding the pathology of IVD degeneration and providing new insights into cell-based therapies for low back pain.

6.4.1 Human IVD under Axial Compression during Stress Relaxation

The objective of this study was to develop a 3D, inhomogeneous FEM for human IVD for analyzing the physical environment and solute transport within the tissue under different mechanical loading conditions. A case of IVD under axial compression was simulated. Because of the complex nature of the problem, the analysis of this simple loading condition is useful for elucidating the effects of changes in material properties (owing to degeneration or growth) on solute (nutrients or growth factors) transport in IVD. It could also serve as a baseline for comparison of different theoretical models as well as for experimentally extracted material properties that may be difficult to measure directly.

6.4.1.1 IVD Geometry, Loading Configuration, and FE Implementation

In this study, the IVD is modeled as an inhomogeneous material with two distinguishing regions, that is, NP and AF regions (Figure 6.4a). Responses of physical signals and solute transport in the human lumbar disc to unconfined compression (stress-relaxation test, Figure 6.4d) were analyzed in this study. The size and geometry of a representative disc are shown in Figure 6.4a [132,153]. The thickness of the disc was $h = 10$ mm. The disc sample was initially equilibrated with a bathing solution of 0.15 M NaCl. An uncharged solute was introduced into the bathing solution at $t = 0$, and the disc was subjected to a ramp compression (10% strain in 10,000 s) between two endplates (Figure 6.4d). For the control case, two endplates were assumed to be perfectly permeable to water and solutes. The effect of endplate calcification on water and solute transport was investigated by assigning

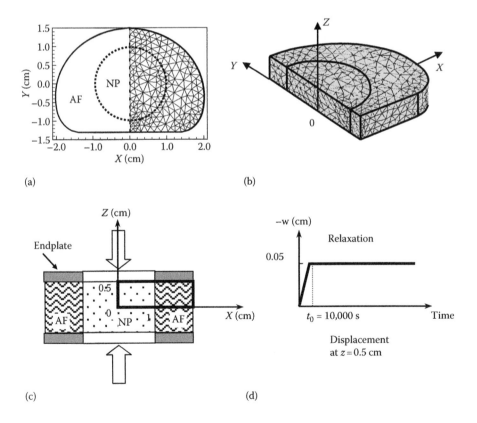

FIGURE 6.4
(a) Disc geometry, (b) mesh, (c) test configuration, and (d) testing protocol. (Adapted from Yao, H. and Gu, W.Y., *Journal of Biomechanics* 40:2071–2077, 2007. With permission.)

impermeable boundary condition to the portion of endplate adjacent to AF or to the portion adjacent to NP (Figure 6.4c). In this study, the human disc was modeled as an isotropic inhomogeneous mixture consisting of an intrinsically incompressible elastic solid (with fixed charge), water, ion (Na^+ and Cl^-), and uncharged solute (uncharged growth factor) phases.

The theoretical model in Section 6.3.1 and the FEM formulation (weak form) in Section 6.3.2 were used in this study. In the model, strain-dependent hydraulic permeability and strain-dependent diffusivity were considered using the constitutive relations for the AF and gels [139,140,149]. The formulation of this 3D initial- and boundary-value problem was solved using COMSOL software (COMSOL Inc.).

The upper quadrant of the disc was modeled with a mesh of 4306 second-order, tetrahedral Lagrange elements (Figure 6.4b). The maximum time step of 100 s was used during the ramp phase, and variable maximum time steps from 5 to 1000 s were used during the relaxation phase. The convergence of the numerical model was examined by refining the mesh and tightening the tolerance. The accuracy of the numerical method was also checked with the results of a 3D homogeneous case published in the literature [154].

The following baseline parameters were used in the simulation: temperature $T = 298$ K, bathing solution $c^* = 0.15$ M NaCl, neutral solute concentration (in bathing solution) $c^{o*} = 4 \times 10^{-5}$ mol/m^3, and coupling coefficient $B_w = 0$. The Stokes radii of cation (Na^+) $r_s^+ = 0.197$ nm, anion (Cl^-) $r_s^- = 0.142$ nm, and uncharged solute radius $r_s^o = 1.146$ nm were calculated on the basis of the corresponding diffusivities in the aqueous solution at 25°C using the Stokes–Einstein equation. The diffusivity values in solution for cation, anion, and neutral solute were 1.28×10^{-9} m^2/s, 1.77×10^{-9} m^2/s, and 2.2×10^{-10} m^2/s, respectively. For the uncharged solute, the diffusivity value was similar to that of IGF-1 and the partition coefficient was $\Phi = 0.1$. For small ions, an activity coefficient $\gamma_\pm/\gamma_\pm^* = 1$ and osmotic coefficient $\phi = 1$ were used. The convection coefficients (hindrance factors) H^α ($\alpha = +, -, o$) have not been determined for IVD tissues. In this study, the values of these parameters were assumed to be unity. The inhomogeneous material properties for the AF and NP were listed in Table 6.1 [61,132,155–159].

TABLE 6.1

Inhomogeneous Material Properties

	NP	AF
Darcy permeability (nm^2)	$a_1 = 0.00339$	$a_1 = 0.00044$
$\kappa = a_1(\phi^w/\phi^w)^{b_1}$	$b_1 = 3.24$	$b_1 = 7.193$
Relative diffusivity	$a_2 = 1.25$	$a_2 = 1.29$
	$b_2 = 0.681$	$b_2 = 0.372$
$\dfrac{D^\alpha}{D_0^\alpha} = \exp\left[-a_2\left(\dfrac{r_s^\alpha}{\sqrt{\kappa}}\right)^{b_2}\right]$		
$\alpha = +, -, o$		
Initial water content ϕ_0^w	0.86	0.75
	Low WC: 0.82	
Initial FCD c_0^F (mEq/ml)	0.25	0.15
	Low FCD: 0.15	
Elastic constant λ (MPa)	0.02	0.2
	Soft NP: 0.002	
Elastic constant μ (MPa)	0.015	0.15
	Soft NP: 0.0015	

6.4.1.2 Profiles of Physical Signals

The distribution of physical signals within the disc under axial compression was determined using the triphasic, inhomogeneous FEM. The solute transport was also investigated. Results of this study clearly show that inhomogeneous material properties have a significant effect on the distributions of physical signals in the IVD. The NP presents an interesting phenomenon where the distribution of effective solid stress, fluid pressure, electrical potential, and FCD (or dilatation, not shown) are very uniform compared to those in the AF (Figure 6.5). There are sharp peaks in effective solid stress distribution in the AF near the interface between the AF and NP (Figure 6.5d). This is mainly attributed to the discontinuity in material properties at the interface used in the model. The inhomogeneous model also predicted greater solid displacement in the posterior (negative y) direction than that in the anterior (positive y) direction when the IVD is subjected to axial compression (Figure 6.5e). Mechanical stiffness affected distributions of effective stress and fluid pressure. For example, a decrease in the NP modulus by one order of magnitude (Table 6.1) increased the effective stress in the AF but reduced the effective stress and pressure in the NP region (Figure 6.6a and b). The solid displacement in the y-direction also increased (Figure 6.6c). These results are important for understanding load-sharing mechanisms in the IVD as well as disc failure under axial compression.

6.4.1.3 Effects of Porosity and FCD

The most significant biochemical change seen in a degenerated disc is the loss of PG, resulting in the decrease in FCD and tissue hydration [43]. A reduction of water content (porosity) in the NP from 86% to 82% slightly increased the fluid pressure in the NP (Figure 6.7a) but slightly reduced the magnitude of electrical potential (Figure 6.7b). It also slightly increased the solid displacement (Figure 6.7c) and effective stress (not shown). The distribution of electrical potential varied significantly when the FCD of the NP was reduced from 0.25 to 0.15 mEq/ml, as shown in Figure 6.8a. Thus, the measurement of this electrical signal might be used as an indicator for disc degeneration. A decrease in FCD also reduces the contribution of osmotic pressure to the fluid pressure, as shown in Figure 6.8b.

6.4.1.4 Solute Transport

Changes in the NP properties (water content, FCD, modulus) affected the distributions of uncharged solute concentration within the tissue (Figure 6.9a and b). A reduction of endplate permeability in the NP region decreased the solute concentration dramatically (Figure 6.9a and b). A decrease in tissue water content will reduce its hydraulic permeability, leading to higher fluid pressurization as well as a reduced solute diffusivity, as shown in Figure 6.7a [149]. Consequently, a lower value of water content reduces both convection and diffusion effects, resulting in a lower solute concentration (Figure 6.9). The mechanism of dynamic mechanical loading on the solute transport has been investigated numerically [160,161]. In the present study, the effect of endplate boundary conditions on the transport of uncharged solute in the IVD under static compression was analyzed. The results indicate that the permeability of the endplate affects the solute transport rate into the tissue as well as its concentration distributions (Figure 6.9).

It is known that the mechanical interaction between solute and matrix may restrict solute transport in cartilaginous tissue for both diffusion and convection [162]. For diffusion, the intratissue diffusivities (D^α) were always smaller than their corresponding values in

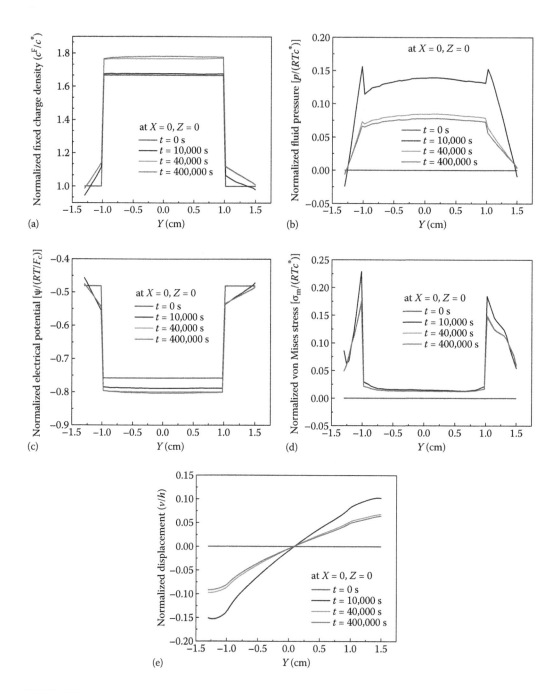

FIGURE 6.5
Transient response of FCD (a), fluid pressure (b), electrical potential (c), effective (von Mises) stress (d), and tissue displacement in the z-direction (e) during stress relaxation.

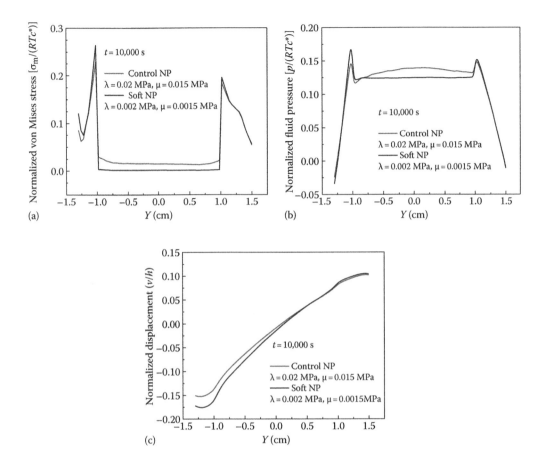

FIGURE 6.6
Effect of NP stiffness on effective stress (a), fluid pressure (b), and tissue displacement in the y-direction (c).

free solution $\left(D_0^\alpha\right)$, and its value is compression dependent [163,164]. For convection, the restriction effect is considered by the convection coefficient (H^α) of the solutes. The value of H^α should be in the range of $\left(D^\alpha/D_0^\alpha\right) \leq H^\alpha \leq 1$ [160]. Note that H^α might be significantly less than 1 for large solutes [165], while its value is close to unity for small solutes. In this study, the value of $H^\alpha = 1$ was used for both small and large solutes, since there are no data available for IVD tissue. Consequently, the concentration of large solute may be overestimated in our results. This is one of the limitations of this study.

6.4.1.5 Summary

This is the first report of 3D inhomogeneous triphasic finite element analysis of mechanical, chemical, and electrical signals within the human disc under axial compression. The effects of tissue porosity, FCD, and modulus on physical signals and fluid transport have been investigated parametrically. The effect of endplate permeability on solute transport and its concentration has also been studied. The results of this study provide additional insights into physical signals and solute transport within the human disc under mechanical loading.

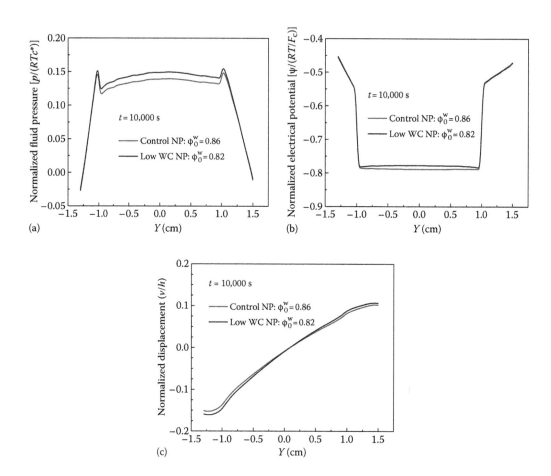

FIGURE 6.7
Effect of NP water content on fluid pressure (a), electrical potential (b), and tissue displacement in the y-direction (c).

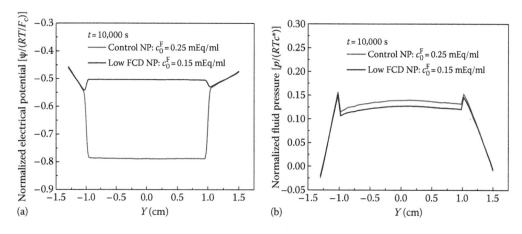

FIGURE 6.8
Effect of FCD on the distribution of electrical potential (a) and fluid pressure (b) in IVD.

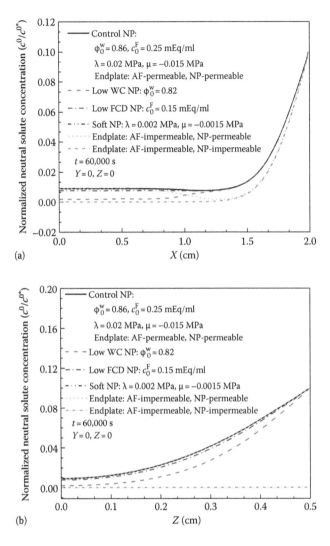

FIGURE 6.9
Effects of NP stiffness, water content, and FCD on solute concentration. A decrease in endplate permeability reduces solute concentration. (a) Concentration distribution in the x-direction. (b) Concentration distribution in the z-direction.

6.4.2 Human IVD under Physiological Diurnal Cyclic Loading

The objective of this study was to further develop a multiphasic mechano-electrochemical 3D FEM of human IVD by considering the disc cell energy metabolism. In comparison with earlier models [129,131,153,154,166–170], the present study is the first to compute the 3D concentration profiles of oxygen, glucose, and lactate in a human lumbar disc under physiological diurnal cyclic loading. This model was then applied to examine the effects of endplate calcification and the injection of IVD cells on the nutrition environment inside the human IVD under physiological loading conditions. The effect of endplate calcification was simulated by a reduction of the tissue porosity (i.e., water volume faction). The effect of a cell injection was simulated by increasing the cell density in the NP region. The role of physiological mechanical loading in regulating the disc nutrient environment was also clarified by considering strain-dependent transport properties (e.g., hydraulic permeability and solute diffusivities). This study is important for understanding the pathology of IVD degeneration and provided new insights into cell-based therapies for low back pain.

6.4.2.1 Nutrient Consumption Rate and Metabolite Production Rate

The energy metabolic rates of the disc cells were taken into consideration by adding the metabolic source term (Q^o) in the mass conservation equation (Equation 6.5) for nutrient solutes.

$$\partial(\phi^w c^o)/\partial t + \nabla \cdot (J^o + \phi^w c^o v^s) = Q^o. \tag{6.33}$$

The consumption rate of oxygen depended on oxygen concentration, as well as the pH value. The rate of production of lactate was based on that of NP cells in the literature [171,172]. A linear relationship between the pH value and lactate concentration was used to calculate the pH values in the disc [170,171]. The glucose is primarily consumed through the process of glycolysis, in which one molecule of glucose is broken down into two lactate molecules [173,174]. Thus, the consumption rate of glucose was set as half of the lactate production rate in this study. The following constitutive relations for the disc cell metabolic rates were used in this study:

$$Q^{Oxy} = -\frac{V'_{max}(pH-4.95)c^{Oxy}}{K'_m(pH-4.59)+c^{Oxy}}\rho_{cell}, \tag{6.34}$$

$$Q^{Lac} = \exp(-2.47 + 0.93pH + 0.16[O_2] - 0.0058[O_2]^2)\rho_{cell}, \tag{6.35}$$

$$pH = -0.092c^{Lac} + 7.33, \tag{6.36}$$

$$Q^{Glu} = -\frac{1}{2}Q^{Lac}, \tag{6.37}$$

where the unit of oxygen consumption rate Q^o (o = glucose, lactate, and oxygen) is nmol/l/h, the unit of oxygen concentration c^{Oxy} is μM, and V'_{max} is 5.27 nmol/million cells/h in the NP region and 3.64 nmol/million cells/h in the AF region. K'_m is 3.4 μM in the NP region and 12.3 μM in the AF region; the unit of oxygen tension [O_2] is kPa, which could be converted into to μM using oxygen solubility in water (1.0268 μmol/kPa-100 ml); the unit of lactate concentration c^{Lac} is mM; the units of lactate production rate Q^{Lac} and glucose consumption rate Q^{Glu} are nmol/l/h. Note that the single cell metabolic rates in the CEP were assumed to be equal to the values in the NP owing to the lack of experimental data in the CEP.

The human lumbar IVD was modeled as an inhomogeneous material with three distinct regions: NP, AF, and CEP (Figure 6.10a; Ref. [175]). The size and geometry of the human IVD in the simulation are based on previous experimental results [132,153]. The thickness of the IVD sample was 10 mm. The thickness of the CEP was 0.6 mm [74,176]. To investigate the effect of the CEP thickness on the nutrient environment, a thin calcified CEP with a thickness of 0.3 mm was also defined and simulated. The IVD sample was initially

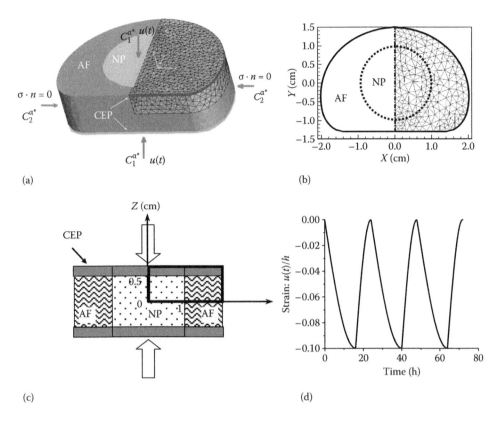

FIGURE 6.10
Geometry of the human lumbar IVD model and loading protocol in the simulation. (a) 3D view of the disc model, (b) disc geometry, (c) test configuration, and (d) cyclic loading on the top and bottom of the disc (Strain = cyclic displacement $u(t)$/initial height of the disc h). (Adapted from Wu, Y. et al., *Molecular and Cellular Biomechanics* 10(2):159–182, 2013. With permission.)

equilibrated under preloaded conditions to maintain the original disc thickness. The solute concentrations at the boundaries were as follows: c^{NaCl} is 0.15 M, c^{Glu} is 4 mM at the CEP boundary and 5 mM at the lateral AF surface, c^{Lac} is 0.8 mM at the CEP boundary and 0.9 mM at the lateral AF surface, and c^{Oxy} is 5.1 kPa at the CEP boundary and 5.8 kPa at the lateral AF surface. The IVD sample was then subjected to a cyclical loading between the two endplates (Figure 6.10d). The amplitude of the compressive strain on the whole disc for the cyclical loading was 10%. The cyclic loading included 16-h compression and 8-h recovery to mimic the physiological diurnal disc height changes [129]. The boundary of the CEP was permeable to both water and solutes.

The 3D weak form of the finite element formulation was solved by COMSOL software in the weak form mode (Version 3.4, COMSOL Inc.). The upper right quadrant of the disc was modeled with 7016 second-order, tetrahedral Lagrange elements (Figure 6.10a). As for the cyclic loading, the maximum time step for beginning each ramp compression was 10 s. The time step used in cyclic loading ranged from 5 to 100 s. The convergence of the numerical model was examined by refining the mesh and tightening the tolerance. The numerical accuracy of this study was validated with the results of the 3D stress relaxation cases published in the literature [154].

TABLE 6.2

Disc Tissue Properties Used in the Numerical Model

	CEP	NP	AF
Parameter for hydraulic permeability $\kappa = a_1(\phi^w/\phi^w)^{b_1}$	$a_1 = 0.0248$ nm[2a] $b_1 = 2.154$[a]	$a_1 = 0.00339$ nm[2b] $b_1 = 3.24$[b]	$a_1 = 0.00044$ nm[2c] $b_1 = 7.193$[c]
Parameter for diffusivity $\dfrac{D^\alpha}{D_0^\alpha} = \exp\left[-a_2\left(\dfrac{r_s^\alpha}{\sqrt{\kappa}}\right)^{b_2}\right]$ α ions and nutrient solutes	$a_2 = 1.29$ nm[d] $b_2 = 0.372$[d]	$a_2 = 1.25$ nm[d] $b_2 = 0.681$[d]	$a_2 = 1.29$ nm[d] $b_2 = 0.372$[d]
Initial water content ϕ_0^w (Water content: $\phi^w = (\phi_0^w + e)/(1+e)$)	0.6[e] Calcified: 0.45	0.86[f]	0.75[f]
Elastic constant λ (MPa)	0.1[g]	0.02[h]	0.2[h]
Elastic constant μ (MPa)	0.2[g]	0.015[h]	0.15[h]
Cell density (cells/mm³)	15,000[i]	4000[i] Therapy: 6000, 8000, 10,000	9000[i]

Source: [a]Maroudas, A., *Biorheology* 12:233–248, 1975; Yao, H. and Gu, W.Y., *Annals Biomed Eng* 32:380–390, 2004. [b]Gu, W.Y. and Yao, H., *Annals Biomed Eng* 31(10):1162–1170, 2003, from agarose gels. [c]Gu, W.Y. and Yao, H., *Annals Biomed Eng* 31(10):1162–1170, 2003, from porcine AF tissue. [d]Gu, W.Y. et al., *Annals Biomed Eng* 32:1710–1717, 2004, from porcine AF tissue and agarose gels. [e]Roberts, S. et al., *Spine* 14(2):166–174, 1989; Setton, L.A. et al., *J Orthopae Res* 11(2):228–239, 1993. [f]Yao, H. and Gu, W.Y., *J Biomech* 40:2071–2077, 2007. [g]Yao, H. and Gu, W.Y., *Annals Biomed Eng* 32:380–390, 2004. [h]Yao, H. and Gu, W.Y., *Biorheology* 43:325–335, 2006. [i]Maroudas, A. et al., *J Anat* 120(1):113–130, 1975.

Note: r_s^α is the hydrodynamic radius of ions and nutrient solutes ($r_s^+ = 0.197$ nm; $r_s^- = 0.142$ nm; $r_s^{Oxy} = 0.1$ nm; $r_s^{Lac} = 0.255$ nm; $r_s^{Glu} = 0.3$ nm), D_0^α is the diffusivity of ions and nutrient solutes in aqueous solution ($D_0^+ = 1.28 \times 10^{-9}$ m²/s, $D_0^- = 1.77 \times 10^{-9}$ m²/s, $D_0^{Oxy} = 3.0 \times 10^{-9}$ m²/s, $D_0^{Lac} = 1.28 \times 10^{-9}$ m²/s, $D_0^{Glu} = 0.92 \times 10^{-9}$ m²/s).

In this study, the effect of endplate calcification on nutrient solute transport was simulated by a reduction of the tissue porosity (i.e., water volume faction). This is feasible since the hydraulic permeability and solute diffusivity are related to the tissue water content, as shown in Table 6.2 [7,93,131,139,149,153,154,176,177]. The tissue porosity of normal CEP was 0.6, while this value in calcified endplate was 0.48 (i.e., a 20% reduction) [77,176]. In addition, the cell density in the NP region was increased by 50%, 100%, and 150% in order to analyze the effect of cell injections in cell-based therapies for low back pain treatment. The material properties for the AF, NP, and CEP were summarized in Table 6.2. The biomechanical response (strain, stress, water flux, and water pressure), electrical signals (ion concentrations and ion current/potential), and nutrient solutes transport (oxygen, glucose, and lactate concentration) in the human IVD under the physiological loading were simultaneously obtained from this multiphasic FEM of the IVD. Only the results for the oxygen, glucose, and lactate concentration profiles were reported here.

6.4.2.2 Concentration Profiles of Nutrient and Metabolite

The nutrition concentration distributions were not uniform in the human IVD. Generally, the glucose and oxygen concentrations decreased when moving away from the blood supply at the margin of the disc. In contrast, the lactate concentration increased toward the center of the disc. Significant nutrient concentration gradients existed inside the disc. The computed minimum oxygen concentration of 0.3 kPa at the center region of the disc falls within the measured range of 0.3–1.1 kPa [173]. The computed minimum glucose concentrations of 0.54 mM in the inner AF is in agreement with the measured range of 0.5–2.5 mM in the AF of scoliotic discs [14]. The computed maximum lactate concentration of 5.21 mM also falls within the measured range of 2–6 mM [178]. These agreements between the model predictions and experimental measurements validated the present FEM of the human IVD to a certain extent.

6.4.2.3 Impact of Cyclical Loading

The human IVD experiences a diurnal cyclic loading in vivo [129]. In this study, a cyclical loading (compression during the day then recovery during the night) was considered to mimic the physiological loading on the IVD, including a 16-h compression and 8-h recovery. The glucose, lactate, and oxygen concentration distributions in the normal IVD at the end of the day (i.e., the end of compression), as well as at the beginning of the day (i.e., the end of recovery), are shown in Figure 6.11. It was apparent that the nutrient concentration profiles remained almost identical during the day and night. The changes in concentration profiles were less than 1% under the diurnal cyclic loading.

The result indicates that cyclical loading–induced fluid flow does not alter the nutrient transport and maintains a stable nutrient environment inside the IVD under the physical diurnal loading condition. Previous studies [179–181] have proposed that fluid flow induced by the mechanical loading may enhance or hinder the solute transport in the disc. However, for small solutes such as glucose, lactate, and oxygen, diffusion is a dominant transport mechanism inside the disc since the convective contribution of *pumping* small solutes is relatively small [78,129,160,173] Although several studies have shown that the long-term sustained static compression may change the nutrient concentration distribution inside the IVD [131,154,168,169,182], the present study further confirmed that the nutrient environment maintains a stable state under the physiological diurnal loading condition. With a stable nutrient environment, the disc cell energy metabolism also keeps a constant rate during the day and night under the physiological condition. This may be beneficial to disc cell homeostasis.

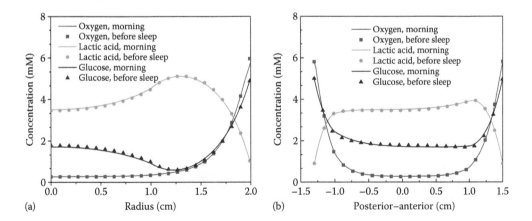

FIGURE 6.11
Nutrient solute (glucose, lactate, and oxygen) concentration distributions inside the human IVD in the morning (end of the recovery) and at night (end of the compression): (a) in the x-direction from the center to the lateral and (b) in the y-direction from the posterior to the anterior.

6.4.2.4 Effects of CEP Calcification

Along with the aging process, calcification of the CEP may appear and alter its transport properties [77,78]. The reduction of the fluid and solute permeability owing to CEP calcification may impede nutrition supply to the disc [183–185]. As shown in our results, the calcification of the CEP dramatically decreased the glucose and oxygen concentrations and increased the lactate concentration inside the IVD (Figure 6.12). There were 69.3% and 33.9% decreases in minimum glucose and oxygen concentrations in the disc with a calcified endplate, respectively. In contrast, there was a 7.3% increase in maximum lactate concentration in the disc with the calcified endplate. Moreover, the nutrient concentration levels in the NP region, compared to the AF region, were more significantly affected by the calcified CEP (Figure 6.13). There were 23.0% and 23.7% decreases in the mean concentrations of oxygen and glucose in the NP region, while 5.1% and 8.2% decreases were found in the AF region. Meanwhile, a 16.5% increase of mean lactate concentration was found in

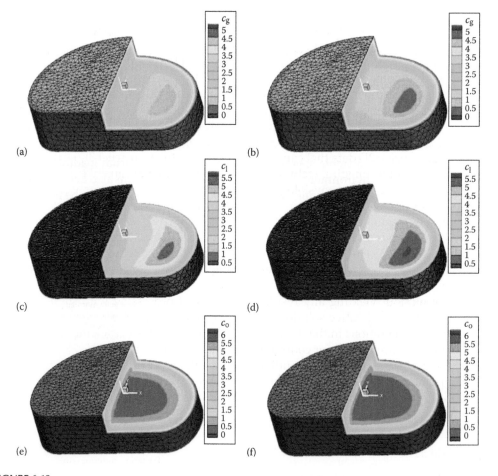

FIGURE 6.12

Effect of CEP calcification on 3D nutrient solute (glucose c_g, lactate c_l, and oxygen c_o) concentration distributions inside the human IVD: (a, c, e) with a normal CEP, and (b, d, f) with a calcified CEP (concentration unit: mM). (Adapted from Wu, Y. et al., *Molecular and Cellular Biomechanics* 10(2):159–182, 2013. With permission.)

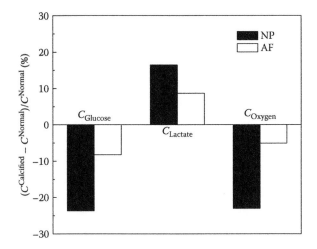

FIGURE 6.13
Effect of CEP calcification on mean concentrations in the NP and AF regions. The change of the concentration was normalized by the concentration with a normal CEP.

the NP region while an 8.7% increase was found in the AF region. The mean concentration was calculated by $c_{mean}^o = \iiint_V c^o \, dx \, dy \, dz \Big/ \iiint_V dx \, dy \, dz$, o = glucose, lactate, and oxygen.

Calcification of the CEP significantly changes the nutrient solute distribution inside the human IVD, including a significant fall of the minimum oxygen and glucose concentrations and a significant increase of maximum lactate concentration (Figure 6.12). Moreover, the effect of CEP calcification is more significant in the NP region (Figure 6.13), as the main source of nutrition supply for the NP is from capillaries and canals in the vertebral bodies adjacent to the endplate [72–74]. Our results also showed that the CEP calcification significantly increased the size of the critical zone (Figure 6.14; Ref. [186]). Note that the critical zone is defined as a disc region in which the glucose concentration is lower than 0.5 mM. The glucose concentration is a limiting factor for the disc cell viability. A previous cell culture study has shown that disc cell death occurs if the glucose concentration is lower than 0.5 mM for more than 3 days [16]. Therefore, the CEP calcification results in a decrease in nutrient supply to the disc. This may lead to changes in the disc cell viability and cellular metabolism, which in turn alters the ECM homeostasis (breakdown/synthesize). The imbalance of the matrix synthesis and degradation implies the onset of disc degeneration.

6.4.2.5 *Effects of NP Cell Injection in Cell-Based Therapy*

In order to develop new treatments for IVD degeneration–associated low back pain, injection of autologous NP/chondrocyte cells or mesenchymal stem cells to the degenerated disc has been proposed for disc regeneration [80–82]. Our results showed that the increase in cell density within the NP region attributed to NP cell injection significantly decreased the extreme oxygen and glucose concentrations (lowest concentration inside the disc), while increasing the extreme lactate concentration (highest concentration inside the disc), as shown in Figure 6.14. The magnitude of the change of the extreme concentrations attributed to the cell injection also depended on the conditions of the CEP (i.e., normal, calcified, and thin calcified). Moreover, the condition of the CEP had a more significant impact on the extreme glucose concentration than on the extreme lactate and oxygen concentrations.

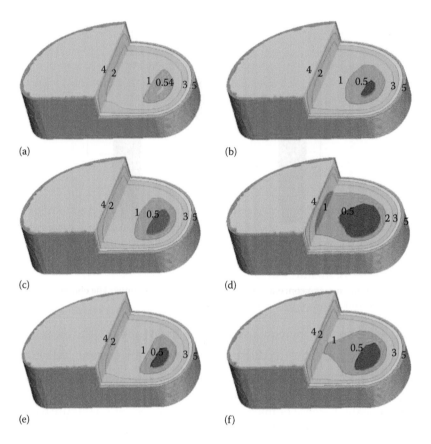

FIGURE 6.14
Effect of increase in cell density on 3D glucose concentration distribution in the disc with a normal CEP (a and b), calcified CEP (c and d), and thin calcified CEP (e and f). The gray color regions indicate the critical zones in which the glucose concentration is lower than 0.5 mM. (Adapted from Wu, Y. et al., *Molecular and Cellular Biomechanics* 10(2):159–182, 2013. With permission.)

Specifically, the extreme glucose concentration sharply reached zero (Figure 6.15) when the NP cell density increased only 50% with the calcified CEP. Glucose concentration is a limiting factor for disc cell viability [14,16,186]. A critical zone was defined as a disc region in which the glucose concentration is lower than 0.5 mM [186]. With the normal CEP, a small volume critical zone (0.016 cm³) appeared in the AF region when the NP cell density increased 50% (Figure 6.14a and b). With the calcified CEP, a 50% increase of the NP cell density caused a 105.6% increase in the volume of the critical zone (Figure 6.14c and d). With the thin calcified CEP, the increase in the volume of the critical zone was reduced to 75.8% (Figure 6.14e and f).

Our results indicated that increasing the cell density in the NP region may increase cellular metabolism, which in turn causes further deterioration of the nutrient environment in the degenerated disc. Even in a disc with a normal CEP, a critical zone appeared immediately once the cell density in the NP region increased by 50% (Figure 6.14b). The critical zone was doubled with the presence of a calcified CEP. Interestingly, after cutting down the calcified CEP to half of its thickness, the volume of the critical zone was decreased to half of its volume compared with the full-thickness CEP. Our results suggested that the nutrient supply is an essential factor that needs to be considered in cell-based therapies for

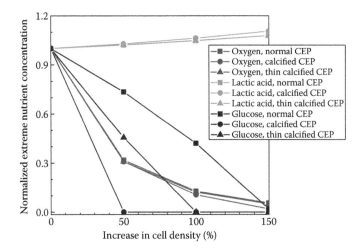

FIGURE 6.15

Effect of increase in cell density on the extreme nutrient concentrations inside human IVD. Cell density in the NP region is increased by 50%, 100%, and 150%. The simulated cases include disc with a normal CEP, calcified CEP, and thin calcified CEP (50% of the full thickness).

human IVD regeneration. Unless it can be assured that a degenerate disc has a nutrient supply that can support the implanted cells, treatment using a cell therapy approach is both pointless and unethical [187]. Our results also suggested that reducing the thickness of the calcified CEP could be an option to restore the nutrient environment in degenerative discs for cell-based therapies. In addition, in order to address the nutrition supply concern, large animal species will be a more appropriate model for testing this approach.

6.4.2.6 Summary

This is the first report of 3D nutrient solute distribution within the human disc under physiological loading conditions using the triphasic FEM. We found that the nutrient solute distribution inside the disc is maintained at a stable state during the day and night. The physiological diurnal cyclic loading does not change the nutrient environment in the human IVD. The CEP plays a significant role in the nutrient supply to the human IVD. Calcification of the CEP significantly reduces the nutrient levels in the human IVD. Therefore, in cell-based therapies for IVD regeneration, the increased nutrient demand by cell injection needs to be seriously considered. Excessive amounts of injected cells may cause further deterioration of the nutrient environment in the degenerated disc. This study provides additional insights into load-supporting mechanisms and physical signals within the human disc under mechanical loading. It is also important for understanding the pathology of IVD degeneration and providing new insights into cell-based therapies for low back pain.

6.5 Conclusion and Future Perspective

Knowledge of the mechano-electrochemical behavior of cartilaginous tissues is crucial for understanding the physiological phenomena of those tissues, such as load-supporting mechanisms, nutrition, and the biological response of cells to their physicochemical environment (signal transduction mechanisms). This knowledge is also important for elucidating the biomechanical etiology of tissue failure (e.g., osteoarthritis and disc degeneration), as well as developing strategies for tissue repair (in vivo) and tissue engineering (in vitro). Especially, since cartilaginous tissues are avascular tissues, poor nutritional supply is believed to be one of the mechanisms of tissue degeneration.

Because of the unique composition and structure of the materials and the complexity of the mechano-electrochemical coupling phenomena in cartilaginous tissues, realistic strain-dependent constitutive relationships of fluid and solute transport properties that were determined in our previous experimental studies were incorporated into our numerical model. The energy metabolic rates of the cells were also taken into consideration on the basis of the experimental results in the literature [170–174]. Therefore, our mechano-electrochemical FEM could systematically predict the physical signals and the transport of fluid and solutes (nutrients and metabolites) in response to mechanical loading.

A specialized formulation of the triphasic theory was presented for charged hydrated soft tissues containing uncharged solutes (such as glucose, lactate, oxygen, and growth factors). The basic variables chosen were as follows: solid displacement $\mathbf{u}$, water chemical potential ε^w, ion electrochemical potentials ε^+ and ε^-, and chemical potential for uncharged solute ε^o. This formulation can satisfy the discontinuous conditions between elements and across the interface boundaries. The corresponding weak formulation for finite element implementation was also derived using the standard Galerkin weight residual method. The finite element formulation was numerically implemented using COMSOL software (COMSOL Inc.).

A 3D isotropic FEM was also developed to analyze the mechanical, chemical, and electrical signals within the human IVD under the physiological loading condition. 3D inhomogeneous physical signals and nutrient solute distribution inside the IVD were investigated. The effects of tissue porosity and FCD on physical signals and fluid transport were investigated parametrically. The mechanism of uncharged solute transport within the IVD was also elucidated. We also found that the physiological diurnal cyclic loading does not significantly change the nutrient environment in the human IVD. Calcification of the CEP significantly reduces the nutrient levels in the human IVD. Moreover, in cell-based therapies for IVD regeneration, we found that excessive amounts of injected cells may cause further deterioration of the nutrient environment in the degenerated disc. This study provides additional insights into load-supporting mechanisms and physical signals within the human disc under mechanical loading. It is also important for understanding the pathology of IVD degeneration and providing new insights into cell-based therapies for low back pain.

The ultimate research goals of our numerical simulation are to help elucidate the etiology of human disc degeneration and develop strategies for restoring tissue function or retarding further disc degeneration. There are several limitations of the studies presented here. In order to improve the accuracy of the simulation, more information about the geometry of the CEP and the region of calcification is needed. The simplified geometry of CEP in this study may overestimate the size of the CEP. The mechanical and transport properties (Table 6.1) used in this study were mainly from animal data. These properties for the human IVD, especially for the CEP, are largely unavailable from the literature. In addition, mechanical properties in normal and calcified endplates were assumed to be the same in this study owing to the lack of experimental data in the literature. In the future, the changes in mechanical properties of CEP attributed to the calcification process should also be incorporated into the numerical model. Experiments regarding the mechanical parameters (lame constants or aggregate modulus) in both normal and calcified human endplates need to be conducted.

Because of the lack of experimental data, the mechanical properties (elastic modulus) and transport properties (hydraulic permeability and solute diffusivities) were assumed to be isotropic in this study. However, because of the unique structure of collagen lamellae in the AF region, the anisotropy of the mechanical and transport properties of the human IVD needs to be considered in our future work [188–190]. As for energy metabolism properties in the NP and AF, there are limited data available for the human IVD. Consequently, bovine and porcine cell data were used in this study. Moreover, the glucose consumption rate was assumed to be half of the lactic production rate based on the glycolysis assumption. The glucose consumption rate may also depend on the oxygen level [16]. Meanwhile, the cell viability needs to be considered in future studies by correlating it with the pH value and glucose concentration. The development of a new constitutive relation for IVD cell viability, based on experiment data, is needed to further improve our model.

The effect of mechanical strain on FCD was incorporated in this model, as shown in Equations 6.19 and 6.20. Mechanical loading could alter the extracellular osmotic environment by changing the FCD in the ECM. Moreover, disc degeneration will induce loss of PG content from the matrix, resulting in a change of FCD and the extracellular osmotic environment. Previous studies have found that cellular responses such as gene expression and collagen synthesis were significantly affected by the osmotic environment [191,192]. Therefore, the energy metabolic activities of IVD cells may also be changed because of the change in the extracellular osmotic environment. A more accurate prediction of the nutrient distribution in the human IVD could be expected once the effects of osmolarity on energy metabolic activities of IVD cells are quantitatively characterized in the future.

Acknowledgments

This study was supported by National Institutes of Health grants AR055775, DE018741, and DE021134; a grant (SCIRF0307) from the South Carolina Spinal Cord Injury Research Fund; a National Science Foundation (NSF) RII grant fellowship (EPS-00903795) to YW; and an NSF graduate research fellowship to SEC.

References

1. Grodzinsky AJ (1983) Electromechanical and physicochemical properties of connective tissue. *Crit Rev Biomed Eng* 9(2):133–199.
2. Maroudas A (1979) Physicochemical properties of articular cartilage. In *Adult Articular Cartilage*, ed. Freeman MAR (Pitman Medical, Philadelphia, PA), Vol. 2, pp. 215–290.
3. Mow VC, Ratcliffe A, and Poole AR (1992) Cartilage and diarthrodial joints as paradigms for hierarchical materials and structures. *Biomaterials* 13(2):67–97.
4. Muir H (1980) The chemistry of the ground substance of joint cartilage. In *The Joints and Synovial Fluid*, ed. Sokolff L (Academic Press, New York), Vol. 2, pp. 27–94.

5. Muir H (1983) Proteoglycons as organizers of the extracellular matrix. *Biochem Soc Trans* 11(6):613–622.
6. Stockwell RA (1979) *Biology of Cartilage Cells* (Cambridge University Press, Cambridge, UK).
7. Maroudas A, Stockwell RA, Nachemson A, and Urban J (1975) Factors involved in the nutrition of the human lumbar intervertebral disc: Cellularity and diffusion of glucose in vitro. *J Anat* 120(1):113–130.
8. Liebscher T, Haefeli M, Wuertz K, Nerlich AG, and Boos N (2011) Age-related variation in cell density of human lumbar intervertebral disc. *Spine* 36(2):153–159.
9. Mow VC, Wang CC, and Hung CT (1999) The extracellular matrix, interstitial fluid and ions as a mechanical signal transducer in articular cartilage. *Osteoarthritis Cartilage* 7(1):41–58.
10. Urban JP (2000) Present perspectives on cartilage and chondrocyte mechanobiology. *Biorheology* 37(1–2):185–190.
11. Grodzinsky AJ, Levenston ME, Jin M, and Frank EH (2000) Cartilage tissue remodeling in response to mechanical forces. *Annu Rev Biomed Eng* 2:691–713.
12. Levenston ME, Frank EH, and Grodzinsky AJ (1999) Electrokinetic and poroelastic coupling during finite deformations of charged porous media. *J Appl Mech* 66(2):323–333.
13. Mow VC, Sun DN, Guo XE, Likhitpanichkul M, and Lai WM (2002) Fixed negative charges modulate mechanical behavior and electrical signals in articular cartilage under unconfined compression—A triphasic paradigm. In *Porous Media: Theory, Experiments and Numerical Application*, eds. Ehlers W, and Bluhm J (Springer, Berlin), pp. 227–247.
14. Bibby SR, Fairbank JC, Urban MR, and Urban JP (2002) Cell viability in scoliotic discs in relation to disc deformity and nutrient levels. *Spine* 27(20):2220–2228.
15. Holm S, and Nachemson A (1982) Nutritional changes in the canine intervertebral disc after spinal fusion. *Clin Orthop* 169:243–258.
16. Horner HA, and Urban JP (2001) 2001 Volvo Award Winner in Basic Science Studies: Effect of nutrient supply on the viability of cells from the nucleus pulposus of the intervertebral disc. *Spine (Phila Pa 1976)* 26(23):2543–2549.
17. Nachemson A, Lewin T, Maroudas A, and Freeman MA (1970) In vitro diffusion of dye through the end-plates and the annulus fibrosus of human lumbar inter-vertebral discs. *Acta Orthop Scand* 41(6):589–607.
18. Urban JP (2001) The role of the physicochemical environment in determining disc cell behaviour. *Biochem Soc Trans* 30(6):858–864.
19. Buckwalter JA (1995) Aging and degeneration of the human intervertebral disc. *Spine (Phila Pa 1976)* 20(11):1307–1314.
20. Eyre DR et al. (1989) Intervertebral disk: Basic science perspectives. In *New Perspectives on Low Back Pain*, eds. Frymoyer JW, and Gordon SL (American Academy of Orthopaedic Surgeons, Park Ridge, IL), pp. 147–207.
21. Gruber HE, and Hanley EN, Jr. (2002) Ultrastructure of the human intervertebral disc during aging and degeneration: Comparison of surgical and control specimens. *Spine (Phila Pa 1976)* 27(8):798–805.
22. Kelsey JL, Pastides H, and Bisbee GE (1978) *Musculoskeletal Disorders: Their Frequency of Occurrence and Their Impact on the Population of the United States* (Prodist, New York).
23. Kelsey JL, Mundt DF, and Golden AL (1992) Epidemiology of low back pain. In *The Lumbar Spine and Back Pain*, ed. Malcolm JIV (Churchill Livingstone, New York), Vol. 4, pp. 537–549.
24. Nerlich AG, Boos N, Wiest I, and Aebi M (1998) Immunolocalization of major interstitial collagen types in human lumbar intervertebral discs of various ages. *Virchows Arch* 432(1):67–76.
25. White AA, & Panjabi MM (1978) Physical properties and functional biomechanics of the spine. In *Clinical Biomechanics of the Spine*, eds. White AA, and Panjabi MM (JB Lippincott, Philadelphia, PA).
26. White AA (1981) Biomechanics of lumbar spine and sacroiliac articulation: Relavance to idiopathic low back pain. In *Symposium on Idiopathic Low Back Pain*, eds. White AA, and Gordon SL (CV Mosby Co., St. Louis, MO), pp. 296–322.

27. Lundon K, and Bolton K (2001) Structure and function of the lumbar intervertebral disk in health, aging, and pathologic conditions. *J Orthop Sports Phys Ther* 31(6):291–303.
28. Guiot BH, and Fessler RG (2000) Molecular biology of degenerative disc disease. *Neurosurgery* 47(5):1034–1040.
29. Hickey DS, and Hukins DWL (1980) Relation between the structure of the anulus fibrosus and the function and failure of the intervertebral disc. *Spine* 5:106–116.
30. Marchand F, and Ahmed AM (1990) Investigation of the laminate structure of lumbar disc anulus fibrosus. *Spine* 15(5):402–410.
31. Ebara S et al. (1996) Tensile properties of nondegenerate human lumbar anulus fibrosus. *Spine* 21(4):452–461.
32. Fujita Y, Lotz JC, and Soejima O (1995) Site specific radial tensile properties of the lumbar annulus fibrosus. *Trans Orthop Res Soc* 20:673.
33. Galante JO (1967) Tensile properties of the human lumbar annulus fibrosus. *Acta Orthop Scand* 100 Suppl:1–91.
34. Marchand F, and Ahmed AM (1989) Mechanical properties and failure mechanisms of the lumbar disc annulus. *Trans Orthop Res Soc* 14:355.
35. Kraemer J, Kolditz D, and Gowin R (1985) Water and electrolyte content of human intervertebral discs under variable load. *Spine* 10(1):69–71.
36. Pearce RH (1993) Morphologic and chemical aspects of aging. In *Musculoskeletal Soft-Tissue Aging: Impact on Mobility*, eds. Wood DO, Goldberg VM, and Woo SL (American Academy of Orthopaedic Surgeons, Rosemont, IL), pp. 363–379.
37. Panagiotacopulos ND, Pope MH, Krag MH, and Block R (1987) Water content in human intervertebral discs. Part I. Measurement by magnetic resonance imaging. *Spine* 12(9):912–917.
38. Gu WY et al. (1999) The anisotropic hydraulic permeability of human lumbar anulus fibrosus. Influence of age, degeneration, direction, and water content. *Spine* 24(23):2449–2455.
39. Hendry NGC (1958) The hydration of the neuclous pulposus and its relation to intervertebral disc derangement. *J Bone Joint Surg* 40B:132–144.
40. Johnstone B, Urban JP, Roberts S, and Menage J (1992) The fluid content of the human intervertebral disc. Comparison between fluid content and swelling pressure profiles of discs removed at surgery and those taken postmortem. *Spine* 17(4):412–416.
41. Cole TC, Ghosh P, and Taylor TK (1986) Variations of the proteoglycans of the canine intervertebral disc with ageing. *Biochim Biophys Acta* 880(2–3):209–219.
42. Jahnke MR, and McDevitt CA (1988) Proteoglycans of the human intervertebral disc. Electrophoretic heterogeneity of the aggregating proteoglycans of the nucleus pulposus. *Biochem J* 251(2):347–356.
43. Lyons G, Eisenstein SM, and Sweet MB (1981) Biochemical changes in intervertebral disc degeneration. *Biochim Biophys Acta* 673(4):443–453.
44. Roberts S, Caterson B, Evans H, and Eisenstein SM (1994) Proteoglycan components of the intervertebral disc and cartilage endplate: An immunolocalization study of animal and human tissues. *Histochem J* 26(5):402–411.
45. Weidenbaum M, Iatridis JC, Setton LA, Foster RJ, and Mow VC (1996) Mechanical behaviors of the intervertebral disc and the effects of degeneration. In *Low Back Pain: A Scientific and Clinical Overview*, eds. Weinstein SL, and Gordon SL (American Academy of Orthopaedic Surgeons, Rosemont, IL), pp. 557–582.
46. Antoniou J et al. (1996) The human lumbar intervertebral disc: Evidence for changes in the biosynthesis and denaturation of the extracellular matrix with growth, maturation, ageing, and degeneration. *J Clin Invest* 98(4):996–1003.
47. Urban JPG, and Maroudas A (1980) The chemistry of the intervertebral disc in relation to its physiological function and requirements. *Clin Rheum Dis* 6:51–77.
48. Donnan FG (1924) The theory of membrane equilibria. *Chem Rev* 1:73–90.
49. Eisenberg SR, and Grodzinsky AJ (1985) Swelling of articular cartilage and other connective tissues: Electromechanochemical forces. *J Orthop Res* 3(2):148–159.

50. Eisenberg SR, and Grodzinsky AJ (1987) The kinetics of chemically induced nonequilibrium swelling of articular cartilage and corneal stroma. *J Biomech Eng* 109(1):79–89.
51. Frank EH, Grodzinsky AJ, Koob TJ, and Eyre DR (1987) Streaming potentials: A sensitive index of enzymatic degradation in articular cartilage. *J Orthop Res* 5(4):497–508.
52. Frank EH, and Grodzinsky AJ (1987) Cartilage electromechanics—I. Electrokinetic transduction and the effects of electrolyte pH and ionic strength. *J Biomech* 20(6):615–627.
53. Gu WY, Lai WM, and Mow VC (1993) Transport of fluid and ions through a porous-permeable charged-hydrated tissue, and streaming potential data on normal bovine articular cartilage. *J Biomech* 26(6):709–723.
54. Gu WY (1994) A study of mechano-electrochemical properties of charged-hydrated-soft tissues and biomechanics of articular cartilage. Columbia University, New York.
55. Gu WY, Lai WM, and Mow VC (1997) A triphasic analysis of negative osmotic flows through charged hydrated soft tissues. *J Biomech* 30(1):71–78.
56. Gu WY, Lai WM, and Mow VC (1998) A mixture theory for charged-hydrated soft tissues containing multi-electrolytes: Passive transport and swelling behaviors. *J Biomech Eng* 120(2):169–180.
57. Gu WY et al. (1999) Streaming potential of human lumbar anulus fibrosus is anisotropic and affected by disc degeneration. *J Biomech* 32(11):1177–1182.
58. Lai WM, Hou JS, and Mow VC (1991) A triphasic theory for the swelling and deformation behaviors of articular cartilage. *J Biomech Eng* 113(3):245–258.
59. Urban JP, and Maroudas A (1981) Swelling of the intervertebral disc in vitro. *Connect Tissue Res* 9(1):1–10.
60. Urban JP, and McMullin JF (1985) Swelling pressure of the intervertebral disc: Influence of proteoglycan and collagen contents. *Biorheology* 22(2):145–157.
61. Urban JP, and McMullin JF (1988) Swelling pressure of the lumbar intervertebral discs: Influence of age, spinal level, composition, and degeneration. *Spine (Phila Pa 1976)* 13(2):179–187.
62. Charnley J (1952) The imbibition of fluid as a cause of herniation of the nucleus pulposus. *Lancet* 1:124–127.
63. Gu WY, Lewis B, Saed-Nejad F, Lai WM, and Ratcliffe A (1997) Hydration and true denstiy of normal and PG-depleted bovine articular cartilage. *Trans Orthop Res Soc* 22:826.
64. Gu WY, Justiz MA, and Yao H (2002) Electrical conductivity of lumbar annulus fibrosis: Effects of porosity and fixed charge density. *Spine* 27:2390–2395.
65. NIH (1997) Research on low back pain and common spinal disorders. *NIH Guide* 26(16).
66. Kelsey JL, White AA, III, Pastides H, and Bisbee GE, Jr. (1979) The impact of musculoskeletal disorders on the population of the United States. *J Bone Joint Surg Am* 61(7):959–964.
67. Kelsey JL, and White AA (1980) Epidemiology and impact of low-back pain. *Spine* 5:133–142.
68. Boos N, Wallin A, Gbedegbegnon T, Aebi M, and Boesch C (1993) Quantitative MR imaging of lumbar intervertebral disks and vertebral bodies: Influence of diurnal water content variations. *Radiology* 188(2):351–354.
69. Miller JAA, Schmatz C, and Schultz AB (1988) Lumbar disc degeneration: Correlation with age, sex, and spine level in 600 autopsy specimens. *Spine* 13:173–178.
70. Urban JPG, and Roberts S (2003) Degeneration of the intervertebral disc. *Arthritis Res Ther* 5(3):120–130.
71. Adams MA, McNally DS, and Dolan P (1996) Stress distributions inside intervertebral discs. The effects of age and degeneration. *J Bone Joint Surg Br* 78(6):965–972.
72. Ayotte DC, Ito K, and Tepic S (2001) Direction-dependent resistance to flow in the endplate of the intervertebral disc: An ex vivo study. *J Orthop Res* 19(6):1073–1077.
73. Ayotte DC, Ito K, Perren SM, and Tepic S (2000) Direction-dependent constriction flow in a poroelastic solid: The intervertebral disc valve. *J Biomech Eng* 122(6):587–593.
74. Accadbled F et al. (2008) Influence of location, fluid flow direction, and tissue maturity on the macroscopic permeability of vertebral end plates. *Spine (Phila Pa 1976)* 33(6):612–619.
75. Urban JP, Smith S, and Fairbank JC (2004) Nutrition of the intervertebral disc. *Spine* 29(23):2700–2709.
76. Urban JP, and Winlove CP (2007) Pathophysiology of the intervertebral disc and the challenges for MRI. *J Magn Reson Imaging* 25(2):419–432.

77. Roberts S, Menage J, and Eisenstein SM (1993) The cartilage end-plate and intervertebral disc in scoliosis: Calcification and other sequelae. *J Orthop Res* 11(5):747–757.
78. Roberts S, Urban JP, Evans H, and Eisenstein SM (1996) Transport properties of the human cartilage endplate in relation to its composition and calcification. *Spine* 21(4):415–420.
79. Urban MR et al. (2001) Electrochemical measurement of transport into scoliotic intervertebral discs in vivo using nitrous oxide as a tracer. *Spine (Phila Pa 1976)* 26(8):984–990.
80. Sakai D et al. (2005) Differentiation of mesenchymal stem cells transplanted to a rabbit degenerative disc model: Potential and limitations for stem cell therapy in disc regeneration. *Spine (Phila Pa 1976)* 30(21):2379–2387.
81. Watanabe K et al. (2003) Effect of reinsertion of activated nucleus pulposus on disc degeneration: An experimental study on various types of collagen in degenerative discs. *Connect Tissue Res* 44(2):104–108.
82. Ganey T et al. (2003) Disc chondrocyte transplantation in a canine model: A treatment for degenerated or damaged intervertebral disc. *Spine (Phila Pa 1976)* 28(23):2609–2620.
83. de Boer R (2000) Contemporary progress in porous media theory. *Appl Mech Rev* 53(12):323–370.
84. Buschmann MD, and Grodzinsky AJ (1995) A molecular model of proteoglycan-associated electrostatic forces in cartilage mechanics. *J Biomech Eng* 117(2):179–192.
85. Ehlers W, and Markert B (2001) A linear viscoelastic biphasic model for soft tissues based on the theory of porous media. *J Biomech Eng* 123(5):418–424.
86. Eisenberg SR, and Grodzinsky AJ (1988) Electrokinetic micromodel of extracellular-matrix and other poly-electrolyte networks. *Physicochem Hydrodyn* 10(4):517–539.
87. Huyghe JM, and Janssen JD (1997) Quadriphasic mechanics of swelling incompressible porous media. *Int J Eng Sci* 35(8):793–802.
88. Huyghe JM, and Janssen JD (1999) Thermo-chemo-electro-mechanical formulation of saturated charged porous solids. *Transport Porous Media* 34:129–141.
89. Levenston ME, Eisenberg SR, and Grodzinsky AJ (1998) A variational formulation for coupled physicochemical flows during finite deformations of charged porous media. *Int J Solids Struct* 35(34–35):4999–5019.
90. Mow VC, Kuei SC, Lai WM, and Armstrong CG (1980) Biphasic creep and stress relaxation of articular cartilage in compression: Theory and experiments. *J Biomech Eng* 102(1):73–84.
91. Huang CY et al. (1999) Anisotrpy, inhomogeneity, and tension-compression nonlinearity of human gelnohumeral cartilage in finite deformation. *Trans Orthop Res Soc* 24:95.
92. Huang CY, Mow VC, and Ateshian GA (2001) The role of flow-independent viscoelasticity in the biphasic tensile and compressive responses of articular cartilage. *J Biomech Eng* 123(5):410–417.
93. Setton LA, Zhu W, Weidenbaum M, Ratcliffe A, and Mow VC (1993) Compressive properties of the cartilaginous end-plate of the baboon lumbar spine. *J Orthop Res* 11(2):228–239.
94. Soltz MA, and Ateshian GA (2000) A Conewise Linear Elasticity mixture model for the analysis of tension-compression nonlinearity in articular cartilage. *J Biomech Eng* 122(6):576–586.
95. Katchalsky A, and Curran PF (1975) *Nonequilibrium Thermodynamics in Biophysics* (Harvard University Press, Cambridge, MA).
96. Trusdell C, and Noll W (1965) Non-linear field theories of mechanics. In *Handbuch der physik*, ed. Flugge S (Springer, Berlin), pp. 537–541.
97. Gu WY, Lewis B, Lai WM, Ratcliffe A, and Mow VC (1996) A technique for measuring volume and true density of the solid matrix of cartilaginous tissues. *Adv Bioeng, ASME* BED33:89–90.
98. Gu WY, Hung CT, Lai WM, and Mow VC (1997) Analysis of transient swelling of isolated cells. *Ann Biomed Eng* 25/S.1:S-80.
99. Gu WY, Lai WM, and Mow VC (1999) Transport of multi-electrolytes in charged hydrated biological soft tissues. *Transport Porous Media* 34:143–157.
100. Lai WM, Gu WY, and Mow VC (1994) Flows of electrolytes through charged hydrated biologic tissue. *Appl Mech Rev* 47(Part 2):277–281.
101. Lai WM, Gu WY, and Mow VC (1998) On the conditional equivalence of chemical loading and mechanical loading on articular cartilage. *J Biomech* 31(12):1181–1185.

102. Lai WM, Mow VC, Sun DD, and Ateshian GA (2000) On the electric potentials inside a charged soft hydrated biological tissue: Streaming potential versus diffusion potential. *J Biomech Eng* 122(4):336–346.

103. Lai WM, Sun DD, Ateshian GA, Guo XE, and Mow VC (2002) Electrical signals for chondrocytes in cartilage. *Biorheology* 39(1,2):39–45.

104. Mow VC, Ateshian GA, Lai WM, and Gu WY (1998) Effects of fixed charge density on the stress-relaxation behavior of hydrated soft tissues in a confined compression problem. *Int J Solids Struct* 35:4945–4962.

105. Sun DN, Gu WY, Guo XE, Lai WM, and Mow VC (1999) A mixed finite element formulation of triphasic mechano-electrochemical theory for charged, hydrated biological soft tissues. *Int J Numer Methods Eng* 45:1375–1402.

106. Gu WY, Sun DN, Lai WM, and Mow VC (2004) Analysis of the dynamic permeation experiment with implication to cartilaginous tissue engineering. *J Biomech Eng* 126(4):485–491.

107. Chammas P, Federspiel WJ, and Eisenberg SR (1994) A microcontinuum model of electrokinetic coupling in the extracellular matrix: Perturbation formulation and solution. *J Colloid Interface Sci* 168:526–538.

108. Cowin SC (1999) Bone poroelasticity. *J Biomech* 32(3):217–238.

109. Weinbaum S, and Curry FE (1995) Modelling the structural pathways for transcapillary exchange. *Symp Soc Exp Biol* 49:323–345.

110. Zeng Y, Cowin SC, and Weinbaum S (1994) A fiber matrix model for fluid flow and streaming potentials in the canaliculi of an osteon. *Ann Biomed Eng* 22(3):280–292.

111. Hung CT, Gu WY, and Mow VC (1998) Quantification of transient swelling behvaior in cultured chondrocytes to osmotic loading. *Trans Orthop Res Soc* 23:870.

112. Belytschko T, Kulak RF, Schultz AB, and Galante JO (1974) Finite element stress analysis of an intervertebral disc. *J Biomech* 7(3):277–285.

113. Kanayama M et al. (1995) A cineradiographic study on the lumbar disc deformation during flexion and extension of the trunk. *Clin Biomech* 10:193–199.

114. Kasra M, Shirazi-Adl A, and Drouin G (1992) Dynamics of human lumbar intervertebral joints. Experimental and finite-element investigations. *Spine* 17(1):93–102.

115. Kulak RF, Belyschko TB, and Schultz AB (1976) Nonlinear behavior of the human intervertebral disc under axial load. *J Biomech* 9:377–386.

116. Laible JP, Pflaster DS, Krag MH, Simon BR, and Haugh LD (1993) A poroelastic-swelling finite element model with application to the intervertebral disc. *Spine* 18(5):659–670.

117. Lin HS, Liu YK, Ray G, and Nikiavesh P (1978) Systems identification for material properties of the intervertebral joint. *J Biomech* 11:1–14.

118. Lu YM, Hutton WC, and Gharpuray VM (1996) Do bending, twisting, and diurnal fluid changes in the disc affect the propensity to prolapse? A viscoelastic finite element model. *Spine* 21(22):2570–2579.

119. Lu YM, Hutton WC, and Gharpuray VM (1998) The effect of fluid loss on the viscoelastic behavior of the lumbar intervertebral disc in compression. *J Biomech Eng* 120(1):48–54.

120. Shirazi-Adl SA, Shrivastava SC, and Ahmed AM (1984) Stress analysis of the lumbar disc-body unit in compression: A three dimensional nonlinear finite element study. *Spine* 9:120–134.

121. Shirazi-Adl SA, Ahmed AM, and Shrivastava SC (1986) A finite element study of a lumbar motion segment subjected to pure sagittal plane moments. *J Biomech* 19:331–350.

122. Simon BR, Wu JSS, Carlton MW, Evans JH, and Kazarian LE (1985) Structural models for human spinal motion segments based on a poroelastic view of the intervertebral disk. *J Biomech Eng* 107:327–335.

123. Simon BR, Liable JP, Pflaster D, Yuan Y, and Krag MH (1996) A poroelastic finite element formulation including transport and swelling in soft tissue structures. *J Biomech Eng* 118(1):1–9.

124. Snijders H et al. (1992) Triphasic material parameters of canine anulus fibrosus. In *Computer Methods in Biomechanics and Biomedical Engineering*, eds. Middleton J, Pande GN, and Williams KR (Books and Journals International, Ltd., Swansea, UK), pp. 220–229.

125. Spilker RL (1980) Mechanical behavior of a simple model of an intervertebral disk under compressive loading. *J Biomech* 13(10):895–901.
126. Spilker RL, Daugirda DM, and Schultz AB (1984) Mechanical response of a simple finite element model of the intervertebral disc under complex loading. *J Biomech* 17(2):103–112.
127. Ueno K, and Liu YK (1987) A three-dimensional nonlinear finite element model of lumbar intervertebral joint in torsion. *J Biomech Eng* 109:1987.
128. Whyne CM, Hu SS, and Lotz JC (2001) Parametric finite element analysis of vertebral bodies affected by tumors. *J Biomech* 34(10):1317–1324.
129. Ferguson SJ, Ito K, and Nolte LP (2004) Fluid flow and convective transport of solutes within the intervertebral disc. *J Biomech* 37:213–221.
130. Sun DN, Guo XE, Likhitpanichkul M, Lai WM, and Mow VC (2004) The influence of the fixed negative charges on mechanical and electrical behaviors of articular cartilage under unconfined compression. *J Biomech Eng* 126:6–16.
131. Yao H, and Gu WY (2004) Physical signals and solute transport in cartilage under dynamic unconfined compression: Finite element analysis. *Ann Biomed Eng* 32:380–390.
132. Iatridis JC, Laible JP, and Krag MH (2003) Influence of fixed charge density magnitude and distribution on the intervertebral disc: Applications of a poroelastic and chemical electric (PEACE) model. *J Biomech Eng* 125:12–24.
133. Jackson GW, and James DF (1986) The permeability of fibrous porous media. *Can J Chem Eng* 64:364–374.
134. Drummond JE, and Tahir MI (1984) Laminar viscous flow through regular arrays of parallel solid cylinders. *Int J Multiphase Flow* 10:515–540.
135. Happel J (1959) Viscous flow relative to arrays of cylinders. *AIChE J* 5:174–177.
136. Kuwabara S (1959) The forces experienced by randomly distributed parallel circular cylinders or spheres in a viscous flow at small Reynolds number. *J Phys Soc Jpn* 14:527–532.
137. Sangani AS, and Acrivos A (1982) Slow flow past periodic arrays of cylinders with application to heat transfer. *Int J Multiphase Flow* 8:193–206.
138. Spielman L, and Goren SL (1968) Model for predicting pressure drop and filtration efficiency in fibrous media. *Environ Sci Technol* 2:279–287.
139. Gu WY, and Yao H (2003) Effects of hydration and fixed charge density on fluid transport in charged hydrated soft tissue. *Ann Biomed Eng* 31(10):1162–1170.
140. Gu WY, Yao H, Huang CY, and Cheung HS (2003) New insight into deformation-dependent hydraulic permeability of gels and cartilage, and dynamic behavior of agarose gels in confined compression. *J Biomech* 36:593–598.
141. Mackie JS, and Meares P (1955) The diffusion of electrolytes in a cation-exchange resin. I. Theoretical. *Proc Roy Soc London* A232:498–509.
142. Ogston AG, Preston BN, and Wells JD (1973) On the transport of compact particles through solutions of chain-polymers. *Proc Roy Soc London* A333:297–316.
143. Brinkman HC (1947) A calculation of the viscous force exerted by a flowing fluid in a dense swarm of particles. *Appl Sci Res* A1:27–34.
144. Phillips RJ, Deen WM, and Brady JF (1989) Hindered transport of spherical macromolecules in fibrous membranes and gels. *AIChE J* 35:1761–1769.
145. Perrins WT, McKenzie DR, and McPhedran RC (1979) Transport properties of regular arrarys of cylinders. *Proc Roy Soc London A* 369:207–225.
146. Johansson L, and Lofroth JE (1993) Diffusion and interaction in gels and solutions. 4. Hard sphere Brownian dynamics simulations. *J Chem Phys* 98:7471–7479.
147. Johnson EM, Berk DA, Jain RK, and Deen WM (1996) Hindered diffusion in agarose gels: Test of effective medium model. *Biophys J* 70:1017–1026.
148. Burstein D, Gray ML, Hartman AL, Gipe R, and Foy BD (1993) Diffusion of small solutes in cartilage as measured by nuclear magnetic resonance (NMR) spectroscopy and imaging. *J Orthop Res* 11(4):465–478.
149. Gu WY, Yao H, Vega AL, and Flagler D (2004) Diffusivity of ions in agarose gels and intervertebral disc: Effect of porosity *Ann Biomed Eng* 32:1710–1717.

150. Biot MA (1941) General theory of three-dimensional consolidation. *J Appl Phys* 12:155–164.
151. Bowen RM (1980) Incompressible porous media models by use of the theory of mixtures. *Int J Eng Sci* 18:1129–1148.
152. Deen WM (1987) Hindered transport of large molecules in liquid-filled pores. *AIChE J* 33(9):1409–1425.
153. Yao H, and Gu WY (2007) Three-dimensional inhomogeneous triphasic finite element analysis of physical signals and solute transport in human intervertebral disc under axial compression. *J Biomech* 40:2071–2077.
154. Yao H, and Gu WY (2006) Physical signals and solute transport in human intervertebral disc during compressive stress relaxation: 3D finite element analysis. *Biorheology* 43:325–335.
155. Iatridis JC, Setton LA, Blood DC, Weidenbaum M, and Mow VC (1995) Mechanical behavior of the human nucleus pulposus in shear. *Trans Orthop Res Soc* 20:675.
156. Iatridis JC et al. (1998) Degeneration affects the anisotropic and nonlinear behaviors of human anulus fibrosus in compression. *J Biomech* 31(6):535–544.
157. Iatridis JC, Setton LA, Weidenbaum M, and Mow VC (1997) The viscoelastic behavior of the non-degenerate human lumbar nucleus pulposus in shear. *J Biomech* 30(10):1005–1013.
158. Iatridis JC, Setton LA, Weidenbaum M, and Mow VC (1997) Alterations in the mechanical behavior of the human lumbar nucleus pulposus with degeneration and aging. *J Orthop Res* 15(2):318–322.
159. Iatridis JC, Weidenbaum M, Setton LA, and Mow VC (1996) Is the nucleus pulposus a solid or a fluid? Mechanical behaviors of the nucleus pulposus of the human intervertebral disc. *Spine (Phila Pa 1976)* 21(10):1174–1184.
160. Yao H, and Gu WY (2006) Convection and diffusion in charged hydrated soft tissues: A mixture theory approach. *Biomech Model Mechanobiol* 6:63–72.
161. Huang CY, and Gu WY (2007) Effects of tension-compression nonlinearity on solute transport in charged hydrated fibrous tissues under dynamic unconfined compression. *J Biomech Eng* 129(3):423–429.
162. Garcia AM, Frank EH, Grimshaw PE, and Grodzinsky AJ (1996) Contributions of fluid convection and electrical migration to transport in cartilage: Relevance to loading. *Arch Biochem Biophys* 333(2):317–325.
163. Quinn TM, Morel V, and Meister JJ (2001) Static compression of articular cartilage can reduce solute diffusivity and partitioning: Implications for the chondrocyte biological response. *J Biomech* 34(11):1463–1469.
164. Leddy HA, and Guilak F (2003) Site-specific molecular diffusion in articular cartilage measured using fluorescence recovery after photobleaching. *Ann Biomed Eng* 31(7):753–760.
165. Evans RC, and Quinn TM (2006) Solute convection in dynamically compressed cartilage. *J Biomech* 39(6):1048–1055.
166. Selard E, Shirazi-Adl A, and Urban JP (2003) Finite element study of nutrient diffusion in the human intervertebral disc. *Spine* 28(17):1945–1953.
167. Soukane DM, Shirazi-Adl A, and Urban JP (2007) Computation of coupled diffusion of oxygen, glucose and lactic acid in an intervertebral disc. *J Biomech* 40(12):2645–2654.
168. Jackson AR, Huang CY, Brown MD, and Gu WY (2011) 3D finite element analysis of nutrient distributions and cell viability in the intervertebral disc: Effects of deformation and degeneration. *J Biomech Eng* 133(9):091006.
169. Huang CY, and Gu WY (2008) Effects of mechanical compression on metabolism and distribution of oxygen and lactate in intervertebral disc. *J Biomech* 41(6):1184–1196.
170. Soukane DM, Shirazi-Adl A, and Urban JP (2005) Analysis of nonlinear coupled diffusion of oxygen and lactic acid in intervertebral discs. *J Biomech Eng* 127(7):1121–1126.
171. Bibby SR, Jones DA, Ripley RM, and Urban JP (2005) Metabolism of the intervertebral disc: Effects of low levels of oxygen, glucose, and pH on rates of energy metabolism of bovine nucleus pulposus cells. *Spine (Phila Pa 1976)* 30(5):487–496.
172. Huang CY et al. (2007) Effects of low glucose concentrations on oxygen consumption rates of intervertebral disc cells. *Spine (Phila Pa 1976)* 32(19):2063–2069.

173. Holm S, Maroudas A, Urban JP, Selstam G, and Nachemson A (1981) Nutrition of the intervertebral disc: Solute transport and metabolism. *Connect Tissue Res* 8(2):101–119.

174. Ishihara H, and Urban JP (1999) Effects of low oxygen concentrations and metabolic inhibitors on proteoglycan and protein synthesis rates in the intervertebral disc. *J Orthop Res* 17(6):829–835.

175. Wu Y, Cisewski S, Sachs BL, and Yao H (2013) Effect of cartilage endplate on cell based disc regeneration: A finite element analysis. *Mol Cell Biomech* 10(2):159–182.

176. Roberts S, Menage J, and Urban JP (1989) Biochemical and structural properties of the cartilage end-plate and its relation to the intervertebral disc. *Spine* 14(2):166–174.

177. Maroudas A (1975) Biophysical chemistry of cartilaginous tissues with special reference to solute and fluid transport. *Biorheology* 12:233–248.

178. Bartels EM, Fairbank JC, Winlove CP, and Urban JP (1998) Oxygen and lactate concentrations measured in vivo in the intervertebral discs of patients with scoliosis and back pain. *Spine (Phila Pa 1976)* 23(1):1–7; discussion 8.

179. Urban JP, Holm S, Maroudas A, and Nachemson A (1982) Nutrition of the intervertebral disc: Effect of fluid flow on solute transport. *Clin Orthop Relat Res* (170):296–302.

180. O'Hara BP, Urban JP, and Maroudas A (1990) Influence of cyclic loading on the nutrition of articular cartilage. *Ann Rheum Dis* 49(7):536–539.

181. McMillan DW, Garbutt G, and Adams MA (1996) Effect of sustained loading on the water content of intervertebral discs: Implications for disc metabolism. *Ann Rheum Dis* 55(12):880–887.

182. Zhu Q, Jackson AR, and Gu WY (2012) Cell viability in intervertebral disc under various nutritional and dynamic loading conditions: 3D finite element analysis. *J Biomech* 45(16):2769–2777.

183. Mokhbi Soukane D, Shirazi-Adl A, and Urban JP (2009) Investigation of solute concentrations in a 3D model of intervertebral disc. *Eur Spine J* 18(2):254–262.

184. Shirazi-Adl A, Taheri M, and Urban JP (2010) Analysis of cell viability in intervertebral disc: Effect of endplate permeability on cell population. *J Biomech* 43(7):1330–1336.

185. Jackson AR, Huang CY, and Gu WY (2011) Effect of endplate calcification and mechanical deformation on the distribution of glucose in intervertebral disc: A 3D finite element study. *Comput Methods Biomech Biomed Eng* 14(2):195–204.

186. Bibby SR, and Urban JP (2004) Effect of nutrient deprivation on the viability of intervertebral disc cells. *Eur Spine J* 13(8):695–701.

187. Kandel R, Roberts S, and Urban JP (2008) Tissue engineering and the intervertebral disc: The challenges. *Eur Spine J* 17 Suppl 4:480–491.

188. Travascio F, and Gu WY (2007) Anisotropic diffusive transport in annulus fibrosus: Experimental determination of the diffusion tensor by FRAP technique. *Ann Biomed Eng* 35(10):1739–1748.

189. Jackson AR, Yuan TY, Huang CY, Travascio F, and Yong Gu W (2008) Effect of compression and anisotropy on the diffusion of glucose in annulus fibrosus. *Spine (Phila Pa 1976)* 33(1):1–7.

190. Shi C, Kuo J, Bell PD, and Yao H (2010) Anisotropic solute diffusion tensor in porcine TMJ discs measured by FRAP with spatial Fourier analysis. *Ann Biomed Eng* 38(11):3398–3408.

191. Wuertz K et al. (2007) Influence of extracellular osmolarity and mechanical stimulation on gene expression of intervertebral disc cells. *J Orthop Res* 25(11):1513–1522.

192. Oswald ES et al. (2011) Effects of hypertonic (NaCl) two-dimensional and three-dimensional culture conditions on the properties of cartilage tissue engineered from an expanded mature bovine chondrocyte source. *Tissue Eng Part C, Methods* 17(11):1041–1049.

7

Multiscale Modeling of Cardiovascular Flows

Alison L. Marsden and Ethan Kung

CONTENTS

ABSTRACT Simulations of blood flow in the cardiovascular system offer investigative and predictive capabilities to augment current clinical tools. Using image-based modeling, the Navier–Stokes equations can be solved to obtain detailed three-dimensional (3D) hemodynamics in patient-specific anatomical models. Relevant parameters such as wall shear stress and particle residence times can then be calculated from the 3D results and correlated with clinical data for treatment planning and device evaluation. Reduced-order models such as open- or closed-loop 0D lumped-parameter models can simulate the dynamic behavior of the circulatory system using an analogy to electrical circuits. When coupled to 3D simulations as boundary conditions, they produce physiologically realistic pressure and flow conditions in the 3D domain. We describe fundamentals and current state of the art of patient-specific, multiscale computational modeling approaches applied to cardiovascular disease. These tools enable investigations of hemodynamics reflecting individual patients' physiology, and we provide several illustrative case studies. These methods can supplement current clinical measurement and imaging capabilities and provide predictions of patient outcomes for surgical planning and risk stratification.

7.1 Introduction to Cardiovascular Simulation

Simulations of blood flow in the cardiovascular system offer a means to augment current medical imaging modalities and physician experience to potentially improve treatment outcomes for a range of cardiovascular diseases. Perhaps more importantly, simulations offer predictive capabilities to test new surgical concepts, medical devices, and postoperative surgical outcomes. Recent advances in computing technology and efficient algorithms have led to increasingly realistic and accurate simulations, which now capture physiologic levels of blood pressure, detailed anatomy, feedback mechanisms of the circulatory system, and vessel wall deformations [1–4].

Early work in fluid mechanics of blood flow produced analytical solutions of the Navier–Stokes equations for pulsatile flow in rigid and elastic tubes. These solutions were derived by J.R. Womersley in the 1950s and are now widely used, in particular as boundary conditions for large-scale flow simulations [5–10]. Following this, starting in the 1960s, lumped-parameter models of the circulatory system were developed by analogy to electrical circuits [11–13]. These models have the advantage that they are governed by ordinary differential equations (ODEs) and can be readily solved in near real time on a desktop computer. While they do not provide spatial information, they can be quite complex, providing a surprisingly realistic representation of circulatory dynamics. The one-dimensional (1D) equations of blood flow (introduced by Hughes and others in the 1970s) also offer an attractive means to obtain near real-time solutions of circulatory flow dynamics and can be coupled to three-dimensional (3D) solvers as boundary conditions [14,15].

The advent of patient-specific modeling in the 1990s paved the way for increasingly detailed flow and pressure information to be solved on an individualized basis. Starting from patient image data (typically magnetic resonance imaging [MRI] or computed tomography [CT]), a 3D model is constructed to represent a portion of the anatomy, often including a diseased region of interest [16–20]. Since only a portion of a patient's anatomy can be included in the 3D model, attributed to both computational expense and limits of image resolution, boundary conditions must be applied at inlets and outlets of the model to accurately represent the vascular network outside. Patient-specific modeling has been applied to a wide range of cardiovascular disease applications, including abdominal aortic aneurysms, cerebral aneurysms, coronary artery disease, heart valves, and congenital heart disease [3,4,21,22]. In this chapter, we first outline the procedures for patient-specific modeling and available methods for flow simulations. We then outline the basic mathematical formulations for boundary conditions and multiscale modeling methods used in computational fluid dynamics (CFD) simulations of blood flow.

7.2 Governing Equations for Hemodynamics

Blood flow is governed by the Navier–Stokes equations, which are, for an incompressible, Newtonian fluid,

$$\frac{\partial u}{\partial t} + u \cdot \nabla u = -\frac{1}{\rho}\nabla p + \mu \nabla^2 u,$$

$$\nabla u = 0.$$

While non-Newtonian effects are known to be important in specific scenarios, for example in capillary flow, we focus here on Newtonian flows, which is a widely accepted assumption for large vessel hemodynamics [23].

These equations can be solved numerically using finite volume or finite element methods (FEMs), among others, with appropriate boundary and initial conditions. This typically requires high-performance parallel computing, with significant computational requirements. Issues that must be addressed when choosing a numerical method for the CFD solver include mesh resolution, complex geometry, use of artificial dissipation, and ability to resolve small-scale structures in the flow.

7.3 Current Methods for Patient-Specific Modeling

7.3.1 Patient-Specific Model Construction

Patient-specific simulations are typically performed on 3D models of vascular anatomy that are derived from patient image data. Depending on the disease application, either CT or MRI data are typically used. Image data may be segmented using two-dimensional (2D) or 3D level set or thresholding methods [24–26]. Common packages for image segmentation include open source packages such as SimVascular (simvascular.org) or ITK-SNAP, or commercial packages such as Mimics (Materialise, Leuven, Belgium). The typical steps for model construction using 2D methods are as follows: (1) create paths along vessels of interest, (2) manually or automatically draw segmentations of the vessel lumen at discrete locations along the paths, (3) loft (interpolate) the segmentations together to create a 3D solid model, and (4) mesh the model for use with a CFD solver. The typical steps for model construction using a 2D method are shown in Figure 7.1 for a patient-specific model of the normal cerebral vasculature. Advantages of 2D methods are the ability to smoothly represent vascular tree-like branching patterns, such as occur in the pulmonary arteries. Advantages of 3D methods include the ability to more readily capture details of local complex geometry, particularly in aneurysms or complex surgical connections. Ultimately, it is likely a combination of both methods that will prove most advantageous in future work. While automated methods do exist for both 2D and 3D segmentation, noise in the image data often leads to significant user intervention and the need for manual segmentation. Improvements in automated segmentation methods, for example, by applying machine learning algorithms, would greatly improve efficiency, reduce user input, and enable high-throughput model construction for clinical applications [27].

7.3.2 Computational Methods for Blood Flow Simulation

Both finite element and finite volume methods have been used to solve the Navier–Stokes equations in cardiovascular applications. FEMs, which are most widely used, are well suited to complex geometries with unstructured meshes. Most recent work has used

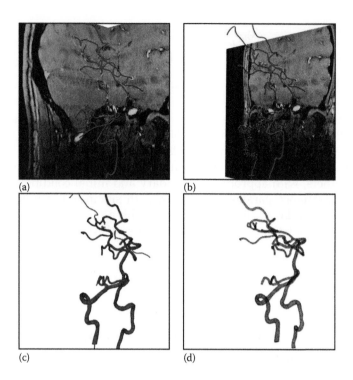

FIGURE 7.1
The steps in model construction using the SimVascular software package with 2D segmentation methods:
(a) creation of pathlines down the center of vessels of interest, (b) 2D segmentation of the vessel lumen, (c) lofting the segmentations to construct a 3D model, and (d) creation of an unstructured mesh for use in a flow solver.
Example shown is construction of a patient-specific model of the vertebral vasculature from MRI data. (Image
courtesy of CVET.)

stabilized (SUPG) methods with linear elements, but higher-order elements have also been
employed [28–30]. In the FEM approach, the weak form of the Navier–Stokes equations
is solved. While commercial solvers can be used on a limited basis, custom solvers offer
more flexibility and control over boundary condition implementation, which is essential
for obtaining an accurate solution.

Immersed boundary methods, introduced by Peskin in the 1970s, offer an attractive
alternative in many situations and have been successfully applied to heart mechanics and
device design [31–33]. These methods offer the advantage of using structured grids for
improved solver efficiency, but the disadvantage of limited mesh resolution in key areas
such as near-wall boundary layers. They are particularly attractive for fluid–structure
interaction problems. Unstructured finite volume methods also offer an attractive alternative to FEM methods, particularly with noncommercial codes that do not require additional stabilization terms. These methods have been shown to more accurately capture
cycle-to-cycle variations in unsteady flow in aneurysms, showing surprising evidence of
turbulence at low Reynolds numbers [34,35].

7.3.3 Fluid–Structure Interaction

Deformation of the vessel walls can be included via fluid–structure interaction simulations, in which the solid and fluid domain problems are solved simultaneously using

either iterative coupling or strong coupling, as in arbitrary Lagrangian–Eulerian methods. Strongly coupled methods are particularly attractive for large deformation problems, including membrane buckling, valves, and ventricular mechanics [36,37]. However, their computational cost can make them prohibitively expensive for some applications. Immersed boundary methods offer an attractive alternative, which allows for use of structured mesh solvers in problems with complex geometries. Other approaches to reduce computational cost include the coupled momentum method of Figueroa and Taylor, which relies on a small deformation approximation based on Womersley theory to impose forces on the fluid domain without requiring mesh motion [1,38].

7.4 The Importance of Boundary Conditions

The choice of boundary conditions is of paramount importance in cardiovascular simulations, as the local flow dynamics are greatly influenced by conditions upstream and downstream of the 3D model. Numerous studies have demonstrated drastic differences in flow solutions, even with simple geometries, and particularly in models with multiple outlets [2,39,40]. Commonly used outlet boundary conditions such as zero pressure or zero traction, while easiest to implement, are well known to lead to unrealistic solutions, in part because of their inability to capture physiologic levels of pressure. These methods should not be used for fluid–structure interaction problems where the wall deformation depends directly on the pressure level in the vessel.

7.4.1 Inflow Boundary Conditions

A typical model with inlets and outlets requiring a variety of boundary conditions is shown in Figure 7.2. Inflow boundary conditions are typically enforced at the inlet of the 3D model, and three choices are commonly available. The simplest choice is to use a plug flow condition, applying a uniform velocity profile. However, this assumption is known to be invalid for flow in a pipe, particularly in unsteady flow. A more realistic choice is to impose a parabolic flow profile using the Poiseuille solution for flow in a circular pipe, a well-known analytical solution of the Navier–Stokes equations in cylindrical coordinates where the axial component of velocity u_z is

$$u_z = -\frac{dp}{dz}\frac{1}{4\mu}(R^2 - r^2).$$

Further improvement can be made by using the analytical solution for pulsatile flow in a pipe of Womersley, which is given by

$$u_z(r,t) = \frac{A}{i\rho\omega}\left[1 - \frac{J_0\left(i^{\frac{3}{2}}r\sqrt{\frac{\omega}{\nu}}\right)}{J_0\left(R\sqrt{\frac{\omega}{\nu}}i^{\frac{3}{2}}\right)}\right]e^{i\omega t},$$

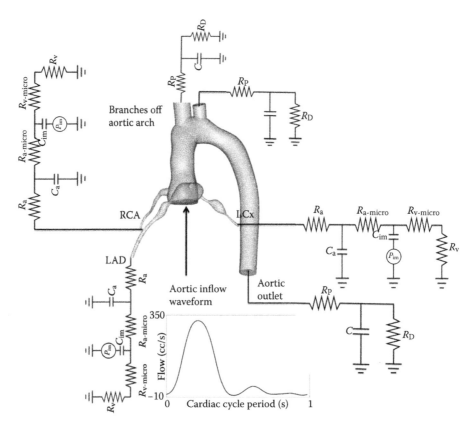

FIGURE 7.2

A typical patient-specific model of the aorta and coronary arteries in a patient with Kawasaki disease, illustrating the application of inflow and outflow boundary conditions. The model requires application of an aortic inflow condition, and lumped RCR models for the aorta and aortic branch vessels, with a specialized lumped coronary model.

where A is the amplitude of sinusoidal pressure oscillation, ω is the frequency, J_0 is the tabulated Bessel function of the first kind, and R is the vessel radius. Full derivation of this solution as well as the solution for a general waveform and for an elastic tube has been presented by Zamir and others [5,41,42].

7.4.2 Outflow Boundary Conditions

The choice of outflow boundary conditions in cardiovascular modeling is a much more complex issue compared to the choice of inflow conditions. Typical choices include zero-pressure or zero-traction conditions applied at the outlet, resistance or impedance conditions, reduced-order models that can be open or closed loop, or reduced-order 1D wave propagation equations. It is desirable to choose a boundary condition that can capture physiologic levels of pressure, particularly for applications involving deformable walls. In this section, we outline several common choices for outflow boundary condition prescription using zero-pressure or lumped-parameter models and illustrate their effects on simulation results.

The vascular resistances in the arterioles and capillaries are largely responsible for producing the blood pressures observed in the large arteries. The same vascular resistances are also responsible for regulating the distribution of blood flow into different regions of the body. A fluid dynamic simulation of large arteries alone, without consideration of the smaller downstream vessels, neglects this important effect of vascular resistance.

Figure 7.3a shows an example of such a scenario, where a zero-pressure outflow boundary condition is used. The pressure in the 3D domain is much lower than normal physiological levels, and the amount of flow through the two different outlets is solely determined by the vessel geometry. Without any downstream resistances, small variations in the conduit resistance in the 3D domain lead to drastic flow bias. In the example shown, the average flow rates through the main and branch outlet are 43 and 2 mL/s, respectively, meaning that almost no flow is passing through the branch outlet. Also, as a result of near-zero pressure, the outlet flows are artificially sensitive to small pressure perturbations in the 3D domain from accelerations of fluid. This artifact is seen in the example as the branch outlet exhibiting reverse flow during the deceleration phase of the inflow waveform. This is inconsistent with most physiological scenarios where the larger branch is more likely to exhibit reversed flow. Due to various artifacts and the lack of ability to mimic realistic vascular impedances, the resulting pressure, flow, and flow split from using a zero-pressure boundary condition usually cannot reflect realistic physiological conditions.

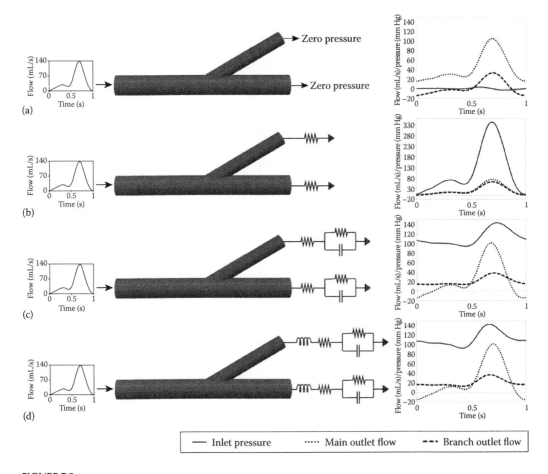

FIGURE 7.3
Examples of outflow BC prescriptions and effects on simulation results. (a) Zero pressure. (b) Resistance. (c) Resistance–capacitance–resistance. (d) Inductance–resistance–capacitance–resistance.

Resistance outflow boundary conditions are a simple approach to partially capture the effects of downstream vasculature, thereby achieving appropriate flow split between the outlets. Figure 7.3b shows an example simulation with the same 3D geometry as Figure 7.3a but with resistance outflow boundary conditions. The ratio between the resistances at the two outlets was adjusted to vary the flow split; the average flow rates through the main and branch outlet are now 24 and 21 mL/s, respectively. The flows through the outlets are now governed principally by the outflow resistances and no longer by small resistance and pressure perturbations in the 3D domain. Note that with resistance outlet boundary condition prescription, there is a direct linear relationship between the flow and pressure. The pressure waveform and the flow waveforms through the two outlets all have the same shape and no phase lag relative to each other. More importantly, this direct linear relationship can lead to large swings in pressure as flow varies over time. In the example shown, the average pressure over the cardiac cycle is 112 mm Hg, which is physiologically realistic, but the pressure peak is unrealistically high because of the pulsatile inflow. In summary, resistance outflow boundary conditions can be useful in steady or near-steady flow cases, but for pulsatile flow conditions, a more complicated lumped-parameter model outflow boundary condition should be used.

Due to blood vessel compliance, wave propagation occurs in the vasculature, leading to pressure and flow waveforms with different shapes and phases. Outflow boundary condition prescription using a Windkessel model containing a capacitance element can account for the downstream vessel compliance and add another level of realism to the simulation. Using the same outlet resistances as in Figure 7.3b, we now add in a capacitance element to observe the resulting effect in Figure 7.3c. The pressure and flows through the outlets averaged across the cardiac cycle (112 mm Hg, 24 mL/s through the main outlet, 21 mL/s through the branch outlet) are the same as in the case represented in Figure 7.3b, but we can see that there are now waveform shape and phase differences between pressure and flow, as well as between the flows through the different outlets. In addition, the energy storage of the capacitor allows the pressure oscillation to be dampened and results in more realistic pressure peaks. This enables greater flexibility for the simulation to capture desired physiological scenarios.

The momentum of the flowing blood presents another variable that affects the relationship between pressure and flow. We can capture the blood momentum effects in the downstream vasculature by incorporating inductance elements in the outflow boundary Windkessel model. Keeping the same outlet resistance and capacitance values, Figure 7.3d shows an example simulation with Windkessel outflow boundary conditions now containing inductances. Note that there is an additional phase difference between pressure and flow due to the inductance elements. Compared with Figure 7.3c, the pressure waveform is shifted forward in time and now peaks before the flow peak. The phase difference between the outlet flows can also be adjusted via the ratio of the outlet inductance values. In a practical situation, the inductance offers another degree of adjustment to achieve correct pressure and flow phase differences.

Using resistance, capacitance, and inductance elements in lumped-parameter circuits, we can fully capture the important relevant phenomena occurring in the downstream vasculature and achieve realistic boundary condition prescription for the fluid dynamic simulation.

7.5 Modeling the Circulation with a Lumped-Parameter Network

Here we present the mathematical formulations for some of the aforementioned lumped-parameter boundary conditions, as well as for a heart and a coronary circulation model.

In lumped-parameter networks, we *lump* the resistive, elastic, and inertial properties of blood flow through vessels into elements analogous to those in an electric circuit. We then solve the associated set of ODEs governing the electrical circuit. The values of circuit elements are tuned to match physiologically realistic values for flow, pressure, and other quantities.

We use the basic circuit element relations defining a resistor, capacitor and inductor, with appropriate analogies to fluid dynamics as follows:

$$V = IR \Leftrightarrow \Delta P = QR \text{ (resistor)}$$

$$V = \frac{d}{dt} LI \Leftrightarrow P = \frac{d}{dt} LQ \text{ (inductor)}$$

$$I = \frac{d}{dt} CV \Leftrightarrow Q = \frac{d}{dt} CP \text{ (capacitor)}$$

Blood viscosity acts to resist flow for a given pressure drop so that, from above,

$$Q = \frac{\Delta P}{R}.$$

Hence, increasing resistance leads to a lower flow rate for a fixed pressure gradient. We recall that for Poiseuille flow, resistance to flow is

$$R = \frac{8\mu l}{\pi a^4},$$

where a is the vessel radius and l is the vessel length, so that resistance drops dramatically with increasing vessel radius.

7.5.1 Windkessel Models

A basic lumped model is a simple three-element Windkessel model containing two resistors and a capacitor. This model accounts for the energy loss owing to viscosity and energy storage owing to vessel distensibility of the vasculature. Windkessel in German means *air chamber*, but is generally taken to imply an elastic reservoir. In the realm of the cardiovascular system, the vessel compliances act as this elastic reservoir.

Applying Kirchhoff's current law (conservation of mass) to the three-element model shown in Figure 7.4, we have

$$Q = Q_r = Q_C + Q_R$$

and the element relations are given by

$$Q_C = C \frac{dp_d}{dt}$$

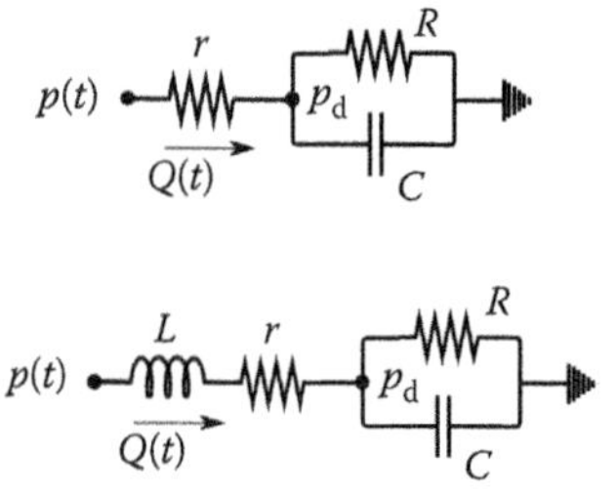

FIGURE 7.4
Lumped-parameter models.

$$p - p_d = Qr$$

$$p_d = Q_R R,$$

where $p - p_d$ is the pressure drop across the proximal resistor. The above relations can be combined into a single ODE, together with conservation of mass, and time constant $\tau = RC$ to obtain

$$\frac{dp}{dt} + p\frac{1}{\tau} = r\frac{dQ}{dt} + \frac{1}{\tau}(r+R)Q,$$

which has solution

$$p(t) = e^{-\frac{t}{\tau}}\left[\int_0^t e^{\frac{s}{\tau}}\left[r\frac{dQ(s)}{ds} + \frac{1}{\tau}(r+R)Q(s)\right]ds + p(0)\right].$$

Referring again to Figure 7.2, we note that the RCR circuit can be used as a boundary condition for large vessels such as the aorta and branch vessels going to the head and neck. In this case, the RCR circuit models the proximal and distal resistance and capacitance of the vasculature distal to the outlet of the model.

The four-element Windkessel model incorporates the inertia of blood in the proximal circulation by adding an inductor to the three-element model. Conservation of mass for this circuit implies

$$Q = Q_r = Q_L = Q_C + Q_R$$

and the element relations are given as

$$p - p_d = L\frac{dQ_L}{dt} + Q_r r,$$

$$Q_C = C\frac{dp_d}{dt},$$

$$p_d = Q_R R.$$

Continuity combined with the last two element relations produces the ODE

$$\frac{dp_d}{dt} + \frac{p_d}{RC} = \frac{Q}{C}.$$

Continuity combined with the first element relation produces

$$p = L\frac{dQ}{dt} + Qr + p_d,$$

which can then be solved using the solution from the first ODE.

7.5.2 A Sample Heart Model

A simple ventricle model can be assembled using the resistor, capacitor, and inductor components described above, with the addition of a diode to represent the heart valve and an elastance function to model ventricular contraction, as shown in Figure 7.5. Given variables P_u, L_u, R_d, E_d, V_{d0}, we model the inductor with

$$\frac{dQ_v}{dt} = \frac{1}{L_u}(P_u - P_d),$$

the capacitor with

$$P_d = \frac{1}{C_d}(V_d - V_{d0}),$$

where V_{d0} is the volume of the downstream chamber at zero pressure, and the resistor with

$$P_d = Q_d R_d.$$

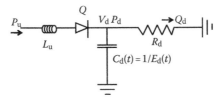

FIGURE 7.5
Sample heart model circuit.

We require that flow goes only one direction through the valve, such that we must have $P_u > P_d$ for an open valve. We wish to derive a set of ODEs to govern this model. We start by relating pressure to elastance by

$$P_d = E_d(t)[V_d - V_{d0}].$$

Substituting this into the inductor equation above, we have

$$\frac{dQ_v}{dt} = \frac{1}{L_u}\left\{P_u - E_d(t)[V_d - V_{d0}]\right\},$$

and substituting this into the equation for resistance, we have

$$Q_d = \frac{E_d[V_d - V_{d0}]}{R_d}.$$

The difference in flow through the valve and downstream is

$$\frac{dV_d}{dt} = Q_v - Q_d = Q_v - \frac{E_d(V_d - V_{d0})}{R_d}$$

from the equation above. This results in two ODEs for ventricular volume and flow

$$\frac{dQ_v}{dt} = \frac{1}{L_u}\left\{P_u - E_d[V_d - V_{d0}]\right\}$$

$$\frac{dV_d}{dt} = Q_v - \frac{E_d(V_d - V_{d0})}{R_d},$$

which can be solved for two scenarios: (1) valve closed such that $P_d \geq P_u$ and $Q_v = 0$, and (2) valve open such that $P_u > P_d$ and we evaluate Q_v.

7.5.3 A Coronary Artery Lumped Model

The coronary arteries are particularly challenging to model because of the interaction of coronary resistance with heart contraction. Coronary flow peaks during diastole, when aortic flow is at a minimum, because coronary vascular resistance is reduced with ventricular relaxation. On the other hand, during systole, coronary resistance is high because of ventricular contraction, and coronary flow is at a minimum. This is particularly pronounced in the left coronary artery. A lumped model for use as a coronary artery boundary condition was proposed by Kim et al. and is shown in Figure 7.6 [43,44]. This circuit is governed by the following second-order ODE:

$$p_2 \frac{d^2P}{dt^2} + p_1 \frac{dP}{dt} + p_0 P = q_2 \frac{d^2Q}{dt^2} + q_1 \frac{dQ}{dt} + q_0 Q + b_1 \frac{dP_{im}}{dt},$$

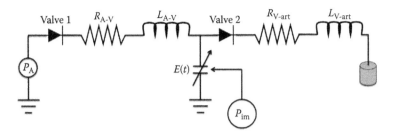

FIGURE 7.6
Sample coronary lumped model circuit.

where $P(t)$ and $Q(t)$ are the time-varying pressure and flow, the constants are functions of the resistances and compliances of the lumped model, and $P_{im}(t)$ is the intramyocardial pressure. This ODE has analytic solution

$$P(t) = \left(RQ(t) + \int_0^t e^{\lambda_1(t-s)} Z_1 Q(s)\, ds \right) - \int_0^t e^{\lambda_2(t-s)} Z_2 Q(s)\, ds$$
$$+ (Ae^{\lambda_1 t} - Be^{\lambda_2 t}) + \left(\int_0^t e^{\lambda_1(t-s)} Y_1 P_{im}(s)\, ds - \int_0^t e^{\lambda_2(t-s)} Y_2 P_{im}(s)\, ds \right),$$

where the constants are obtained from coefficients of the ODE and initial conditions, as described previously by Kim et al. Now directing our attention back to Figure 7.2, we observe that these coronary lumped models can be coupled to a 3D model. Because there is a known analytic solution to this ODE, coupling can be done monolithically using the multidomain method introduced by Vignon et al. and following the work of Kim et al. [2,43].

7.6 Modeling the Circulation with the 1D Equations of Blood Flow

An alternative to the lumped-parameter approach is to solve the 1D equations of blood flow, which offers a compromise between full 3D models and 0D lumped-parameter networks with no spatial dimension. Derivations of the 1D equations can be found in previous work, along with details of coupling algorithms [14].

7.7 Closed-Loop Multiscale Simulations

To capture the interaction between the 3D domain and the circulatory system, it is necessary to couple 3D simulations to reduced-order models such as 1D equations or lumped-parameter models that capture circulatory dynamics [45]. The open-loop lumped-parameter models described above can be expanded to full closed-loop networks that can then be coupled to the 3D domain [3,46–48].

A closed-loop lumped-parameter model has the advantage that the effects from all parts of the circulation are fully coupled together to influence the overall simulated physiology. Figure 7.7 shows an example of a closed-loop multiscale simulation setup. Compared to the open-loop examples presented in Figure 7.3, there is no longer any prescribed fixed inflow to the 3D domain, but rather the boundary conditions result from solving the 0D model equations, which describe the responses of the heart as well as different parts of the circulation to pressure and flow. We have discussed the importance of the boundary conditions provided by reduced-order models in a simulation. In a closed-loop scenario, the 3D domain presents itself to the 0D model as a time-varying resistance, inductance, and capacitance (in the case of deformable wall simulation) that are functions of the flow patterns within the 3D domain. The 0D model behavior is affected by this 3D model behavior and thus provides boundary conditions that are fully coupled to the 3D domain, forming a complete feedback loop.

Closed-loop multiscale models have been particularly useful in modeling coronary flows, as well as complex surgeries in pediatric cardiology applications [3]. For example,

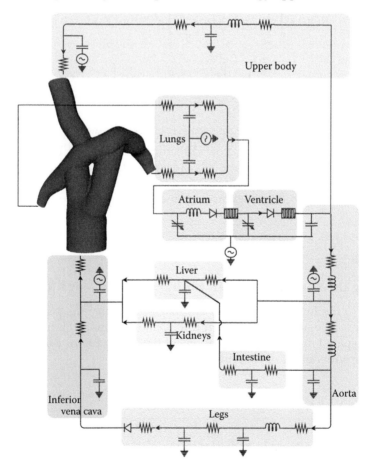

FIGURE 7.7
Sample closed-loop 3D/0D coupled simulation setup.

the effects of a surgical shunt in single ventricle patients can be investigated using such a model, which enables considerations of how the shunt resistance influences the balance of blood flow through various pathways in light of other systemic resistances and heart behavior [47,49,50].

7.8 Example Case Studies

7.8.1 Virtual Surgeries of the Superior Cavopulmonary Connection

In this case study, we demonstrate the application of patient-specific computational modeling to the virtual planning of surgical procedures. We demonstrate the power and potential of modeling to predict vascular surgical outcomes and obtain detailed hemodynamic information at zero risk to the patient, through a case study of a patient-specific model of a single ventricle stage 2 procedure.

Single ventricle congenital defects result in a heart that has only one functional pumping chamber. Palliation for these conditions typically requires a three-staged operative process, where a shunt is placed between the systemic and pulmonary arteries in stage 1, and the superior venous return is connected to the pulmonary circulation in stage 2. The stage 2 palliative surgery has two options: the *Glenn* or *Hemi-Fontan* procedures [51]. The Glenn procedure involves directly connecting the superior vena cava to the right pulmonary artery, and the Hemi-Fontan procedure involves reconstruction of the right atrium and pulmonary artery to allow for an enlarged confluence with the superior vena cava. Various degrees of pulmonary stenosis are also common among these patients, and additional surgical steps are often taken to remove the stenosis during the stage 2 procedure. Using a multiscale blood flow simulation, we can computationally investigate the hemodynamic differences between the Glenn and the Hemi-Fontan surgical options, as well as the necessity of pulmonary stenosis (if one is present) palliation during the stage 2 surgery.

The computational model is created using the preoperative imaging and clinical data acquired in the patient. From the patient imaging data, we can construct a preoperative 3D model that is a representation of the patient's preoperative anatomy. Then, based on the preoperative 3D model, we perform *virtual* Glenn or Hemi-Fontan surgeries by computationally modifying the preoperative 3D model. Additionally, we add a *virtual* left pulmonary stenosis to create different 3D models representing various stage 2 scenarios (Figure 7.8). Using the preoperative clinical data, we also tune the closed-loop lumped-parameter network (0D model) to represent the systemic circulation of the patient and couple the network to the 3D model to complete a multiscale simulation setup (Figure 7.9).

Using commercial mesh generation software (MESHSIM, Simmetrix, Inc., New York), the 3D models are discretized into isotropic finite-element meshes with a maximum edge size of 0.3 mm and containing 864,000 to 1.3 million linear tetrahedral elements. We couple the 3D anatomical model to the lumped-parameter network and numerically compute the coupled system using custom stabilized FEM solving the incompressible Navier–Stokes equations (SimVascular; http://simtk.org) while assuming nonmoving vessel walls [45,52]. Neumann boundary conditions are applied between the 3D and 0D models, in which the 3D model receives pressure information from the 0D model and returns flow information to the 0D model. Flow and pressure in the 0D model are computed from a set of

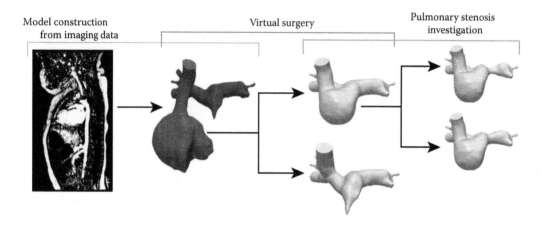

FIGURE 7.8

The process of preoperative 3D anatomical model construction from imaging data, virtual stage 2 surgery, and virtual pulmonary stenosis.

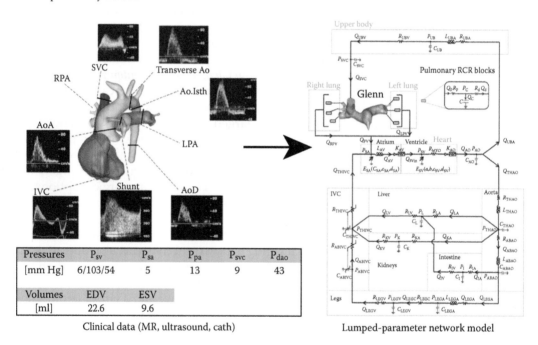

Pressures	P_{sv}	P_{sa}	P_{pa}	P_{svc}	P_{dao}
[mm Hg]	6/103/54	5	13	9	43

Volumes	EDV	ESV
[ml]	22.6	9.6

Clinical data (MR, ultrasound, cath)   Lumped-parameter network model

FIGURE 7.9

Preoperative clinical data, and the 0D lumped-parameter network model coupled to the 3D anatomical model.

algebraic and ODEs derived from the lumped-parameter network, using a fourth-order Runge–Kutta method.

We extract clinically relevant information from the results of these multiscale simulations, such as the 3D pressure and flow in the anatomical model (Figure 7.10), time tracings of various quantities in the circulation (Figure 7.11), measures of power loss in the surgical junction relative to other systemic powers (Figure 7.12), and so on. From the results of this case study, we see that the different surgical options and pulmonary palliation would not greatly affect the physiologies at the systemic level. However, local fluid dynamics differences do exist in

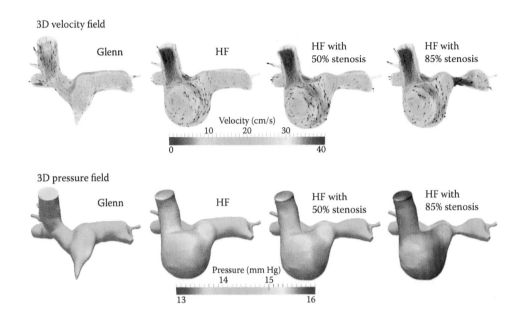

FIGURE 7.10
3D domain simulation results.

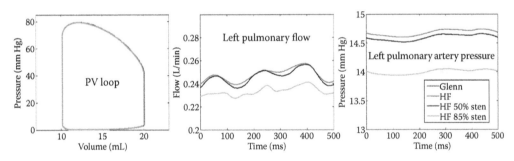

FIGURE 7.11
Time tracing of various physiological parameters.

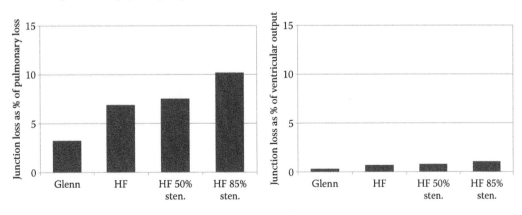

FIGURE 7.12
Power loss in the surgical junction as a fraction of other systemic powers.

the surgical junction, and the 3D hemodynamics data can be used to consider clinical issues such as thrombotic risk. In addition, the analysis of power loss within the surgical junction relative to systemic power can be used to provide pulmonary stenosis palliation decision support. In this particular example case and under the physiology investigated, it appears that a 50% or 85% area stenosis would not introduce a significant load to the cardiovascular system as a whole or significantly affect overall physiology. The results extracted from these simulations suggest that hemodynamic differences between the surgical options for this particular patient may be small and that surgical considerations could place higher priorities to other factors such as procedural risk or the confidence of the surgeon toward different procedures.

7.8.2 Thrombotic Risk in Kawasaki Disease Aneurysms

In this example, we show how blood flow simulation is applied to investigate hemodynamics in coronary artery aneurysms caused by Kawasaki disease (KD) and how they differ from the hemodynamics in healthy coronary arteries [4].

KD is an acute vasculitis occurring primarily in young children. The acute phase of the disease can damage the coronary arteries and leave coronary aneurysms in approximately 25% of untreated cases [53] and 3%–5% of intravenous immunoglobulin-treated cases [54]. These coronary aneurysms elevate the risk of thrombosis, which can then lead to myocardial infarction and sudden death [55]. Without a thrombotic episode, patients with KD coronary aneurysms are typically asymptomatic, and patient selection for treatments such as systemic anticoagulation and coronary artery bypass surgery [56] is challenging. Hemodynamic parameters from blood flow simulations may ultimately provide an estimate for the risk of thrombosis and help guide patient management.

Based on clinical imaging data from a 10-year-old patient who had suffered KD at age 3, and developed giant coronary artery aneurysms, we constructed a 3D computational model of the patient anatomy (Figure 7.13a). Another 3D model was created to represent a normal healthy coronary artery anatomy by replacing the aneurysmal regions with normal coronary geometry (Figure 7.13b). This allows for a direct comparison of hemodynamic differences between the normal and pathological states of the same patient. We construct a finite element mesh for each model using commercial software (Symmetrix, Inc., Troy, New York). Adaptive meshing with a minimum mesh size of 0.2 mm is then

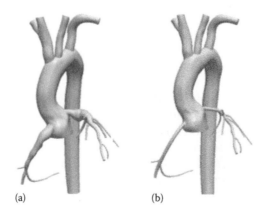

(a)   (b)

FIGURE 7.13
3D models of aorta and coronary arteries (a) with and (b) without aneurysms. (From Sengupta D et al., *Biomechanics and Modeling in Mechanobiology*, 11(6):915–932, 2012.)

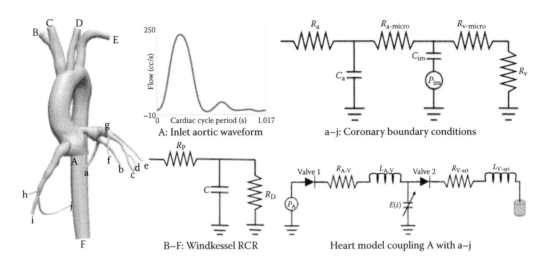

FIGURE 7.14

Multiscale simulation setup for modeling coronary flow. (From Sengupta D et al., *Biomechanics and Modeling in Mechanobiology*, 11(6):915–932, 2012.)

applied based on the Hessian of the velocity field. The resulting meshes have more than 3.5 million elements for both the normal and the KD model.

Figure 7.14 represents the multiscale simulation setup using these 3D anatomical models coupled to reduced-order 0D models. We prescribe an inflow boundary condition at the aortic root, coronary boundary conditions at the coronary artery outlets, and RCR boundary conditions at all other outlets of the model. Readers may refer to Sections 7.4 and 7.5 for detailed descriptions of these types of boundary conditions. The parameters in the 0D models are tuned using a combination of clinical data measured in the patient and literature knowledge of flow and resistances. Computation of the coupled system is then performed using the methods described in the previous case study.

From simulated pressure and flow results, we compute wall shear stress and particle residence times. Figure 7.15 compares the spatially averaged wall shear stress between the KD and normal cases at different locations. It is clear that the aneurysmal coronary arteries exhibit much lower wall shear stresses compared to normal ones. Particle tracking analysis also demonstrates differences between normal and aneurysmal coronaries. In the aneurysmal case, 30% of particles released at the aortic root circulate in the aneurysms for one full cardiac cycle, and some particles remain in the domain for as long as 5 cardiac cycles. In the normal coronary artery model, all particles exit the domain within 1.3 cardiac cycles. With continual improvement in the understanding of how hemodynamic parameters specifically correlate with thrombotic risk, these blood flow simulation results will provide increasingly valuable information toward clinical support of KD patient management.

7.8.3 Hepatic Blood Flow Distribution in the Fontan Junction

In this case study, we demonstrate how blood flow simulations are used to evaluate the performance of different Fontan surgical geometries, using hepatic flow distribution to each lung as a metric of performance [57].

As presented in Section 7.8.1, palliation for single ventricle defects typically requires a three-staged operative process. Here we focus on the stage 3 Fontan completion procedure, in which

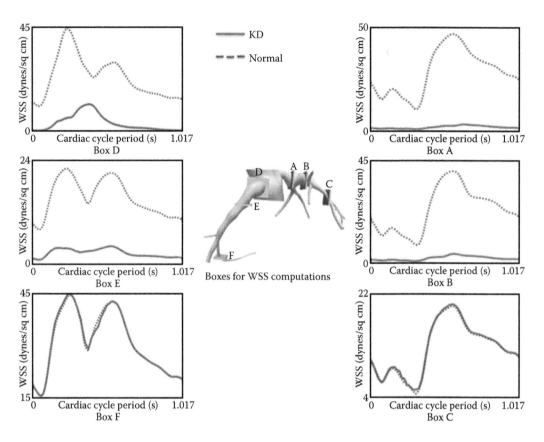

FIGURE 7.15

Comparison of spatially averaged wall shear stress (WSS) between the KD and normal cases at different locations. (From Sengupta D et al., *Biomechanics and Modeling in Mechanobiology*, 11(6):915–932, 2012.)

the inferior vena cava (IVC) is connected to the pulmonary arteries, restoring an in-series systemic-to-pulmonary circulation. One clinical consideration regarding this physiology is the development of pulmonary arteriovenous malformations, which is known to correlate with hepatic flow distribution, i.e., the fractional split of the blood returning from the liver through the IVC entering each lung. Studies have revealed a clear link between the absence of hepatic venous return and the development of pulmonary arteriovenous malformations, suggesting that the hepatic blood flow may contain factors required for proper lung development [58]. It is therefore important to consider the maintenance of an even hepatic flow distribution while designing a Fontan surgical geometry, to ensure the proper development of both lungs.

There are various surgical options for the stage 3 procedure, including the T-junction option where the IVC is anastomosed to the pulmonary arteries via a straight vascular graft, the offset option where a curved graft is anastomosed to the left pulmonary artery, and the Y-graft option where a bifurcated Y-shaped graft is anastomosed to the left and right pulmonary arteries separately [59,60]. For each surgical option, there can also be variations in the geometrical design.

In this case study, we evaluate the performance of various surgical alternatives in terms of hepatic distribution in five patients. Starting from a preoperative 3D anatomical model constructed based on clinical imaging data of each patient, we perform virtual stage 3 surgeries to construct various Fontan surgical junction geometries based on different surgical alternatives (Figure 7.16). Following common clinical practice, the virtual surgeries adapt Y-grafts with a 20-mm-diameter trunk and 15-mm-diameter branches and T-junction and offset grafts with a 20-mm-diameter trunk. The anatomical models are then processed via isotropic tetrahedral mesh generation and anisotropic mesh adaptation, resulting in final finite element meshes consisting of approximately 1 to 1.5 million elements.

Based on preoperative phase-contrast MRI acquired in each patient, we prescribe inflow boundary conditions to the superior vena cava and IVC faces of each anatomical model. Because of the anatomical differences pre- and postsurgery affecting the IVC flow waveform shape, the amplitude of the IVC flow waveform is scaled to match that of a typical Fontan patient. For the pulmonary outlet branches, we prescribe RCR boundary conditions tuned to preoperative pressure and flow split, assuming that they do not change in the immediate postoperative scenario.

From the 3D simulation results, we perform Lagrangian particle tracking to quantify the hepatic flow distribution. Massless particles are computationally released at the IVC face and tracked until they exit the domain through a pulmonary outlet (Figure 7.17). The

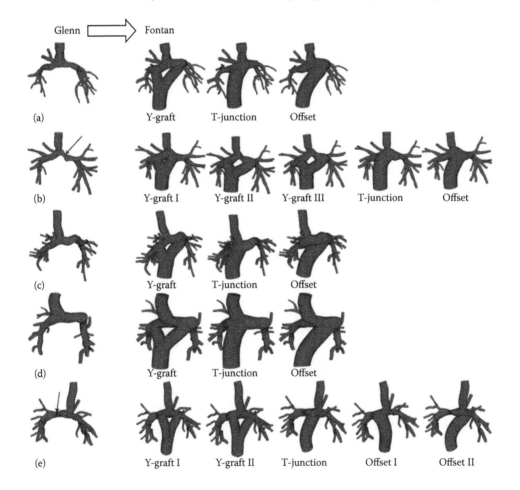

FIGURE 7.16
Preoperative patient models and variations of Fontan geometries for five patients. Patients B and E have stenoses in the preoperative anatomy denoted by arrows. (a–e) are the anatomies for the different patients (Patients A–E).

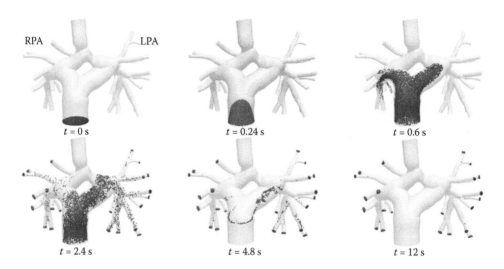

FIGURE 7.17
An example visualization of the particle tracking computation. LPA, left pulmonary artery; RPA, right pulmonary artery.

fraction of IVC flow that enters the left and right pulmonary arteries for different surgical alternatives for each patient is then obtained and shown in Figure 7.18. The theoretical optimum hepatic distribution is calculated based on conservation of mass and the total amount of flow entering each lung.

We can see from these results that the different surgical alternatives can indeed return drastically different hepatic distribution performances in each patient. Surgical alternatives can be selected with these considerations in mind. The blood flow simulation analyses presented in this case study provide means to predict surgical outcomes and to aid in surgical decision support for the Fontan stage 3 procedure.

7.9 Future Perspective

Simulation technology for cardiovascular disease has now advanced to the point of successful clinical adoption in select studies, with more widespread adoption likely to follow in the near future. Most notably, simulations led to the development and clinical pilot studies of the Fontan Y-graft surgery and recent favorable comparisons of simulation-derived fractional flow reserve (FFR_{CT}) with catheter measurements in adult coronary artery disease patients [61].

There are several roadblocks currently preventing wider adoption of simulation tools and application to large-scale clinical studies. First, there is a pressing need for clinical validation data and statistical correlation with patient outcomes. Unlike other traditional engineering fields, acquisition of in vivo validation data is often hindered by ethical considerations and imaging limitations. However, this is likely the single most important factor currently hindering the adoption of simulation methods in the clinic. Second, there is a need for a numerical framework to handle uncertainty propagation from simulation inputs (e.g., clinical data and noisy images) to outputs (e.g., simulation predictions of patient risk).

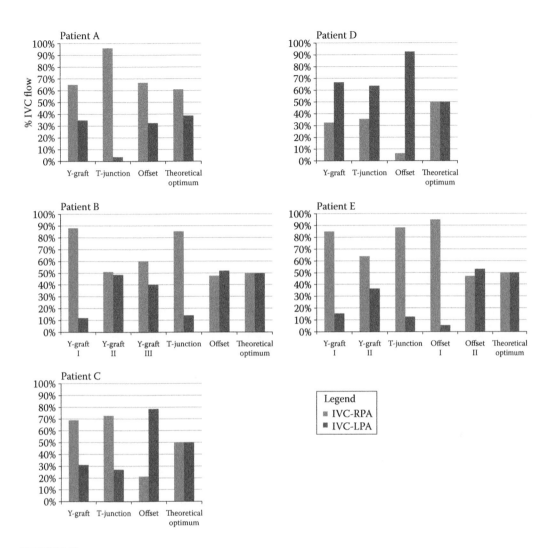

FIGURE 7.18

Hepatic flow distribution results. IVC, inferior vena cava; RPA, right pulmonary artery; LPA, left pulmonary artery.

Together with uncertainties, parameter identification should be used to automatically tune models to match available clinical data in the presence of uncertainties. Third, there is a pressing need for accelerated image segmentation tools to automate the model construction process. Without these tools to reduce laborious user input, simulations will remain limited to small-scale clinical studies.

In addition to overcoming the above roadblocks, there are several important new areas of research that will enhance the future scientific and clinical value of cardiovascular simulations. First, there is a need to couple simulations with models of vascular growth and remodeling. This would enable fluid solid growth simulations, in which vessels would adapt in silico to changing flow and pressure conditions. Second, there is a need to couple simulations with biochemical models of the thrombosis process. This would allow for improved prediction of thrombotic risk attributed to aneurysms, for stroke patients, or inside medical devices. Finally, fluid–structure interaction simulations should be improved to fully model the vessel wall, including variable properties and external tissue support, and better characterization of patient-specific material properties.

References

1. Figueroa CA, Vignon-Clementel IE, Jansen KE, Hughes TJR, Taylor CA: A coupled momentum method for modeling blood flow in three-dimensional deformable arteries. *Computer Methods in Applied Mechanics and Engineering* 2006, 195(41–43):5685–5706.
2. Vignon-Clementel IE, Figueroa CA, Jansen KE, Taylor CA: Outflow boundary conditions for three-dimensional finite element modeling of blood flow and pressure in arteries. *Computer Methods in Applied Mechanics and Engineering* 2006, 195(29–32):3776–3796.
3. Sankaran S, Moghadam ME, Kahn AM, Tseng EE, Guccione JM, Marsden AL: Patient-specific multiscale modeling of blood flow for coronary artery bypass graft surgery. *Annals of Biomedical Engineering* 2012, 40(10):2228–2242.
4. Sengupta D, Kahn AM, Burns JC, Sankaran S, Shadden SC, Marsden AL: Image-based modeling of hemodynamics in coronary artery aneurysms caused by Kawasaki disease. *Biomechanics and Modeling in Mechanobiology* 2012, 11(6):915–932.
5. Womersley JR: Mathematical theory of oscillating flow in an elastic tube. *The Journal of Physiology* 1955, 127(2):37–38P.
6. Womersley JR: Method for the calculation of velocity, rate of flow and viscous drag in arteries when the pressure gradient is known. *Journal of Physiology-London* 1955, 127(3):553–563.
7. Womersley JR: Oscillatory motion of a viscous liquid in a thin-walled elastic tube. 1. The linear approximation for long waves. *Philosophical Magazine* 1955, 46(373):199–221.
8. Womersley JR: Oscillatory flow in arteries—The constrained elastic tube as a model of arterial flow and pulse transmission. *Physics in Medicine and Biology* 1957, 2(2):178–187.
9. Womersley JR: Oscillatory flow in arteries. 2. The reflection of the pulse wave at junctions and rigid inserts in the arterial system. *Physics in Medicine and Biology* 1958, 2(4):313–323.
10. Womersley JR: Oscillatory flow in arteries. 3. Flow and pulse-velocity formulae for a liquid whose viscosity varies with frequency. *Physics in Medicine and Biology* 1958, 2(4):374–382.
11. Thiry PS, Roberge FA: Analogs and models of systemic arterial blood-flow. *Revue Canadienne De Biologie* 1976, 35(4):217–238.
12. Westerhof N, Bosman F, De Vries CJ, Noordergraaf A: Analog studies of human systemic arterial tree. *Journal of Biomechanics* 1969, 2(2):121–134.
13. Westerhof N, Lankhaar JW, Westerhof BE: The arterial Windkessel. *Medical & Biological Engineering & Computing* 2009, 47(2):131–141.
14. Hughes TJR, Lubliner J: On the 1 dimensional theory of blood flow in the larger vessels. *Mathematical Biosciences* 1973, 18(1–2):161–170.
15. Formaggia L, Gerbeau JF, Nobile F, Quarteroni A: On the coupling of 3D and 1D Navier-Stokes equations for flow problems in compliant vessels. *Computer Methods in Applied Mechanics and Engineering* 2001, 191(6–7):561–582.
16. Taylor CA, Hughes TJR, Zarins CK: Finite element modeling of blood flow in arteries. *Computer Methods in Applied Mechanics and Engineering* 1998, 158(1–2):155–196.
17. Taylor CA, Hughes TJR, Zarins CK: Finite element modeling of three-dimensional pulsatile flow in the abdominal aorta: Relevance to atherosclerosis. *Annals of Biomedical Engineering* 1998, 26(6):975–987.
18. Taylor CA, Draney MT, Ku JP, Parker D, Steele BN, Wang K, Zarins CK: Predictive medicine: Computational techniques in therapeutic decision-making. *Computer Aided Surgery* 1999, 4:231–247.

19. Milner JS, Moore JA, Rutt BK, Steinman DA: Hemodynamics of human carotid artery bifurcations: Computational studies with models reconstructed from magnetic resonance imaging of normal subjects. *Journal of Vascular Surgery* 1998, 28(1):143–156.

20. Steinman DA: Image-based computational fluid dynamics modeling in realistic arterial geometries. *Annals of Biomedical Engineering* 2002, 30(4):483–497.

21. Castro MA, Putman CM, Cebral JR: Patient-specific computational fluid dynamics modeling of anterior communicating artery aneurysms: A study of the sensitivity of intra-aneurysmal flow patterns to flow conditions in the carotid arteries. *American Journal of Neuroradiology* 2006, 27(10):2061–2068.

22. Whitehead KK, Pekkan K, Kitajima HD, Paridon SM, Yoganathan AP, Fogel MA: Nonlinear power loss during exercise in single-ventricle patients after the Fontan—Insights from computational fluid dynamics. *Circulation* 2007, 116(11):I165–I171.

23. Gijsen FJH, van de Vosse FN, Janssen JD: The influence of the non-Newtonian properties of blood on the flow in large arteries: Steady flow in a carotid bifurcation model. *Journal of Biomechanics* 1999, 32(6):601–608.

24. Malladi R, Sethian JA, Vemuri BC: Shape modeling with front propagation—A level set approach. *IEEE Transactions on Pattern Analysis and Machine Intelligence* 1995, 17(2):158–175.

25. Malladi R, Sethian JA, Vemuri BC: A fast level set based algorithm for topology-independent shape modeling. *Journal of Mathematical Imaging and Vision* 1996, 6(2–3):269–289.

26. Wang K: *Level Set Methods for Computational Prototyping with Application to Hemodynamic Modeling*. Stanford, CA: Stanford University; 2001.

27. Dollár P, Tu Z, Belongie S: Supervised learning of edges and object boundaries. In: *CVPR*. New York City; 2006.

28. Hughes TJR, Mallet M, Mizukami A: A new finite-element formulation for computational fluid-dynamics. 2. Beyond SUPG. *Computer Methods in Applied Mechanics and Engineering* 1986, 54(3):341–355.

29. Peiro J, Sherwin SJ, Giordana S: Automatic reconstruction of a patient-specific high-order surface representation and its application to mesh generation for CFD calculations. *Medical & Biological Engineering & Computing* 2008, 46(11):1069–1083.

30. Sherwin SJ, Karniadakis GE: Tetrahedral spectral elements for CFD. In: *Fourteenth International Conference on Numerical Methods in Fluid Dynamics Proceedings of the Conference*. Edited by Deshpande SM, Desai SS, Narasimha R, New York: Springer-Verlag; 1995: 429–434.

31. Peskin CS: Flow patterns around heart valves: A numerical method. *Journal of Computational Physics* 1972, 10(2):252–271.

32. Peskin CS: Numerical-analysis of blood-flow in heart. *Journal of Computational Physics* 1977, 25(3):220–252.

33. Zheng X, Seo JH, Vedula V, Abraham T, Mittal R: Computational modeling and analysis of intracardiac flows in simple models of the left ventricle. *European Journal of Mechanics B-Fluids* 2012, 35:31–39.

34. Valen-Sendstad K, Mardal K-A, Mortensen M, Reif BAP, Langtangen HP: Direct numerical simulation of transitional flow in a patient-specific intracranial aneurysm. *Journal of Biomechanics* 2011, 44(16):2826–2832.

35. Ford MD, Piomelli U: Exploring high frequency temporal fluctuations in the terminal aneurysm of the basilar bifurcation. *Journal of Biomechanical Engineering-Transactions of the ASME* 2012, 134(9):091003.

36. Long CC, Hsu MC, Bazilevs Y, Feinstein JA, Marsden AL: Fluid-structure interaction simulations of the Fontan procedure using variable wall properties. *Communications in Numerical Methods in Engineering* 2012, 28(5):513–527.

37. Bazilevs Y, Hsu MC, Zhang Y, Wang W, Kvamsdal T, Hentschel S, Isaksen JG: Computational vascular fluid-structure interaction: Methodology and application to cerebral aneurysms. *Biomechanics and Modeling in Mechanobiology* 2010, 9(4):481–498.

38. Kung EO, Les AS, Figueroa CA, Medina F, Arcaute K, Wicker RB, McConnell MV, Taylor CA: In vitro validation of finite element analysis of blood flow in deformable models. *Annals of Biomedical Engineering* 2011, 39(7):1947–1960.

39. Balossino R, Pennati G, Migliavacca F, Formaggia L, Veneziani A, Tuveri M, Dubini G: Computational models to predict stenosis growth in carotid arteries: Which is the role of boundary conditions? *Computer Methods in Biomechanics and Biomedical Engineering* 2009, 12(1):113–123.

40. Vignon IE, Taylor CA: Outflow boundary conditions for one-dimensional finite element modeling of blood flow and pressure waves in arteries. *Wave Motion* 2004, 39(4):361–374.

41. Duan B, Zamir M: Approximate solution for pulsatile flow in tubes of slightly noncircular cross-sections. *Utilitas Mathematica* 1991, 40:13–26.

42. Hodis S, Zamir M: Mechanical events within the arterial wall under the forces of pulsatile flow: A review. *Journal of the Mechanical Behavior of Biomedical Materials* 2011, 4(8):1595–1602.

43. Kim HJ, Vignon-Clementel IE, Figueroa CA, Jansen KE, Taylor CA: Developing computational methods for three-dimensional finite element simulations of coronary blood flow. *Finite Elements in Analysis and Design* 2010, 46(6):514–525.

44. Kim HJ, Vignon-Clementel IE, Coogan JS, Figueroa CA, Jansen KE, Taylor CA: Patient-specific modeling of blood flow and pressure in human coronary arteries. *Annals of Biomedical Engineering* 2010, 38(10):3195–3209.

45. Esmaily Moghadam M, Vignon-Clementel IE, Figliola R, Marsden AL, MOCHA: A modular numerical method for implicit 0D/3D coupling in cardiovascular finite element simulations. *Journal of Computational Physics* 2013, 244:63–79.

46. Baretta A, Corsini C, Yang W, Vignon-Clementel IE, Marsden AL, Feinstein JA, Hsia TY, Dubini G, Migliavacca F, Pennati G et al: Virtual surgeries in patients with congenital heart disease: A multi-scale modelling test case. *Philosophical Transactions of the Royal Society A-Mathematical Physical and Engineering Sciences* 2011, 369(1954):4316–4330.

47. Corsini C, Cosentino D, Pennati G, Dubini G, Hsia T-Y, Migliavacca F: Multiscale models of the hybrid palliation for hypoplastic left heart syndrome. *Journal of Biomechanics* 2011, 44(4):767–770.

48. Kung E, Baretta A, Baker C, Arbia G, Biglino G, Corsini C, Schievano S, Vignon-Clementel IE, Dubini G, Pennati G et al: Predictive modeling of the virtual Hemi-Fontan operation for second stage single ventricle palliation: Two patient-specific cases. *Journal of Biomechanics* 2013, 46(2):423–429.

49. Moghadam ME, Migliavacca F, Vignon-Clementel IE, Hsia T-Y, Marsden AL, Modeling Congenital Hearts A: Optimization of shunt placement for the Norwood surgery using multi-domain modeling. *Journal of Biomechanical Engineering-Transactions of the ASME* 2012, 134(5):051002.

50. Migliavacca F, Balossino R, Pennati G, Dubini G, Hsia TY, de Leval MR, Bove EL: Multiscale modelling in biofluidynamics: Application to reconstructive paediatric cardiac surgery. *Journal of Biomechanics* 2006, 39(6):1010–1020.

51. Norwood JWI: Hypoplastic left heart syndrome. *The Annals of Thoracic Surgery* 1991, 52(3):688–695.

52. Schmidt JP, Delp SL, Sherman MA, Taylor CA, Pande VS, Altman RB: The Simbios National Center: Systems biology in motion. *Proceedings of the IEEE* 2008, 96(8):1266–1280.

53. Kato H, Sugimura T, Akagi T, Sato N, Hashino K, Maeno Y, Kazue T, Eto G, Yamakawa R: Long-term consequences of Kawasaki disease—A 10- to 21-year follow-up study of 594 patients. *Circulation* 1996, 94(6):1379–1385.

54. Newburger J, Takahashi M, Beiser A, Burns J, Bastian J, Chung K, Colan S, Duffy C, Fulton D, Glode M et al: A single intravenous-infusion of gamma-globulin as compared with 4 infusions in the treatment of acute Kawasaki syndrome. *New England Journal of Medicine* 1991, 324(23):1633–1639.

55. Gordon J, Kahn A, Burns J: When children with Kawasaki disease grow up myocardial and vascular complications in adulthood. *Journal of the American College of Cardiology* 2009, 54(21):1911–1920.

56. Newburger JW, Takahashi M, Gerber MA, Gewitz MH, Tani LY, Burns JC, Shulman ST, Bolger AF, Ferrieri P, Baltimore RS et al: Diagnosis, treatment, and long-term management of Kawasaki disease: A statement for health professionals from the Committee on Rheumatic Fever, Endocarditis, and Kawasaki Disease, Council on Cardiovascular Disease in the Young, American Heart Association. *Pediatrics* 2004, 114(6):1708–1733.

57. Yang WG, Vignon-Clementel IE, Troianowski G, Reddy VM, Feinstein JA, Marsden AL: Hepatic blood flow distribution and performance in conventional and novel Y-graft Fontan geometries: A case series computational fluid dynamics study. *Journal of Thoracic and Cardiovascular Surgery* 2012, 143(5):1086–1097.

58. Pike NA, Vricella LA, Feinstein JA, Black MD, Reitz BA: Regression of severe pulmonary arteriovenous malformations after Fontan revision and *hepatic factor* rerouting. *Annals of Thoracic Surgery* 2004, 78(2):697–699.

59. Marsden AL, Bernstein AJ, Reddy VM, Shadden SC, Spilker RL, Chan FP, Taylor CA, Feinstein JA: Evaluation of a novel Y-shaped extracardiac Fontan baffle using computational fluid dynamics. *Journal of Thoracic and Cardiovascular Surgery* 2009, 137(2):394–403.

60. Dubini G, deLeval MR, Pietrabissa R, Montevecchi FM, Fumero R: A numerical fluid mechanical study of repaired congenital heart defects. Application to the total cavopulmonary connection. *Journal of Biomechanics* 1996, 29(1):111–121.

61. Min J, Berman D, Shaw L, Mauri L, Koo BK, Erglis A, Leipsic J: Fractional Flow Reserved Derived From Computed Tomographic Angiography (FFRCT) for Intermediate Severity Coronary Lesions: Results from the DeFACTO Trial (Determination of Fractional Flow Reserve by Anatomic Computed Tomographic Angiography). *Journal of the American College of Cardiology* 2012, 60(17):B6.

8

Computational Fluid Modeling of Heart Valves

Manuel Salinas and Sharan Ramaswamy

CONTENTS

ABSTRACT Heart valve disease (HVD) requiring surgical intervention can be broadly classified as a condition that may be congenital or acquired later in life. The latter can result from a combination of genetic and environmental factors (e.g., rheumatic fever). Recent advances in the treatment of HVD have been focused on either minimally invasive percutaneous approaches for prosthesis implantation or the understanding of fundamental insights toward development of completely autologous and living biological valves, known as tissue-engineered heart valves, usually grown from progenitor cell sources. In either scenario, the complex hemodynamics that are present in the vicinity of the valve and time-varying stresses on the leaflets are likely to provide valuable information in terms of surgical planning and preoperative, postoperative, and temporal, longitudinal functional assessment. Today, advances in computational fluid dynamics (CFD) have reached a point of accuracy where very complex flow scenarios can be modeled in a straightforward manner provided that three-dimensional geometry and boundary conditions are representative of the actual, physical states. Here, we provide a review of the role that CFD has and will play in guiding technologies toward treatment of HVD.

8.1 Background

8.1.1 Heart Valves

Healthy heart valves are essential for proper blood circulation. Their role is to ensure unidirectional blood flow in the circulatory system. They consist of different tissue layers and are capable of adapting and remodeling their tissue composition according to the hemodynamic environments surrounding them [1–3]. The mitral and tricuspid valves are located between the atria and ventricles while the pulmonary valve is found intersecting the right ventricle and the pulmonary artery. The aortic valve resides between the left ventricle and the aorta.

When blood enters the heart through the vena cava into the right atrium, it creates an increase in intrachamber pressure. When the right atrial pressure exceeds the pressure in the right ventricle, the tricuspid valve opens, thereby allowing blood to flow into the right ventricle. Simultaneously, the mitral valve also opens and permits blood to flow from the left atrium into the left ventricle. When the right ventricular pressure exceeds the pressure of the pulmonary arteries, the pulmonary valve opens, allowing blood to flow toward the lungs, permitting exchange of oxygen and carbon dioxide. Concurrently, the aortic valve allows oxygen-rich blood to flow to the aorta and toward systemic organs and tissues. It closes once the pressure in the aorta exceeds the ventricular pressure.

Over the course of the average human lifespan, native heart valves (NHVs) open and close an estimated 3 billion times [4]. During each heartbeat, they are subjected to different hemodynamic loads in the form of flow, stretch, and flexure [5–7]. In past decades, NHVs have been thought to be passive structures. However, recent studies have shown tremendous cell and tissue activity occurring on its surface and within its layered structure [5–9].

8.1.2 Heart Valve Disease

For simplicity, we refer from this point forward to any aberrant condition caused by anomalous structures or disease manifestation on heart valves as heart valve disease (HVD). HVD can be caused by immune disorders, trauma to the valve or surrounding tissues, hypertension, degenerative valve calcification, endocarditis, rheumatic fever, and congenital birth defects [2,3,10–21]. It can be diagnosed by listening to the opening and closing of the valves through a stethoscope for the identification of heart murmurs. Other methods of detection include echocardiography, electrocardiogram, chest x-ray, cardiac catheterization, stress testing, or magnetic resonance imaging [12,13,15,16,20,21].

Common symptoms of HVD include aortic valve regurgitation, wherein one or more of the three leaflets do not close properly, thereby causing blood to flow back through the valve into the left ventricle [10–12,22]. When regurgitation fractions are large, the left ventricle will overwork to pump more blood out of the heart, which may result in left ventricular hypertrophy and possibly heart failure, if left untreated. Another condition, aortic valve stenosis, is a state in which the valve leaflets become stiff or even fuse together, resulting in narrowing of the aortic valve [3,19,21]. This in turn causes a reduction in the valve orifice area, which exhibits disturbances in the normal hemodynamics [2,3,15–17,20,21]. Valve stenosis can be congenital or be caused later in life owing to, for example, onset of calcification of leaflets. Importantly, the workload on the left ventricle increases considerably, which can result in serious complications, as mentioned previously.

8.1.3 Valve Prosthetics and Substitutes

8.1.3.1 Mechanical Valves

Mechanical heart valves (MHVs) are prosthetic devices made of high-strength artificial materials such as titanium and pyrolytic carbon [17,19,23]. The most common MHV designs include the ball and cage, tilting disk, and the bileaflet MHV (BMHV) [1,19,24,25]. The bileaflet design (e.g., bileaflet valve from St. Jude Medical) is currently very popular because of its superior hemodynamics, such as the ability to exhibit low transvalvular pressure gradients [16,17,19].

MHVs have shown to be reliable and long lasting. However, there are some serious limitations that tend to exclude several segments of the population affected by severe HVD. One problem is a predisposition to hemolysis and platelet activation that can trigger thrombus nucleation that could potentially cause blood flow disturbances [26–28]. Furthermore, blood clots could potentially separate from the valve surface and cause a stroke if the clot migrates to the vasculature in the brain. Anticoagulation therapy (e.g., heparin) is required for as long as the MHV is implanted. The use of MHVs are mainly suggested for adults and are not recommended for young children who are prone to injury, women who wish to have children, individuals who cannot tolerate anticoagulation medication (e.g., heparin), and other subpopulation groups who are at risk for traumatic episodes of bleeding [21,22].

8.1.3.2 Bioprosthetic Valves

Bioprosthetic valves (BPVs) are created by forming the native tissue found in animals [18,29] into a valve-shaped construct. Sources of animal tissue include the porcine aortic valve and the bovine pericardium [1,18]. BPVs offer superior hemodynamics over any mechanical valve including the bileaflet design. However, they are predisposed to leaflet calcification and early structural breakdown [5,7].

Homografts, derived from human cadavers, serve as allografts [19,30]. The first aortic valve replacement with a homograft occurred in 1962 by Ross [31]. These substitutes do not pose a risk of coagulation problems, thereby eliminating the need for anticoagulation therapies [30]. Other advantages include an absence of hemolysis, very good hemodynamics, good implant integration, resistance to infection, and a low transvalvular pressure [19,30]. However, homografts are also calcification prone and are very limited in supply.

8.1.3.3 Autografts

Valve autografts are valve implants wherein a pulmonary valve is dissected and secured in the aortic position to compensate for a malfunctioning aortic valve. Meanwhile, a homograft is implanted in the pulmonary artery to substitute for the native valve that is removed. This process, clinically known as the Ross procedure, has demonstrated extensive benefits [31–41] such as (i) no necessity for lifelong coagulation therapy, (ii) minimal risk of calcification, (iii) durability, (iv) minimal scarring, (v) adequate hemodynamics, (vi) growth potential, and (vii) a low risk of infections and tissue rejection. However, the critical shortcomings [31,33–41] that restrict this approach are that (i) it requires a high level of technical skill from the surgeon, (ii) data to support long-term outcomes are limited, (iii) homograft in pulmonary circulation will likely require replacement over human lifetime, (iv) it cannot be used in children with structural abnormalities on their pulmonary valve (owing to Marfan syndrome, systemic lupus erythematosus, and juvenile rheumatoid arthritis).

8.1.3.4 Emerging Technologies

8.1.3.4.1 Polymer Valves

Development of polymer heart valves was investigated several years ago. However, the main challenge presented at that time was material durability, and this caused an abandonment of these technologies [42]. Recently, this area of research has been revisited because of more advanced state-of-the-art polymer manufacturing technologies and the development of stronger, biocompatible polymers and polymer composite materials [42–45]. There is also a need for developing valve substitutes that can be integrated with minimal invasive techniques, such as percutaneous valve technologies, which polymer valves are thought to be able to meet [19,46,47].

Polymeric implants can be produced in large quantities and in multiple sizes with low manufacturing cost. The polymers of preference are highly biocompatible elastomers that can be formed to resemble valve-like structures and are able to mimic the deformation of native valve leaflets [42,44]. However, much needs to be done in development to ensure that these types of valves are durable long-term and this remains a subject of ongoing research. To date, no polymer valve implant has been approved by the US Food and Drug Administration. A critical limitation of polymer valves, even if thrombosis, calcification, lack of functionality, and weak structural properties can be overcome, is that they cannot account for somatic growth in children who have severe HVD; in other words, the replacement valve cannot grow and remodel with the overall growth of the child. This means that multiple surgical procedures will still be needed for the pediatric patient with severe congenital HVD.

8.1.3.4.2 Tissue-Engineered Heart Valves

The purpose of heart valve tissue engineering is to obtain an in vitro graft with mechanical properties and anatomical-like structures similar to those of native valves as well as to accommodate somatic growth [5–7,48]. This can be potentially achieved by seeding biomaterial scaffolds with autologous cells such as bone marrow–derived stem cells (BMSCs) [5–7,49–51] and subjecting them to mechanical conditioning paradigms until sufficient heart valve cells and tissue growth in vitro has been achieved [52]. Suitable cell sources for tissue-engineered heart valves (TEHVs) are primary endothelial cells and smooth muscle cells from a vein that can be harvested without compromise to the vasculature (e.g., saphenous vein in the leg) [53,54] as well as progenitor cell sources such as periodontal ligament cells derived from wisdom teeth [55]. Stem cells such as BMSCs offer the advantage of being obtained in a much less invasive approach and are accessible whenever needed [5,56].

In terms of the scaffolding components, common biodegradable polymers such as polylactic acid, polyglycolic acid (PGA), and blends or copolymers of these two materials, for example, a 50:50 blend (by weight) of PGA:PLLA nonwoven fabric or poly(lactic-co-glycolic acid), PLGA, have been utilized for heart valve tissue engineering purposes because of their biocompatibility and biodegradable properties [50,57,58]. However, as cell sources are being identified and as mechanical conditioning protocols are being optimized, it is also critical, at the same time, to tailor scaffold properties that will demonstrate resilience to cyclic tensile, bending, and fluid-induced stress states, while still permitting adequate levels of opening and closing dynamics [50,57,58]. In this regard, scaffolds made of decellularized animal valves have been utilized [59], but unfavorable interactions between the colonizing cells and tissue proteins such as collagen have persisted [24,60]. Recent work has also focused on the idea of using elastomeric substrates that can recapitulate native valve deformation [5–7]. Many challenges need to yet be overcome in optimizing in vitro grown TEHVs that are capable of withstanding in vivo hemodynamic challenges and concomitantly permit growth and tissue remodeling. These technical barriers need to be addressed in order to bring TEHVs from the current research state to that of clinical reality [24,61,62].

8.1.4 Computational Models

Heart valves are subjected to a complex hemodynamic environment. The loading states on native valves during healthy, diseased, pre- and postsurgical interventional states as well as prosthetic valves and emerging tissue-engineered constructs can be delineated using computational predictive models. Valuable insights on how these results may translate to long-term functionality can be made. In this context, computational fluid dynamics (CFD) and finite element (FE) model development in the heart valve arena remain a vibrant area of research. FE models are generally applied to evaluate solid surface strains attributed to cyclical stretching and bending. On the other hand, CFD models examine the effects of fluid-induced stresses on the leaflet surfaces. In this chapter, we focus on CFD models. However, we also present fluid–structure interaction (FSI) approaches, which essentially combine both CFD and FE approaches to delineate both the fluid and solid mechanical responses of the leaflets.

CFD processes for heart valve analyses are based on two numerical methods: the finite element method (FEM) and finite volume method (FVM) [63–65]. Both of these techniques subdivide the flow domain into a large number of finite entities, elements in the case of the FEM, and control volumes in the case of FVM [63–65]. Later, an iterative method is used to obtain the solution for each spatial element or volume. The overall goal is to solve the governing equations of the fluid given by the three-dimensional (3D) Navier–Stokes equations, by simplifying large complex partial differential equations for the flow physics into algebraic equations [66–68]. Through this approach, CFD can numerically predict a solution for the nonlinear Navier–Stokes equations, which allows the uncovering of the blood flow field surrounding a heart valve [60,69].

The usage of CFD to study heart valves can be traced back to the early 1970s. The first models accounted only for two-dimensional (2D) analysis with oversimplified geometries. 3D models were constructed several years later in the late 1980s and early 1990s. We summarize some important milestones in CFD of heart valves and heart valve prostheses here: The flow through a tilting disk in a permanently half-open position was simulated using a FEM approach by Shim and Chang [70]. Ge et al. [71,72] performed computer simulations for mechanical valves at Reynolds numbers (Re) describing laminar and turbulent flow, specifically at Reynolds numbers of 750 and 6000, respectively. The leaflets of this simplified valve were fixed at a completely open state. McQueen and Peskin [73] described how computer modeling can be used to study design criteria in bileaflet valves with flat and curved leaflets. Lei et al. [74] developed a 2D flow model around a Björk–Shiley tilting disk valve under steady-state conditions. Simultaneously, Lei et al. [74] conducted laser Doppler anemometry (LDA) on an experimental Björk–Shiley tilting disk valve setup that used a mixture of oil and kerosene as the fluid. However, helical vortices observed in the experimental data could not be predicted through the computational results.

Kiris et al. [75] focused on flow past a tilting disk in a fixed position of 30° while ranging the Re value between 2000 and 6000. This study used the FVM and solved the 3D Reynolds-averaged Navier–Stokes equations that also accounted for turbulence. King et al. [76] described the presence of orifice jets during systole in a CarboMedics valve. The jet regions were observed to merge toward the aortic walls, and there was evidence of jets in the central flow downstream of the valve leaflets. Experimental results from this study by means of flow visualization and LDA reasonably supported these observations.

King et al. [77] used a commercially available FEM-based software called FIDAP (Fluent, Lebanon, New Hampshire) to simulate a simplified one-quarter model of a fixed valve at Re = 1500. Different leaflet opening angles were used, and it was shown that downstream flow became more centralized and maximum velocity and maximum shear rate increased as well.

8.1.4.1 General CFD Steps

Presently, there are a wide variety of commercially available software packages such as CFX (Ansys, Canonsburg, Pennsylvania), CFD-ACE (ESI Group, France), COMSOL (Burlington, Massachusetts), FLEX PDE (Scientific Software Solutions Int, GR - Europe), FLUENT (Ansys), and so on. The operating stages of any of these software packages can be described in three basic steps: preprocessing, solving, and postprocessing. The preprocessing stage deals with the construction of geometry; meshing parameters such as grid type and cell size; boundary conditions for all inlets, outlets, walls, and interfaces; coupling of equations; and incorporation of physical, mechanical, and chemical properties (if needed) into the system. The solving stage involves the setting up of the numerical model, selection of the most appropriate solver, and monitoring the computed solution. The postprocessing stage mainly deals with the creation of 2D and 3D plots as well as videos in order to present and interpret the results. If general, revisions and updates to the model will need to be done if the results are erroneous owing to lack of numerical accuracy. As a result, a large part of the modeling process will require validation of the computational results with a corresponding experiment.

8.1.4.2 Moving Boundary Problems

Presently, simulations involving moving interfaces between flowing or deforming media are some of the most challenging problems in computational science [78–80]. In the body, the movement of heart valves represents an active dynamic system [65,81]. From a modeling perspective, the challenges are linked directly to the numerous differential equations that need to be satisfied for different components within the system (e.g., blood, vessel wall, moving leaflets, etc.), and that these solutions need to also be satisfied through mathematical relationships and appropriate boundary conditions that must hold at the interface of the two components [23,79,82]. As the name implies, moving boundary methods alludes to techniques that incorporate the movement of a solid component with the movement of the fluid in evaluating the fluid and, in some cases, the solid stresses as well, as a function of the motion of the solid. In particular, FSI techniques comprise scenarios where the movement of the solid–liquid interface is unknown in advance and must be determined as part of the solution. However, to date, the ability to solve FSI problems efficiently on a regular basis is limited largely to idealized cases, as it is not straightforward and is computationally expensive. As FSI techniques in heart valve research are generally time-consuming, during the study planning stage, their usage has to be weighed against the added amount of accuracy that will be provided and level of additional insights that can be gained to benefit the clinical problem at hand.

Initial algorithmic methods included the Eulerian and Lagrangian approach. In the Eulerian case, the velocity field is provided for a fixed control volume. The generated grid is fixed and therefore has a grid velocity, $V_g = 0$. It is suitable for scenarios with small displacement and conversely is not suitable for systems with massive boundary movement such as those that occur in valve leaflets [8,83,84].

In the Lagrangian method, the generated grid can move and therefore has a grid velocity equal to the velocity of the fluid, $V_g = V_f$. It is suitable when the system can be easily identified (e.g., elastic solid) [85], but it is not appropriate for systems with randomized boundary movement as it cannot treat arbitrary motion that can occur, for example, in HVD states (e.g., severe mitral valve prolapse) [8,84].

Two moving boundary algorithms used for the modeling of flow in deforming heart valves include the arbitrary Lagrangian–Eulerian (ALE) and the immersed body method (IBM). The ALE formulation can be used to solve problems where the velocity of the grid V_g is arbitrary and has no relation to the velocity of the fluid V_f. Although the ALE approach has been extensively used, it presents the disadvantage that the mesh needs to be continuously deformed and updated as the control volume travels through the complete system. Given this fact, using the ALE approach could result in a large computational expense, especially for 3D FSI problems. This is why this method is limited to relatively small time steps (e.g., simulating the dynamics that occurs between a series of contiguous phases within a cardiac cycle as opposed to the entire cycle itself) as it requires frequent remeshing. The ALE method is most suitable when the definition of a fixed control volume is not sufficient, for example, when dealing with large-displacement moving walls and, in some cases, when the grid velocity can be accurately prescribed a priori (e.g., from patient-specific medical images) [23].

IBM allows for accurate interpolations at the fluid–structure interface. This method is efficient as it requires lesser to no mesh update. It is flexible and it can be extended to multiphase flows, which makes it suitable for various applications [86,87]. Here, the entire fluid computational domain is discretized as an independent mesh. Similarly, the solid computational domain is also discretized as an independent mesh that is immersed inside the fluid domain. Although both domains are independently meshed, their governing equations are coupled by adding body forces to the Navier–Stokes equations that describe the fluid domain [81,86–88]. This creates a no-slip boundary effect at the boundary between the fluid and the solid, and the system accounts for these body forces at the start of the simulation until all iterations have been run. In view of the fact that the grid used to discretize the fluid domain is independent and does not have to be deformed or updated, the IBM is mostly appropriate for large structural displacements such as MHV modeling.

Hong et al. [82] developed an FSI model using the FLUENT commercial CFD package to create a moving grid with remeshing techniques based on the ALE approach. They wanted to observe the physical interactions of MHVs to investigate flows interacting with the moving leaflets. Different rotating positions and tilting angles of the bileaflet valves were considered. It was shown that the valve rotation had a significant effect on the transvalvular pressure drop and that valve tilting greatly affects the flow direction.

Ge and Sotiropoulos [71] were the first to successfully use direct numerical simulations of pulsatile flow through BMHVs. They simulated blood flow through a BMHV embedded within a straight aortic segment using an IBM approach, and they conducted in vitro studies using a similar experimental setup. Specifically, they discretized the computational fluid domain with a curvilinear mesh, and the immersed bodies inside the mesh were treated as sharp-interface boundaries that were subsequently discretized using an unstructured meshing scheme. The IBM-based model was able to closely match flow data from in vitro laboratory tests. Sotiropoulos and Borazjani [23] also used the IBM to perform high-resolution FSI simulations of a physiologic pulsatile flow through a BMHV in an anatomically realistic aorta and through an identical BMHV implanted in a straight aorta. The 3D aortic geometries were reconstructed from stacks of magnetic resonance imaging (MRI) 2D images. The comparisons showed that although some of the salient features of the flow remained the same, the specific geometry of the aorta (e.g., from patient to patient) could have a major effect on both the flow patterns and the motion of the valve leaflets. It was also shown that higher leaflet shear stresses were observed in the anatomical-like aorta rather than in the straight idealized case.

TABLE 8.1
Summary of the Advantages and Disadvantages of Different CFD Methodologies for Moving Boundary Problems

Method	Advantages	Disadvantages
Eulerian	• Good for fixed system analysis with low/no boundary movement • Computationally feasible	• Function of space only • Bad for large deformations • No adaptive mesh refinement
Lagrangian	• Neglects convective terms • Easy to solve • Computationally feasible	• Function of time only • Bad for large deformations • No adaptive mesh refinement
ALE	• Adaptive mesh ($f(x)$ or $f(t)$) • Good for FSI with low boundary movement • Adaptive mesh refinement if needed	• Frequent mesh conformation • Takes long time • Expensive for large 3D systems • Computationally challenging
Immersed body	• Versatile • Adequate for large structural displacement • Adaptive mesh refinement	• Requires deep understanding of CFD • Computationally challenging

When the valve material is flexible, there is higher complexity in CFD simulations and therefore it becomes more challenging because the deformation is localized and motions of the leaflets are highly spatially varying. This is the case in the computational modeling of polymer tissue-engineered valves. In 1972, Peskin [65] developed the first successful 2D model of a simplified MHV inside an artery in order to capture the movement of two solid leaflets embedded in a fluid domain. This was achieved by using an IBM approach. Peskin et al. continued to work on improving this method based on a finite difference scheme and later demonstrated its suitability in capturing interactions between deforming bodies in fluids [64,65].

Table 8.1 summarizes the advantages and disadvantages of different CFD methods for moving boundary problems.

8.1.4.3 CFD Usage for Emerging Technologies in Heart Valve Research

Driessen et al. [80] employed a mathematical model to study the mechanical properties of a TEHV. Engelmayr et al. [89] utilized GAMBIT (v2.1) and FLUENT (v6.2) (Ansys) to study flow behavior through a novel bioreactor for heart valve tissue engineering. Computational studies on the flow physics on and around the housed bioreactor specimens [89] were subsequently evaluated further by Ramaswamy et al. [5]. The commercially available software FLUENT (Ansys) was employed on a structured grid composed of 1.43 million hexahedral elements and 1.54 million nodes. They hypothesized that the oscillatory shear stresses (OSSs) that were created during specimen, valve-like bending were involved in engineered heart valve tissue formation [5]. Ramaswamy et al. [52] also developed a u-shaped novel bioreactor. Its design permitted the in vitro recapitulation of physiologically relevant shear stress magnitudes.

8.2 Recent Advances in CFD Applications for Heart Valve Research

8.2.1 From Imaging to Meshing to CFD

Blood flow physics that occur in the neighborhood of native or prosthetic valves can be a key indicator of the functionality of the valve [23]. It can reveal disease in native valves [90,91] and performance issues in the case of prosthetic ones [23]. In order to develop a strong, accurate CFD model, the incorporation of these flow physics as boundary or initial conditions is paramount [92,93]. Equally important is the usage of geometry structures that correctly depict valve and surrounding tissues in vivo [92]. This represents a key challenge owing to the light scattering nature of blood, which excludes the usage of some imaging techniques [94]. It is also important to be able to compare computational results with experimental data, and this can be achieved only if the valvular flow physics can be sufficiently captured in vivo.

Doppler echocardiography and cardiac magnetic resonance (CMR) have typically been used to obtain mainly unidirectional 2D velocity profiles [94,95]. More advanced versions such as the four-dimensional flow CMR can provide temporal and 3D spatial information [94] with resolution in the order of 50 ms and 3 mm^3, respectively [94]. Color Doppler echocardiography has been used to observe abnormal flow patterns and superimposed turbulence [90,91]. It does so via application of an ultrasonic beam that can be used to compute axial velocities [90,96]. It can also provide radial velocities, but the integration of both radial and axial velocities, necessary for obtaining the true flow field is not usually obtained in routine clinical management [94].

Particle image velocimetry (PIV) is a popular technique for the characterization of the flow field through in vitro models of heart valves and chambers [94]. It is capable of capturing a highly physiologically similar flow field by using tiny particles that light up in response to the presence of a laser light. PIV does not track the individual particle displacement; it tracks the alignments of the particles as a group [97]. Imaging technologies such as computed tomography (CT) scans, ultrasound, and MRI can help in the virtual geometry reconstruction of cardiovascular component such as heart valves, chambers, and vessels [92–94,98,99]. For instance, CT consists of acquiring multiple 2D cross-section images that can be later stacked together for 3D reconstruction [94]. Presently, the accuracy and acceptability of CFD models greatly rely on these types of imaging techniques, which are capable of acquiring extensive 2D data that can be later processed to reconstruct 3D structures [92].

The advancement in imaging technologies and computational capabilities and a better understanding of the electrophysiology of the heart and its interactions with neighboring tissues and organs have infused new hope for the development of a virtual model that can closely resemble the heart and its valves [92,94,95,98]. Meshing geometries with high-density elements and nodes can be promptly accomplished through supercomputers [6,7,60,100]. Geometry remeshing can be triggered by setting tolerance levels for specific parameters such as element volume or element angle deformation, thereby delaying negative volume sectors, which will cause computational errors that will terminate the iteration process without yielding any results [101]. Parallel processing with state-of-the-art processors makes the iterative solution process more efficient. It is a common practice to set the number of iterations in the thousands. It also helps achieve academic and research standard convergence criteria for continuity and momentum equations [5–7].

In the following paragraphs, we outline a few of the most up-to-date efforts in heart valve computational fluid modeling that were able to leverage accurate geometric reconstructions derived from original medical imaging data sets. We discuss some specific case studies with visual illustrations.

8.2.1.1 Case #1

Le and Sotiropoulos [92] employed the curvilinear immersed boundary method and developed an FSI model of a left ventricle and a MHV. The 3D reconstruction of the ventricle geometry was obtained by merging 2D MRI images from a healthy individual. The results were found to be in good agreement with clinical observations. This work revealed complex

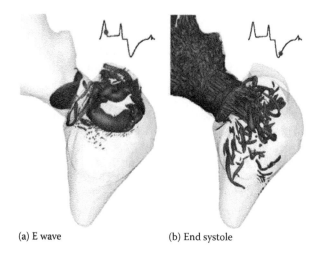

(a) E wave   (b) End systole

FIGURE 8.1

(a) The formation of coherent structures inside the left ventricular chamber during diastole. (b) The small-scale structures are advected into the aorta during systole. The dot in the inset shows the time instance in the cardiac cycle. (Reprinted from *J Comput Phys.* (244), Le TB, Sotiropoulos F, Fluid–structure interaction of an aortic heart valve prosthesis driven by an animated anatomic left ventricle, 41–62, Copyright 2013, with permission from Elsevier.)

valve leaflet kinematics and emphasized the importance of patient-specific simulations for heart valve prostheses and other cardiac devices. In Figure 8.1, it can be seen that there was the formation of coherent structures at different time points during the cardiac cycle. Coherent structures are well-developed zones within the flow that exhibit a characteristic flow pattern such as vortices. Studying the formation and transient life of such structures could help in understanding damage to blood cells as well as prosthetic valve dynamics.

Pelliccioni et al. [102] utilized the Lattice–Boltzmann (LB) method in a flow simulation past a mechanical valve in the aortic position. Other efforts that have utilized the same approach include the work of Krafczyk et al. [103,104]. These efforts showed that the LB method was capable of predicting blood flow physics accurately.

8.2.1.2 Case #2

Shahriari et al. [105] developed a model for a BMHV flow study. The model employed a smoothed particle hydrodynamics mesh-free approach. This study was the first of its kind to use this technique in the area of heart valve research and was originally developed for the astrophysics arena. Essentially, the fluid is represented by interacting particles that obey the Navier–Stokes equation using an interpolation function. The particles can move freely in the reference frame with a Lagrangian configuration. The trajectory of the particles was used to correlate flow patterns with damage to blood components. In addition, large recirculation regions were found to be present in the dysfunctional BMHVs as shown in Figure 8.2.

8.2.1.3 Case #3

Borazjani [106] developed a 3D FSI model for both mechanical valves and BPVs. He used a Fung model to capture the soft tissue response and validated his results using flow measurements from a MHV. Figures 8.3 through 8.5 show the comparison of shear stress, 3D wake structure formation, and the nondimensional second Piola–Kirchhoff stress, respectively. It

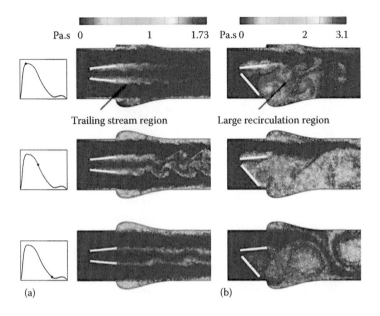

FIGURE 8.2
The patterns associated with accumulative shear stress applied on particles passing through (a) a normal BMHV and (b) a dysfunctional BMHV. (Reprinted from *J Biomech.* 45(15), Shahriari S et al., Evaluation of shear stress accumulation on blood components in normal and dysfunctional BMHVs using smoothed particle hydro-dynamics, 2637–2644, Copyright 2012, with permission from Elsevier.)

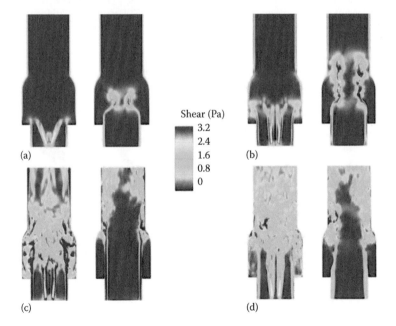

FIGURE 8.3
FSI simulations with peak Re = 6000: Comparison of instantaneous local maximum shear stress contours over the midplane of the valve for a MHV versus BPV implanted in a straight aorta at time (a) t = 52 ms, (b) t = 93 ms, (c) t = 186 ms, and (d) t = 334 ms within the cardiac cycle. (Reprinted from *Comput Methods Appl Mech Eng.*, 257, Borazjani I, Fluid–structure interaction, immersed boundary-finite element method simulations of biopros-thetic heart valves, 103–116, Copyright 2013, with permission from Elsevier.)

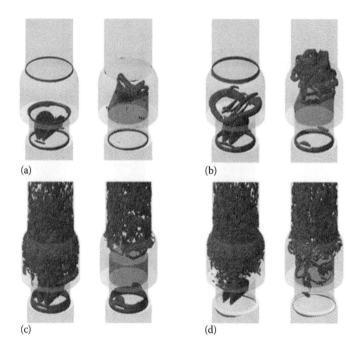

FIGURE 8.4

FSI simulations with peak Re = 6000: 3D wake structure visualized by the iso-surfaces of q-criteria for a MHV versus BPV implanted in a straight aorta at time (a) $t = 52$ ms, (b) $t = 93$ ms, (c) $t = 186$ ms, and (d) $t = 334$ ms within the cardiac cycle. (Reprinted from *Comput Methods Appl Mech Eng.*, 257, Borazjani I, Fluid–structure interaction, immersed boundary-finite element method simulations of bioprosthetic heart valves, 103–116, Copyright 2013, with permission from Elsevier.)

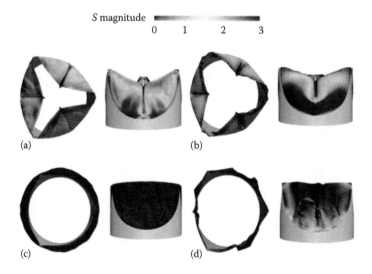

FIGURE 8.5

FSI simulations of BPV: The shape of the BPV and the magnitude of the nondimensional second Piola–Kirchhoff stress S on the BPV at time (a) $t = 52$ ms, (b) $t = 93$ ms, (c) $t = 186$ ms, and (d) $t = 334$ ms within the cardiac cycle. (Reprinted from *Comput Methods Appl Mech Eng.*, 257, Borazjani I, Fluid–structure interaction, immersed boundary-finite element method simulations of bioprosthetic heart valves, 103–116, Copyright 2013, with permission from Elsevier.)

can be seen that shear stress acting on blood components was higher in the mechanical valve. Other efforts have shown a correlation between higher shear stress and thrombus nucleation [98,107]. The nondimensional second Piola–Kirchhoff stress was used to identify the points of maximum stress that were found to occur when flow pushed the valve toward the open position.

8.2.2 Our Recent Experience

8.2.2.1 Case #4

We performed computational simulations of flow in a custom-made bioreactor [52] capable of imparting physiologically relevant shear stresses onto rectangular scaffolds (Figure 8.6). The rationale for replicating native valve flow physics on rectangular surfaces was previously documented [5].

The movement of the samples was assumed to follow a parabolic profile during cyclic flexure deformation [6,7]. In this study, we wanted to observe the effects of flow pulsatility versus sample movement on OSS. OSS has been shown to be important in the differentiation pathways of BMSCs [108–110]. Our interests were in BMSC differentiation to support

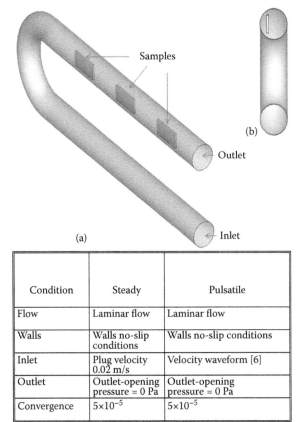

Condition	Steady	Pulsatile
Flow	Laminar flow	Laminar flow
Walls	Walls no-slip conditions	Walls no-slip conditions
Inlet	Plug velocity 0.02 m/s	Velocity waveform [6]
Outlet	Outlet-opening pressure = 0 Pa	Outlet-opening pressure = 0 Pa
Convergence	5×10^{-5}	5×10^{-5}

FIGURE 8.6
(a) U-shaped bioreactor showing the three samples. (b) Front view of the bioreactor inlet, outlet, and sample position. The table indicates the parameters for steady and pulsatile flow simulations.

the heart valve phenotype, as it is a popular cell choice utilized in heart valve tissue engineering studies. We performed a quasi-static analysis on steady flow simulations at different sample bending positions. Pulsatile flow simulations were performed for fixed sample positions as described by Salinas et al. [6,7]. All the simulations were carried out using CFX (Ansys) software with parameters described in Figure 8.6.

An oscillatory shear index (OSI) [111] was used to quantify the OSS along the centerline of the specimens. OSI was overall found to be the most uniform along both walls (inner and outer) for straight specimens that underwent pulsatile flow (Figure 8.7). In addition, mean OSI distribution was highest along both the inner and outer walls when specimens ($n = 3$) were held fixed in a straight configuration (average specimen OSI = 0.26, inner wall; average specimen OSI = 0.27, outer wall). Thus, these types of analyses illustrate an example of deriving insights from computational efforts without building complex CFD models (e.g., FSI), in aiding the design of experiments. In this case, the models guided the planning of maximizing OSS levels in BMSC-seeded scaffolds uniformly. Subsequent evaluation of OSS-induced mechanobiology could thus be accomplished in a clear-cut fashion, purely through a physiological pulsatile waveform, maintaining the samples in a straight configuration, without the need for moving the specimens [6,7].

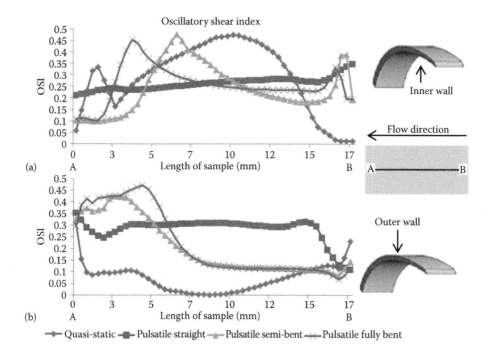

FIGURE 8.7
OSI distribution along the centerline of samples for (a) the inner wall and (b) the outer wall. Notice how the OSI variability was lowest along the inner and outer walls of straight samples ($n = 3$) subjected to pulsatile flow. The average OSI in the inner surface was found to be 0.2627, 0.2121, 0.2396, and 0.1009 for straight, semi-bent, fully bent, and quasi-static, respectively. In that same order, the outer wall values were 0.2689, 0.1859, 0.2159 and 0.2485. (From Salinas M et al., *Comput Methods Biomech Biomed Eng.*, 17:728–739, 2004; Salinas M et al., *Comput Methods Biomech Biomed Eng.*, 17:932, 2014.)

8.3 Conclusions and Future Outlook

The advent of new technologies such as TEHVs and percutaneously deployed valves are areas that are still relatively understudied using CFD. In this regard, several insights may be gained even from very straightforward modeling approaches (e.g., laminar flow, static models) provided that accurate depiction of the geometric features can be reproduced. On the other hand, the culmination of CFD research over the last several years has enabled streamlining of more advanced methodologies such as FSI-based approaches to the extent that research groups that utilize their in-house developed code are able to simulate very complex dynamic states of heart valves in a highly efficient fashion. While these approaches are also available in commercial CFD packages, direct control of localized deformation states is still tedious. In the years to come, it is expected that these packages will begin to offer more flexibility in the prescription of mesh movement, thereby allowing for more direct control of the simulations by the end user.

Irrespective of whether the usage of an advanced CFD technique becomes commonplace, or if several insights on the flow physics can be uncovered in emerging heart valve therapeutics using CFD, we expect that the findings resulting from CFD simulations in the heart valve research area will now, perhaps more than ever before, play a central role in the research or clinical process. This can be by way of, for example, enhancing the design features of a TEHV or a prosthetic valve, or alternatively, towards more rigorous quantitative evaluation of in vivo valve functionality, thereby better guiding the surgeon in selecting the next course of treatment for the patient.

References

1. Zilla P, Brink J, Human P, Bezuidenhout D. Prosthetic heart valves: Catering for the few. *Biomaterials.* 2008;29(4):385–406.
2. Westhoff-Bleck M, Girke S, Breymann T et al. Pulmonary valve replacement in chronic pulmonary regurgitation in adults with congenital heart disease: Impact of preoperative QRS-duration and NT-proBNP levels on postoperative right ventricular function. *Int J Cardiol.* 2011;151(3):303–306.
3. Waterbolk TW, Hoendermis ES, den Hamer IJ, Ebels T. Pulmonary valve replacement with a mechanical prosthesis: Promising results of 28 procedures in patients with congenital heart disease. *Eur J Cardio-Thorac.* 2006;30(1):28–32.
4. Schoen FJ. Evolving concepts of cardiac valve dynamics the continuum of development, functional structure, pathobiology and tissue engineering. *Circulation.* 2008;118(18):1864–1880.
5. Ramaswamy S, Gottlieb D, Engelmayr Jr. GC et al. The role of organ level conditioning on the promotion of engineered heart valve tissue development in-vitro using mesenchymal stem cells. *Biomaterials.* 2010;31(6):1114–1125.
6. Salinas M, Schmidt DE, Libera M, Lange RR, Ramaswamy S. Oscillatory shear stress created by fluid pulsatility versus flexed specimen configurations. *Comput Methods Biomech Biomed Eng.* 2014;17:728–739.
7. Salinas M, Schmidt DE, Libera M, Lange RR, Ramaswamy S. Corrigendum. *Comput Methods Biomech Biomed Eng.* 2014;17:932.
8. Sacks MS, David Merryman W, Schmidt DE. On the biomechanics of heart valve function. *J Biomech.* 2009;42(12):1804–1824.

9. Sacks MS, Schoen FJ, Mayer JE. Bioengineering challenges for heart valve tissue engineering. *Annu Rev Biomed Eng*. 2009;11:289–313.

10. Bernard I. Mitral stenosis still a concern in heart valve diseases. *Arch Cardiovasc Dis*. 2008;101(10):597–599.

11. Dal Pan F, Donzella G, Fucci C, Schreiber M. Structural effects of an innovative surgical technique to repair heart valve defects. *J Biomech*. 2005;38(12):2460–2471.

12. Elkayam U, Bitar F. Valvular heart disease and pregnancy: Part II: Prosthetic valves. *J Am Coll Cardiol*. 2005;46(3):403–410.

13. Elkayam U, Bitar F. Valvular heart disease and pregnancy: Part I: Native valves. *J Am Coll Cardiol*. 2005;46(2):223–230.

14. Frederick JS. New frontiers in the pathology and therapy of heart valve disease: 2006 Society for Cardiovascular Pathology, Distinguished Achievement Award Lecture, United States–Canadian Academy of Pathology, Atlanta, GA, February 12, 2006. *Cardiovasc Pathol*. 2006;15(5):271–279.

15. Iyengar SS, Pontefract DE, Barlow CW. Heart valve surgery. *Surgery (Oxford)*. 2004;22(6): 135–138.

16. Lorna S. Surgery for valve disease in young people-beyond morbidity and mortality. *Int J Cardiol*. 2010;145(3):411–412.

17. Mohammadi H, Mequanint K. Prosthetic aortic heart valves: Modeling and design. *Med Eng Phys*. 2011;33(2):131–147.

18. Neuenschwander S, Hoerstrup SP. Heart valve tissue engineering. *Transpl Immunol*. 2004; 12(3–4):359–365.

19. Shahbudin HR. Choice of prosthetic heart valve in adults: An update. *J Am Coll Cardiol*. 2010;55(22):2413–2426.

20. Siu SC, Silversides CK. Bicuspid aortic valve disease. *J Am Coll Cardiol*. 2010;55(25):2789–2800.

21. Talwar S, Rajesh MR, Subramanian A, Saxena A, Kumar AS. Mitral valve repair in children with rheumatic heart disease. *J Thorac Cardiovasc Surg*. 2005;129(4):875–879.

22. Baig K, Punjabi P. Heart valve surgery. *Surgery (Oxford)*. 2008;26(12):491–495.

23. Sotiropoulos F, Borazjani I. A review of state-of-the-art numerical methods for simulating flow through mechanical heart valves. *Med Biol Eng Comput*. 2009;47(3):245–256.

24. Gandaglia A, Bagno A, Naso F, Spina M, Gerosa G. Cells, scaffolds and bioreactors for tissue-engineered heart valves: A journey from basic concepts to contemporary developmental innovations. *Eur J Cardio-Thorac*. 2011;39(4):523–531.

25. Butcher JT, Mahler GJ, Hockaday LA. Aortic valve disease and treatment: The need for naturally engineered solutions. *Adv Drug Deliv Rev*. 2011;63(4–5):242–268.

26. Arcidiacono G, Corvi A, Severi T. Functional analysis of bioprosthetic heart valves. *J Biomech*. 2005;38(7):1483–1490.

27. David T, Hsu CH. Dynamic analysis and geometry models for the design of bi-leaflet prosthetic mechanical heart valves. *Med Eng Phys*. 1996;18(6):463–476.

28. David T, Hsu CH. The integrated design of mechanical bi-leaflet prosthetic heart valves. *Med Eng Phys*. 1996;18(6):452–462.

29. Sha P. Tricuspid and pulmonary valve disease evaluation and management. *Rev Esp Cardiol*. 2010;63(11):1349–1365.

30. Anastasiadis K, Kambouroglou D, Spanos P. The use of valve homografts and autografts in adult cardiac surgery. *Hellenic J Cardiol*. 2004;45:36–41.

31. Ungerleider RM, Ootaki Y, Shen I, Welke KF. Modified Ross procedure to prevent autograft dilatation. *Ann Thorac Surg*. 2010;90(3):1035–1037.

32. Athanasiou T, Cherian A, Ross D. The Ross II procedure: Pulmonary autograft in the mitral position. *Ann Thorac Surg*. 2004;78(4):1489–1495.

33. Brown JW, Ruzmetov M, Turrentine MW, Rodefeld MD. Mitral valve replacement with the pulmonary autograft: Ross II procedure with kabanni modification. *Semin Thorac Cardiovasc Surg Pediatr Card Surg Annu*. 2004;7(1):107–114.

34. Gamez A, Castillo JC, Bonilla JL, Anguita MP. Infective endocarditis after the Ross procedure. *Int J Cardiol.* 2011;147(3):e53–e54.

35. Jaggers J, Harrison JK, Bashore TM, Davis RD, Glower DD, Ungerleider RM. The Ross procedure: Shorter hospital stay, decreased morbidity, and cost effective. *Ann Thorac Surg.* 1998;65(6):1553–1558.

36. Khwaja S, Nigro JJ, Starnes VA. The Ross procedure is an ideal aortic valve replacement operation for the teen patient. *Semin Thorac Cardiovasc Surg Pediatr Card Surg Annu.* 2005;8(1):173–175.

37. Pretorius V, Jones A, Taylor D, Coe Y, Ross DB. Percutaneous valved stent repair of a failed homograft: Implications for the Ross procedure. *Can J Cardiol.* 2008;24(8):S54–S55.

38. Rus C, Mesa D, Concha M et al. Short-term results with the Ross procedure. Does the etiology of aortic valvulopathy affect the outcome? *Rev Esp Cardiol.* 2004;57(6):531–537.

39. Sarioglu T, Erek E, Yalçınbas YK, Salihoğlu E, Sarioglu A, Tekin S. Pericardial collar modification for Ross procedure. *Cardiovasc Surg.* 2003;11(3):229–230.

40. Slater M, Shen I, Welke K, Komanapalli C, Ungerleider R. Modification to the Ross procedure to prevent autograft dilatation. *Semin Thorac Cardiovasc Surg Pediatr Card Surg Annu.* 2005;8(1):181–184.

41. Stelzer P. The Ross procedure: State of the art 2011. *Semin Thorac Cardiovasc Surg.* 2011; 23(2):115–123.

42. Ghanbari H, Viatge H, Kidane AG, Burriesci G, Tavakoli M, Seifalian AM. Polymeric heart valves: New materials, emerging hopes. *Trends Biotechnol.* 2009;27(6):359–367.

43. Di Martino E, Pietrabissa R, Mantero S. The computational approach applied to the design and structural verification of a trileaflet polymeric heart valve. *Adv Eng Software.* 1997;28(6):341–346.

44. Kidane AG, Burriesci G, Edirisinghe M, Ghanbari H, Bonhoeffer P, Seifalian AM. A novel nanocomposite polymer for development of synthetic heart valve leaflets. *Acta Biomater.* 2009;5(7):2409–2417.

45. Ramaswamy S, Salinas M, Carrol R et al. Protocol for relative hydrodynamic assesment of trileaflet polymer valves. *J Vis Exp.* 2013;17(80):e50335.

46. Vyavahare P, Chen P, Joshi P et al. Current progress in anticalcif ication for bioprosthetic and polymeric heart valves. *Cardiovasc Pathol.* 1997;6(4):219–229.

47. Ramaswamy S, Schmidt D, Kassab G. Biomechanics of heart valves. In: Navia JL, Al-Ruzzeh S, eds. *Percutaneous Valve Technology: Present and Future.* New York: Nova Science Publishers, Inc.; 2012:175–194.

48. Martinez C, Rath S, Van Gulden S et al. Periodontal ligament cells cultured under steady flow environments demonstrate potential for use in heart valve tissue engineering. *Tissue Eng.* 2012;19:458–466.

49. Kadner A, Hoerstrup SP, Zund G et al. A new source for cardiovascular tissue engineering: Human bone marrow stromal cells. *Eur J Cardio-Thorac.* 2002;21(6):1055–1060.

50. Leor J, Amsalem Y, Cohen S. Cells, scaffolds, and molecules for myocardial tissue engineering. *Pharmacol Ther.* 2005;105(2):151–163.

51. Perry TE, Kaushal S, Sutherland FWH et al. Bone marrow as a cell source for tissue engineering heart valves. *Ann Thorac Surg.* 2003;75(3):761–767.

52. Ramaswamy S, Boronyak S, Le T, Holmes A, Sotiropoulos F, Sacks MS. A novel bioreactor for mechanobiological studies of engineered heart valve tissue formation under pulmonary arterial physiological flow conditions. *J Biomech Eng.* 2014;136(12):121009.

53. Siepe M, Akhyari P, Lichtenberg A, Schlensak C, Beyersdorf F. Stem cells used for cardiovascular tissue engineering. *Eur J Cardio-Thorac.* 2008;34(2):242–247.

54. Schmidt D, Dijkman PE, Driessen-Mol A et al. Minimally-invasive implantation of living tissue engineered heart valves: A comprehensive approach from autologous vascular cells to stem cells. *J Am Coll Cardiol.* 2010;56(6):510–520.

55. Huang CY, Pelaez D, Dominguez-Bendala J, Garcia-Godoy F, Cheung HS. Plasticity of stem cells derived from adult periodontal ligament. *Regen Med.* 2009;4(6):809–821.

56. Engelmayr GC, Sales VL, Mayer JE, Sacks MS. Cyclic flexure and laminar flow synergistically accelerate mesenchymal stem cell-mediated engineered tissue formation: Implications for engineered heart valve tissues. *Biomaterials.* 2006;27(36):6083–6095.

57. Fong P, Shin'oka T, Lopez-Soler RI, Breuer C. The use of polymer based scaffolds in tissue-engineered heart valves. *Prog Pediatr Cardiol.* 2006;21(2):193–199.
58. Chen G, Wu Q. The application of polyhydroxyalkanoates as tissue engineering materials. *Biomaterials.* 2005;26(33):6565–6578.
59. Lichtenberg A, Breymann T, Cebotari S, Haverich A. Cell seeded tissue engineered cardiac valves based on allograft and xenograft scaffolds. *Prog Pediatr Cardiol.* 2006;21(2):211–217.
60. Kleinstreuer C. *Biofluid Dymamics: Principles and Applications.* Boca Raton, FL: CRC Press; 2006:472–478.
61. El-Hamamsy I, Chester AH, Yacoub MH. Cellular regulation of the structure and function of aortic valves. *J Adv Res.* 2010;1(1):5–12.
62. Sutherland FW, Perry TE, Yu Y et al. From stem cells to viable autologous semilunar heart valve. *Circulation.* 2005;111(21):2783–2791.
63. Krause E. Computational fluid dynamics: Its present status and future direction. *Comput Fluids.* 1985;13(3):239–269.
64. Peskin CS, McQueen DM. Modeling prosthetic heart valves for numerical analysis of blood flow in the heart. *J Comput Phys.* 1980;37(1):113–132.
65. Peskin C. Flow patterns around heart valves: A numerical method. *J Comput Phys.* 1972;10:252–271.
66. Storti MA, Nigro NM, Paz RR, Dalcínm LD. Dynamic boundary conditions in computational fluid dynamics. *Comput Method Appl M.* 2008;197(13–16):1219–1232.
67. Hose DR, Narracott AJ, Penrose JMT, Baguley D, Jones IP, Lawford PV. Fundamental mechanics of aortic heart valve closure. *J Biomech.* 2006;39(5):958–967.
68. Onate E, Idelsohn SR, Del Pin F, Aubry R. The particle finite element method. An overview. *Int J Comput M.* 2004:307.
69. Chandran KB, Yoganathan AP, Rittgers SE. *Bio-Fluid Mechanics: The Human Circulation,* 2nd ed. CRC Press, Boca Raton, FL, 2012.
70. Shim E, Chang K. Three-dimensional vortex flow past a tilting disc valve using a segregated finite element scheme. *Comput Dyn J.* 1994;3:205.
71. Ge L, Jones C, Sotiropoulos F, Healy TM, Yoganathan AP. Numerical simulation of flow in mechanical heart valves: Grid resolution and the assumption of flow symmetry. *J Biomech Eng-T ASME.* 2003;125(5):709–718.
72. Ge L, Fellow P, Leo HL, Student PD, Sotiropoulos F, Yoganathan AP. Flow in a mechanical bileaflet heart valve at laminar and near-peak systole flow rates: Cfd simulations and experiments. *J Biomech Eng.* 2005;127:782.
73. McQueen DM, Peskin CS. Computer-assisted design of butterfly bileaflet valves for the mitral position. *Scand J Thorac Cardiovasc Surg.* 1985;19(2):139–148.
74. Lei M, Van-Steenhoven A, Van-Campen D. Experimental and numerical analyses of the steady flow field around an aortic bjork-shiley standard valve prostheses. *J Biomech.* 1992;3:213–222.
75. Kiris C, Kwak D, Rogers S, Chang ID. Computational approach for probing the flow through artificial heart devices. *J Biomech Eng.* 1997;119:452–460.
76. King MJ, Corden J, David T, Fisher J. A three-dimensional, time-dependent analysis of flow through a bileaflet mechanical heart valve: Comparison of experimental and numerical results. *J Biomech.* 1996;29(5):609–618.
77. King M, David T, Fisher J. Three-dimensional study of the effect of two leaflet opening angles on the time-dependent flow through a bileaflet mechanical heart valve. *Med Eng Phys.* 1997;19(5):235–241.
78. Nobili M, Morbiducci U, Ponzini R et al. Numerical simulation of the dynamics of a bileaflet prosthetic heart valve using a fluid–structure interaction approach. *J Biomech.* 2008;41(11):2539–2550.
79. Vierendeels J, Dumont K, Verdonck PR. A partitioned strongly coupled fluid-structure interaction method to model heart valve dynamics. *J Comput Appl Math.* 2008;215(2):602–609.
80. Driessen NJB, Mol A, Bouten CVC, Baaijens FPT. Modeling the mechanics of tissue-engineered human heart valve leaflets. *J Biomech.* 2007;40(2):325–334.

81. Gilmanov A, Sotiropoulos F. A hybrid cartesian/immersed boundary method for simulating flows with 3D, geometrically complex, moving bodies. *J Comput Phys*. 2005;207(2):457–492.

82. Hong T, Choeng-Ryul C, Chang-Nyung K. Characteristics of hemodynamics in a bileaflet mechanical heart valve using an implicit FSI method. *Eng Tech*. 2009;49:679–684.

83. Kukreja N, Onuma Y, Daemen J, Serruys PW. The future of drug-eluting stents. *Pharmacol Res*. 2008;57(3):171–180.

84. Oshima M, Torii R, Kobayashi T, Taniguchi N, Takagi K. Finite element simulation of blood flow in the cerebral artery. *Comput Method Appl M*. 2001;191(6–7):661–671.

85. Nguyen MC, Lim YL. Benefits of drug-eluting stents in coronary heart disease treatment with emphasis on the diabetic subgroup. *Heart Lung Circ*. 2007;16(1):7–9.

86. Zhang LT, Gay M. Immersed finite element method for fluid-structure interactions. *J Fluid Struct*. 2007;23(6):839–857.

87. Kim D, Choi H. Immersed boundary method for flow around an arbitrarily moving body. *J Comput Phys*. 2006;212(2):662–680.

88. Tai CH, Liew KM, Zhao Y. Numerical simulation of 3D fluid–structure interaction flow using an immersed object method with overlapping grids. *Comput Struct*. 2007;85(11–14):749–762.

89. Engelmayr GC, Soletti L, Vigmostad SC et al. A novel flex-stretch-flow bioreactor for the study of engineered heart valve tissue mechanobiology. *Ann Biomed Eng*. 2008;36(5):1–13.

90. Ryan LP, Salgo IS, Gorman RC, Gorman III JH. The emerging role of three-dimensional echo-cardiography in mitral valve repair. *Semin Thorac Cardiovasc Surg*. 2006;18(2):126–134.

91. Schlosshan D, Aggarwal G, Mathur G, Allan R, Cranney G. Real-time 3D transesophageal echocardiography for the evaluation of rheumatic mitral stenosis. *JACC Cardiovasc Imaging*. 2011;4(6):580–588.

92. Le TB, Sotiropoulos F. Fluid-structure interaction of an aortic heart valve prosthesis driven by an animated anatomic left ventricle. *J Comput Phys*. 2013;244:41–62.

93. Wong KKL, Sun Z, Tu J, Worthley SG, Mazumdar J, Abbott D. Medical image diagnostics based on computer-aided flow analysis using magnetic resonance images. *Comput Med Imaging Graph*. 2012;36(7):527–541.

94. Sengupta PP, Pedrizzetti G, Kilner PJ et al. Emerging trends in CV flow visualization. *JACC Cardiovasc Imaging*. 2012;5(3):305–316.

95. Cavalcante JL, Rodriguez LL, Kapadia S, Tuzcu EM, Stewart WJ. Role of echocardiography in percutaneous mitral valve interventions. *JACC Cardiovasc Imaging*. 2012;5(7):733–746.

96. Leopaldi AM, Vismara R, Lemma M et al. In vitro hemodynamics and valve imaging in passive beating hearts. *J Biomech*. 2012;45(7):1133–1139.

97. Lim WL, Chew YT, Chew TC, Low HT. Steady flow dynamics of prosthetic aortic heart valves: A comparative evaluation with PIV techniques. *J Biomech*. 1998;31(5):411–421.

98. De Bartolo L, Leindlein A, Hofmann D et al. Bio-hybrid organs and tissues for patient therapy: A future vision for 2030. *Chem Eng Process: Process Intensif*. 2012;51:79–87.

99. Lantz J, Karlsson M. Large eddy simulation of LDL surface concentration in a subject specific human aorta. *J Biomech*. 2012;45(3):537–542.

100. Haj-Ali R, Dasi LP, Kim H, Choi J, Leo HW, Yoganathan AP. Structural simulations of prosthetic tri-leaflet aortic heart valves. *J Biomech*. 2008;41(7):1510–1519.

101. Ansys. Ansys cfx solver theory guide. *Release 14.1*. 2012.

102. Pelliccioni O, Cerrolaza M, Herrera M. Lattice Boltzmann dynamic simulation of a mechanical heart valve device. *Math Comput Simul*. 2007;75(1–2):1–14.

103. Krafczyk M, Tolke J, Rank E, Schulz M. Two-dimensional simulation of fluid-structure interaction using lattice-boltzmann methods. *Comput Struct*. 2001;79:2031–2037.

104. Krafczyk M, Cerrolaza M, Schulz M, Rank E. Analysis of 3D transient bloodflow passing through and artificial aortic valve by Lattice–Boltzmann methods. *J Biomech*. 1998;31:453–462.

105. Shahriari S, Maleki H, Hassan I, Kadem L. Evaluation of shear stress accumulation on blood components in normal and dysfunctional bileaflet mechanical heart valves using smoothed particle hydrodynamics. *J Biomech*. 2012;45(15):2637–2644.

106. Borazjani I. Fluid–structure interaction, immersed boundary-finite element method simulations of bio-prosthetic heart valves. *Comput Methods Appl Mech Eng*. 2013;257:103–116.
107. Banerjee R. *Fatigue Analysis of Arteries Using Finite Element Method*. M.S. North Dakota State University, Fargo, ND, 2013.
108. Jacobs CR, Yellowley CE, Davis BR, Zhou Z, Cimbala JM, Donahue HJ. Differential effect of steady versus oscillating flow on bone cells. *J Biomech*. 1998;31(11):969–976.
109. Arnsdorf EJ, Tummala P, Jacobs CR. Non-canonical wnt signaling and N-cadherin related b-catenin signaling play a role in mechanically induced osteogenic cell fate. *PLoS One*. 2009;4(4):e5388.
110. Arnsdorf E, Tummala P, Kwon R, Jacobs C. Mechanically induced osteogenic differentiation—The role of RhoA, ROCKII and cytoskeletal dynamics. *J Cell Sci*. 2009;122(Pt 4):546–553.
111. He X, Ku DN. Pulsatile flow in the human left coronary artery bifurcation: Average conditions. *J Biomech Eng*. 1996;118(1):74–82.

9

Mathematical Modeling of Cancer Metastases

Marc D. Ryser and Svetlana V. Komarova

CONTENTS

ABSTRACT Most cancer types develop the ability to leave their site of origin and spread to distant organs to form metastases, also called secondary cancers. Metastases are the most common cause of death among cancer patients, and hence there is an immense clinical interest to understand the underlying biological mechanisms and to develop preventive and therapeutic measures. Over the past decades, an increasing number of applied mathematicians and biomedical engineers have taken on the challenge to design models and devise in silico tools for the study of cancer and cancer metastases. The goals of this chapter are to introduce to the reader the important challenges in the field of metastases and to give an overview of the existing modeling tools. Guided by pertinent biological questions, we review a number of deterministic and stochastic approaches and discuss their potential and limitations.

9.1 Introduction

Cancer is a complex disease, extremely diverse and heterogeneous at virtually all levels. Not only can two patients with the same cancer type experience different disease evolution and outcomes, but also within a single patient, the tumor is likely to consist of several subtypes. These facts render targeted treatment a tough challenge, and to date, many cancer types are at best manageable, rather than curable. In view of the overwhelming complexity, modern cancer research is an interdisciplinary effort involving a multitude of disciplines, including medicine, molecular biology, genetics, epidemiology, and biostatistics, to name just a few. In addition to these more traditional branches of cancer research, a steadily growing number of applied mathematicians and biomedical engineers are entering the field of cancer research. Over the past two decades, we have seen a veritable boom in mathematical modeling of the various aspects of disease progression. Needless to say, diversity and complexity in the biological system lead to diversity and complexity in the corresponding modeling approaches. Nowadays, the mathematical tools used in the study of cancer range from ordinary differential equations (ODEs) to partial differential equations (PDEs), from branching processes to interacting particle systems, from evolutionary games to cellular automata, and more and more researchers base their efforts on multiscale hybrid models. Since we do not intend to review the field of mathematical cancer modeling in its entirety—such an endeavor would fill an entire book at the very least, we will discuss some relevant references on the modeling of cancer. Over the past few years, several books have been published. For example, Komarova and Wodarz provide a general review of computational methods in cancer biology [1], and the whole spectrum of continuum, discrete, and hybrid models is reviewed by Cristini and Lowengrub [2]. Furthermore, a broad range of contributions from leading researchers in the field is compiled in recent books edited by Deisboeck and Stamatakos [3] and Bellomo and de Angelis [4]. A review of mathematical modeling with a focus on breast cancer is given by Chauviere et al. [5], and the state of the art of hybrid models is summarized by Rejniak and Anderson [6]. Michor et al. reviewed the physics side of cancer research [7], and Blair et al. discussed mathematical modeling from the perspective of systems biology [8].

The goal of this chapter is to focus on the modeling efforts directed at one of the key aspects of cancer research: formation and evolution of metastases, the last and most lethal stage of cancer evolution. When writing about an interdisciplinary subject, it is always difficult to cater to audiences on both sides. Here, and in the spirit of the encapsulating book, we focus on the reader who has a good working knowledge of the mathematical tools, and aim to highlight different areas of cancer research where such knowledge can be applied. A particular challenge of this approach is that we only have limited space to provide an overview of the biological processes in question. We selected examples of modeling studies based on their mathematical approaches, and as a result, these studies spotlight a wide variety of different cancer types, including breast, prostate, ovarian, and colorectal, as well as their metastases to different sites. While it is clear that many cancer types progress similarly, it is important to keep in mind that each type has a distinct underlying biology. Because of space limitations, we cannot provide an in-depth description of the biological processes, but we will provide references to recent reviews for the interested reader. We start with a short overview of the underlying biology of cancer metastases in Section 9.2 and then discuss how different research questions have been approached from the mathematical modeling perspective in Sections 9.3 through 9.6. To conclude, we provide an overview of the challenges and open questions in the field in Section 9.7. Finally, we apologize to all colleagues whose work is not cited in this review—either for reasons of space or because of the limitation of our own knowledge of the literature.

9.2 Brief Overview of the Biology of Cancer Metastases

Cancer starts with healthy tissue cells that randomly acquire genetic or epigenetic mutations during cell division. While most mutations are deleterious and lead to programmed cell death, there are a number of mutations that can increase the fitness of the affected cell, leading to more aggressive growth. Once a growth advantage has been acquired, the mutated cell can give rise to a subpopulation of abnormally proliferating tissue cells, which in turn develop an increasingly malignant phenotype by means of further mutations. Premalignant and malignant cells exhibit critical differences from their normal counterparts in their increased ability to divide, decreased death rate, lack of differentiation, and shift in bioenergetics [9–11]. However, even though the primary tumor represents a dangerous pathology, the most detrimental part of cancer is the development of metastases— spreading of cancer to distant sites where numerous new tumors can be established [12–14]. It is believed that acquisition of the metastatic capacity by primary cancer cells is once more attributed to (epi)genetic mutations. Both the activation of metastasis-enabling oncogenes and inactivation of metastasis suppressor genes (MSGs) have been proposed to drive metastases [15,16]. Metastatic spread of malignant cancer cells from the primary location (e.g., breast, prostate, skin) usually starts with the nearby lymph nodes and eventually reaches distant organs (e.g., bone, liver, lung) via the blood and lymphatic systems [17]. Several tasks generally need to be accomplished by the metastasizing cancer cells (Figure 9.1). First, some cells within the primary tumor need to acquire a sufficiently motile phenotype to escape the primary location [18,19]. For many cancer types, this is achieved through epithelial-to-mesenchymal transition, in which cells lose the molecular apparatus required for their adhesion to other cells (prominent in epithelial tissues) and acquire a motile mesenchymal phenotype [19]. Next, cancer cells need to access the circulation and survive the journey to the secondary site [20]. Thereby, preferential homing of cancer cells to specific secondary organs has long been recognized: each cancer type has a specific propensity to arrive and thrive in different organs [21,22]. When circulating cancer cells reach their target organ, they need to leave the circulation and survive in the foreign microenvironment of a metastatic site [23]. Once metastases have started growing, cure is usually out of reach, and most cancer patients die from the consequences of metastatic growth rather than the primary cancer itself. Metastatic spread is a complex process, still generating more questions than answers. Here is a selection of pertinent questions, which are relevant both biologically and clinically.

- What is the relationship between intratumor heterogeneity and metastatic potential?
- What are the mechanisms that enable cancer cells in the primary site to leave their origin and migrate to distant locations?
- Is there a relationship between the growth dynamics of the primary tumor and secondary metastases? Can it be used for clinical decision making?

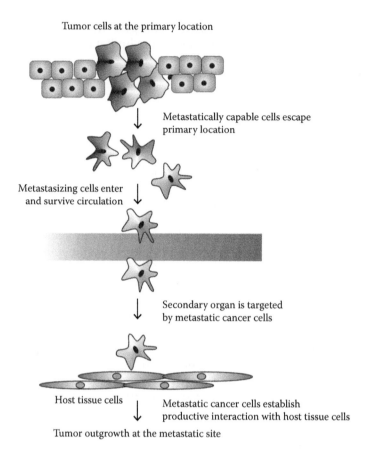

Tumor cells at the primary location

Metastatically capable cells escape
primary location

Metastasizing cells enter
and survive circulation

Secondary organ is targeted
by metastatic cancer cells

Host tissue cells

Metastatic cancer cells establish
productive interaction with host tissue cells

Tumor outgrowth at the metastatic site

FIGURE 9.1
Schematic representation of the process of metastasis formation. Cancer cells at the primary site develop the capacity to migrate and enter the circulation. They leave the circulation at the secondary organ, establish a productive interaction with host tissue cells, and start growing at the metastatic site.

- What is the expected time for onset of metastases? Is there an optimal screening window to detect the cancer before it spreads to distant sites and becomes incurable?

- What are the mechanisms of preferential localization of different cancer cells to common metastatic sites such as lung, liver, and bone?

- How do the cancer cells co-opt and take advantage of the local microenvironment?

In the subsequent sections, we will provide examples of how these questions can be addressed using mathematical modeling.

9.3 Acquiring the Metastatic Phenotype

The metastatic phenotype, that is, the capacity to metastasize, is acquired by dividing cells in the primary cancer through genetic and epigenetic mutations [15,16,24]. To leave its site of origin and metastasize to a distant organ is a nontrivial task for a cancer cell and requires acquisition of traits not present in the parental population, such as motility, rheological properties to circulate through small capillaries and survive large sheer stresses of arterial circulation, and the ability to interact with and influence resident cells at the metastatic site. Because of this layered complexity, the success rate for each cell that leaves the primary tumor is very small, and even though primary tumors can shed large quantities of potentially metastasis-enabled cells, only a few eventually give rise to new metastatic colonies [25,26]. While there is an ever-growing amount of data collected on these issues, it remains difficult to disentangle the underlying mechanisms and obtain reliable estimates on quantities such as the rate and number of metastasis-enabling genetic mutations, the relative fitness of metastatic cells with respect to primary cancer cells, the export probability, and the survival probability. As we are going to discuss in the remainder of this section, stochastic modeling provides a powerful tool in the quest for a deeper understanding of these issues.

To analyze the dynamics of metastasis-enabling genetic and epigenetic mutations, Michor et al. [27] developed a stochastic model that describes the acquisition of a single metastasis-enabling oncogene mutation, such as RAS [28]. The authors assume that there is a fixed number N of cancer cells, each of which is either a parental cancer cell of fitness 1, or a mutated cell of fitness $r > 0$. The cell dynamics are described by a discrete-time Markov chain, and at each time step, a cell is chosen for proliferation with probability proportional to its relative fitness. For example, if the current number of parental cells is j, then with probability $p = j/(j + r(N - j))$, the chosen cell is a parental cell, and with probability $1 - p$, it is a mutated cell. In either case, the offspring cell then replaces an arbitrary cell, that is, the latter is assumed to die. In addition, during each cell division, the offspring of a parental cell can acquire a metastasis-enabling mutation with probability u. A crucial role in these Markov dynamics is played by the relative fitness of the mutated cells: if $r < 1$, the metastasis-enabled cells have a selective disadvantage compared to parental cells; that is, they proliferate less frequently. If $r > 1$, the mutated cells proliferate at a higher rate than parental cells, and at $r = 1$, both cell types are equally fit. Starting with all parental cells, once a mutated cell is born, there are two possible outcomes: either the progeny of the mutant will linger at a low frequency and eventually die out or it will take over the whole population. As expected, the higher the relative fitness r, the higher the probability that it will take over the population. Starting with only parental cells, the authors then study the evolution of the mutated cancer cell population $z(t)$, both numerically and analytically. Assuming that only a fraction q of mutated cells actually leave the tumor and successfully metastasize, the formation of new metastatic colonies is an inhomogeneous Poisson process of rate $q\,z(t)$. The authors show that because of increased probability of taking over the whole population, advantageous mutations ($r > 1$) are much more successful (several orders of magnitude) at creating metastases than neutral or disadvantageous mutations ($r \leq 1$). This study provides insights into the question, "Is metastatic potential the property of the majority of cells in the primary tumor or only the property of a small subset of cells?" and concludes that while it is possible for a cell type with extremely high metastatic potential to metastasize despite a disadvantage in the primary tumor, metastases are more likely derived from advantageous mutations that take over a large part of the tumor.

To address the scenario where the metastatic phenotype is acquired through inactivation of an MSG, Michor and Iwasa [29] generalized the above model from a single mutation to two mutations, therefore accounting for inactivation of both MSG alleles. Similarly to the results in Ref. [27], the authors conclude that it is more likely for metastases to stem from mutants with an increased relative fitness $r > 1$. The authors provide numerical estimates and show that in order for deleterious mutations to be as efficient for metastasis formation as advantageous mutations, they need to be accompanied by an export probability that is 10^8-fold higher than that of advantageous mutations.

The above models ignore the physical departure of metastasizing cancer cells. However, once a mutant cell leaves the tumor, it decreases the number of remaining mutant cells in the primary tumor. To show that departure does indeed have an influence on the fraction of mutated cells in the evolving primary tumor, Dingli et al. [30] extended the single mutation model by Michor et al. [27]. More precisely, the authors assume that upon division of a mutated cell, the offspring cell leaves the primary tumor with probability q. Note that if the offspring cell does leave the primary site, then no cell has to be chosen for death as the total number is automatically conserved. The authors show that there exists a critical export probability q_{crit}, depending on the mutation rate u and the fitness r only, such that if $q > q_{crit}$, the growth of the mutated cell population in the primary site is reduced, hence leading to a primary tumor where the mutated population makes up for a small fraction rather than the majority of the tumor. In other words, large export probabilities can lead to an increase in tumor heterogeneity. In the second part of the article, the authors relax the assumption of a conserved number of cancer cells in the primary tumor and introduce branching process dynamics to account for exponential growth of the tumor population. Even though the populations of parental and mutated cancer cells grow over time, and the detailed dynamics are quite different, the relative frequency of metastasis-enabled cells is affected by the export probability q in the same way as for the case of a constant tumor size. In particular, the critical value q_{crit} is the same as in the case of a constant tumor size.

9.4 Growth Dynamics of Metastases

Assume for instance that a primary cancer is detected and successfully treated at an early stage, and that there is no clinical evidence of metastatic activity elsewhere in the body. Unfortunately, a promising clinical history of this sort might be misleading and does not necessarily imply definite recovery of the patient [31]. In addition to the risk of a relapse at the primary site, there is the problem of occult metastases (also called micrometastases), that is, dormant or slowly growing metastatic colonies that are too small to be detected at the time of treatment of the primary cancer [32]. In the clinical setting, the issue of such occult metastases can be addressed by continuous treatment to kill potential undetectable micrometastases before they can grow into a macroscopic tumor. However, most cancer therapies have a significant burden of side effects. Therefore, the therapeutic intervention needs to be designed in such a way that it is aggressive enough to kill any residual malignant cells in the body, while at the same time only minimally affecting the functionality and well-being of the patient [33]. To strike this optimal balance, knowledge about preferred locations of potential metastases, expected number and size of currently present occult metastases, and growth dynamics and aggressiveness of potential metastatic colonies is extremely valuable for the oncologist. Unfortunately, the amount of available information at the time of excision is usually very limited, and much more than the size of the primary tumor, and the number of detectable metastases is rarely known. In particular, direct information about occult metastases and dynamics of the metastatic process is usually missing. This leads us to a clinically relevant and mathematically challenging question: given a set of basic measurements, how much can we infer regarding the underlying metastasis dynamics? Over the past two decades, this problem has been approached from different angles, three of which we are now going to discuss in more detail.

9.4.1 Stochastic Mechanistic Models

To elucidate the correlation between local cancer relapse at the primary site and incidence of metastases, Yorke et al. introduce a stochastic model in their study [34]. Guided by the underlying biology, the authors develop a simple mechanistic model, capturing the main stages in the process of metastasis formation. The primary cancer cell population, n, is assumed to grow according to a deterministic Gompertzian growth law, and a subset $\mu(n)$ of the primary cancer cells is metastatically capable; that is, they can potentially leave the primary tumor to form metastatic foci at a distant site. Assuming furthermore that only a small fraction η of these metastatically capable cells actually leave the primary site to successfully colonize the secondary site, the authors describe the metastasis formation by means of an inhomogeneous Poisson process of rate $\eta\mu(n(t))$. Based primarily on computer simulations, the authors perform in silico comparisons of patients with and without local relapse and find that local relapse has a great impact on emergence of metastases in the long run. In particular, Yorke et al. conjectured that by preventing relapse at the primary site, the long-term metastasis-free survival of patients who are initially free of detectable metastases could be substantially improved. Notably, their hypothesis was confirmed later on in the work by Zelefsky et al. [35], where it is shown that local tumor control is associated with a decrease in distant metastases and prostate cancer mortality.

A generalized version of the Yorke et al. model is rigorously studied and analyzed by Hanin et al. [36]. In particular, their framework allows for arbitrary growth laws of the cancer population, and migrating cancer cells are subject to a random promotion time between shedding from the primary tumor to inoculation at the secondary site. Exploiting the mathematical properties of Poisson processes, the authors compute the probability density function p such that conditioned on their number n, the sizes $X_1 < X_2 < \ldots X_n$ of metastases are given by the order statistics of n p-distributed samples (see their Theorem on page 410). Hanin et al. explicitly apply their results to special cases of growth laws and promotion time distributions and carefully discuss the amount of parameter information that can be inferred from clinical observations. Finally, they evaluate their model and possible implications on the specific example of breast cancer.

Haeno and Michor [37] rendered the above model fully stochastic by replacing the deterministic Gompertzian growth model by a branching process model. Similarly to the models discussed in Section 9.3, they distinguish between parental cells and metastases-enabled cells with differing relative fitness, and they account for mutations from parental to metastasis-enabled cells, as well as the export rate of metastatic phenotypes. Using a combination of analytical results and numerical simulations, the authors study quantities such as probability of presence of metastases and expected number of undetectable metastases at diagnosis. Because of the relatively large number of model parameters, their approach will benefit from future experimental assessment of the different rates and probabilities involved.

9.4.2 Deterministic Mechanistic Models

It is known that metastases do not necessarily originate from the primary site but can also arise from already existing metastases in the body. These so-called secondary metastases can lead to metastatic cascades and rapid progression of the disease [38]. To study the contribution of secondary metastases, Iwata et al. [39] introduced an extended deterministic version of the previously described mechanistic model. More precisely, the authors study the evolution of $\rho(x,t)$, the colony size distribution of metastatic tumors with x cells at time t. Based on conservation of tumor mass, they show that the evolution of $\rho(x,t)$ is described by the following hyperbolic PDE:

$$\frac{\partial \rho(x,t)}{\partial t} + \frac{\partial (g(x)\rho(x,t))}{\partial x} = 0,$$

with initial condition $\rho(x,0) = 0$ (initially, no metastases are present) and boundary condition

$$g(1)\rho(1,t) = \int_1^\infty \beta(x)\rho(x,t)\,\mathrm{d}x + \beta(x_\mathrm{p}(t)),$$

where $g(x)$ is the size-dependent growth rate of cancer cell populations, $\beta(x)$ is the rate at which a population of size x sheds cells with metastatic potential, and $x_\mathrm{p}(t)$ is the size of the primary cancer population, that is, solution to the initial value problem

$$\frac{\mathrm{d}x_\mathrm{p}}{\mathrm{d}t} = g(x_\mathrm{p}), \quad x_\mathrm{p}(0) = 1.$$

Assuming $\beta(x) = Cx^\alpha$, for $C > 0$ a constant, Iwata et al. solve the PDE for exponential, power law, and Gompertzian growth rates $g(x)$, respectively. In the case of Gompertzian tumor growth, they fit their model to data from a primary liver cancer. Since the analytic expression of $\rho(x,t)$ involves an infinite series, they use asymptotics, but nevertheless find a good agreement between data and model.

In what provides a nice example of the multifaceted nature of applied mathematics, the model proposed by Iwata et al. was later on revisited by Barbolosi et al. [40] for a rigorous mathematical analysis of the PDE and the design of a numerical scheme. Besides establishing existence and uniqueness of solutions to the PDE, the authors devise a suitable numerical method and establish convergence results. Furthermore, they show that the differential operator of the problem,

$$-\frac{\partial}{\partial x}(g(x)\cdot)$$

has a unique positive real eigenvalue λ, and that this parameter, the so-called Malthus parameter, determines the large time asymptotics of the total number of metastatic cells as $N(t) \approx e^{\lambda t}$.

The results and insights gained by Barbolosi et al. [40] and Iwata et al. [39] are further explored by Benzekry et al. [41]. Modifying the growth dynamics by adapting $g(x)$, the authors model the effects of drugs used in antiangiogenic and cytotoxic chemotherapy. Based on in silico experiments, they first show that the model recapitulates clinical data and then use the model as a predictive tool to propose optimal therapeutic schedules.

9.4.3 Phenomenological Markov Chain Model

An interesting approach to quantify pathways of metastatic progression for lung cancer is adopted by Newton et al. [42]. Motivated by the fact that the metastatic process is intrinsically stochastic, and assuming that secondary metastases arise in the same way as primary metastases do, they model the temporal evolution of the metastatic distribution as a discrete-time Markov chain. Given N potential metastatic sites in the body, they describe the state of the system at time step t_k by an N-dimensional vector v_k, where $(v_k)_j$ is the probability that a metastasis is present at location j. They assume that the dynamics of the natural history can be cast by means of an N by N transition matrix A such that $v_{k+1} = v_k A$. Of course, the main challenge here is that the transition matrix A is a priori unknown and has to be inferred from clinical data. Assuming that by the time of autopsy (i.e., the patient's death), the Markov chain has reached a stationary state, that is, $v_\infty = v_\infty A$, they use a stochastic optimization algorithm to find a suitable matrix A. The performance of the algorithm is assessed on the specific case of a primary lung cancer with detailed information on metastases at time of autopsy. We note that the model is rather phenomenological than mechanistic in nature. To attempt a mechanistic interpretation, we follow the suggestion of the authors and consider the Markov chain as a statistical ensemble of random walkers on the network, that is, the complete graph of potential secondary sites. However, it is important to realize that the number of walkers is not conserved over time owing to the stochastic processes of proliferation and death. Note that in the special case of state-independent proliferation and killing rates, the relative frequency of metastatic cells at different sites would approximately coincide with the relative frequency in the case of conserved walkers (conditioned on survival). However, it seems very likely that proliferation and death rates of cells vary substantially with organ site. Also questionable is the assumption that the chain has reached its steady state by the time of death of the patient. As highlighted by the above stochastic and mechanistic models, many metastases lie dormant or remain very small for a long time, after which they literally explode. Death of the patient is presumably happening in the midst of this exploding regime, and hence it is hard to see this as a stationary state. Nevertheless, the Markov chain approach highlights some interesting aspects of the dynamics. Based on the matrix A, the authors are able to distinguish between first-order and second-order metastases, depending on whether the cancer cells are more likely to get to a specific location directly from the primary site or by passing through another secondary site, respectively. Furthermore, the diagonal entries of A can be interpreted as self-seeding probabilities, a concept that has attracted attention in recent years [43]. Overall, this model calls attention to the importance of the complex, subtle, and heterogeneous connections among the many potential metastatic locations that may be critical in the understanding of cancer progression.

9.5 Beat the Metastasis: Screening Window Estimates

Most cancer patients die from the consequences of metastatic disease rather than the primary tumor, and it is therefore crucial to detect and treat a growing cancer before it leaves the primary site. Striking evidence for this is apparent in the numbers [44]: whereas cancers that are commonly caught in nonmetastatic stages (93% for both breast and prostate cancers) have a relatively high 5-year survival rate (89.1% for breast, 99.4% for prostate), cancers that are more often detected in metastatic stages (68% for ovarian cancer) have a much lower 5-year survival rate (45% for ovarian cancer). In an ideal world, such numbers would lead to systematic, high-frequency screening programs for the entire population—however, in the real-world this does not work out: screening procedures are very expensive, they have a nonnegligible error rate, and false positives can lead to unnecessary invasive treatments with an adverse impact on the patient's health. These limitations lead to several optimization problems for the screening procedures, including the following: how big is the time window between the onset of a detectable primary tumor and the onset of metastases? This question can be approached from different angles: Danesh et al. [44] used a multitype branching process together with epidemiological data, whereas Jones et al. [45] combined mathematical modeling with genetic sequencing.

9.5.1 Multitype Branching Process

The evolution of cancer is intrinsically stochastic: transformation of normal tissue into first a benign neoplasm, then an invasive carcinoma, and finally a metastasizing cancer is caused by relatively rare genetic mutations. In their study [44], Danesh et al. model this multistage progression in the case of ovarian cancer by means of a multitype branching process. Their model captures the three stages of disease progression (not corresponding to the standard stage classification of ovarian cancer):

- Stage 1: primary cancer confined to the ovary of origin;
- Stage 2: detached cells accumulating in the peritoneal fluid;
- Stage 3: reattached cells growing at a metastatic site. In stage i, a cell divides to create an offspring cell at rate a_i, and it dies at rate b_i.

To capture the genetic mutation dynamics, each cell of type i can transition to stage $i + 1$ at a very small rate μ_i. More precisely, a primary cancer cell mutates at rate μ_1 into a detached peritoneal cell, which can then mutate at rate μ_2 into a cell that can attach and grow at the secondary site. A key feature of this model is its mechanistic nature that captures the biological essence at the mesoscopic level. In particular, introduction of the disease stages—primary, diffuse, and secondary—allows a model calibration based on epidemiological data. Danesh et al. use analytical results from their model combined with data from the SEER database to determine unknown parameter values and then compute the

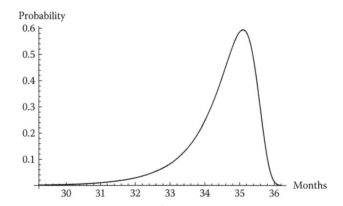

FIGURE 9.2

Narrow screening window for ovarian cancer is predicted by a multitype branching process model. Probability density function for the time between emergence of a detectable primary tumor and onset of metastases. This provides the window of opportunity for ovarian cancer screening. (Reproduced from Danesh K et al., *Journal of Theoretical Biology*, 2012, 314:10–15. With permission.)

distribution of the time between emergence of a detectable primary cancer and onset of metastasis. More precisely, they estimate the window of opportunity for ovarian cancer screening to be approximately 2.9 years (Figure 9.2).

9.5.2 Comparative Lesion Sequencing

A different approach to estimate the time to metastasis is based on the use of molecular information gained from individual tumor sequencing, a method developed by Jones et al. [45]. Thereby, the key idea is to compare the genetic fingerprints of the primary and metastatic cells. On the basis of the number of mutations that are present in the metastasis, but not in the primary tumor, the authors deduce the expected amount of time between onset of invasive cancer and emergence of metastases. Applied to the example of colorectal carcinogenesis, the authors estimate that it takes approximately 17 years for a benign pre-cancer to become invasive, but less than 2 years for this invasive carcinoma to become meta-static. Therefore, and similarly to the case of ovarian cancer, the window of opportunity is rather small. The mathematical model by Jones et al. [45] is based on some rather stringent assumptions; for example, the mutation rate is assumed to be constant during carcinogenesis, and mutations that confer a positive or negative growth advantage are neglected. While the authors are able to justify these restrictions in the current case of colorectal cancer, the method might not be suitable, for example, for cancer types with mutator phenotypes such as breast cancer. A similar sequencing approach is applied to the case of pancreatic cancer in the work of Yachida et al. [46], and there the time window from onset of the primary tumor to the emergence of metastases is estimated to be at least 10 years.

9.6 Tumor–Stroma Interactions

In both primary and secondary tumors, cancer cells interact to a varying degree with the microenvironment, including both the connective network of supporting stromal cells and organ-specific functional cells [47]. By actively altering and co-opting their environment, cancer cells can increase their relative fitness and hence grow more aggressively. In this section, we will discuss mathematical modeling of the tumor–stroma interactions using as an example the case of bone metastases, a disease state associated with high morbidity and increased mortality, especially in breast and prostate cancer patients [48]. We will discuss two types of cancer–bone cross-talk: (1) the bone marrow is very rich in growth factors and nutrients, and cancer cells can increase their fitness drastically if they are able to co-opt stromal cells; and (2) cancer cells face the spatial constraint of inelastic bone tissue, and hence they rely on osteoclasts, the only cells able to resorb mineralized bone matrix [49]. In addition to bone metastases of solid primary cancers, we include multiple myeloma (MM)–induced bone disease in our discussion. By definition, the latter is not a proper metastasis: MM is a plasma cell malignancy and its natural history is significantly different from the one of solid tumors [50]. The initiating genetic aberrations in the plasma cells can occur anywhere in the lymphatic system, rather than in a specific primary site, and the result-ing malignant MM cells move freely across the lymphatic and cardiovascular systems. However, circulating MM cells tend to accumulate and thrive in the bone environment [51], and the preferential attachment to bone as well as the MM–bone cross-talk are both reminiscent of the formation of bone metastases in solid tumors.

To prepare the reader for the mathematical models presented below, we provide a brief overview of the relevant bone biology [52]. Despite the fact that the total bone volume in the human body remains—in absence of disease—constant, bone tissue is far from being static. Global bone homeostasis is the result of a well-balanced remodeling mechanism executed by the bone cells: osteoclasts that resorb old and damaged bone and osteoblasts that form new and sound tissue (Figure 9.3a). Upon arrival in the marrow, cancer cells start interfering with and destabilizing the bone cell dynamics (Figure 9.3b). In general, we distinguish between two types of cancer-induced bone pathologies: osteolytic lesions (e.g., breast cancer metastases and MM), where the balance is shifted toward resorption, and osteoblastic lesions (e.g., prostate cancer metastases), where the balance is shifted toward formation. It is important to stress that even if the overall disease burden is osteoblastic, there is an active osteolytic component owing to the coupling of osteoclasts and osteoblasts. In either case, the osteolytic part of metastatic or MM-induced bone disease is particularly detrimental because of the so-called *vicious cycle* of cancer–bone interactions: cancer-derived growth factors enhance bone resorption, which in turn provides more space for cancer cells, which then produce even more growth factors, causing the balance to shift even more toward resorption, and so forth [48]. Improvement of our understanding

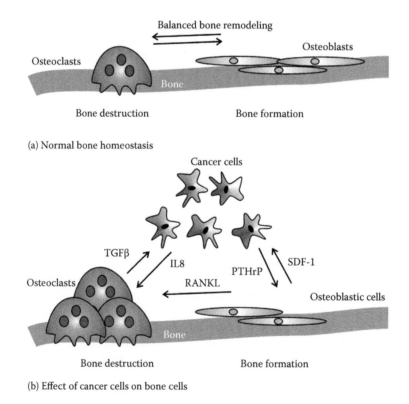

(a) Normal bone homeostasis

(b) Effect of cancer cells on bone cells

FIGURE 9.3
Schematic representation of bone remodeling and interactions between cancer and bone cells. (a) During physiological bone remodeling, osteoclasts resorb old and damaged tissue, while osteoblasts replace the resorbed tissue with new bone matrix. The overall bone balance is neutral. (b) In the presence of cancer cells, this balance is shifted toward resorption. Cancer cells stimulate osteoclasts and inhibit osteoblasts, leading to a negative bone balance.

of the key steps in this destructive feedback loop and design of suitable therapeutic measures are the subject of ongoing research.

9.6.1 Mechanistic ODE Modeling

Over the past 10 years, various mathematical models of physiological and pathological bone remodeling have been developed; see, for example, Refs. [53] and [54] for reviews. One modeling approach is to explicitly describe the cytokine pathways and cell population dynamics, leading to a system of ODEs [55,56]. On the basis of this approach, it is conceptually straightforward to incorporate the cancer dynamics by adding equations capturing the cancer cell population and the cancer-relevant pathways. In the case of MM-induced bone disease, such a strategy is adopted by Wang et al. [57]. The authors develop a mechanistic bottom–up approach, explicitly modeling the bone cells and their precursors, the MM cells, the chemokine concentrations, and the bone volume. On the basis of the resulting model, the authors investigate the different molecular mediators of cross-talk between MM and bone cells. By means of numerical simulations, they find that there are several pathways by which MM cells can co-opt bone cells to their own advantage. By systematically muting specific parts of the model, they are then able to gain insight into the relative importance of different pathways for cancer growth. While such detailed mechanistic models are able to disentangle intricate pathways in silico, they come with the drawback of complexity: the complete model by Wang et al. entails 44 parameters, of which only approximately 2/3 can be derived from the literature—the remaining parameters have to be estimated or calibrated using least-square optimization. Furthermore, the resulting system of nonlinear ODEs cannot be studied analytically, and only systematic numerical simulations can provide insights into stability, bifurcations, parameter sensitivity, and the existence of different dynamical regimes.

9.6.2 Evolutionary Game Approach

An alternative to the bottom–up approach as described above is the use of evolutionary game theory (EGT). Originally introduced in the context of ecology (see, e.g., Ref. [58]), EGT has recently been used to study MM–bone cell interactions by Dingli et al. [59] and cancer–stroma interactions by Basanta et al. [60]. Dingli et al. [59] consider a three-player game between MM cells, osteoclasts, and osteoblasts, based on the idea that the cell dynamics are governed by the fitness of each cell: if a cell has high fitness relative to its surrounding cells, it tends to proliferate, and if it has low relative fitness, it tends to die. Importantly, the fitness is not intrinsic to each cell but depends on the type and number of surrounding cells [48]. For example, in the presence of MM cells, osteoclasts experience an increase in fitness because of the expression of osteoclast-stimulating growth factors by MM cells. On the other hand, osteoblasts will see their fitness reduced in the presence of MM cells because the latter express osteoblast-inhibiting factors. In this manner, one can systematically determine the relative fitness of each player in the presence of another one. Denoting by x_1, x_2, and x_3 the relative frequencies of MM cells, osteoclasts, and osteoblasts, respectively, we can describe the fitness f_i of the type i population by means of a 3×3 payoff matrix $A = (a_{ij})$ as $f_i = (Ax)_i$, where $x = (x_1; x_2; x_3)$ and a_{ij} is the fitness of a cell of type i in the presence of a cell of type j. The proliferative potential of each subtype depends on its relative fitness compared to the average fitness of the entire population, and hence we can describe the dynamics as

$$\dot{x}_i(t) = x_i(t)[(Ax)_i - x^T Ax],$$

where $x^T A x$ is easily seen to correspond to the average fitness in the population. The EGT approach has several advantages. First, using biological information and an appropriate mathematical transformation, Dingli et al. were able to reduce the number of parameters from 9 (i.e., the number of entries in A) to 5. Second, the specific structure of the nonlinear replicator equations renders it easy to determine the fixed points analytically, and the authors show that their stability depends on only two parameters. The possibility of a detailed analysis without having to resort to simulations makes EGT an attractive tool. In particular, thanks to explicit expressions of the fixed points, it is possible to determine which parts of the cross-talk between different cell types affect the overall outcome of the game most significantly. Ideally, thereby gained insights can then help designing therapeutic protocols.

Another application of EGT to the study of prostate cancer metastases is found in the work of Basanta et al. [60]. The authors study a three-player game between (1) stromagenic cancer cells that co-opt the stroma to their advantage, (2) stroma-independent cancer cells, and (3) stroma cells themselves. Rather than working with continuous-time replicator equations, the authors use a discrete-time analogue of the dynamics. The discrete-time dynamics render a direct analysis cumbersome, and the authors resort to systematic simulations in order to elucidate the role of the different parameters. With an eye on therapeutic implications, they highlight interesting model properties. Consider, for example. the scenario depicted in Figure 9.4: a slight change in the environment's resource richness (after 20 iterations) has significant repercussions on the tumor content: an initially mostly stromagenic tumor turns into an exclusively stroma-independent cancer. Furthermore, the authors illustrate the importance of therapeutic timing: start time (relative to the natural history of the disease) and length of intervention can drastically change the outcome of therapy. In comparison to the mechanistic approach, the complexity of the EGT approach is minimal: 44 parameters in the ODE model [57] versus 5 in the EGT model [59].

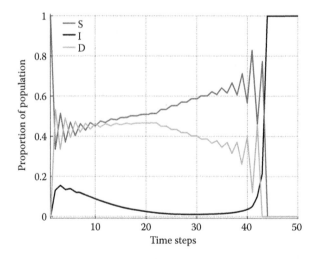

FIGURE 9.4

Evolutionary game-based model demonstrates transition from stroma-dependent to stroma-independent metastasis. Evolution of stroma cells (S), stroma-independent cells (I), and stroma-dependent cells (D). At $t = 20$, the cost of resource extraction for stroma-dependent cells is increased from 0.7 to 0.8; in consequence, the dynamics are shifted from a dwindling I-population to a regime of I-cell dominance. (Reproduced from Basanta D et al., *British Journal of Cancer*, 2011, 106(1):174–181. With permission.)

In addition, analytic considerations help understand the dynamics. On the other hand, the EGT approach is heuristic rather than mechanistic: for example, investigating isolated links in a signaling pathway as done by Wang et al. [57] would not be possible in the framework used by Dingli et al. [59].

9.6.3 PDE Modeling

We note that all the above models are purely temporal and neglect the spatial aspects of the metastatic process. However, spatial considerations are integral to the biology of cancer growth and metastases. Consider, for example, cells in the core of a growing tumor: they cannot directly interact with stromal cells on the outside of the tumor, and they only have limited access to diffusing nutrients. Similarly, at the metastatic site, the picture is an intrinsically spatial one; for example, cancer cells grow directionally into the healthy tissue, and molecular factors diffuse and form gradients. In many instances, the homogenously mixing models behave similarly to their spatial counterparts—however, there are various scenarios where the spatial distribution of the agents does play a role [61]. Thus, even though models taking into account the spatial anisotropy associated with cancer growth are more involved mathematically, they can provide unique insights into tumor progression.

A concrete problem where space plays a crucial role has recently been investigated by Ryser et al. [62]. The authors derive a system of nonlinear PDEs to study the role of the RANKL (receptor activator of nuclear factor kappa B ligand)–OPG (osteoprotegerin) pathway in the *vicious cycle* of osteolytic bone metastases (Figure 9.5a). The cytokine RANKL is a potent stimulator of osteoclast activity. By inducing the expression of RANKL on stromal cells and osteocytes via production of PTHrP, cancer cells can enhance bone resorption to their own advantage. OPG on the other hand is a decoy receptor of RANKL and hence provides means to reduce the RANKL-mediated osteoclast stimulation by cancer cells. However, based on in silico experiments, the authors show that OPG production by cancer cells does not necessarily lead to the anticipated decrease in tumor burden: there is an

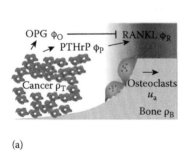
(a)

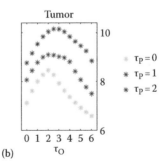
(b)

FIGURE 9.5

Spatiotemporal model suggests a novel role for OPG in promoting cancer metastases in bone. (a) Spatial distribution of cells and chemokine fields in bone metastases. Cancer cells produce PTHrP, which diffuses and induces RANKL expression by cells in the bone tissue. Osteoclasts move along the resulting RANKL gradient, away from the tumor and into the bone. By producing OPG, cancer cells can alter the RANKL gradient. (b) Tumor burden after 90 days as a function of OPG production (τ_O). Independent of the PTHrP expression level (τ_P), there is an intermediate regime where OPG enhances resorption and tumor burden. (From Ryser MD et al., *PLOS Computational Biology* 8(10):e1002703, 2012. Reproduced under the Creative Commons Attribution License.)

intermediate regime of expression levels where OPG production enhances bone resorption, and hence tumor growth, by altering the chemotactic gradients responsible for osteoclast movement (Figure 9.5b). The modeling results provide an explanation for seemingly contradictory experimental results [63,64] and constitute an example where the dynamics can only be understood in a spatial framework.

PDE models suffer from similar disadvantages as ODE models, and results are usually derived from simulations rather than analytic considerations. However, whereas it is straightforward to integrate ODEs with existing software packages, the numerical solution to nonlinear—potentially stiff and multiscale—PDEs can be much more delicate. For example, Ryser et al. had to resort to fractional multistep methods for their simulations. Nevertheless, since taking into account spatial considerations is critical and provides unique insights into the underlying biological mechanisms, further development of PDE-based modeling platforms is necessary.

9.7 Conclusions and Outlook

Mathematical oncology is a rapidly growing field of research that uses diverse modeling approaches to investigate complex problems related to the formation, progression, and growth of primary cancers and metastases. Oncology in general is one of the most active fields of study in biomedical sciences. However, despite substantial progress over the past decades, many questions remain unanswered. These open questions range from aspects of basic molecular and cell biology all the way to clinical problems in screening, diagnosis, prognosis, and treatment of patients. We are convinced that employing mathematical tools has the potential to greatly improve our understanding of cancer, and a lot of work is still in front of us.

Cancer development and progression represent biologically complex processes that attract a wide variety of modeling approaches. There is not a single field in the natural sciences where a one-suits-all mathematical model can capture the entire story—and cancer modeling is not an exception. The mathematical modeler will always have to gauge the optimal degree of complexity required: a complex, mechanistic model might be able to capture a subset of the underlying processes explicitly, but complexity may obscure important features of the system in question. In addition, parameter estimation quickly turns into a tedious exercise of uncertainty quantification. On the other hand, a simplistic, heuristic model may be more tractable analytically, but at the same time, it might be too far removed from the physical or biological reality. To find the right balance of complexity, to determine whether stochastic effects play a significant role, to assess whether space matters, to choose the suitable mathematical tool—these are the main challenges and should be evaluated carefully on a case-by-case basis.

Mathematical modeling can be of great help in the design and evaluation stages of experimental studies and clinical trials—let us illustrate this on a specific example. To figure out which therapeutic strategies are most efficient for the treatment of a specific cancer type and its metastases, pharmaceutical companies perform lengthy and expensive clinical trials. However, the steadily growing number of therapeutic possibilities for every given type of cancer comes with an even bigger number of possible combinations and temporal permutations of these treatments. In view of this development, mathematical oncology has a lot of potential, because once a reliable in silico model has been established and tested, the modeler can experiment with possible drug and therapy combinations—and even though the clinical trial will never be replaced by a computer, its efficiency can be optimized if adequately combined with the predictive power of simulations.

In the medical world, mathematical modeling is still greeted with skepticism. This has several reasons, including the fact that clinicians and biomedical researchers often do not receive the mathematical training necessary to fully appreciate the modeling work. On the other hand, mathematicians and biomedical engineers often lack appreciation for complex biology and the level of uncertainty that prevails in experimental and clinical sciences. It also does not help that assumptions used by biomedical scientists are often not fully verbalized and different experts may have conflicting opinion [65]. In addition, we believe that a large part of the disparity between the theoretical and experimental communities is caused by a gap between model analysis and experimental data. If mathematical modeling wants to make its way into the clinic—be it to assist the design of trials, to address patient-specific issues, or to guide therapeutic approaches—then it has to get closer to data. Together with a rigorous mathematical analysis of established models, it is important to spend time and effort to bridge the gap between the clinical and experimental worlds. We are convinced that this would greatly improve the credibility of mathematical modeling in the medical world.

Acknowledgments

M.D.R. is grateful for fruitful discussions with Rick Durrett. M.D.R. is partially supported by National Institutes of Health grant R01-GM096190-02. S.V.K. holds a Canada Research Chair in Osteoclast Biology.

References

1. Wodarz D, Komarova DWNL: *Computational Biology of Cancer: Lecture Notes and Mathematical Modeling.* Singapore: World Scientific; 2005.
2. Cristini V, Lowengrub J: *Multiscale Modeling of Cancer: An Integrated Experimental and Mathematical Modeling Approach.* Cambridge, UK, Cambridge University Press; 2010.
3. Deisboeck TS, Stamatakos GS: *Multiscale Cancer Modeling.* Boca Raton, FL, CRC Press; 2010.
4. Bellomo N, de Angelis E: *Selected Topics in Cancer Modeling: Genesis, Evolution, Immune Competition, and Therapy.* Boston, MA, Birkhäuser; 2008.
5. Chauviere AH, Hatzikirou H, Lowengrub JS, Frieboes HB, Thompson AM, Cristini V: Mathematical oncology: How are the mathematical and physical sciences contributing to the war on breast cancer? *Current Breast Cancer Reports* 2010, 2(3):121–129.
6. Rejniak KA, Anderson ARA: Hybrid models of tumor growth. *Wiley Interdisciplinary Reviews: Systems Biology and Medicine* 2010, 3(1):115–125.
7. Michor F, Liphardt J, Ferrari M, Widom J: What does physics have to do with cancer? *Nature Reviews Cancer* 2011, 11(9):657–670.
8. Blair RH, Trichler DL, Gaille DP: Mathematical and statistical modeling in cancer systems biology. *Frontiers in Physiology* 2012, 3:227.

9. Chan KS, Koh CG, Li HY: Mitosis-targeted anti-cancer therapies: Where they stand. *Cell Death & Disease* 2012, 3:e411.

10. Zuckerman V, Wolyniec K, Sionov RV, Haupt S, Haupt Y: Tumour suppression by p53: The importance of apoptosis and cellular senescence. *The Journal of Pathology* 2009, 219(1):3–15.

11. Zhang Y, Yang JM: Altered energy metabolism in cancer: A unique opportunity for therapeutic intervention. *Cancer Biology & Therapy* 2012, 14(2):81–89.

12. Lianidou ES, Markou A, Strati A: Molecular characterization of circulating tumor cells in breast cancer: Challenges and promises for individualized cancer treatment. *Cancer Metastasis Reviews* 2012, 31(3–4):663–671.

13. Brinton LT, Brentnall TA, Smith JA, Kelly KA: Metastatic biomarker discovery through proteomics. *Cancer Genomics & Proteomics* 2012, 9(6):345–355.

14. Spano D, Heck C, De Antonellis P, Christofori G, Zollo M: Molecular networks that regulate cancer metastasis. *Seminars in Cancer Biology* 2012, 22(3):234–249.

15. Pylayeva-Gupta Y, Grabocka E, Bar-Sagi D: RAS oncogenes: Weaving a tumorigenic web. *Nature Reviews Cancer* 2011, 11(11):761–774.

16. Smith SC, Theodorescu D: Learning therapeutic lessons from metastasis suppressor proteins. *Nature Reviews Cancer* 2009, 9(4):253–264.

17. Sundar SS, Ganesan TS: Role of lymphangiogenesis in cancer. *Journal of Clinical Oncology: Official Journal of the American Society of Clinical Oncology* 2007, 25(27):4298–4307.

18. Kandouz M: The Eph/Ephrin family in cancer metastasis: Communication at the service of invasion. *Cancer Metastasis Reviews* 2012, 31(1–2):353–373.

19. Polyak K, Weinberg RA: Transitions between epithelial and mesenchymal states: Acquisition of malignant and stem cell traits. *Nature Reviews Cancer* 2009, 9(4):265–273.

20. Vande Broek I, Vanderkerken K, Van Camp B, Van Riet I: Extravasation and homing mechanisms in multiple myeloma. *Clinical & Experimental Metastasis* 2008, 25(4):325–334.

21. Paget S: The distribution of secondary growths in cancer of the breast. *Lancet* 1889, 133(3421):571–573.

22. Langley RR, Fidler IJ: The seed and soil hypothesis revisited—the role of tumor-stroma interactions in metastasis to different organs. *International Journal of Cancer Journal International du Cancer* 2011, 128(11):2527–2535.

23. Joyce JA, Pollard JW: Microenvironmental regulation of metastasis. *Nature Reviews Cancer* 2009, 9(4):239–252.

24. You JS, Jones PA: Cancer genetics and epigenetics: Two sides of the same coin? *Cancer Cell* 2012, 22(1):9–20.

25. Cristofanilli M, Budd GT, Ellis MJ, Stopeck A, Matera J, Miller MC, Reuben JM, Doyle GV, Allard WJ, Terstappen LW et al: Circulating tumor cells, disease progression, and survival in metastatic breast cancer. *The New England Journal of Medicine* 2004, 351(8):781–791.

26. Bednarz-Knoll N, Alix-Panabieres C, Pantel K: Clinical relevance and biology of circulating tumor cells. *Breast Cancer Research: BCR* 2011, 13(6):228.

27. Michor F, Nowak MA, Iwasa Y: Stochastic dynamics of metastasis formation. *Journal of Theoretical Biology* 2006, 240(4):521–530.

28. Deb M, Sengupta D, Patra SK: Integrin-epigenetics: A system with imperative impact on cancer. *Cancer Metastasis Reviews* 2012, 31(1–2):221–234.

29. Michor F, Iwasa Y: Dynamics of metastasis suppressor gene inactivation. *Journal of Theoretical Biology* 2006, 241(3):676–689.

30. Dingli D, Michor F, Antal T, Pacheco JM: The emergence of tumor metastases. *Cancer Biology & Therapy* 2007, 6(3):383–390.

31. Paez D, Labonte MJ, Bohanes P, Zhang W, Benhanim L, Ning Y, Wakatsuki T, Loupakis F, Lenz HJ: Cancer dormancy: A model of early dissemination and late cancer recurrence. *Clinical Cancer Research: An Official Journal of the American Association for Cancer Research* 2012, 18(3):645–653.

32. Pantel K, Alix-Panabières C, Riethdorf S: Cancer micrometastases. *Nature Reviews Clinical Oncology* 2009, 6(6):339–351.

33. Heidenreich A, Pfister D: Management of patients with clinical stage I nonseminomatous testicular germ cell tumours: Active surveillance versus primary chemotherapy versus nerve sparing retroperitoneal lymphadenectomy. *Archivos espanoles de urologia* 2012, 65(2):215–226.

34. Yorke E, Fuks Z, Norton L, Whitmore W, Ling C: Modeling the development of metastases from primary and locally recurrent tumors: Comparison with a clinical data base for prostatic cancer. *Cancer Research* 1993, 53(13):2987–2993.

35. Zelefsky MJ, Reuter VE, Fuks Z, Scardino P, Shippy A: Influence of local tumor control on distant metastases and cancer related mortality after external beam radiotherapy for prostate cancer. *The Journal of Urology* 2008, 179(4):1368.

36. Hanin L, Rose J, Zaider M: A stochastic model for the sizes of detectable metastases. *Journal of Theoretical Biology* 2006, 243(3):407–417.

37. Haeno H, Michor F: The evolution of tumor metastases during clonal expansion. *Journal of Theoretical Biology* 2010, 263(1):30–44.

38. Klein CA: Parallel progression of primary tumours and metastases. *Nature Reviews Cancer* 2009, 9(4):302–312.

39. Iwata K, Kawasaki K, Shigesada N: A dynamical model for the growth and size distribution of multiple metastatic tumors. *Journal of Theoretical Biology* 2000, 203(2):177–186.

40. Barbolosi D, Benabdallah A, Hubert F, Verga F: Mathematical and numerical analysis for a model of growing metastatic tumors. *Mathematical Biosciences* 2009, 218(1):1–14.

41. Benzekry S, André N, Benabdallah A, Ciccolini J, Faivre C, Hubert F, Barbolosi D: Modeling the impact of anticancer agents on metastatic spreading. *Mathematical Modelling of Natural Phenomena* 2012, 7(1):306–336.

42. Newton PK, Mason J, Bethel K, Bazhenova LA, Nieva J, Kuhn P: A stochastic Markov chain model to describe lung cancer growth and metastasis. *PLoS One* 2012, 7(4):e34637.

43. Norton L, Massagué J: Is cancer a disease of self-seeding? *Nature Medicine* 2006, 12(8):875–878.

44. Danesh K, Durrett R, Havrilesky L, Myers E: A branching process model of ovarian cancer. *Journal of Theoretical Biology* 2012, 314:10–15.

45. Jones S, Chen W, Parmigiani G, Diehl F, Beerenwinkel N, Antal T, Traulsen A, Nowak MA, Siegel C, Velculescu VE: Comparative lesion sequencing provides insights into tumor evolution. *Proceedings of the National Academy of Sciences* 2008, 105(11):4283–4288.

46. Yachida S, Jones S, Bozic I, Antal T, Leary R, Fu B, Kamiyama M, Hruban RH, Eshleman JR, Nowak MA: Distant metastasis occurs late during the genetic evolution of pancreatic cancer. *Nature* 2010, 467(7319):1114–1117.

47. Mueller MM, Fusenig NE: Friends or foes—Bipolar effects of the tumour stroma in cancer. *Nature Reviews Cancer* 2004, 4(11):839–849.

48. Roodman GD: Mechanisms of bone metastasis. *New England Journal of Medicine* 2004, 350(16):1655–1664.

49. Teitelbaum SL: Bone resorption by osteoclasts. *Science* 2000, 289(5484):1504–1508.

50. Mahindra A, Hideshima T, Anderson KC: Multiple myeloma: Biology of the disease. *Blood Reviews* 2010, 24:S5–S11.

51. Raje N, Roodman GD: Advances in the biology and treatment of bone disease in multiple myeloma. *Clinical Cancer Research* 2011, 17(6):1278–1286.

52. Robling AG, Castillo AB, Turner CH: Biomechanical and molecular regulation of bone remodeling. *Annual Review of Biomedical Engineering* 2006, 8:455–498.

53. Pivonka P, Komarova SV: Mathematical modeling in bone biology: From intracellular signaling to tissue mechanics. *Bone* 2010, 47(2):181–189.

54. Webster D, Müller R: In silico models of bone remodeling from macro to nano—From organ to cell. *Wiley Interdisciplinary Reviews: Systems Biology and Medicine* 2011, 3(2):241–251.

55. Komarova SV, Smith RJ, Dixon SJ, Sims SM, Wahl LM: Mathematical model predicts a critical role for osteoclast autocrine regulation in the control of bone remodeling. *Bone* 2003, 33(2):206–215.

56. Lemaire V, Tobin FL, Greller LD, Cho CR, Suva LJ: Modeling the interactions between osteoblast and osteoclast activities in bone remodeling. *Journal of Theoretical Biology* 2004, 229(3):293–309.

57. Wang Y, Pivonka P, Buenzli PR, Smith DW, Dunstan CR: Computational modeling of interactions between multiple myeloma and the bone microenvironment. *PLoS One* 2011, 6(11):e27494.
58. Smith JM: *Evolution and the Theory of Games*. Cambridge, UK, Cambridge University Press; 1982.
59. Dingli D, Chalub F, Santos F, Van Segbroeck S, Pacheco J: Cancer phenotype as the outcome of an evolutionary game between normal and malignant cells. *British Journal of Cancer* 2009, 101(7):1130–1136.
60. Basanta D, Scott JG, Fishman MN, Ayala G, Hayward SW, Anderson ARA: Investigating prostate cancer tumour–stroma interactions: Clinical and biological insights from an evolutionary game. *British Journal of Cancer* 2011, 106(1):174–181.
61. Durrett R, Levin S: The importance of being discrete (and spatial). *Theoretical Population Biology* 1994, 46(3):363–394.
62. Ryser MD, Qu Y, Komarova SV: Osteoprotegerin in bone metastases: Mathematical solution to the puzzle. *PLoS Computational Biology* 2012, 8(10):e1002703.
63. Corey E, Brown LG, Kiefer JA, Quinn JE, Pitts TE, Blair JM, Vessella RL: Osteoprotegerin in prostate cancer bone metastasis. *Cancer Research* 2005, 65(5):1710–1718.
64. Fisher JL, Thomas-Mudge RJ, Elliott J, Hards DK, Sims NA, Slavin J, Martin TJ, Gillespie MT: Osteoprotegerin overexpression by breast cancer cells enhances orthotopic and osseous tumor growth and contrasts with that delivered therapeutically. *Cancer Research* 2006, 66(7):3620–3628.
65. Divoli A, Mendonca EA, Evans JA, Rzhetsky A: Conflicting biomedical assumptions for mathematical modeling: The case of cancer metastasis. *PLoS Computational Biology* 2011, 7(10):e1002132.

10

Dynamic Processes in Photodynamic Therapy

Timothy C. Zhu, Baochang Liu, and Michele M. Kim

CONTENTS

ABSTRACT Photodynamic therapy (PDT) is an emerging cancer treatment modality that uses visible light to activate photosensitizers to generate cytotoxic oxygen radicals to kill cancer cells. PDT employs the photochemical interaction of three components: light, photosensitizer, and oxygen. Tremendous progress has been made in the last three decades to understand quantitatively the basic biophysical mechanisms describing all three components, as well as their interactions. This chapter provides a complete description of the most important photochemical models describing the transport of light, the diffusion of photosensitizer drug, and the diffusion of oxygen through vasculature in human tissue (a turbid medium, where scattering dominates over absorption in the near-infrared region), as well as their interactions. At the current stage of development, it is still impossible to model the heterogeneities of the microscopic vascular structures completely to provide a comprehensive description of the dynamic process during PDT. However, it is practical to develop a macroscopic model that ignores underlying microscopic details to describe the light transport, the oxygen consumption, and singlet oxygen generation during PDT.

List of Symbols

a	Albedo, $a = \mu_s/(\mu_s + \mu_a)$
c	Speed of light in medium (cm/s)
C_H	Hemoglobin concentration in blood (μM), see Equation 10.33 and Table 10.1
C_{HR}	Hemoglobin concentration in red blood cell (μM), see Equation 10.27 and Table 10.1
D	Diffuse coefficient (cm^2/s), see Equations 10.19 and 10.38
D_c	$^3O_2$ diffusion coefficient in capillary (μm^2/s), see Equations 10.32 and 10.37 and Table 10.1
D_H	Hemoglobin diffusion coefficient (μm^2/s), see Equation 10.33
D_R	$^3O_2$ diffusion coefficient in red blood cell (μm^2/s), see Equation 10.30
D_t	$^3O_2$ diffusion coefficient in tissue (μm^2/s), see Equations 10.35 and 10.37 and Table 10.1
f	Scattering phase function, see Equations 10.2 and 10.12
g	Scattering anisotropy, see Equation 10.3
J	Photon flux/current density (mW/cm^2)
k	Oxygen dissociation rate constant (1/s), see Equation 10.28 and Table 10.1
k_0	Photon absorption rate of photosensitizer per photosensitizer concentration (1/s), $k_0 = \varepsilon\phi/h\nu$, see Table 10.2
k_1	Bimolecular rate for $^1O_2$ reaction with ground-state photosensitizer (1/μM/s), see Table 10.2
k_2	Bimolecular rate of triplet photosensitizer quenching by $^3O_2$ (1/μM/s), see Table 10.2
k_3	Fluorescence decay rate of first excited singlet-state photosensitizer to ground-state photosensitizer (1/s), see Table 10.2
k_4	Phosphorescence rate of monomolecular decay of the photosensitizer triplet state (1/s), see Table 10.2
k_5	Intersystem crossing rate of first excited photosensitizer to triplet-state photosensitizer (1/s), see Table 10.2
k_6	$^1O_2$ to $^3O_2$ phosphorescence decay rate (1/s), see Table 10.2
k_7	Bimolecular rate of reaction of $^1O_2$ with biological substrate [A] (1/μM/s), see Table 10.2
L	Radiance (mW/cm^2/sr), see Equation 10.1
l	Length of capillary (μm), see Table 10.1
n	Hill constant, see Equation 10.29 and Table 10.1
P	Oxygen partial pressure (mm Hg), see Equation 10.25
P_{50}	Half maximum hemoglobin saturation (mm Hg), see Equation 10.29 and Table 10.1
P_m	Half maximum oxygen consumption (mm Hg), see Equation 10.35 and Table 10.1
q_0	$^3O_2$ maximum metabolic consumption rate (μM/s), see Equation 10.35 and Table 10.1

R_c	Capillary radius (μm), see Table 10.1
R_t	Tissue radius (μm), see Table 10.1
$\vec{r}$	Position vector (cm), see Equation 10.1
S	Source term (mW/cm³/sr), see Equation 10.1
$\hat{s}$	Angular unit vector, see Equation 10.1
S_Δ	Fraction of triplet-state photosensitizer–$^3O_2$ reactions to produce $^1O_2$, see Table 10.2
$Sa(SaO_2)$	Hemoglobin oxygen saturation, see Equation 10.27
t	Photon step size (cm), see Equation 10.5
$\vec{v}(v)$	Vector (and value) of velocity of blood flow (μm/s), see Equations 10.32 and 10.33 and Table 10.1
α	$^3O_2$ solubility (μM/mm Hg), see Equations 10.25 and 10.31
α_c	$^3O_2$ solubility in capillary (μM/mm Hg), see Equations 10.30, 10.32, and 10.37 and Table 10.1
α_R	$^3O_2$ solubility in red blood cell (μM/mm Hg), see Equation 10.30
α_t	$^3O_2$ solubility in tissue (μM/mm Hg), see Equation 10.35 and Table 10.1
β	k_4/k_2 (μM), see Table 10.2
Γ	Rate of the oxygen unloading (μM/s), see Equations 10.27 and 10.28
δ	Low concentration correction (μM), see Table 10.2
ε	Extinction coefficient (1/cm/μM), see Table 10.2
ζ	Uniformly distributed random number, see Equation 10.4
$\eta(\eta_x,\eta_y,\eta_z)$	Directional cosine between vectors, $\cos\theta$, see Equation 10.6
μ_a	Absorption coefficient (1/cm), see Equation 10.1
μ_s	Scattering coefficient (1/cm), see Equation 10.1
μ_s'	Reduced scattering coefficient (1/cm), $\mu_s(1-g)$, see Equation 10.14
μ_t	Total attenuation coefficient (1/cm), see Equation 10.1
ξ	$S_\Delta\left(\dfrac{k_5}{k_5+k_3}\right)\dfrac{\varepsilon}{h\nu}\dfrac{k_7[A]/k_6}{k_7[A]/k_6+1}$ (cm² mW^{-1} s^{-1}), see Table 10.2
σ	$k_1/k_7\,[A]$ (μM^{-1}), see Table 10.2
ϕ	Fluence rate (mW/cm²), see Equations 10.13, 10.17–10.19

10.1 Introduction

10.1.1 Photodynamic Therapy

Photodynamic therapy (PDT) is a cancer treatment modality that uses visible light to activate photosensitizers to generate cytotoxic oxygen radicals to kill cancer cells. PDT has been approved by the US Food and Drug Administration for the treatment of microinvasive lung cancer, obstructing lung cancer, and obstructing esophageal cancer, as well as for premalignant actinic keratosis and age-related macular degeneration [1].

10.1.2 Dynamic Processes of PDT

PDT is inherently a dynamic process. There are three principal components: photosensitizer, light, and oxygen, all of which interact on time scales relevant to a single treatment. The distribution of light is determined by the light source characteristics and the tissue optical properties. The tissue optical properties, in turn, are influenced by the concentration of the photosensitizer and the concentration and oxygenation of the blood. The distribution of oxygen is altered by the photodynamic process, which consumes oxygen, as well as the diffusion process where the oxygen gets diffused to tissue. The distribution of photosensitizer can be modeled as a diffusion process through the vasculature. Finally, distribution of the photosensitizer may change as a result of photobleaching, the photodynamic destruction of the photosensitizer itself. To account for these interactions, a dynamic model of the photodynamic process is required.

A photosensitizer is classified as type I or type II depending on the types of reactive oxygen species generated. For type I photosensitizers, the triplet-state photosensitizer reacts directly with the substrate to produce a radical ion both in the photosensitizer (PS–) and the substrate (S+). In the presence of oxygen, the photosensitizer radical anion (PS–) can undergo autoxidation with oxygen (O_2) to generate a superoxide anion radical (O_2^-) and then regenerate to the ground-state photosensitizer. Most photosensitizers are of type II. For type II photosensitizers, singlet oxygen is the main photocytotoxic agent that causes cell death and therapeutic effects [1]. During PDT, as shown in Figure 10.1, the sensitizer is excited by light at a certain wavelength matching the absorption energy gap to the excited state (S_1) from its ground state (S_0). Both this state and the ground state are spectroscopic singlet states. One essential property of a good photosensitizer is a high intersystem crossing yield, that is, a high probability of transition from S_1 to an excited triplet state (T_1). In the T_1 state, the photosensitizer can transfer energy to molecular oxygen ($^3O_2$), exciting it to its highly reactive singlet state ($^1O_2$).

In this chapter, we present an integrated approach to model the dynamic process between light, photosensitizer, and oxygen to generate singlet oxygen. In Section 10.2, we will describe the Boltzmann equation and various approximations used to solve the light transport equation in tissue; in Section 10.3, we will describe the oxygen diffusion models and vasculature; in Section 10.4, we will briefly describe the diffusion for photosensitizer through the vasculature; and finally, in Section 10.5, we will solve the coupled equations for the generation of singlet oxygen. We will summarize the chapter and discuss the future prospective in Section 10.6.

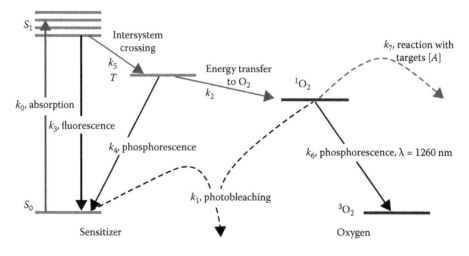

FIGURE 10.1
Energy level diagram for a typical type II sensitizer and oxygen. The sensitizer in its ground state (S_0) absorbs a photon and is excited to its first singlet state (S_1). It spontaneously decays to its excited triplet state (T_1) via intersystem crossing. From T_1, energy is transferred to ground-state molecular oxygen ($^3O_2$), creating reactive singlet oxygen ($^1O_2$). (From Zhu, T.C. et al., *Proc. SPIE*, 6427: 1–12, 2007.)

10.2 Light Transport in Turbid Medium

Light propagates in turbid medium very differently compared to a clear medium. In regions of near infrared, that is, the 600–800 nm wavelength region, the scattering dominates for light propagation in tissue rather than absorption, which is determined by the hemoglobin concentration in tissue [2]. Light dosimetry is one of the three critical quantities to accurately predict photodynamic therapeutic effects.

10.2.1 Radiation Transport Equation

Radiative transport theory provides a mathematical model for the propagation of light through scattering and absorbing media. The radiance, $L(\vec{r}, \hat{s})$, is defined as the power per unit area per unit solid angle in direction $\hat{s}$ at position $\vec{r}$ [3,4]. $L(\vec{r}, \hat{s})$ is described by the time-independent Boltzmann equation, also referred to as the radiation transport equation [5]:

$$\frac{1}{c}\frac{\partial L(\vec{r}, \hat{s}, t)}{\partial t} = -\nabla \cdot L(\vec{r}, \hat{s}, t)\hat{s} - \mu_t L(\vec{r}, \hat{s}, t) + \mu_s \int_{4\pi} L(\vec{r}, \hat{s}', t)f(\hat{s}, \hat{s}')d\Omega' + S(\vec{r}, \hat{s}, t). \quad (10.1)$$

The absorption coefficient (μ_a) is the probability of absorption per unit distance and the scattering coefficient (μ_s) is the probability of scattering per unit distance, μ_t is given by $\mu_a + \mu_s$, and $S(\vec{r}, \hat{s})$ represents the source term. The $f(\hat{s}, \hat{s}')$ term is the scattering phase function, which describes the probability that a photon incident in direction $\hat{s}'$ will be scattered into direction $\hat{s}$. The right side of Equation 10.1 describes the gradient in radiance distribution (first term), the decrease of $L(\vec{r}, \hat{s})$ by absorption and photons that are scattered away from direction $\hat{s}$ (second term), and the increase of radiance by photons scattered into $\hat{s}$ (third term) and by the light source $S(\vec{r}, \hat{s})$ (the remaining terms). The source term $S(\vec{r}, \hat{s})$ is represented in many ways depending on the light source used. For planar geometries, the light can be a wide beam with collimated incidence (often referred to as a pencil beam or a wide beam with diffuse incidence). If the source is an isotropic point source, $S_0\delta(r)$, the solution to Equation 10.1 is also called Green's function and the solution for any other source can be obtained by a convolution of the source and Green's function.

The scattering phase function $f(\hat{s}, \hat{s}')$ is assumed to depend only on the deflection angle θ between $\hat{s}$ and $\hat{s}' \cdot f(\hat{s}, \hat{s}')$ becomes a complicated function in biological media owing to the high particle density and inhomogeneity of tissue. An accepted approximation for $f(\hat{s}, \hat{s}')$ is the Henyey–Greenstein phase function [6,7]

$$f_{HG}(\cos\theta) = \left(\frac{1}{4\pi}\right)\frac{1 - g^2}{(1 + g^2 - 2g\cos\theta)^{3/2}}, \quad (10.2)$$

where g is the scattering anisotropy given by

$$g = \int_{4\pi} f(\hat{s}, \hat{s}')d\Omega. \quad (10.3)$$

This quantity, g, is equal to the average of the scattering cos θ. The scattering anisotropy ranges from −1 to 1, corresponding to backward and forward scattering, respectively. If $g = 0$, then there is no preference for forward or backward scattering. In tissue, g, is estimated to be in the range of 0.7–0.9 but is commonly taken to be equal to 0.9 [6,8].

At the boundary of two different media (L_1 and L_2) with different indexes of refraction, the boundary condition can be specified by following the reflection and transmission attributed to Fresnel's law [9]:

$$L_1(\hat{s})\hat{s} \cdot \hat{n} = R_{\text{Fresnel}}(\hat{s})L_1(\hat{s})\hat{s} \cdot (-\hat{n}) + T_{\text{Fresnel}}(\hat{s})L_2(\hat{s})\hat{s} \cdot \hat{n}$$
$$L_2(\hat{s})\hat{s} \cdot \hat{n} = R_{\text{Fresnel}}(\hat{s})L_2(\hat{s})\hat{s} \cdot (-\hat{n}) + T_{\text{Fresnel}}(\hat{s})L_1(\hat{s})\hat{s} \cdot \hat{n}'$$

(10.4)

where $\hat{n}$ is the normal direction of the boundary, $\hat{s}$ is the direction of the irradiance under consideration, and R_{Fresnel} and $T_{\text{Fresnel}} = 1 - R_{\text{Fresnel}}$ are the reflectance and transmission coefficients according to Fresnel's law [10].

10.2.2 Monte Carlo Simulation

In a light transport problem, the Monte Carlo (MC) method consists of recording photons' histories as they are scattered and absorbed. The Monte Carlo method begins by launching a photon into the tissue. If a collimated beam normally incident on a slab is simulated, then the photon's initial direction is chosen to be downward into the tissue. If an isotropic diffuse irradiance is simulated, then the photon's direction is chosen randomly from all possible directions in the downward hemisphere [11].

The MC method of calculating light distributions in turbid media, such as tissue, has become the gold standard, especially in complex geometries and heterogeneous tissue. MC simulations can be made arbitrarily accurate by increasing the total number of incident photons, and they do not need any additional approximations beyond assuming each step is the same and equal to the mean free path, as they are based purely on fundamental interaction properties of the media. The most significant disadvantage of the MC method is the high computational intensity (or computational time). A macroscopic model can be adapted to reduce the time and computational intensity needed to perform these calculations [12]. Another common technique to speed up the calculation is to use graphics processing units [13].

Most MC methods used for tissue optics simulations trace individual photons or *photon packets* through many scattering and absorption events. Each photon is scattered tens or hundreds of times before leaving the sample since the tissue or region of interest being simulated are orders of magnitude greater than the scattering mean free path in the sample [12].

A photon is launched in a user-specific direction from a given location. To achieve an isotropic point source, each photon is launched in a random direction ranging from 0 to 2π from the center of the cavity. The length to the first scattering event is calculated using an exponential distribution. Photon absorption is determined by decreasing the photon weight by $\exp(-\mu_a L)$, where L is the length the photon travels [14]. The Henyey–Greenstein phase function (Equation 10.2) is used to determine the scattering angle. The new scattering length of the photon is then determined from an exponential distribution, as before. The photon has propagated this new length in the new direction. This propagation process continues until the photon exits the medium or the photon has traveled for 10 ns, which is which its weight can be regarded as negligible. When a photon encounters a medium boundary, the probability of reflection is calculated using Fresnel's equation. If the photon is reflected back into the cavity, the multiple scattering treatment determines the photon's path [15].

After a photon is launched, the step size of the photon packet is calculated based on a sampling of the photon's free path. This becomes its step size t, and it is determined by

$$t = -\ln (\zeta)/\mu_t, \tag{10.5}$$

where ζ is a uniformly distributed random number and μ_t is the interaction coefficient. Once this step size is determined, the photon is moved by updating the position of the photon packet with the following equations:

$$
\begin{aligned}
x' &= x + \eta_x t \\
y' &= y + \eta_y t \\
z' &= z + \eta_z t,
\end{aligned} \tag{10.6}
$$

where η_x, η_y, and η_z are the directional cosines to describe the traveling direction of a photon packet. After a photon packet has reached an interaction site, and its weight has decreased because of absorption, the scattering (deflection) angle is determined. The probability distribution for the cosine of the deflection angle is described by the Henyey–Greenstein function (Equation 10.2). The choice for $\cos \theta$ is then expressed as a function of the random number ζ:

$$
\cos \theta =
\begin{cases}
\dfrac{1}{2g}\left\{ 1+g^2 - \left[\dfrac{1-g^2}{1-g+2g\zeta}\right]^2 \right\} & \text{if } g \neq 0 \\[4mm]
2\zeta - 1 & \text{if } g = 0.
\end{cases} \tag{10.7}
$$

The azimuthal angle is uniformly distributed over the interval 0 to 2π and is given by

$$\psi = 2\pi\zeta. \tag{10.8}$$

The new direction is then calculated with the deflection and azimuthal angles

$$
\begin{aligned}
\eta'_x &= \sin\theta(\eta_x \eta_z \cos\psi - \eta_y \sin\psi)\big/\sqrt{1-\eta_z^2} + \eta_x \cos\theta \\
\eta'_y &= \sin\theta(\eta_y \eta_z \cos\psi + \eta_x \sin\psi)\big/\sqrt{1-\eta_z^2} + \eta_y \cos\theta \\
\eta'_z &= -\sin\theta \cos\psi \sqrt{1-\eta_z^2} + \eta_z \cos\theta.
\end{aligned} \tag{10.9}
$$

This process continues until the photon meets a boundary or is completely absorbed [14,16]. A flow chart of MC simulation of light is shown in Figure 10.2 [11].

The boundary conditions for simulations will depend on the geometries used and are similar to those described by Equation 10.4 for each photon [9]. During a step of size t, the

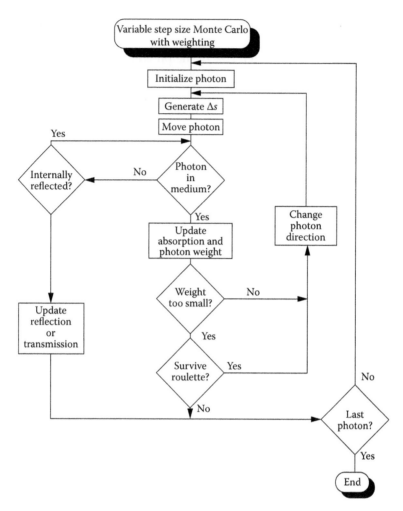

FIGURE 10.2
Flow chart of an MC simulation. (From Prahl, S.A. et al., *Proc. SPIE*, IS5: 102–111, 1989.)

photon packet may hit a boundary, which can either be an interface between the tissue and the ambient medium or an interface between the current layer of tissue and another layer of tissue. The photon packet is then either internally reflected by the boundary or it will transmit across. Snell's law will describe the angle of transmission across such a boundary [10].

Figure 10.3 shows the result of MC simulations for circular fields of various radius incident on a semi-infinite surface of tissue with various optical properties [17]. Good agreement is observed between MC simulation and measurement. On the tissue surface, the actual light fluence rate is always larger than that calculated based on the incident irradiance (also called the in-air fluence rate), $\phi_{air} = S/A$, where S is the total laser power and $A = \pi r^2$ is the area of the entire laser beam incident on the tissue surface. This is because of photon backscattering to the tissue surface. In general, $\phi/\phi_{air} = 1 + 2R_d$, where R_d is the diffuse reflectance. Inside the tissue, the light fluence rate will rise up to as high as six times that of the in-air fluence rate and then decrease exponentially following the effective

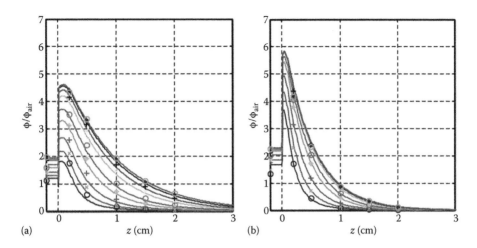

FIGURE 10.3

Comparison of measured (symbols) and MC calculated (lines) ϕ/ϕ_{air}, in a semi-infinite turbid medium as a function of depth for different tissue optical properties: (a) $\mu_a = 0.1$ cm^{-1}, $\mu_s = 40$ cm^{-1}, $g = 0.9$, $n = 1.4$; (b) $\mu_a = 0.1$ cm^{-1}, $\mu_s = 130$ cm^{-1}, $g = 0.9$, $n = 1.4$. Curves are for different radii: from bottom to top: $R = 0.25$, 0.35, 0.5, 0.75, 1, 1.5, 2, 3, and 8 cm. (From Zhu, T.C. et al., *Proc. SPIE*, 4952: 56–67, 2003.)

attenuation coefficient $\mu_{eff} = \sqrt{3\mu_a \cdot (\mu_a + \mu_s')}$ for a sufficiently large radius beam ($R > 2$ cm). The effective attenuation coefficient increases with decreasing radius. Oblique incidence has limited effect on the light fluence distribution [18].

10.2.3 Analytical Solutions, P_1 and P_3 Approximations

Equation 10.1 can be approximated by using a series of spherical harmonics. The most common approximation is the first-order (P_1) and the third-order (P_3) approximation [6,19]. It is possible to obtain analytical solutions for the P_1 and P_3 approximations of the radiation transport equation.

The radiance and source terms can be expanded as a series of spherical harmonics, and the scattering phase function can be expanded as a series of Legendre polynomials [6,8,19]

$$L(\vec{r}, \hat{s}) = \sum_{l=0}^{N} \sum_{m=-1}^{l} \sqrt{\frac{2l+1}{4\pi}} \, \phi_{lm} Y_{lm}(\hat{s}) \tag{10.10}$$

$$S(\vec{r}, \hat{s}) = \sum_{l=0}^{N} \sum_{m=-1}^{l} \sqrt{\frac{2l+1}{4\pi}} \, q_{lm} Y_{lm}(\hat{s}) \tag{10.11}$$

$$f(\hat{s}, \hat{s}') = \sum_{l=0}^{N} \frac{2l+1}{4\pi} g_l P_l(\hat{s} \cdot \hat{s}'). \tag{10.12}$$

In general, $Y_{lm}(\theta,\phi) = \sqrt{\dfrac{2l+1}{4\pi}\dfrac{(l-m)!}{(l+m)!}} P_{lm}(\cos\theta)e^{im\phi}$ [10].* By expanding the radiance, phase function, and source terms of the transport equation (Equation 10.1) in spherical harmonics and evaluating the integral over the solid angle and using the orthogonality relations for the spherical harmonics, $\int Y_{lm}(\theta,\phi)Y_{l'm'}(\theta,\phi)d\Omega = \delta(l-l')\delta(m-m')$, the transport equation can be rewritten as [19]

$$\sum_{l,m}\left[\frac{1}{c}\frac{\partial\phi_{l,m}}{\partial t}+\mu_t^{(l)}\phi_{l,m}-q_{l,m}\right]Y_{l,m}(\hat{s})+\nabla\cdot(\phi_{l,m}Y_{l,m}(\hat{s})\hat{s})=0, \qquad (10.13)$$

where $\mu_t^{(l)}=\mu_s(1-g_l)+\mu_a$ (note: $\mu_t^{(0)}=\mu_a)/g_l$ is the coefficient for the lth moment of the normalized phase function. For the Henyey–Greenstein phase function, $g_l=g^l$, where g is the average cosine of the scattering angle [6]. The P_N approximation is obtained by truncating the expansions in Equations 10.10 through 10.12 at $l=N$, where N is the order of the approximation. The resulting set of coupled differential equations can be solved to determine the corresponding moments of the radiance.

The P_1 approximation, also known as the diffusion approximation, has been widely used to model photon transport in tissue. With this approximation, only $l = 0, 1$ is considered. Thus, the radiance can be written as [8,9]

$$L(\vec{r},\hat{s},t)=\frac{1}{4\pi}\phi(\vec{r},t)+\frac{3}{4\pi}J(\vec{r},t)\cdot\hat{s}, \qquad (10.14)$$

where the fluence rate is given by $\phi(\vec{r})=\displaystyle\int_{4\pi} L(\vec{r},\hat{s},t)d\Omega$ and has units of mW/cm^2, and the photon flux, or current density, is given by $J(\vec{r},t)=\displaystyle\int_{4\pi} L(\vec{r},\hat{s},t)\hat{s}\,d\Omega$ and has units of mW/cm^2.

The source term can be written as [8,9]

$$S(\vec{r},\hat{s},t)=\frac{1}{4\pi}S_0(\vec{r},t)+\frac{3}{4\pi}S_1(\vec{r},t)\cdot\hat{s}, \qquad (10.15)$$

where $S_0(\vec{r},t)$ and $S_1(\vec{r},t)$ are the monopole (isotropic) and dipole moments of the source, respectively. By inserting Equations 10.14 and 10.15 into Equation 10.1 and integrating over $\hat{s}$, we can get [9]

$$\frac{1}{c}\frac{\partial}{\partial t}\phi(\vec{r},t)+\mu_a\phi(\vec{r},t)+\nabla\cdot J(\vec{r},t)=S_0(\vec{r},t). \qquad (10.16)$$

---

* The associated Legendre function, $P_{lm}(x)$, with positive or negative values of $m = -l, \dots , l$ is given by the following formula: $P_{lm}(x)=\dfrac{(-1)^m}{2^l l!}(1-x^2)^{m/2}\dfrac{\mathrm{d}^{l+m}}{\mathrm{d}x^{l+m}}(x^2-1)^l$. The Legendre polynomials, P_l, are given by Rodrigues' formula, $P_l(x)=\dfrac{1}{2^l l!}\dfrac{\mathrm{d}^l}{\mathrm{d}x^l}(x^2-1)^l$.

By inserting Equations 10.14 and 10.15 into Equation 10.1 and multiplying by $\hat{s}$ and then integrating over $\hat{s}$, we can get [9]

$$\frac{1}{c}\frac{\partial}{\partial t}J(\vec{r},t)+(\mu'_s+\mu_a)J(\vec{r},t)+\frac{1}{3}\nabla\cdot\varphi(\vec{r},t)=S_1(\vec{r},t).$$ (10.17)

By decoupling Equations 10.16 and 10.17 for $\phi(\vec{r},t)$, we can get the P_1 equation [9]

$$-D\nabla^2\phi(\vec{r},t)+\mu_a\phi(\vec{r},t)+\frac{1}{c}\cdot\frac{\partial\phi(\vec{r},t)}{\partial t}+\frac{3D}{c}\left[\mu_a\frac{\partial\phi(\vec{r},t)}{\partial t}+\frac{1}{c}\frac{\partial^2\phi(\vec{r},t)}{\partial t^2}\right]$$

$$=S_0(\vec{r},t)+\frac{3D}{c}\frac{\partial S_0}{\partial t}-3D\nabla\cdot S_1(\vec{r},t),$$ (10.18)

where the diffuse coefficient is $D=\dfrac{1}{3(\mu_a+\mu'_s)}$, and the reduced scattering coefficient is given by $\mu'_s=(1-g)\mu_s$. The standard photon diffusion equation for the P_1 approximation is obtained when certain terms are dropped from Equation 10.18. The dipole moment term of the source can be dropped by assuming an isotropic source. Collimated sources are treated as isotropic sources displaced one transport mean free path into the scattering medium from the collimated source, thus supporting this assumption. The last term on the left-hand side of the equation is dropped as well. In the frequency domain, the time dependence of the source is taken as $\exp(-i\omega t)$. When the intensity of the source is sinusoidally modulated, the photon fluence becomes $\phi(\vec{r})\exp(-i\omega t)$. The time derivative can be replaced by $-i\omega$ and the rest of the term can be ignored when $3D\omega/c^2 \ll 1$ [9]. This is equivalent to $c\mu'_s/\omega \gg 1$, which means that the scattering frequency $(c\mu'_s)$ must be much larger than the modulation frequency (ω). Given these assumptions, the photon diffusion equation can be rewritten as the following:

$$-D\nabla^2\phi(\vec{r},t)+\mu_a\phi(\vec{r},t)+\frac{1}{c}\cdot\frac{\partial\phi(\vec{r},t)}{\partial t}=S_0(\vec{r},t).$$ (10.19)

The even-order approximations do not significantly change the degree of anisotropy in the radiance that is modeled, and inconsistencies arise at the boundaries with the solutions [6,19,20]. Therefore, the odd-order approximations are widely used. This approximation is good when the albedo, $a = \mu_s/(\mu_s + \mu_a)$, is close to 1, the phase function is not too anisotropic, and the source–detector separation is large compared with $1/(\mu_s(a - g_1))$ [19].

In the tissue-nonscattering medium interface, the boundary condition consistent with P_1 approximation is obtained by integrating Equation 10.4 over all angles Ω over 2π [9]:

$$\phi(\vec{r})-2AD\hat{n}\cdot\nabla\phi=0,$$ (10.20)

where $\hat{n}$ is the normal direction of the boundary, D is the diffusion coefficient, and A is a dimensionless internal reflection coefficient that accounts for the reflectance and transmission because of the mismatch of the indexes of refraction between the two media ($A = 1$ for matching interface and $A = 2.95$ for an air–tissue interface) [6]. In the scattering–scattering medium boundary with mismatching indexes of refraction, the boundary condition consistent with P_1 approximation can be expressed as discontinuous fluence rate, $\phi_1/\phi_2 = (n_1/n_2)^2$, and continuous flux, $D_1\hat{n}\cdot\nabla\phi_1 = D_2\hat{n}\cdot\nabla\phi_2$ [21].

For a point source in an infinite homogenous medium, the source term becomes $S_0(\vec{r}) = S_0\delta(\vec{r})$, where $\vec{r}$ is the position at which fluence rate is measured and the position of the source is at 0, the origin. The steady-state solution of the fluence rate becomes [6,22]

$$\phi(\vec{r}) = \frac{S_0}{4\pi Dr}\exp(\mu_{\text{eff}}r), \tag{10.21}$$

where r is the distance to the point source and $\mu_{\text{eff}} = \sqrt{3\mu_a\cdot(\mu_a+\mu_s')}$.

The P_3 approximation is often necessary in regions of high tissue absorption of proximity to the light source position. For the P_3 approximation, moments greater than $l = 3$ are ignored, so $\phi_{l,m} = 0$ for $l > 3$ in Equation 10.13. Equations 10.10 through 10.12 can be simplified as $L(\vec{r},\hat{s}) = \sum_{l=0}^{3}\frac{2l+1}{4\pi}\phi_l(r)P_l(\vec{r}\cdot\hat{s})$, $S(\vec{r},\hat{s}) = \sum_{l=0}^{3}\frac{2l+1}{4\pi}q_l(r)P_l(\vec{r}\cdot\hat{s})$, $f(\hat{s},\hat{s}') = \sum_{l=0}^{3}\frac{2l+1}{4\pi}g_lP_l(\hat{s}\cdot\hat{s}')$ for a point source in steady-state condition since only the $m = 0$ term needs to be considered because of spherical symmetry. Inserting them into Equation 10.1 and ignoring the time dependent term resulted in Equation 10.13 with $m = 0$ only. Multiplying the resulting equation (Equation 10.13) by P_l and integrating over all solid angles yields the following equation set for ϕ_l in an infinite homogeneous medium [6,23,24]:

$$\frac{1}{2l+1}\cdot\left\{\left[(l+1)\frac{\partial\phi_{l+1}}{\partial r}+l\frac{\partial\phi_{l-1}}{\partial r}\right]+\frac{1}{r}\left[(l+1)(l+2)\phi_{l+1}(r)-l(l-1)\phi_{l-1}(r)\right]\right\}$$
$$+\mu_t^{(l)}\phi_l(r) = q_l. \tag{10.22}$$

Here, $l = 0, 1, 2, 3$, and the orthogonality properties of the Legendre polynomials were used: $\int P_l(x)P_{l'}(x)\,\mathrm{d}x = \frac{2}{2l+1}\delta(l-l')$. This equation set yields 4-coupled differential equations ($\phi_{-1} = \phi_4 = 0$). The right-hand side of Equation 10.22 has the moments of the source distribution. If we are a few scattering lengths from the source, we can assume that the source is an isotropic point source such that $q_l = 0$ for $l > 0$. For an infinite medium, the solution of Equation 10.22 for ϕ_0, that is, the light fluence rate, has been solved by Hull and Foster for an isotropic point source at the origin $q_0 = \delta(r)$ as [6]

$$\phi_0(r) = \left[\frac{-C_-(v^-)^2}{2\pi}\right]\frac{\exp(-v^-r)}{(-v^-r)} + \left[\frac{-C_+(v^+)^2}{2\pi}\right]\frac{\exp(-v^+r)}{(-v^+r)}, \tag{10.23}$$

where

$$C_- = \frac{v^{-3}\left(3\mu_a\mu_t^{(1)}-v^{+2}\right)}{6\mu_a^2\mu_t^{(1)}(v^{-2}-v^{+2})}$$

$$C_+ = \frac{v^{-3}\left(3\mu_a\mu_t^{(1)}-v^{-2}\right)}{6\mu_a^2\mu_t^{(1)}(v^{+2}-v^{-2})}$$

$$v^{\pm} = \left(\frac{\beta \pm \sqrt{\beta^2 - \gamma}}{18} \right)^{1/2} \tag{10.24}$$

$$\beta = 27\mu_a\mu_t^{(1)} + 28\mu_a\mu_t^{(3)} + 35\mu_t^{(2)}\mu_t^{(3)}$$

$$\gamma = 3780\mu_a\mu_t^{(1)}\mu_t^{(2)}\mu_t^{(3)}.$$

Here, $\mu_t^{(l)} = \mu_s(1-g_l)+\mu_a$ (note: $\mu_t^{(0)}=\mu_a$). Unlike the analytical solution for the P_1 approximation (Equation 10.21), the analytical solution for the P_3 approximation includes two exponential terms: one rapidly decaying term with an attenuation coefficient v^- and another slower decaying term with an attenuation coefficient v^+ that is corresponding to the solution for the P_1 approximation. Under the condition that $\beta^2 \gg \gamma$ and $\mu_t^{(l)} \ll \mu_t^1, l = 2, 3,$ one has $v^+ = \mu_{\text{eff}}$ and $C_+ = \mu_{\text{eff}}/2\mu_a$ so that the second term takes the same form as Equation 10.21. (The first term disappears since $v^- = 0$ under the condition.) For this reason, the second term in Equation 10.23 is also called the asymptotic solution of P_3 approximation according to Hull and Foster [6].

Figure 10.4 shows the comparison between P_1, P_3, asymptotic P_3, and MC simulation results as calculated by Hull and Foster [6]. Clearly, the P_3 approximation is only necessary for turbid medium with a high absorption coefficient in regions close to the point source (Figure 10.4a). In general, the solution in a homogeneous medium can be treated as a sum of point sources with appropriate weight.

The boundary conditions for P_3 approximation can be obtained by integrating Equation 10.4 multiplied by P_l over all angles over 2π and insisting the terms belong to different P_l to be equal for the moment l [6].

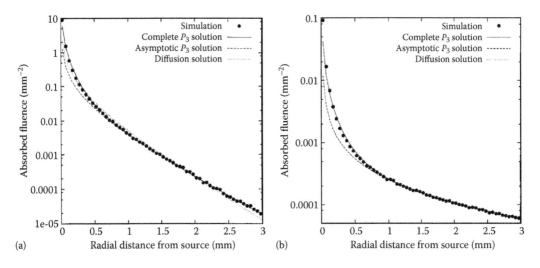

FIGURE 10.4
Comparisons of the diffusion (P_1) solution, P_3 solution, asymptotic P_3 solution, and MC simulation for a point isotropic source in an infinite medium for (a) $\mu_a = 10$ cm^{-1}, $\mu_s = 100$ cm^{-1}, and $g = 0.9$ and (b) $\mu_a = 0.1$ cm^{-1}, $\mu_s = 100$ cm^{-1}, and $g = 0.9$. (From Hull, E.L. and T.H. Foster., *J. Opt. Soc. Am. A*, 18(3): 584–599, 2001.)

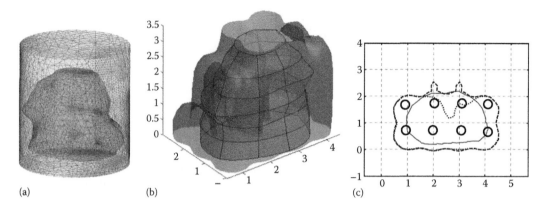

FIGURE 10.5
(a) Mesh plot of the prostate geometry with a cylindrical outer layer. (b) Isofluence rate surface of 150 mW/cm^2 obtained by FEM using heterogeneous optical properties. (c) Isofluence rate lines in a slice of prostate at $z = 2$ cm. Solid line, prostate contour; dashed line, 150 mW/cm^2 isofluence rate line using homogeneous optical properties; dotted line, 150 mW/cm^2 isofluence rate line using heterogeneous optical properties. (From Li, J. et al., *Proc. SPIE*, 6139: 61390, 2006M.)

Figure 10.5 shows the calculation of light fluence rate distribution inside a prostate during prostate PDT with heterogeneous optical properties using the diffusion approximation [25]. The prostate geometry along with a cylinder outer layer is meshed based on the transrectum ultrasound images (Figure 10.5a). Linear light sources covering the entire prostate gland were used to treat the prostate (see *circles* in Figure 10.5c). The steady-state diffusion equation (Equation 10.19 without the time differential term) was solved using a finite-difference method (FEM) using the heterogeneously distributed optical properties (for details, see Ref. [25]). The resulting isofluence rate surface is shown in Figure 10.5b. For comparison, isofluence rate lines are shown in Figure 10.5c, where the dotted line used clinically measured heterogeneous optical properties while the dashed line used homogeneous optical properties based on the patient average ($\mu_a = 0.3$ cm^{-1} and $\mu_s' = 14$ cm^{-1}). Clearly, the isofluence rate line taking into account heterogeneous optical properties missed the top portion of the prostate owing to increased absorption in that region while the isofluence rate line that did not take into account the optical property heterogeneity can cover the entire prostate. This example illustrates the importance of optical property distribution on the light fluence rate distribution during PDT. The FEM of the P_1 approximation is currently the predominant method for calculating the light fluence rate in conditions of arbitrary geometry and heterogeneous optical properties.

10.2.4 Deterministic Solutions

The Boltzmann equation can be solved either analytically or numerically; they are so-called the deterministic solutions. Analytical methods involve the applications of a Green's function (often called a kernel). Green's function is the solution when the source is a δ function, and the solution for any other source can be obtained by convolution of the source and Green's function. Figure 10.6 shows Green's function for a pencil-beam incident at 45° on a semi-infinite tissue surface [18]. A P_3 hybrid solution with two sources gives good agreement with the MC simulation except for near the pencil beam at the surface. For isolines less than 0.1 or for locations far away from the point of entrance of the pencil beam, Green's function for the 45° incidence is almost identical to that of normal incidence,

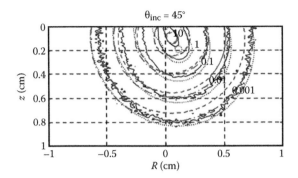

FIGURE 10.6

Comparisons of Green's functions calculated by MC simulation and analytical calculation for a 45° incident pencil photon beam on a semi-infinite medium with optical properties $\mu_a = 5$ cm^{-1}, $\mu_s = 40$ cm^{-1}, $g = 0.9$, and $n = 1.4$. The MC simulation results are represented by the dark solid line; the analytical calculation uses P_1 approximation with one source (dashed lines), P_3 hybrid with one source (dashed–dotted lines), and P_3 hybrid with two sources (dotted lines). (From Zhu, T.C. et al., *Proc. SPIE*, 5315: 113–124, 2004.)

provided a lateral shift of $2AD\sin\theta$ is made, where θ (=45°) is the angle of incidence, $D = 1/3\ D = 1/3\mu'_s$ is the diffusion coefficient, and A is the internal reflection coefficient. In general, a convolution formalism using Green's function is not suitable to be used in regions where there are heterogeneities of optical properties, which can often happen in humans. In these cases, a superposition formalism is needed [26]. One possible method is to determine the form of Green's function in a heterogeneous medium directly for locations with known intensities of point sources, and then the final solution is a superposition of the heterogeneous Green's function and the intensities distribution of the sources. An analytical kernel suitable for an interstitial light source in a heterogeneous medium is demonstrated elsewhere [26].

The Boltzmann equation can be solved numerically by approximating each term in Equation 10.1 as a numerical difference term based on either a rectangular grid (finite difference method [FDM]) or a more complex mesh element (FEM).

The FDM is a standard technique to solve a partial differential equation. A regular grid is established in the problem domain and differential operators are replaced by discrete differences. This method can be used to solve elliptic equations to be applied in optical tomography [27]. The FDM can solve the transport equation when the angular integral over scattering directions is discretized [28].

The FEM is slightly more versatile than the FDM in regard to complex geometries and for modeling boundary effects. The general problem is reduced to that of finding an approximate solution that lies in the vector space spanned by a finite number of basis functions. Then, the forward problem becomes one of matrix algebra for a finite size [28–30].

Compared with the MC simulation described earlier, deterministic methods often provide a solution more quickly with one key advantage that the solution in the interface region where the light fluence is low can be determined very accurately without worrying too much about increased statistical uncertainties in these regions from MC simulation. The disadvantage of the deterministic method is the increased computer memory requirement for a large number of grid (or mesh) elements, which can quickly reach more than 16 GB for a problem containing over 0.5 million mesh elements. If a larger mesh size is used to reduce the total number of mesh elements, then the solution accuracy in regions with a large mesh element size will decrease.

There are limited number of commercial codes [31,32] and open source codes [33,34] that can solve the Boltzmann equation using FEM or FDM methods. All of these current codes solve the transport of megavoltage photons and electrons and have not been directly applied to light transport in turbid media. As more commercial codes become available, utilization of this method is expected to explode in the future for transport of light in turbid media.

10.3 Oxygen Diffusion and Transport during PDT

10.3.1 Cylinder Model

10.3.1.1 Introduction

As described in Section 10.1, one essential component in PDT is ground-state molecular tissue oxygen, which is used to generate the cytotoxic species, singlet oxygen, in PDT. Hence, it becomes apparent that tissue oxygenation in the target volume is one of the critical factors that determine the efficacy of PDT. Many studies have been conducted and are undergoing to investigate a variety of aspects of tissue oxygenation in PDT, such as oxygen diffusion and perfusion in tissue and blood vessel, tissue reoxygenation during fractional PDT, oxygen consumption, and depletion in PDT [35–40].

Most of the oxygen supplied to the body tissues is transported via systemic circulation, specifically the cardiovascular system consisting of arteries, capillaries, and veins. Oxygen-rich blood enters the blood vessels through the aorta and then branches into smaller arteries via the contraction of the heart's left ventricle. These many blood vessel branches deliver oxygen-rich blood to every part of the body such as the brain, kidneys, and limbs. The *destination* of most oxygen-rich blood is normally the smallest vessels of the vascular system, called capillaries, where the oxygen and nutrients are released. The waste products and carbon dioxide are collected in the meantime. This waste-rich blood flows into the veins and circulates back to the heart. Then, it exchanges gases in the lungs through pulmonary circulation and becomes oxygen-rich blood again. In the literature, a spectrum of theoretical models have been developed to model the transport of oxygen, ranging from the transport from alveolar gas to the red blood cells (RBCs) in the lungs to that from the RBCs to tissue [41–45].

For the purposes of understanding oxygen supply and consumption in PDT, modeling oxygen transport in the blood vessels such as capillaries and in the tissue becomes more important. Hence, the main focus of this section is to introduce the simplified but commonly adopted models for oxygen transport within capillaries, from capillary into tissue, and within the target tissue. The section will be discussed in two parts. The first part is to provide readers with some fundamental knowledge of oxygen in the blood and RBCs; the second part is to introduce a cylindrical model for modeling oxygen transport.

10.3.1.2 Oxygen in the RBCs

For modeling oxygen transport in the blood, it is reasonable to simplify blood into two phases: RBCs and plasma. The volume percentage of RBCs in blood is usually referred to as hematocrit, which is approximately 45% for male and 40% for female human adults [46]. Second, oxygen in the blood is normally present in two forms: (1) chemically bound to hemoglobin in the RBCs and (2) free molecules dissolved in the plasma and RBC water.

Under normal physiological conditions, only a small fraction of oxygen is dissolved in the plasma as free molecules because of its low solubility. However, these free oxygen molecules can impinge on the measuring oxygen electrode, which results in the measured partial pressure of oxygen (PaO_2 or P for simplicity hereafter). According to Henry's law, the concentration of oxygen dissolved in the plasma is directly proportional to P. This relation is expressed in Equation 10.25, in which α is the solubility of oxygen and $[^3O_2]$ denotes the concentration of the free ground-state oxygen molecules.

$$[^3O_2] = \alpha \times P \qquad (10.25)$$

Oxygen in the RBCs is either dissolved in the water content or reversibly bound to hemoglobin. Hemoglobin bound with oxygen is usually known as oxyhemoglobin (HbO); in contrast, hemoglobin without bound oxygen is deoxyhemoglobin (Hb). Since approximately 98% of oxygen is carried by HbO, hemoglobin is usually considered as the main oxygen carrier in the blood [47].

Each hemoglobin molecule is composed of four heme groups. Each heme group has a porphyrin ring structure with an Fe^{++} in its center, which can reversibly bind an oxygen. Hence, four heme sites in a hemoglobin molecule can maximally bind four oxygen molecules. The percentage of all the available heme sites saturated with oxygen is usually referred to as the hemoglobin oxygen saturation (SaO_2). SaO_2 is a function of partial pressure of oxygen P, which has an approximately sigmoidal relationship. A representative relation curve is shown in Figure 10.7. As shown, SaO_2 increases with P until saturation. This curve is also known as the oxygen dissociation curve. When the concentration of oxygen dissolved in the blood decreases, the P decreases, and oxyhemoglobin will release oxygen; that is, SaO_2 decreases.

Typically, oxygen has to be released from oxyhemoglobin before it diffuses from RBCs into the blood plasma and further into tissue. Thus, it is useful to briefly introduce the mathematical model of the oxygen unloading process before discussing the transport of oxygen into tissue. Each hemoglobin has four heme sites available for oxygen, and the binding to one site can potentially influence the binding to other sites; hence, the four-step Adair reaction process is more appropriate to describe it [42]. However, this is more

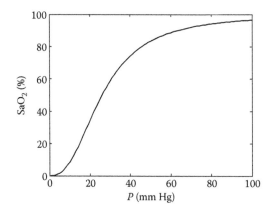

FIGURE 10.7
A representative oxygen saturation curve. The curve is plotted using Equation 10.29 with $P_{50} = 26$ mm Hg and $n = 2.46$.

complex for modeling and beyond the scope of this chapter. For simplicity, a one-step binding process assuming that oxygen reacts with four heme sites with equal probabilities is adopted as described in Equation 10.26.

$$Hb + O_2 \leftrightarrow HbO_2 \tag{10.26}$$

Oxygen saturation SaO_2 (or Sa for simplicity hereafter) represents the percentage of oxyhemoglobin over the total amount of hemoglobin. Within an RBC, the time-dependent differential equation governing bound oxygen (or HbO) can be expressed as Equation 10.27 according to Fick's second law, where Γ represents the rates of the oxygen unloading from HbO [41,43]. The first term on the right-hand side of the equation calculates the diffusion of bound oxygen. In addition, if the oxygen unloading process is assumed to reach equilibrium instantaneously, oxygen saturation, $Sa = h(P)$, is expressed using Hill's equation (Equation 10.29). In this case, the rate of oxygen unloading becomes 0 (see Equation 10.28). A full glossary of all terms used in the mathematical model is given in Table 10.1 [48,49].

$$C_{HR}\frac{\partial Sa}{\partial t} = C_{HR}D_H\nabla^2 Sa - \Gamma \tag{10.27}$$

$$\Gamma = k \cdot C_{HR}\frac{h(P) - Sa}{1 - h(P)} \tag{10.28}$$

$$h(P) = \frac{P^n}{P^n + P_{50}^n}. \tag{10.29}$$

TABLE 10.1

Definition of Symbols and Values for Diffusion of Oxygen in Vasculature

Symbol	Definition	Values
α_c	$^3O_2$ solubility in capillary	1.527 μM/mm Hg
α_t	$^3O_2$ solubility in tissue	1.295 μM/mm Hg
CHR	Hemoglobin concentration in RBC	5000 μM
CH	Hemoglobin concentration in blood	2500 μM
D_c	$^3O_2$ diffusion coefficient in capillary	1240 μm²/s
D_H	Diffusion coefficient of hemoglobin	14 μm²/s
D_t	$^3O_2$ diffusion coefficient in tissue	1700 μm²/s
k	Oxygen dissociation rate constant	44 s⁻¹
l	Length of capillary	300 μm
n	Hill constant	2.46
P_{50}	Half maximum hemoglobin saturation	26 mm Hg
P_m	Half maximum oxygen consumption	0.386 mm Hg
P_{ts}	Supply oxygen pressure at artery	100 mm Hg
R_c	Capillary radius	4–10 μm
R_t	Tissue radius	60 μm
q_0	$^3O_2$ maximum metabolic consumption rate	0.9 μM/s
v	Velocity of blood flow	50–200 μm/s

Source: Zhu, T.C. et al., *Proc. SPIE*, 6427: 1–12, 2007; Liu, B. et al., *Proc. SPIE*, 8568: 856805, 2013.

The time-dependent differential equation for the concentration of free oxygen in the RBCs is given in Equation 10.30. Note that the oxygen concentration term was explicitly expressed using the partial pressure of oxygen based on Henry's law (Equation 10.25) because of its continuity boundary conditions. This conversion will be used in the rest of the section wherever it applies:

$$\alpha_R \frac{\partial P}{\partial t} = \alpha_R D_R \nabla^2 P + \Gamma. \tag{10.30}$$

The initial conditions for two time-dependent differential equations (Equations 10.27 and 10.30) for Sa and P can be strictly defined to mimic the exact biological environments; however, it is unnecessarily complicated. An assumption of uniform distributions of Sa and P inside RBC is sufficient for most studies. Per the boundary conditions, since hemoglobin cannot pass through the RBC membrane, one should have a boundary condition for Sa as given in Equation 10.31. The boundary conditions for P are the continuities of the oxygen flux and the partial pressure P as expressed in Equation 10.31. This is true when the RBC membrane resistance is small. Huxley and Kutchai [50] have confirmed this assumption.

$$\vec{n} \cdot \nabla Sa = 0,$$
$$\begin{cases} \vec{n} \cdot D\alpha \nabla P \big|_{in} = \vec{n} \cdot D\alpha \nabla P \big|_{out} \\ P \big|_{in} = P \big|_{out} \end{cases} \tag{10.31}$$

10.3.1.3 Simplified Cylinder Model for Oxygen Transport in Vascularized Tissue

The unloaded oxygen from hemoglobin can diffuse from the RBC to the blood in response to the gradient in oxygen concentration and even further into surrounding tissue through the blood vessel walls. The vascular structure such as distribution of capillaries in normal healthy tissue is usually varied from location to location. Modeling of the realistic capillary network for a tissue of interest can be complex. This can be even harder for a tumor tissue, as it is well known for its highly heterogeneous vascular structures. For this reason, simplified models are normally used to simulate oxygen transport in vascularized tissue [43].

One of the most commonly used simplified models is the Krogh cylindrical model [51] in which a cylindrical blood vessel is assumed to be surrounded by a cylindrical tissue as shown in Figure 10.8. This single-vessel model can be expanded to a two-dimensional (2D) array of vessels, or a three-dimensional (3D) matrix or bundle of vessels. To demonstrate the concepts of modeling oxygen transport, a 3D single-vessel model is used as an example

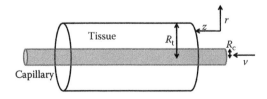

FIGURE 10.8
3D Krogh cylindrical model. The blood is assumed to flow in from the right-hand side with velocity v along the z-direction. The capillary has a radius R_c and the surrounding tissue has a radius R_t. R_t determines the average vascular density (number of capillaries per unit volume) and R_c determines the average capillary dimension.

here. The models with more complex structure can be developed based on the single-vessel model with different boundary conditions. A more realistic microscopic model will be briefly introduced in Section 10.3.2.

In reality, the RBCs are flowing discretely in the blood stream. The membrane of RBC has negligible resistance to oxygen diffusion [52]. Therefore, a few assumptions can be made for this simple model. First, unloaded oxygen from oxyhemoglobin can instantaneously diffuse into blood plasma as if no diffusion barrier is present. Second, RBCs are uniformly distributed in the blood. Hence, the governing equations for bound and free oxygen introduced earlier can be adopted and modified to calculate oxygen in the blood plasma, as summarized in Equations 10.32 and 10.33. Note that the new second terms on the right-hand sides of two equations describe the convection of free and bound oxygen, respectively. Since the concentration of the bound oxygen is calculated in the volume of blood plasma instead of in the RBC, the total hemoglobin concentration C_{HR} in the RBC should be corrected by the hematocrit to account for the concentration of RBC in the blood, and the total hemoglobin concentration per the volume of blood plasma is denoted as C_H.

$$\alpha_c \frac{\partial P}{\partial t} = \alpha_c D_c \nabla^2 P - \vec{v} \cdot \alpha_c \nabla P + \Gamma \tag{10.32}$$

$$C_H \frac{\partial Sa}{\partial t} = C_H D_H \nabla^2 Sa - \vec{v} \cdot C_H \nabla Sa - \Gamma \tag{10.33}$$

By manipulating the above equations, one can derive Equation 10.34, assuming that oxygen and RBC have velocities only along the z-axis, but the diffusion is isotropic.

$$(\alpha_c + KC_H) \frac{\partial P}{\partial t} = \alpha_c D_c \nabla^2 P + C_H D_H \nabla^2 Sa - v_z(\alpha_c + KC_H) \frac{\partial P}{\partial z}, \tag{10.34}$$

where $K = \dfrac{nP^{n-1}P_{50}^n}{\left(P^n + P_{50}^n\right)^2}$ and we have made the assumption that $Sa = f(P)$. The time-dependent differential equation for oxygen in tissue is given in Equation 10.35. The second term on the right-hand side is the Michaelis–Menten-type metabolic oxygen concentration rates [53].

$$\alpha_t \frac{\partial P}{\partial t} = \alpha_t D_t \nabla^2 P - q_0 \frac{\alpha_t P}{\alpha_t P + \alpha_t P_m} \tag{10.35}$$

Two coupled differential equations can be solved using FEM with appropriate boundary conditions and constraints. General boundary conditions are the continuities of partial pressure of oxygen and oxygen flux, insulation boundary condition, and the source oxygen pressure term, as listed in Equation 10.36.

$$\vec{n} \cdot D\alpha \nabla P\big|_- = \vec{n} \cdot D\alpha \nabla P\big|_+$$

$$P\big|_- = P\big|_+$$

$$\nabla P\big|_{boundaries} = 0 \tag{10.36}$$

$$P\big|_{z=0, r\in[0,R_c]} = P\big|_{const}.$$

10.3.1.4 An Example of the Steady-State Krogh Model

This section will demonstrate an example of oxygen diffusion at the steady state. Since the Krogh model is cylindrically symmetric, one can simplify the geometry in Figure 10.8 using a 2D cylindrical model. The definition of the physiological parameters and values in this example model are given in Table 10.1. Briefly, a blood capillary with radius of R_c has the same length (l) as a cylinder-shaped tissue with radius of R_t. R_t actually represents half of the intercapillary distance between two adjacent capillaries, which is considered large enough so that each capillary supplies oxygen only to its immediate concentric surrounding tissue. R_t also represents vascular density; that is, a larger R_t means a smaller vascular density.

Given the assumptions in Section 10.3.1.3, the governing equations for the concentration of the bound and free oxygen in the capillary and tissue at the steady state are obtained by setting Equations 10.34 and 10.35 to zero. The boundary conditions used in this example are mostly the same as Equation 10.36. At $r = R_c$ and all z, both the flux of oxygen and P are continuous. The partial pressure of oxygen, P, at the inflow boundary ($z = 0$) of the capillary is a constant, which is set to be the same pressure as that in an artery, P_{ts}. This boundary condition expressed in Equation 10.37 is considered as a source term in this example. All other boundaries are considered as insulations. Using the FEM in COMSOL (Burlington, Massachusetts), one can derive the spatial distribution of partial pressure of oxygen:

$$P\Big|_{z=0,r\in[0,R_c]} = P_{ts}. \qquad (10.37)$$

Figure 10.9 shows one representative result of the radial distribution of P at $z = 0, 10, 20, 30, 40, 50, 100, 200,$ and 300 µm. One can see that the gradient of P along the radial direction decreases as z increases.

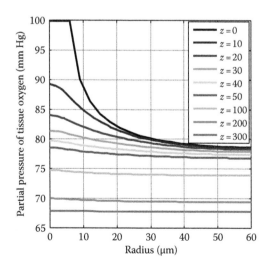

FIGURE 10.9
The radial distribution of partial pressure of tissue oxygen for a capillary radius of 6 µm, a blood flow velocity of 100 µm/s, and at various positions along the capillary. Unit of z: micrometers.

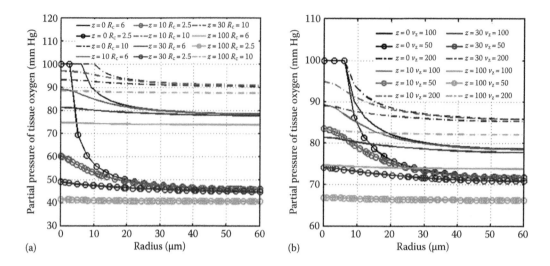

FIGURE 10.10
The radial distributions of P for various capillary radii (a) and various velocities of blood flow (b). z and R_c are expressed in units of micrometers, and v_z is expressed in micrometers per second.

Figure 10.10 shows the radial distribution of partial pressure at positions 0, 10, 30, and 100 μm along the capillary for different capillary radii (Figure 10.10a) and different velocities of blood flow (Figure 10.10b).

10.3.2 Realistic Microscopic Models

The classic Krogh model usually provides a good approximation for simple oxygen transportation studies. It normally requires several assumptions, some of which are introduced in the above section. In a more realistic microcirculation environment, oxygen transportation is usually much more complex because of heterogeneous distribution of microvessels, random directions of blood flow, unevenly spaced vessel densities, and so forth. Hence, a realistic microscopic model for oxygen transport will first require much more input information for the description of the model, boundary, and initial conditions. Second, it will be much more computationally expensive.

In some biological cases, the model of Krogh may serve as a building block for a more complex model. For instance, simulating oxygen transport in the skeletal muscle can be accomplished by expanding a single Krogh cylinder to an array or a bundle of evenly spaced cylinders because capillaries in the skeletal muscle normally are parallel to the muscle fibers and evenly spaced [54].

For an even more realistic microcirculation model, one or a simple array of Krogh cylinders may not be sufficient. A variety of techniques were used to simulate these complex vascular geometries. For instance, the model developed by Secomb et al. [55] simulated oxygen transport from irregularly distributed vessels in a rectangular cuboidal medium. The tissue oxygen distribution was obtained by the superposition of the contribution from each vessel. This irregular distribution of vessel network was obtained via the contracted imaging technique. Secomb et al. [55] used a Green's function method to solve oxygen transport equations. In addition, Beard et al. [56,57] proposed to use the FEM to solve the similar 3D problems.

10.4 Photosensitizer Diffusion and Transport during PDT

Photosensitizers are normally delivered systemically or topically in PDT. The systemic administration involves either oral administration or intravenous injection so that the drug will be circulated through the whole body system, and preferentially more drug will be localized in the target site than in others. An ideal photosensitizer should have low or no toxicities and a fast clearance process. Some systemically delivered photosensitizers are benzoporphyrin derivative (BPD), Photofrin, and HPPH (2-[1-hexyloxyethyl]-2-devinyl pyropheophorbide-a). In contrast with the systemic administration, ALA (5-aminolevulinic acid), a prodrug that reacts with tissue to generate the photosensitizer protoporphyrin IX (PpIX), can also be applied topically to perform more localized delivery, which is commonly used for skin treatment.

A complete mathematical model of photosensitizer transport can be very complicated because of the great heterogeneity of the tissue and the complex pharmacokinetics. However, the diffusion approximation can be a good approach for simulating the spatial and temporal distribution of the photosensitizer. For instance, the diffusion model has been developed to model photosensitizer BPD diffusion from blood vessel [58]. Similar to the oxygen transport simulation discussed above, the distribution of vascular network can be obtained via the contrast agent–enhanced imaging techniques such as fluorescence microscopy, and then each vessel is considered as a source-supplying drug to the surrounding tissue. The diffusion equation, such as Equation 10.38, is solved using the FEM with assumptions on the homogeneous diffusivity in the tissue, where Q is the source term of drug.

$$\frac{\partial [PS]}{\partial t} = D\nabla^2 [PS] + Q \tag{10.38}$$

Figure 10.11 shows the simulated results of BPD diffusion processes at different time intervals after intravenous injection of BPD in two different tumor models: orthotopic (top row) and subcutaneous (bottom row) [58]. The left column shows the BPD distribution at a 15-min interval, and the right column represents that at a 3-h interval. As shown, in the orthotopic tumor model, a more even distribution of BPD (represented by the red color) can be found with a 3-h interval (Figure 10.11b) than that with a 15-min interval (Figure 10.11a). The same results are found in the subcutaneous tumor model, which implies the dynamic diffusion process of BPD.

The diffusion approximation can also be used for modeling the topical administration of a photosensitizer, which may be relatively easier because the vascular network is usually not involved and diffusion is caused mainly by the spatial gradient in the drug concentration. For instance, the prodrug ALA is usually topically applied to treat skin diseases. ALA is called a prodrug because it is not a photosensitizer itself. The actual photosensitive species in ALA-PDT is the induced PpIX. ALA is used to elevate the endogenous production of PpIX. Hence, two additional processes may be needed to model the dynamic process of drug transport in ALA-induced PpIX PDT. The first process is using Fick's second law to calculate the diffusion of the prodrug. A source or reaction consumption term may be added to the diffusion equation. The second step is to use a compartment model to model the conversion of ALA to PpIX [59].

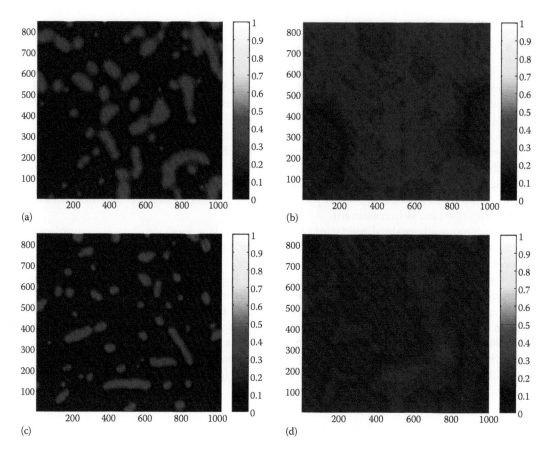

FIGURE 10.11
Simulation results of BPD diffusion distribution at 15 min (a, c) and 3 h (b, d) after BPD intravenous injection in the orthotopic (a, b) and subcutaneous (c, d) tumor models. (a) At 15 min in the orthotopic tumor; (b) at 3 h in the orthotopic tumor; (c) at 15 min in the subcutaneous tumor; (d) at 3 h in the subcutaneous tumor. (From Zhou, X. et al., *Photochem. Photobiol.*, 79: 323–331, 2004.)

10.5 Modeling the Generation of Singlet Oxygen during PDT

During PDT, energy from the triplet-state photosensitizer excited via the absorption of light is transferred to ground-state oxygen, which produces singlet-state oxygen. Singlet oxygen is accepted to be the cytotoxic agent causing therapeutic outcomes in PDT [60]. Mathematical models have been developed to simulate the process of PDT. These models use a set of differential equations describing the major photochemical and photophysical reaction pathways in PDT to calculate temporal and spatial distributions of singlet oxygen, ground-state oxygen, and the photosensitizer. Tissue oxygen replenishment, PDT consumption, and metabolic consumption of oxygen are considered as well.

In the microscopic model, oxygen diffusion into capillaries, from capillaries into tissue, and diffusion within tissue is taken into account [61]. In contrast, oxygen diffusion is not considered in a macroscopic model. Rather, a generalized oxygen supply term is assumed to implicitly include metabolic oxygen consumption [49].

10.5.1 Microscopic Model

In the microscopic model, the tumor has uniformly distributed blood capillaries aligned parallel to the linear light source. The intercapillary distance between two adjacent capillaries is large enough so that each can supply oxygen only to its immediate, concentric surrounding tissue. Therefore, a Krogh cylinder model can be adopted for a single capillary and its surrounding tissue [48]. A 3D Krogh model can be simplified as a 2D cylindrically symmetric model. Normally in blood, hemoglobin is contained in the RBC, in which hemoglobin saturation and desaturation occur. After oxygen unloads from oxyhemoglobin, it diffuses into blood through the RBC cell membrane and then into the tissue. An assumption that is made in the microscopic model is that no oxygen diffusion barrier is in the RBC cell membrane. The distribution of hemoglobin within the capillary is assumed to be uniform.

In capillaries, the governing oxygen transport equations are described by Equations 10.30 through 10.32. Oxygen concentration has been expressed using oxygen partial pressure.

The governing equation for ground-state oxygen in tissue is given by the following equation:

$$\frac{\partial [^3O_2]}{\partial t} + \left(\xi \frac{\phi[S_0][^3O_2](1+\sigma([S_0]+\delta))}{[^3O_2]+\beta} \right) = D_t \nabla^2 [^3O_2] - q_0 \frac{[^3O_2]}{[^3O_2]+\alpha_t P_m}, \tag{10.39}$$

where q_0 is the maximum metabolic oxygen consumption rate in the Michaelis–Menten relationship [62].

In the microscopic model, the velocity of blood flow often decreases with increased treatment time to simulate PDT-induced physiological response [63].

10.5.2 Macroscopic Model

Unless the microscopic vascular structures are known or important for the purpose of the model, it is often unnecessary to model the oxygen diffusion process if they are assumed to be uniformly distributed because the oxygen diffusion typically happens at a spatial scale of less than 50 μm and the details of oxygen diffusion have little impact on light transport or drug distribution, which often happen in the millimeter spatial scale. A macroscopic model can be formulated to obtain the same result as the microscopic model if one includes an oxygen replenishment term and ignores the oxygen diffusion processes. The oxygen replenishment term implicitly includes the metabolic consumption of oxygen in tissue. On the basis of the kinetics equations of the photochemical reactions, a set of coupled differential equations can be used to describe the PDT process [48,64,65].

$$\frac{d[S_0]}{dt} = -k_0[S_0] - k_1[^1O_2]([S_0]+\delta) + k_2[T][^3O_2] + k_3[S_1] + k_4[T] \tag{10.40}$$

$$\frac{d[S_1]}{dt} = -(k_3 + k_5)[S_1] + k_0[S_0] \tag{10.41}$$

$$\frac{d[T]}{dt} = -k_2[T][^3O_2] - k_4[T] + k_5[S_1] \tag{10.42}$$

$$\frac{d[^3O_2]}{dt} = -S_\Delta k_2[T][^3O_2] + k_6[^1O_2] + g\left(1 - \frac{[^3O_2]}{[^3O_2]_0}\right) \tag{10.43}$$

$$\frac{d[^1O_2]}{dt} = -k_1([S_0]+\delta)[^1O_2] + S_\Delta k_2[T][^3O_2] - k_6[^1O_2] - k_7[A][^1O_2] \tag{10.44}$$

$$\frac{d[A]}{dt} = -k_7[A][^1O_2] \tag{10.45}$$

Here, $[S_0]$, $[S_1]$, and $[T]$ are the ground, first excited singlet, and triplet sensitizer concentrations, respectively. $[^3O_2]$ and $[^1O_2]$ are the ground triplet and excited singlet-state oxygen concentrations. $g(1 - [^3O_2]/[^3O_2]_0)$ and $[A]$ are the oxygen supply term and the concentration of $^1O_2$ acceptors excluding the sensitizer molecule, respectively. δ is a low photosensitizer concentration correction term. If one only cares about the dynamic process of PDT in the time scale of a few seconds to hours, then the time derivative in the right-hand sides of Equations 10.41, 10.42, and 10.44 can be set to zero because these processes are known to be very fast (~ microseconds or less). Then, the required photochemical parameters can be reduced from 8 (δ, k_1, ..., k_7) to 4 (δ, β, ξ, σ), with the latter expressed as ratios of the former. A summary of the photochemical parameters is listed in Table 10.2.

With the addition of the light diffusion equation, the coupled differential equations (Equations 10.40 through 10.45) above can be written as [49,64]

$$\mu_a\phi - \nabla \cdot \left(\frac{1}{3\mu_s'}\nabla\phi\right) = S \tag{10.46}$$

$$\frac{d[S_0]}{dt} + \left(\xi\sigma\frac{\phi([S_0]+\delta)[^3O_2]}{[^3O_2]+\beta}\right)[S_0] = 0 \tag{10.47}$$

$$\frac{d[^3O_2]}{dt} + \left(\xi\frac{\phi[S_0]}{[^3O_2]+\beta}\right)[^3O_2] - g\left(1 - \frac{[^3O_2]}{[^3O_2]_{(t=0)}}\right) = 0 \tag{10.48}$$

$$\frac{d[^1O_2]_{rx}}{dt} - \left(\xi\frac{\phi[S_0][^3O_2]}{[^3O_2]+\beta}\right) = 0 \tag{10.49}$$

Here, the reacted singlet oxygen concentration $[^1O_2]_{rx}$ is defined as the fraction of singlet oxygen that interacted with $[A]$ [48]. These equations can be used for any treatment geometry. Furthermore, they can be solved numerically using the FEM. Experiments have been performed to determine the parameters for various photosensitizer drugs [64,66,67].

TABLE 10.2

Parameter List for Photochemical Parameters for Photofrin Singlet Oxygen Generation during PDT

Symbol	Definition	Values for Photofrin	References
β (μM)	k_4/k_2	11.9	[68]
δ (μM)	Low concentration correction	33	[69,70]
ξ (cm^2 mW^{-1} s^{-1})	$S_\Delta \left(\dfrac{k_5}{k_5+k_3} \right) \dfrac{\varepsilon}{h\nu} \dfrac{k_7[A]/k_6}{k_7[A]/k_6+1}$	3.7×10^{-3}	[68,71]
σ (μM^{-1})	$k_1/k_7[A]$	7.6×10^{-5}	[68]
$[A]$ (μM)	Singlet oxygen receptors, considered a constant during PDT because it is too large to be changed during PDT	830	[65]
g (μM/s)	Oxygen perfusion rate	0.76	[64]
k_0 (1/s)	Photon absorption rate of photosensitizer per photosensitizer concentration (in μM), $k_0 = \varepsilon\phi/h\nu$, for $\phi = 100$ mW/cm^2	1.9	[48]
k_1 (1/μM/s)	Bimolecular rate for $^1O_2$ reaction with ground-state photosensitizer	760	a
k_2 (1/μM/s)	Bimolecular rate of triplet photosensitizer quenching by $^3O_2$	1400	[72]
k_3 (1/s)	Fluorescence rate of first excited singlet-state photosensitizer to ground-state photosensitizer	2.9×10^7	[72]
k_4 (1/s)	Phosphorescence rate of monomolecular decay of the photosensitizer triplet state	1.67×10^4	b
k_5 (1/s)	Intersystem crossing rate from first excited photosensitizer to triplet-state photosensitizer	4.94×10^7	c
k_6 (1/s)	$^1O_2$ to $^3O_2$ phosphorescence rate	3.3×10^5	τ_Δ in water[d] [73,74]
$k_7[A]$ (1/s)	Bimolecular rate of reaction of $^1O_2$ with biological substrate $[A]$	1×10^7	τ_Δ in tissue[d] [69]
S_Δ	Fraction of triplet-state photosensitizer–$^3O_2$ reactions to produce $^1O_2$	0.37	e

Source: Zhu, T.C. et al., *Proc. SPIE*, 6427: 1–12, 2007; Liu, B. et al., *Proc. SPIE*, 8568: 856805, 2013; Wang, K.K. et al., *J. Biophoton.*, 3(5–6): 304–318, 2010.
a $k_1 = \sigma^*k_7[A] = 7.6 \times 10^{-5}$ (1/μM) $\times 1 \times 10^7$ (1/s) = 760 (1/μM/s).
b $k_4 = \beta^*k_2 = 11.9$ (μM) $\times 1400$ (1/μM/s) = 1.67×10^4 (1/s).
c $k_5 = \phi_t/(1 - \phi_t) k_3 = 0.63/(1 - 0.63)^*2.9 \times 10^7$ (1/s) = 4.94×10^7 (1/s), where the triplet quantum yield, $\phi_t = k_5/(k_5 + k_3)$ is obtained from Ref. [75].
d τ_Δ is the singlet oxygen lifetime, $\tau_\Delta = 3$ μs in water and 0.1 μs in tissue. $1/\tau_\Delta = k_6 + k_7[A]$.
e $S_\Delta = \xi/\phi_t(\varepsilon/h\nu) = 3.7 \times 10^{-3}$ (cm^2 mW^{-1} s^{-1})/0.63/(0.003(cm^{-1} μM^{-1})/6.022 $\times 10^{14}$(cm^{-3}/μM))*(1.97(eV)* 1.6×10^{-16} (mWs/eV)) = 0.37, where $\varepsilon = 0.003$ cm^{-1} μM^{-1} for Photofrin is obtained from Ref. [76] and $h\nu = 1.97$ eV for the 630-nm red light. Notice that we have used the approximation $k_7[A]/k_6/(k_7[A]/k_6 + 1) \sim 1$.

10.5.3 An Example

Singlet oxygen production depends on the local fluence rate and concentration of drug and tissue oxygen as seen in Equation 10.49. Usually, tissue oxygen is a critical limiting factor in producing singlet oxygen as it can be depleted during PDT. The rate of oxygen depletion is also dependent on fluence rate and replenishment. Hence, first, this section presents a simple example using a wide range of fluence rate from 20 to 200 mW/cm^2 to illustrate the fluence rate–dependent oxygen depletion effects on the cumulative concentration of

singlet oxygen. Second, some results using clinical parameters such as distribution of photosensitizer and tissue optical properties are presented. To better demonstrate the effect
of oxygen depletion, the radius of the capillary in the Krogh model is set to be 2.5 μm, and
all other physiological parameters are the same as listed in Tables 10.1 and 10.2. The initial
concentration of photosensitizer in tissue is 7 μM. Total radiant exposure is 100 J/cm².

The cumulative concentration of reacted singlet oxygen under uniform fluence rate distribution is higher at the lower fluence rate for the same total fluence, resulting from more oxygen
depletion at the higher fluence rate (Figure 10.12a). If the therapeutic outcomes are positively
correlated to the production of singlet oxygen, these results imply that the higher fluence rate
of the treatment light source does not produce as good of an outcome as the lower one does.

Figure 10.12b shows the spatial distributions of cumulative reacted singlet oxygen along
the radial direction perpendicular to the center of a 1-cm-long linear light source at different treatment times (i.e., different total light fluence) at a source strength of 100 mW/cm. As
seen on this logarithmically scaled figure, the radial distribution of the cumulative singlet
oxygen has two different exponential decays with the radial distance, and the changes of
slope occurs around 0.4–0.5 cm, varying with time in this example. Assuming that the
singlet oxygen threshold concentration for Photofrin is 1 mM, that is, tissue damage only
occurs when the singlet oxygen concentration exceeds this limit, Figure 10.12b shows that
the tissue damage will be a maximum of 0.9 cm at 6000 s (or 600 J/cm) while it can already
reach 0.6 cm at 2000 s (or 200 J/cm) according to this model. In contrast, the light fluence
rate distribution (the black solid line) does not have this apparent slope change, which cannot explain the sharp edge between necrotic and nonnecrotic zones for PDT.

In addition to tissue oxygenation, the spatial distribution of photosensitizer and heterogeneous optical properties are another two critical factors determining the production
of singlet oxygen and its coverage for the target volume. Figure 10.13 shows the effects
of different initial distributions of the photosensitizer as well as optical properties [77].

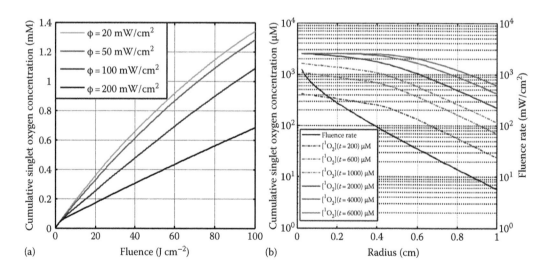

FIGURE 10.12
Temporal and spatial distribution of cumulative singlet oxygen concentration calculated using the microscopic
model. (a) The temporal distribution at different uniform fluence rates. (b) The spatial distributions at different
times of the treatment are plotted on the logarithmic scale from a 1-cm-long linear source with a source strength
of 100 mW/cm. R_c = 2.5 μm and the initial Photofrin drug concentration is 7 μM. The optical properties used for
panel (b) are as follows: μ_a = 0.5 cm⁻¹ and μ_s' = 10 cm⁻¹. The other PDT parameters are given in Table 10.2.

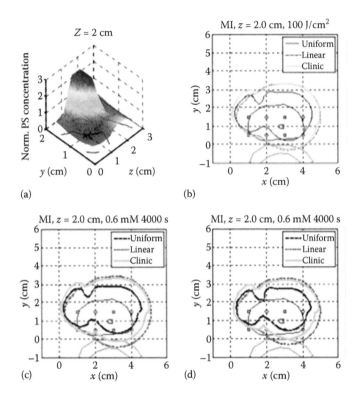

FIGURE 10.13
The simulated dose coverage for different initial distributions of the photosensitizer. (a) A representative clinical distribution of the drug; (b) the isodose distribution of PDT dose (a product of local drug concentration and fluence); (c and d) the isodose distribution of 0.6 mM singlet oxygen concentration for the light dose of 80 and 100 J/cm² at irradiance of 20 and 100 mW/cm², respectively. The three types of initial distribution of the photosensitizer: uniform throughout the target, linear along the x-axis, and the data obtained from clinical studies. (From Zhu, T.C. et al., *Proc. SPIE*, 7551: 75510E, 2010.)

A representative distribution of the photosensitizer determined clinically was shown in Figure 10.13a. Figure 10.13b is the isodose distribution of PDT dose (100 J/cm²) as a product of the local light fluence and photosensitizer concentration, which compares the different PDT dose coverage calculated using three different initial distributions of the drug concentration: uniform, linear along x-axis, and clinical results. The isodose line for the clinical drug distribution does show a relatively full coverage of the target volume; however, since PDT dose does not take into account tissue oxygenation, it will not reflect the effects of the local fluence rate on the production of singlet oxygen. Figure 10.13c and d show the isodose distribution for the reacted singlet oxygen concentration (0.6 mM) for total delivered light doses of 80 and 100 J/cm² at fluence rates of 20 and 100 mW/cm², respectively. At first, as seen in Figure 10.13d, the actual distribution of reacted singlet oxygen calculated using the clinical drug distribution does not cover the entire target, which is unlike the results in Figure 10.13b. This may imply the inadequacy of PDT dose as it does not include the effects of fluence rate on oxygen depletion. Second, the same isodose line for the clinical results in Figure 10.13c provides better coverage than that in Figure 10.13d, which means the distribution of reacted singlet oxygen at a lower fluence rate may be more uniform than that at a higher fluence rate. This can be obtained even with the delivery of less total light dose.

Comparison of the results in Figures 10.5 and 10.13 shows the progress of modeling of the PDT processes in a prostate PDT from a single component (light via fluence [rate]) in Figure 10.5 to two components (light and PS via PDT dose, defined as the light energy absorbed by the photosensitizer) in Figure 10.13b, to, ultimately, all three components (light, PS, and oxygen via reacted singlet oxygen concentration) in Figure 10.13c and d, which reflect better PDT dosimetry and better understanding of the interactions between different components during PDT.

10.6 Summary and Future Perspectives

In this chapter, we have examined the equations governing the dynamic process for the singlet oxygen generation for PDT. Among the three components, light, PS drug, and oxygen, a great deal of work has been done for the light and oxygen transport. There is limited work done in the PS drug transport partly because most PDT is operated at sufficiently long drug–light intervals (DLIs) so that the drug distribution is already in equilibrium. As long as the spatial distribution of the PS drug concentration can be quantified, the practical need for modeling the drug diffusion is limited. However, to understand the PDT process with very short DLI, one needs to explore the PS drug diffusion process more extensively.

At the current stage of development, light transport is of critical importance for determining the efficacy of PDT. The most common situation for light transport in humans can be effectively dealt with using the diffusion (P_1) approximation. The techniques to solve the light transport equation using the diffusion approximation and FEM are very mature. Solving the diffusion equation for a realistically clinical problem requires the quantification of the tissue optical properties distribution, which by itself is challenging to solve as an inverse problem. Inside patient cavities, for example, inside the mouth for head and neck cancer treatments or inside the lung cavity for lung cancer treatments, multiple scattering of light inside the open cavity will be important (the so-called integrating sphere effect). There is still work to be done to completely describe light transport under these conditions. In addition, solving the radiation transport equation (or Boltzmann equation) directly using deterministic methods remains challenging, but it is expected to explode in the next decade because of the great advance of the 64-bit PC, which solves the insufficient memory problem.

Oxygen transport and consumption during PDT remain critically important for the modeling of the singlet oxygen generation during PDT, which is ultimately responsible for the PDT efficacy. At the current state of development, there are no noninvasive methods to directly measure the tissue oxygenation distribution (diffuse optical tomography and BOLD MRI are the closest, but they are still indirect methods for measuring the tissue oxygen concentration distribution). The state-of-the-art technique is the macroscopic modeling of the oxygen consumption process. There is emerging work on the detailed microscopic modeling of the oxygen diffusion when taking into account the 3D vasculature distribution. However, the model is still very computationally challenging.

Although the focus of this chapter is entirely on the biophysical models of the dynamic process during PDT, the importance of biological mechanisms of cell death by PDT should also be emphasized. While this is not included in this chapter, it is crucial to understand the complex processes of biological systems and their responses to PDT. The cell killing mechanism is very different among different photosensitizer drugs, and these differences will change the dynamics of the important variables to model during PDT [78]. We have mentioned that depending on the DLI, the PDT killing mechanism can be predominantly vascular (by shutting down the blood vessels to the tumor) or apoptotic (by direct killing of cellular tissues) [79]. There are also complex biological pathways that can be utilized to enhance PDT efficacy, for example, by combining PDT with other modifiers of microenvironments (e.g., VEGF), by tagging PS drug with antibodies that match a particular cancer tumor to cause tumor seeking PDT, by encapsulating the PS inside nanoparticles to penetrate cell membranes [80], or by utilizing the immunological effect of PDT to enhance the body's immune response to cancer cells [81].

Acknowledgments

This work is supported by grants from the National Institutes of Health (P01 CA87971 and R01 CA 154562). We are grateful for the helpful discussions and insights from Dr. Jarod C. Finlay.

References

1. Zhu, T.C., and J.C. Finlay, The role of photodynamic therapy (PDT) physics. *Med. Phys.*, 2008. **35**(7): pp. 3127–3136.
2. Sandell, J.L., and T.C. Zhu, A review of in-vivo optical properties of human tissues and its impact on PDT. *J. Biophoton.*, 2011. **4**(11–12): pp. 773–787.
3. Star, W.M., Light dosimetry in vivo. *Phys. Med. Biol.*, 1997. **42**: pp. 763–787.
4. Zhu, T.C., C. Bonnerup, V.C. Colussi, M.L. Dowell, J.C. Finlay, L. Lilge, T.W. Slowey, and C.H. Sibata, Absolute calibration of optical power for PDT: Report of AAPM TG140. *Med. Phys.*, 2013. **40**(8): p. 081501.
5. Ishimaru, A., *Wave Propagation and Scattering in Random Media*. 1997, Oxford, UK: Oxford Univ. Press.
6. Hull, E.L., and T.H. Foster, Steady-state reflectance spectroscopy in the P_3 approximation. *J. Opt. Soc. Am. A*, 2001. **18**(3): pp. 584–599.
7. Henyey, L.G., and J.L. Greenstein, Diffuse radiation in the galaxy. *Astrophys. J.*, 1941. **93**: pp. 70–83.
8. Boas, D.A., Diffuse photon probes of structure and dynamic properties of turbid media: Theory and biomedical application, in *Physics*, PhD thesis, 1996, Philadelphia: University of Pennsylvania, p. 260.
9. Haskell, R.C., L.O. Svaasand, T.T. Tsay, T.C. Feng, M.S. McAdams, and B.J. Tromberg, Boundary conditions for the diffusion equation in radiative transfer. *J. Opt. Soc. Am. A*, 1994. **11**(10): pp. 2727–2741.
10. Jackson, J.D., *Classical Electrodynamics*, 2nd ed. 1975, New York: John Wiley & Sons, Inc.
11. Prahl, S.A., M. Keijzer, S.L. Jacquez, and A.J. Welch, A Monte Carlo model of light propagation in tissue. *Proc. SPIE*, 1989. **IS5**: pp. 102–111.
12. Finlay, J.C., and T.C. Zhu, A macro-Monte Carlo method for the simulation of diffuse light transport in tissue. *Proc. SPIE*, 2006. **6139**: p. 613913.
13. Fang, Q., and D.A. Boas, Monte Carlo simulation of photon migration in 3D turbid media accelerated by graphics processing units. *Opt. Exp.*, 2009. **17**(22): pp. 20178–20190.
14. Wang, L., S.L. Jacques, and L. Zheng, MCML-Monte Carlo modeling of light transport in multi-layered tissues. *Comput. Methods Programs Biomed.*, 1995. **47**: pp. 131–146.
15. Sandell, J.L., and T.C. Zhu, Monte Carlo simulation of light fluence calculation during pleural PDT. *Proc. SPIE*, 2013. **8568**: p. 85680U.

16. Jacques, S.L., and L. Wang, Monte Carlo modeling of light transport in tissues, in *Optical-Thermal Response of Laser-Irradiated Tissue*, A.J. Welch, and V. Gemert, Editors. 1995, New York: Plenum.

17. Zhu, T.C., A. Dimofte, S.M. Hahn, and R.A. Lustig, Light dosimetry at tissue surfaces for small circular fields. *Proc. SPIE*, 2003. **4952**: pp. 56–67.

18. Zhu, T.C., J.C. Finlay, A. Dimofte, and S.M. Hahn, Light dosimetry at tissue surfaces for oblique incident circular fields. *Proc. SPIE*, 2004. **5315**: pp. 113–124.

19. Boas, D.A., H. Liu, M.A. O'Leary, B. Chance, and A. Yodh, Photon migration within the P_3 approximation. *Proc. SPIE*, 1995. **2389**: pp. 240–247.

20. Davison, B., *Neutron Tranport Theory*. 1957, Oxford: Oxford Univ. Press.

21. Dehghani, H., B. Brooksby, K. Vishwanath, B.W. Pogue, and K.D. Paulsen, The effects of internal refractive index variation in near-infrared optical tomography: A finite element modelling approach. *Phys. Med. Biol.*, 2003. **48**: pp. 2713–2727.

22. Fishkin, J.B., S. Fantini, M.J. vandeVen, and E. Gratton, Gigahertz photon density waves in a turbid medium: Theory and experiments. *Phys. Rev. E*, 1996. **53**: pp. 2307–2319.

23. Case, K.M., and P.F. Zweifel, *Linear Transport Theory*. 1967, Reading, MA: Addison-Wesley Publishing Company.

24. Dickey, D.J., R.B. Moore, D.C. Rayner, and J. Tulip, Light dosimetry using the P_3 approximation. *Phys. Med. Biol.*, 2001. **45**: pp. 2359–2370.

25. Li, J., T.C. Zhu, and J.C. Finlay, Study of light fluence rate distribution in photodynamic therapy using finite-element method. *Proc. SPIE*, 2006. **6139**: p. 61390M.

26. Li, J., and T.C. Zhu, Determination of in-vivo light fluence distribution in a heterogeneous prostate during photodynamic therapy. *Phys. Med. Biol.*, 2008. **53**: pp. 2103–2114.

27. Pogue, B.W., M.S. Patterson, H. Jiang, and K.D. Paulsen, Initial assessment of a simple system for frequency domain diffuse optical tomography. *Phys. Med. Biol.*, 1995. **40**: pp. 1709–1729.

28. Arridge, S.R., and J.C. Hebden, Optical imaging in medicine: II Modelling and reconstruction. *Phys. Med. Biol.*, 1997. **42**: pp. 841–853.

29. Aydin, E.D., C.R.E. de Oliveira, and A.J.H. Goddard, A finite element-spherical harmonics radiation transport model for photon migration in turbid media. *J. Quant. Spectrosc. Radiat. Trans.*, 2004. **84**(3): pp. 247–260.

30. Aydin, E.D., C.R.E. de Oliveira, and A.J.H. Goddard, A comparison between transport and diffusion calculations using a finite element-spherical harmonics radiation transport method. *Med. Phys.*, 2002. **29**(9): pp. 2013–2023.

31. Gifford, K.A., J.L. Horton Jr., T.A. Wareing, G. Failla, and F. Mourtada, Comparison of a finite-element multigroup discrete-ordinances code with Monte Carlo for radiotherapy calculations. *Phys. Med. Biol.*, 2006. **51**: pp. 2253–2265.

32. Vassiliev, O.N., T.A. Wareing, J.M. McGhee, G. Failla, M.M. Salehpour, and F. Mourtada, Validation of a new grid-based Boltzmann equation solver for dose calculation in radiotherapy with photon beams. *Phys. Med. Biol.*, 2010. **55**: pp. 581–598.

33. Warsar, J.S., T.A. Wareing, J.E. Morel, J.M. McGhee, and R.B. Lahoucq, Krylov subspace integrations for the calculation of k-Eigenvalues with SN transport codes, Nuclear Mathematical and Computational Sciences: A Century in Review, A Century Anew, Gatlinburg, Tennessee, April 6–11, 2003.

34. Evans, T.M., *Denovo-A New Parallel Discrete Transport Code for Radiation Shielding Applications*. 2009, Oak Ridge, TN: Oak Ridge National Laboratory (ORNL).

35. Tyrrell, J., C. Thorn, A. Shore, S. Campbell, and A. Curow, Oxygen saturation and perfusion changes during dermatological methylaminolaevulinate photodynamic therapy. *Br. J. Dermatol*, 2011. **165**(12): pp. 1323–1331.

36. Pogue, B.W., and T. Hasan, A theoretical study of light fractionation and dose-rate effects study in photodynamic therapy. *Radiat. Res.*, 1997. **147**(5): pp. 551–559.

37. Woodhams, J.H., L. Kunz, S.G. Bown, and A.J. MacRobert, Correlation of real-time hemoglobin oxygen saturation monitoring during photodynamic therapy with microvascular effects and tissue necrosis in normal rat liver. *Br. J. Cancer*, 2004. **91**(4): pp. 788–794.

38. Busch, T.M., E.P. Wileyto, M.J. Emanuele, F.D. Piero, L. Marconato, E. Glatstein, and C.J. Koch, Photodynamic therapy creates fluence rate-dependent gradients in the intratumoral spatial distribution of oxygen. *Cancer Res.*, 2002. **62**: pp. 7273–7279.

39. Herman, M.A., D. Fromm, and D. Kessel, Tumor blood-flow changes following protoporphyrin IX-based photodynamic therapy in mice and humans. *J. Photochem. Photobiol. B*, 1999. **52**: pp. 99–104.

40. Wang, H.W., M.E. Putt, M.J. Emanuele, D.B. Shin, E. Glatstein, A.G. Yodh, and T.M. Busch, Treatment-induced changes in tumor oxygenation predict photodynamic therapy outcome. *Cancer Res.*, 2004. **64**: pp. 7553–7561.

41. Whiteley, J.P., D.J. Gavaghan, and C.E. Hahn, Some factors affecting oxygen uptake by red blood cells in the pulmonary capillaries. *Math. Biosci.*, 2001. **169**(2): pp. 153–172.

42. Clark Jr., A., W.J. Federspiel, P.A.A. Clark, and G.R. Cohelet, Oxygen delivery from red cells. *Biophys. J.*, 1985. **47**: pp. 171–181.

43. Whiteley, J.P., D.J. Gavaghan, and C.E.W. Hahn, Mathematical modeling of oxygen transport to tissue. *J. Math. Biol.*, 2002. **44**: pp. 503–522.

44. Tsoukias, N.M., D. Goldman, A. Vadapalli, R.N. Pittman, and A.S. Popel, A computational model of oxygen delivery by hemoglobin-based oxygen carriers in three-dimensional micro-vascular networks. *J. Theor. Biol.*, 2007. **248**(4): pp. 657–674.

45. Zheng, L., A.S. Golub, and R.N. Pittman, Determination of pO2 and its heterogeneity in single capillaries. *Am. J. Physiol.*, 1996. **271**(1): pp. H365–H372.

46. Purves, W.K., D. Sadava, G.H. Orians, and H.C. Heller, *Life: The Science of Biology*, 7th ed. 2004, Sunderland, MA: Sinauer Associates, p. 953.

47. Martin, L., *All You Really Need to Know to Interpret Arterial Blood Gases*, 2nd ed. 1999, Philadelphia, PA: Lippincott Williams & Wilkins.

48. Zhu, T.C., J.C. Finlay, X. Zhou, and J. Li, Macroscopic modeling of the singlet oxygen production during PDT. *Proc. SPIE*, 2007. **6427**: pp. 1–12.

49. Liu, B., M.M. Kim, and T.C. Zhu, A theoretical comparison of macroscopic and microscopic modeling of singlet oxygen during Photfrin and HPPH-mediated PDT. *Proc. SPIE*, 2013. **8568**: p. 856805.

50. Huxley, V.H., and H. Kutchai, Effect of diffusion boundary layers on the initial uptake of O_2 by red cells. Theory versus experiment. *Microvasc. Res.*, 1983. **26**: pp. 89–107.

51. Krogh, A., The number and distribution of capillaries in muscle with the calculation of the oxygen pressure necessary for supplying the tissue. *J. Physiol. (Lond.)*, 1919. **52**: pp. 409–515.

52. Vadapalli, A., D. Goldman, and A.S. Popel, Calculations of oxygen transport by red blood cells and hemoglobin solutions in capillaries. *Artif. Cells Blood Substit. Immobil. Biotechnol.*, 2002. **30**(3): pp. 157–188.

53. Egginton, S., and E. Gaffney, Tissue capillary supply—It's quality not quantity that counts. *Exp. Physiol.*, 2010. **95**(10): pp. 971–979.

54. Middleman, S., *Transport Phenomena in the Cardiovascular System*. 1972, New York: John Wiley.

55. Secomb, T.W., R. Hsu, E.Y.H. Park, and M.W. Dewhirst, Green's function methods for analysis of oxygen delivery to tissue by microvascular networks. *Ann. Biomed. Eng.*, 2004. **32**: pp. 1519–1529.

56. Beard, D.A., and J.B. Bassingthwaighte, Modeling advection and diffusion of oxygen in complex vascular networks, *Ann. Biomed. Eng.*, 2001. **29**: pp. 298–310.

57. Beard, D.A., K.A. Schenkman, and E.O. Feigl, Myocardial oxygenation in isolated hearts predicted by an anatomically realistic micovascular transport model. *Am. J. Physiol. Heart. Circ. Physiol.*, 2003. **285**: pp. 1826–1836.

58. Zhou, X., B.W. Pogue, B. Chen, and T. Hasan, Analysis of effective molecular diffusion rates for Verteporfin in subcutaneous versus orthotopic duning prostate tumors. *Photochem. Photobiol.*, 2004. **79**: pp. 323–331.

59. Star, W.M., M.C.G. Aalders, A. Sac, and H.J.C.M. Sterenborg, Quantitative model calculation of the time-dependent protoporphyrin IX concentration in normal human epidermis after delivery of ALA by passive topical application or iontophoresis. *Photochem. Photobiol.*, 2002. **75**: pp. 424–432.

60. Weishaupt, K.R., C.J. Gomer, and T.J. Dougherty, Identification of singlet oxygen as the cyto-toxic agent in photo-activation of a murine tumor. *Cancer Res.*, 1976. **36**: pp. 2326–2392.

61. Wang, K.K., S. Mitra, and T.H. Foster, A comprehensive mathematical model of microscopic dose deposition in photodynamic therapy. *Med. Phys.*, 2007. **34**(1): pp. 282–293.

62. Hudson, J.A., and D.B. Cater, An analysis of factors affecting tissue oxygen tension. *Proc. R. Soc. Lond. B*, 1964. **161**(983): pp. 247–274.

63. Yu, G., T. Durduran, C. Zhou, H.W. Wang, M.E. Putt, M. Saunders, C.M. Sehgal, E. Glatstein, A.G. Yodh, and T.M. Busch, Noninvasive monitoring of murine tumor blood flow during and after photodynamic therapy provides early assessment of therapeutic efficacy. *Clin. Cancer Res.*, 2005. **11**: pp. 3543–3552.

64. Wang, K.K., J.C. Finlay, T.M. Busch, S.M. Hahn, and T.C. Zhu, Explicit dosimetry for photodynamic therapy: Macroscopic singlet oxygen modeling. *J. Biophoton.*, 2010. **3**(5–6): pp. 304–318.

65. Hu, X.H., Y. Feng, J.Q. Lu, R.R. Allison, R.E. Cuenca, G.H. Downie, and C.H. Sibata, Modeling of a type II photofrin-mediated photodynamic therapy process in a heterogeneous tissue phantom. *Photochem. Photobiol.*, 2005. **81**(6): pp. 1460–1468.

66. Niedre, M.J., M.S. Patterson, and B.C. Wilson, Direct near-infrared luminescence detection of singlet oxygen generated by photodynamic therapy in cells *in vitro* and tissues *in vivo*. *Photochem. Photobiol.*, 2002. **75**(4): pp. 382–391.

67. McMillan, D.D., D. Chen, M.M. Kim, X. Liang, and T.C. Zhu, Parameter determination for singlet oxygen modeling of BPD-mediated PDT. *Proc. SPIE*, 2013. **8568**: p. 856810.

68. Georgakoudi, I., M.G. Nichols, and T.H. Foster, The mechanism of Photofrin photobleaching and its consequences for photodynamic dosimetry. *Photochem. Photobiol.*, 1997. **65**: pp. 135–144.

69. Dysart, J.S., G. Singh, and M.S. Patterson, Calculation of singlet oxygen dose from photosensitizer fluorescence and photobleaching during mTHPC photodynamic therapy of MLL cells. *Photochem. Photobiol.*, 2005. **81**: pp. 196–205.

70. Finlay, J.C., S. Mitra, M.S. Patterson, and T.H. Foster, Photobleaching kinetics of Photofrin *in vivo* and in multicell tumour spheroids indicate two simultaneous bleaching mechanisms. *Phys. Med. Biol.*, 2004. **49**: pp. 4837–4860.

71. Mitra, S., and T.H. Foster, Photophysical parameters, photosensitizer retention and tissue optical properties completely account for the higher photodynamic efficacy of meso-tetra-hydroxyphenyl-chlorin vs photophrin. *Photochem. Photobiol.*, 2005. **81**(4): pp. 849–859.

72. Sterenborg, H.J.C.M. and M.J.C. van Gemert, Photodynamic therapy with pulsed light sources: A theoretical analysis. *Phys. Med. Biol.*, 1996. **41**: p. 835–849.

73. Gorman, A.A. and M.A. Rodgers, Life time and reactivity of singlet oxygen in an acqeous micellar system: A pulsed nigrogen laser study. *Chem. Phys. Lett.*, 1978. **55**: p. 52–4.

74. Redmond, R.W., K. Heihoff, S.E. Braslavski, and T.G. Truscott, Thermal lensing and phosphorescence studies of the quantum yield and life time of singlet molecular oxygen sensitized by hematoporphyrin and related porphyrins in deuterated and non-deuterated ethanols. *Photochem. Photobiol.*, 1987. **45**: p. 209–13.

75. Foster, T.H., R.S. Murant, R.G. Bryant, R.S. Knox, S.L. Gribson, and R. Hilf, Oxygen consumption and diffusion effects in photodynamic therapy. *Radiat. Res.*, 1991. **126**: p. 296–303.

76. Lovell, J.F., T.W. Liu, J. Chen, and G. Zheng, Activatable photosensitizers for imaging and therapy. *Chem. Rev.*, 2010. **110**: pp. 2839–2857.

77. Zhu, T.C., M.D. Altschuler, Y. Hu, K. Wang, J.C. Finlay, A. Dimofte, K. Cengel, and S.M. Hahn, A heterogeneous optimization algorithm for reacted singlet oxygen for interstitial PDT. *Proc. SPIE*, 2010. **7551**: p. 75510E.

78. Kessel, D., M. Castelli, and J. Reiners Jr., On the mechanism of PDT-induced mitochondrial photodamage. *Proc. SPIE*, 2001. **4248**: pp. 157–162.

79. Chen, B., B.W. Pogue, J.M. Luna, R.L. Hardman, P.J. Hoopes, and T. Hasan, Tumor vascular permeabilization by vascular-targeting photosensitization: Effects, mechanism, and therapeutic implications. *Clin. Cancer Res.*, 2006. **12**(3): pp. 917–923.

80. Spring, B., Z. Mai, P. Rai, S. Chang, and T. Hasan, Theranostic nanocells for simultaneous imaging and photodynamic therapy of pancreatic cancer. *Proc. SPIE*, 2010. **7551**: pp. 755104-1–755104-11.

81. Wilson, B.C., and M.S. Patterson, The physics, biophysics, and technology of photodynamic therapy. *Phys. Med. Biol.*, 2008. **53**: pp. R61–R109.

11

Computational Cell Phenotyping in the Lab, Plant, and Clinic

Rahul Rekhi, David T. Ryan, Becky Zaunbrecher,
Chenyue W. Hu, and Amina A. Qutub

CONTENTS

ABSTRACT   Advances in computational cell phenotyping are enabling scientists to characterize and transform biological systems in the lab, industrial plant, and clinical setting
with unprecedented quantitative precision. Coupled to broad advances in computational
bioengineering, the rise of image analysis and development of new *big data* technologies are
pushing the bounds of biological understanding by allowing for predictive assessments of

unique cellular phenotypes in the larger context of physiological or pathological stimuli, multiple cell types, tissues, and organs. The result is a transformation in how biological research is conducted and interpreted in both basic and translational settings. In this chapter, we explore the ways computational cell phenotyping is being employed in three domains: the research laboratory (the lab), the pharmaceutical industry (the plant), and the health care industry (the clinic). Specific examples of phenotyping techniques and usage in each setting are provided. We highlight both the problems these technologies can solve and the new challenges they introduce.

11.1 Cell Phenotyping: A Brief Definition

Computational cell phenotyping, broadly defined, involves the use of computation to parse, measure, and classify cells. The basis for this phenotyping can be nonspatial (e.g., gene or protein arrays) or image based. While genomics- and proteomics-based methods have established themselves as universal analysis tools in the biomedical research field (Cox and Mann 2007; Ludwig and Weinstein 2005; Rosenson 2010; Tyers and Mann 2003), the ability of image-based analyses to provide spatiotemporal details on top of quantitative expression profiles makes them increasingly attractive options for laboratory, industrial, and clinical applications alike (Deckers et al. 2009; Dehmelt and Bastiaens 2010; Wang et al. 2008). As a result, the scope of this chapter is focused on image-based cell phenotyping. In general, the process of image-based computational cell phenotyping can be broken into five main steps: (1) experimental processing, (2) imaging, (3) segmentation/object recognition, (4) automated measurements of key features, and (5) classification of cell phenotypes (Figure 11.1).

11.1.1 Experimental Processing and Imaging

Traditionally, experiments looking to gather information about phenotypic cell behaviors are designed similarly to those used for genomic and proteomic studies. In both cases, investigators monitor responses to specific cellular stimuli, such as drug compounds, growth factors, and altered microenvironments. The most significant difference between image-based and nonspatial studies is that the latter typically use cell lysates, components, or fragments (e.g., in toxicity studies), while phenotyping studies examine whole cells and intact tissue or tissue slices (Clemons 2004; Karr et al. 2012; Sozzani and Benfey 2011). Regardless of scale (two- or three-dimensional) and type (in vitro or in vivo), these cellular assays are inherently more difficult to conduct than nonspatial assays. However, the additional spatiotemporal information offered by image-based studies compels their use in many research applications (Bickle 2010; McCann 2010).

While nonspatial assays leverage such tools as flow cytometry, western blotting, and protein arrays, cellular phenotyping relies heavily on microscopy. Specifically, component labels for both fixed and live cells allow for cellular features to be visualized with fluorescent microscopy (Chung et al. 2008; Ohya et al. 2005). Among the methods used for fixed cells are immunohistochemistry and immunocytochemistry, which use antibody markers to target specific proteins and peptides of interest in cells, sections of biological tissue, and

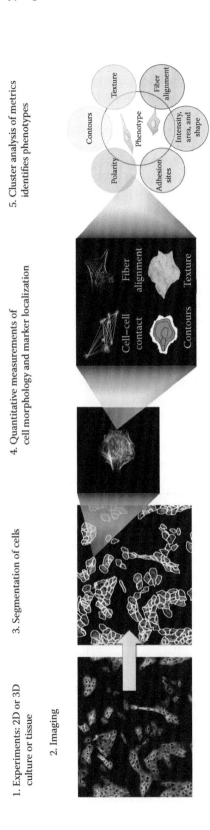

FIGURE 11.1
Overview of steps for computational cell phenotyping.

isolated cell samples. Live cells, on the other hand, can have similar features highlighted and tracked in real time via specialized transfection and labeling techniques. While these live cell methods are subject to drawbacks like photobleaching and potential interference with normal cellular function, their unique ability to provide dynamic cellular information often outweighs these limitations (Chen et al. 2002; Wang et al. 2008).

Currently, standard fluorescent microscope systems remain the most accessible for cellular imaging in phenotypic analyses. However, finer resolution can be captured with confocal units and emerging technologies like superresolution imaging. Furthermore, new nucleic acid–based molecular imaging probes address the problems associated with the limited color real estate of standard three-color or five-color fluorescence systems (Schweller et al. 2012), and the limitations of antibody-based methods are being overcome by mass spectroscopy–based imaging. These two imaging technologies enable dozens if not hundreds of molecules to be studied in the same specimen. Additionally, automated systems that incorporate robotic plate handling, microscope control, and microenvironmental chambers allow for culture and assay automation, eliminating variable handling techniques that contribute to error (Mioulane et al. 2012). Finally, high-throughput units that integrate image analysis platforms provide users with turnkey solutions to streamline the entire experimental process.

11.1.2 Segmentation and Automated Feature Measurements

As cellular phenotyping describes single-cell behavior and interactions, effective analysis methods must include a segmentation step for isolating individual cells in images and videos. Within the field of image segmentation, there exist a number of techniques directly designed for microscopy images. For instance, the most basic tools are built into graphical user interfaces in image-friendly software like Adobe Photoshop, MATLAB®, and ImageJ that allow users to manually outline and segment cells of interest (Brugger et al. 2012; Huth et al. 2011). While this approach functions adequately for a small set of cells and images, its time-consuming and error-prone nature preclude it from being an attractive solution for large image sets.

In contrast, more computationally advanced methods, such as active contours, level sets, the watershed algorithm, and even combination methods like water balloons, are more suitable for image sets containing larger numbers of cells (Tan et al. 2013). These methods also better accommodate automated analyses of variable image sets in large databases (Ryan et al. 2013). After segmentation, the human eye can serve as a useful guide for developing computational image processing methods, as it can quickly focus on unique identifying objects and characteristic features of individual cells—as well as patterns within and across images. Statistically relevant comparisons of cells based on measurements corresponding to these user-observed properties can help distinguish distinct cell behaviors. Of particular significance in these applications is the ability to automatically capture complex patterns by incorporating suites of metrics optimized for cell types of interest, each tailored to consider local microenvironments and cellular communication.

11.1.3 Classification of Cell Phenotypes

After obtaining quantitative information on cell properties, structure, and interactions from image analyses (i.e., a suite of metrics), cells can be placed into groups, or clusters, with other cells that share similar characteristics. These clusters represent specific cellular phenotypes (Lange et al. 2004). Accurate cluster determination can, for example, allow for the identification of similarities in how the morphological and mechanical properties of cells relate to their intracellular activities. Two of the most common clustering methods for such analyses are hierarchical and *k*-means clustering (Lee and Yang 2009). The agglomerative hierarchical clustering starts by setting each cell as one single cluster and then merges pairs of cells and clusters iteratively based on similarity calculations until a specified distance between clusters is reached or there is a sufficiently small number of clusters (Kandemir-Cavas and Nasibov 2009; Murtagh et al. 2011). Different distance metrics (e.g., Euclidean distance) and linkage criteria (e.g., average linkage) are specified to determine how the distance between pairs of cellular metrics should be calculated and how two clusters should be chosen to merge in each step (Tibshirani et al. 2000). Hierarchical clustering generates a dendrogram or tree diagram, where nodes of lower hierarchy near the roots denote closer distance and higher similarity between two branches, and vice versa. The tree can be cut at specified levels to yield different numbers of branches, in which each branch represents a unique cluster.

An alternative method, known as *k*-means clustering, works by iteratively calculating cluster centroids and assigning cells to their closest centroid until a local minimum of within-cluster sum of squares (WCSS) is reached (Wilkin and Huang 2007). With *k*-means, the user must input an estimate for the number of clusters and run the algorithm multiple times with different initiations in order to converge on the global minimum as defined by WCSS. Advanced methods such as gap statistic and cluster stability are usually applied in combination with hierarchical and *k*-means clustering to statistically determine the optimal number of clusters in the data. The completion of clustering yields a set of distinct cell states (or phenotypes) that can be studied further and examined at new levels.

11.2 Computational Cell Phenotyping in the Laboratory

From a survey of historical and recent advances, the tools and methods that computational cell phenotyping provides to biomedical researchers can be subdivided into three broad classifications: image processing, data analysis, and predictive simulation. In this section, we explore each of these thematic elements in more detail, with specific attention paid to the new research approaches developed to catalyze laboratory discovery. As these avenues are the focus of significant laboratory efforts with new explorations in constant development, we highlight recent studies and survey available tools that show the utility of cell phenotyping and offer insight into where the field is headed.

11.2.1 Image Processing

Historically, biological image data have been primarily qualitative in nature, and the limited quantitative measurements obtained were done so manually, or on a small scale. In studies of cellular behavior, this resulted in accordingly qualitative descriptions of cell processes like migration, blebbing, proliferation, or quiescence. Even where quantitative measurements are made (e.g., microns migrated), manual measurements have been unable to keep pace with the rapid expansion in available data that has accompanied the growth of high-throughput microscopy of in vitro and in situ systems. Additionally, qualitative descriptions of cell behaviors lack efficiency and reproducibility in capturing the complexity of biology at the cellular or subcellular level. As a solution, advances in image analysis tools enable rapid, automated, reproducible, high-throughput quantification of a diverse array of biological assays.

Accordingly, image analysis is poised to make a significant impact on understanding cell biology and classifying cells. It has already been used in the lab to classify cells by morphology in key physiological and pathological situations, including cardiovascular disease, cancer, angiogenesis, and stem cell differentiation (Lee et al. 2006; Lloyd et al. 2010; Petushi et al. 2006; Rayment and Williams 2010; Ricci-Vitiani et al. 2010; Ryan et al. 2013; Zanella et al. 2010). As an example, a recent study described an automated image analysis approach for quantifying phenotypes of cardiac myocytes from immunofluorescence images, providing measures of myocyte size, elongation, circularity, sarcomeric organization, and cell–cell contact to better characterize cardiac hypertrophy (Bass et al. 2011). With these metrics, the authors demonstrated an ability to extract measures of key cellular properties from *high-content* imaging of cardiac myocyte hypertrophy, and to tie the resultant information to five key subcellular pathways implicated in cardiac hypertrophy, including those of the signaling molecules IGF-1 (insulin-like growth factor 1) and TNFα (tumor necrosis factor alpha) (Bass et al. 2011). This example study employed an open-source platform, CellProfiler, which, like other image analysis platforms, lends itself to a wide range of laboratory applications (Tables 11.1 and 11.2). In another physiological example, an analogous technique was used to screen neuronal phenotypes via semiautomated image processing software (Narro et al. 2007). The researchers' *NeuronMetrics* approach allowed for the skeletonization of a neuron cell culture image, thereby permitting linear measurements of total neurite length, branch number, primary neurite number, territory (the surface area bounding the neuronal cell body), and a polarity index (defined as the fraction of total length constituted by the longest primary neurite). The authors built their method around modules on the open-source ImageJ tool, which initially required an *extensive* degree of manual editing of the skeletons; however, results demonstrated the algorithm's high fidelity and analysis speed with no statistically significant decrease in precision over a fully manual analysis (Narro et al. 2007). Additionally, it is notable that these two research examples share clinical significance. Alongside better characterizing of myocyte and neuronal biology through quantitative assessments of biochemical pathways that alter cell morphology in vitro, this type of research can provide a means to accelerate cardiovascular and neurological drug discovery by uncovering the link between intracellular signaling and cell phenotypes.

These computational cell phenotyping methods can provide the advantage of scale—allowing researchers to analyze a previously intractable volume of data—and can also uncover subtle, complex morphological phenotypes that have long been inaccessible to standard tools. A study, for instance, developed a technique to automatically compute image-based cytological profiles, which allows cells to be classified on the basis of a desired phenotypic trait (Jones et al. 2009). These profiles consisted of 600 distinct measurements of cell morphology (including texture, intensity, and cell area) to *score* cell populations for specific phenotypes. The authors leverage machine learning algorithms in tandem with manual error correction to piece together the rules tying cell morphology to perturbations in specific biological pathways. For example, the study demonstrated that cells exhibiting blebbing of the actin cytoskeleton also generally possess 4N (tetraploid) DNA content, suggesting a link with peripheral actin structures and cell cycle (Jones et al. 2009). Though these specific rules are assay specific, the automated method itself is applicable between protocols, experiments, and instrumentation.

TABLE 11.1

Image Analysis Software Used in the Lab, Industrial Setting, and Clinic

Tools	Main Features	Benefits	Limitations
Research Tools			
ImageJ	• Supports image stacks • Standard image processing • Geometric transformations • Image enhancement • Multithreaded	• Flexible • Open source • Regularly updated • Platform independent • Speed	• No image modification • Limited 3D visualization • No batch processing
CellProfiler	• Semiautomatic, modular analysis algorithms • Specialized image processing modules • Distributed processing capability	• Open source • Batch processing • Ease of use • Tailored for phenotypic measurements	• Software stability • Heavily dependent on fluorescence microscopy
MATLAB	• Complete coding environment • Script-based functionality • Wide array of built-in toolboxes • Platform independent	• Flexible • Relatively inexpensive • Wide applicability	• Rudimentary image processing toolbox • Lack of native GUI (command line) • No 3D reconstruction
Bitplane Imaris	• 3D and 4D volume rendering • Surface-based segmentation algorithms • Animation/movie creation	• Multithreaded processing and graphics • User-friendly operation • Wide functionality	• Expensive (feature modules sold separately) • Proprietary software • Processor intensive
Neurolucida	• High-fidelity neuronal reconstruction • Serial reconstruction and 3D visualization • Quantitative image analysis • Advanced artifact correction	• Fully automated image tracing • High anatomical accuracy • Wide hardware support and device integration	• Designed specifically for brain applications • Proprietary software • Limited hardware
Research/Industrial/Clinical Tools			
Definiens	• Segmentation/network-based image analysis • Biomarker expression profiling • Built-in machine learning	• Scale flexible (cell through tissue) • Batch processing • Ease of use	• Proprietary • Relatively expensive • Limited set of metrics • Primarily 2D processing
Amira	• 3D data visualization, rendering, and reconstruction • Automatic image segmentation and analysis • Advanced tracing, skeletonization, and analysis toolboxes	• Flexible and friendly user interface • Diverse array of applications • Modular • Virtual-reality display compatible	• Expensive • Proprietary • Relative complexity of software
MetaMorph	• Real-time image processing • Automated acquisition and device control • Multidimensional acquisition • 4D viewing • Standard and advanced image processing/analysis	• Direct device acquisition • Robust array of analysis modules • Macro-friendly • Interfaces with most devices	• Proprietary • Expensive • Steep learning curve

TABLE 11.2

Features of Image Analysis Software for Research Scientists

Feature	ImageJ	CellProfiler	MetaMorph	Definiens	MATLAB	Neurolucida
Price	Free	Free	$$	$$$$	$	$$
Flexible	+	+	+		+	
Optimized for	(Customizable)	*C. elegans* studies	Clinical imaging	Histology	(Customizable)	Neurons
3D, deconvolution algorithms	⊙		⊙			⊙
Speedy		→	→	→	→	
Batch jobs		✓	✓	✓	✓	✓
Friendly user interface	★	★		★		
Segmentation accuracy			↑	↑	↑	↑
Good for advanced programmers			◆		◆	
Good for phase images	✪		✪	✪	✪	✪
Good for fluorescence images	❖	❖	❖	❖	❖	❖

A summary of image analysis tools, including those used in the described example studies, can be found in Tables 11.1 and 11.2. By allowing for the extraction of morphological, spatial, and modular data from existing microscopy, advances in image processing techniques and a growing set of open-source tools open the door for quantitative analyses of cell phenotypes to become part of researchers' standard experimental procedures.

11.2.2 Data Analysis

The preponderance of novel data sets generated through image processing advances necessitates the development of new methods by which to analyze them—to extract from the terabytes of high-dimensional data meaningful biological insights. Fortunately, there also exist a growing number of tools, methods, and techniques within the computational cell phenotyping field to interpret large data sets for meaningful descriptions of cellular behavior.

Perhaps the most prominent example of techniques applied to cell phenotyping is the use of statistical association methods. Broadly, these methods encompass machine learning algorithms, means assessment methods, and network analyses to comb through large data sets to uncover patterns that link specific classes, or clusters, of measurements to cell phenotypes. For instance, a study classified morphological phenotypes of endothelial cells undergoing angiogenic tube formation, through cluster analysis (Parsa et al. 2011). This enabled the researchers to study dynamics of multicellular organization and track contributions of behaviors like cell spreading, cell aggregation, cell elongation, and vascular plexus stabilization and reorganization (Figure 11.2). Similarly, ongoing work in our lab utilizes a diverse collection of image processing metrics—circularity, actin polarity, and so on—on fluorescence imaging of endothelial cells to quantitatively define their cytoskeletal features (Qutub et al. 2013; Ryan et al. 2013). These numerical descriptors are then

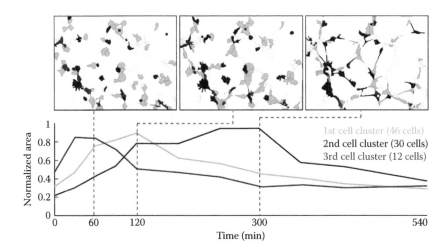

FIGURE 11.2
Endothelial cell community organization is studied by identifying and tracking cells of similar surface area in time. Cell area is represented by three clusters shown in purple, light blue, and dark blue. Cells that were not clustered are shown in white. (From Parsa, H. et al., *Proceedings of the National Academy of Sciences of the United States of America* 108 (12): 5133–5138, 2011.)

analyzed through cluster analysis to identify whether specific patterns in cellular morphology emerge with respect to different exogenous chemical signals or growth factors that play a role in capillary regeneration.

Researchers, like those cited, employ a variety of algorithms for the cluster analysis, including two popular methods, *k*-means and hierarchical clustering. Methods for reducing the dimensional space of image analysis data, like principal component analysis, are also used to identify distinct categories of cells and determine where the greatest variance in the data lies. Leveraging these methods has been shown to uncover biological insights. For example, another recent study demonstrated that tumor stem cells mirror genotypes and phenotypes of primary tumors better than serum-derived cell lines (Lee et al. 2006). An example of hierarchical cluster analysis and principal component analysis applied to classify brain cancer cells is shown in Figure 11.3. While this classification was based on gene expression profiling, morphological phenotypes of the corresponding tumors were also observed by immunohistochemistry. Open-source cluster analysis software packages such as Cluster 3.0 and R, and dendrogram-rendering programs like JavaTree and MATLAB, provide researchers with the means to perform high-throughput cluster analysis and visualization of large data sets, like those performed in these example studies. Integrating additional machine learning algorithms into the cluster analysis can accelerate and optimize large-scale analysis. By tying clusters in fundamental data to cellular- and tissue-level observed patterns of phenotypes, these approaches can help serve as the basis for new theories regarding stem cells, carcinogenesis, angiogenesis, and a variety of other biological systems.

11.2.3 Predictive Simulation

Ultimately, the real power of cell phenotyping techniques lies in their ability to uncover biological insights that were previously unattainable. Image processing methods permit researchers to produce large volumes of data for phenotypic analysis. When these

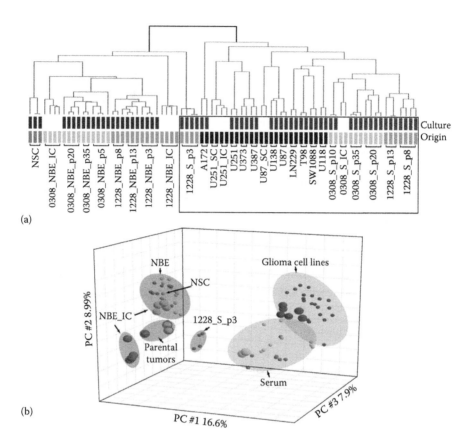

FIGURE 11.3
Unsupervised hierarchical cluster analysis (a) and principal component analysis (b) of 79 in vitro and in vivo xenograph glioma samples show distinct clusters of cell lines (boxed area) versus primary glioblastoma and neural stem cells cultured under neural stem cell conditions (NBE/NSCs), as determined by gene expression. (From Lee, J. et al., *Cancer Cell* 9 (5): 391–403, 2006.)

high-throughput methods are coupled with appropriate statistical analyses and modeling techniques, new hypotheses of biological systems can be both generated and tested.

For instance, building on earlier computational approaches, researchers coupled image processing, confocal microscopy, and mathematical modeling techniques to reconstruct a theory of murine liver regeneration (Hoehme et al. 2010). The power in this approach lies in applying image processing filters—in this case, the technique of adaptive histogram equalization, or the redistribution of image lightness values—to investigate the complex morphological properties of hepatocytes. Likewise, an *assembly-line* image processing approach was adopted, with successive filters applied to images in a batch-job chain, allowing for high-throughput analysis. The team paired this with mathematical modeling, using the image data as inputs in a predictive simulation (Hoehme et al. 2010). The benefits of this coupled imaging–modeling approach included the prediction of a novel biological mechanism, hepatocyte-sinusoid alignment, which was verified in vitro. Moreover, the model outputs served as inputs into image generation software, which allowed for three-dimensional reconstruction of liver lobules in silico. This example highlights how computational techniques can be used in tandem with image analysis to optimally characterize mammalian cells, leading to results that allow scientists to uncover mechanisms on a wide range of spatiotemporal scales. Methods like these for *in silico* hypothesis generation and testing have the potential to catalyze discovery at the bench.

11.2.4 Current Limitations

Despite tremendous progress in computational cell phenotyping, significant obstacles remain. In applications of cell phenotyping to the development of computational models, many in silico models still outpace the resolution of the biological assays they are meant to simulate: some model results cannot be validated by available in vitro and in vivo experimental platforms. Multiscale computational models can encompass predictions that range from the microscale of the cell to the macroscale of human physiology. The sheer range of such a computational experiment is currently impossible to reconstruct, verify, or test at the laboratory bench on all biological levels. Furthermore, despite dramatic gains in the resolving power of microscopy, standard, high-throughput microscopy techniques may still lack the level of subcellular resolution required to characterize links between cellular morphological phenotypes. Currently, most imaging and image processing capabilities allow for investigation of spatial and morphological characteristics at the macromolecular or cellular levels. For instance, a 2003 study examined the localization of focal adhesions around the periphery of the endothelial cell as a phenotypic indicator of the HIF1α (hypoxia-inducible factor 1 alpha) pathway (Yoshigi et al. 2003). Taking this line of research a level further and examining, say, the localization of specific tubulin molecules and relating these to the cell phenotype would require a dramatic increase in image resolution. Similarly, examining specific spatial distributions of key proteins or pathways would necessitate a greater degree of subcellular resolution—facilitated in part by the emergence of ultrahigh-resolution imaging methods. These newer methods, like superresolution imaging, while currently slow, expensive, and complex, can in the future be harnessed to perform the automated, rapid analysis required to phenotype hundreds or thousands of cells at the level of single molecule resolution.

Lastly, thus far, cell phenotyping efforts have centered on in vitro systems, which provide a manageable magnitude of complexity while allowing for experimental validation at the bench. However, the true value of computational cell phenotyping techniques lies in their power to generate insights toward in vivo constructs. Consequently, adapting existing in vitro cell phenotyping techniques for in situ and in vivo study is a prerequisite for continued advancements. Doing so will require the adoption of computational techniques that account for the complexity observed in *in vivo* systems, as well as novel imaging paradigms that can achieve similar resolutions in these constructs.

None of these obstacles is insurmountable. Advances in imaging and image processing that transcend these current limitations can unlock a wellspring of biological understanding, paving the way to novel hypotheses, targeted therapies, and new drugs.

11.2.5 Case Study

In a translational application, Yuan et al. (2012) described the large-scale analysis of biomarkers in breast cancer cells from 564 patients. The authors developed a systematic approach that integrated supervised learning with image analysis of histological samples. Training their image processing approach on a portion of the data set, they found that the distribution of three cell types (lymphocytes, cancer cells, and stroma) was a feature of tumor tissue that correlated to genetic markers and to breast cancer patients' survival duration. Specifically, by identifying lymphocytes, cancer cells, and stroma by their shape and size, and then assessing each cell type's distribution in the histopathological images, they came up with an automated way to grade biopsy samples based on predicted patient outcome. Beyond their utility to identify known biomarkers, techniques such as these can uncover previously unknown pathways or cell features in tumorigenesis, paving the way for more robust prognostic measures in the clinic.

11.3 Computational Cell Phenotyping in Industry

Biological insights gained from cell phenotyping laboratory research offer opportunities for the creation of targeted therapies and drugs. In order for related discoveries to be translated from the laboratory to the clinic, however, they must first pass through and be scaled up in the biopharmaceutical industry. Despite economic struggles in the United States from 2007 to 2013, the American pharmaceutical industry continues to be a prevalent force in industry, with its top four companies (Pfizer, Johnson & Johnson, Novartis, and Bayer) pulling in more than $240 billion combined in 2011 (Agrawal 2012). Even with these lofty revenues, a closer look at recent trends in the biopharmaceutical industry demonstrates that it still misses out on significant sources of profit. For instance, a large portion of this unrealized revenue can be attributed to the high attrition rates of newly developed drugs (Bickle 2010; Contag 2002; Möller and Slack 2010; Shillingford and Vose 2001). Surprisingly, it has been reported that only 0.4% of drugs entering preclinical development and, of those, only 4% reaching clinical development are ever approved, manufactured, and distributed to patients (Shillingford and Vose 2001). This aggregate performance yields a failure rate of at least 90% for drugs in late clinical phases of development (Contag 2002). Not only does this cause companies to miss out on significant sources of income, it also contributes to their current expenditures. Spending on new drug development can easily exceed $500 million (Shillingford and Vose 2001), and with estimated internal rates of return below 10% (David et al. 2009), large portions of these investments can be lost on drugs that fail to reach the market.

Many companies are trying to combat these alarming margins by adjusting the way they conduct drug research and development (R&D). For example, biopharmaceutical companies have focused more on creating high-throughput screens to allow for rapid, abundant accumulation of information about cellular response to aid therapeutic compound evaluation and drug target identification. The goal of these types of tests is to identify issues with drug safety and efficacy at earlier time points and, hence, free up resources and costs invested in later stages of development (Contag 2002). However, even with the advent of these technologies, the number of new, successful drugs and targets coming out of the discovery pipeline has stagnated (David et al. 2009; Möller and Slack 2010).

As a result, the need has become apparent to gather not only high-level data about both target validity and compound safety and efficacy but also detailed information about human cell behavior in their native, complex environments (Möller and Slack 2010). With an understanding of physiologically relevant cellular actions, more conclusive decisions can be made about compound identification and selection in the drug discovery process. This can in turn help eliminate ineffective or limited agents earlier in the pipeline and save biopharmaceutical companies substantial economic resources (Shillingford and Vose 2001).

Because of the inherent complexity of cells, obtaining quantitative descriptors of specific features can lead to a vast array of complex data without an appropriate way of representing the information for easy interpretation. Biopharmaceutical companies use methods like those employed in research lab settings to simplify these analyses; that is, they group/cluster cells on the basis of the information obtained from high-throughput screens (Möller and Slack 2010). Since these groups are built from data on defined, observable characteristics of cells, they can, by definition, be labeled as specific cellular phenotypes. Understanding phenotypic transitions and fates helps companies gain a more thorough understanding of complex cellular behavior that is required for effective R&D. Additionally, this knowledge aids in making succinct, definitive conclusions about the therapeutic potential of a compound or target.

11.3.1 Cellular Phenotyping in Industrial High Content Analysis

The traditional drug discovery process begins with a primary screen focused on identifying targets and determining mechanisms of action. Advances in automated microscopy and data storage and analysis methods have allowed this first step to be conducted rapidly and in bulk. For instance, high-throughput screening (HTS) employs carefully designed assays to detect compounds from large libraries that bind to, inhibit, or enhance designated targets as desired. After these *hits* are discovered, subsequent assays investigate them further, exploring their effects on normal biological functions and conditions in an attempt to confirm their efficacy (Lang et al. 2006). Typically, secondary screening is conducted using cell-based assays in order to demonstrate physiological relevance. After confirming the functionality of hits, secondary screening, or an ensuing process, concludes the in vitro portion of drug discovery by directly analyzing a compound's disposition, as well as its performance and activity in a cellular assay. This process, known as ADME, specifically examines compound absorption, distribution, metabolism, and excretion (Amir-Aslani and Negassi 2006; Bickle 2010; Cottens et al. 2011; Lang et al. 2006; McCann 2010; Shillingford and Vose 2001; Zanella et al. 2010). Toxicity screening may also be included in the process (renaming the process *ADMET*) or it may be conducted at a later stage (Bickle 2010). While this process proves effective in eventually selecting only the best possible candidates for use in clinical trials—and eventually for commercialization—it has traditionally been conducted in separate stages. Needless to say, this prolongs the time to development and maximizes the costs involved. Recently, many companies have attempted to integrate the different screening stages and tests into one step known as high content screening (HCS) or high content analysis (HCA).

The overarching goal of HCA is to combine the concepts of traditional high-throughput compound screening and cellular characterization assays to help improve the success rate for compounds emerging from the discovery pipeline, while simultaneously reducing the costs associated with high attrition rates (Bickle 2010; McCann 2010; Noah 2010). By combining multiple drug discovery stages into a single step that uses cells instead of cellular components or fragments like many primary HTS assays, HCA incorporates physiological relevance into the process as early as possible (McCann 2010). For instance, initial insight can be made about how compounds will affect signal transduction pathways, mechanical and morphological properties, and overall cell health and viability. Additionally, with cellular imaging analyses, off-target effects (i.e., side effects) of compound candidates can be visualized and understood at an earlier stage as a result of the ability to simultaneously observe multiple cellular parameters (McCann 2010). As a result, subsequent predictions and follow-up studies on in vivo behavior will be more relevant with a thorough understanding of the effects and mechanisms of action of compounds on observed cellular phenotypes (Bickle 2010; McCann 2010).

HCA facilitates this simultaneous assessment of multiple parameters in a single cellular assay by incorporating automated microscopy and image processing tools. Typically, specific cellular components or constituents of interest are labeled with fluorescent tags so that they can be highlighted and clearly visualized in fluorescent microscopy images. This allows for these features to be represented and analyzed quantitatively, and then used to answer complex questions about mechanisms, pathways, and overall phenotypic behavior of cells (McCann 2010; Noah 2010). Additionally, HCA presents an advantage over manual image interpretation by using automated microscopy, processing, and evaluating methods, which remove much of the bias from the screening process (Bickle 2010). Finally, with HCA, it is also possible to quantitatively capture the spatiotemporal features of a cell and its responses to compounds being investigated, which was not possible with the traditional end point assays of HTS (Bickle 2010).

Nevertheless, the true value of incorporating quantitative image analyses of cellular assays into drug discovery through HCA lies in the ability to describe phenotypic behavior of cells and group them into distinct phenotypes on the basis of their actions and properties. For instance, in studies and models of angiogenesis, endothelial cells are often classified by actions such as proliferation, migration, elongation, and branching (Bentley et al. 2008; Gerhardt 2008; Liu et al. 2011; Mac Gabhann et al. 2010; Qutub and Popel 2009; Qutub, Liu et al. 2009; Qutub, Mac Gabhann et al. 2009; Wood et al. 2008). Descriptors of these types of cellular characteristics and behaviors are fairly comparable across companies and, as a result, are largely unbiased (Bickle 2010). The most commonly analyzed properties, like cellular shape, area, polarity, and nuclear conformation, are important because they can correspond to intracellular and intercellular molecular events like signaling pathways and protein expression patterns (Bickle 2010).

Like academic research laboratories, companies use a variety of statistical methods to subsequently establish connections between analyzed cellular metrics, that is, cluster analysis and self-organizing maps. Clustering cells according to the quantitative information obtained from image analyses allows for the identification of similarities in how the morphological and mechanical properties of cells relate to their intracellular activities. Therefore, gathering this information allows for structure–activity relationships to define a phenotype fingerprint that can be assigned to cells that display similar patterns (Bickle 2010). Results from these screens are significantly more descriptive and sensitive than those from homogeneous, traditional end point assays, and they allow for important individual cell examination. Thus, phenotyping in HCA at early stages of drug development provides a clear advantage over older methods, which only use whole-cell assays to determine a compound's mode of action at later stages of R&D (Bickle 2010).

In conclusion, by harnessing the wealth of quantitative information imbedded in images of in vitro cellular assays, HCA provides an automated and unbiased method for high-throughput investigation of physiologically relevant cellular responses that is clearly an improvement over HTS methods traditionally used in drug discovery. By grouping examined cells with similar metric information, HCA can also define distinct cellular phenotypes to identify and classify cells with related behaviors in screens. Since phenotypes are normally defined with a number of parameters, fewer false positives occur during drug development with HCA than HTS, leading to a lower attrition rate (Bickle 2010). Additionally, phenotyping permits the effects of compounds on cells to be visualized immediately, without prior knowledge of target specificity. Not only does this further lower the candidate attrition rate, but it also combines previously distinct stages in the pipeline and helps increase the efficiency of compound selection and validation (Bickle

2010). Finally, since HCA establishes biologically relevant phenotypic responses of cells to compounds and conditions, it minimizes the need for excessive animal studies focused on drug toxicity (Bickle 2010). Together, these benefits of cellular phenotypic analyses through HCA in drug discovery allow for significant time and cost savings for biopharmaceutical companies.

11.3.2 Details of Cellular Phenotyping

The advantages of HCA over non-image-based plate readers and fixed end point assays clearly indicate that the use of HCA in industry will only continue to increase in the coming years. With steadily increasing demands from biopharmaceutical companies, the imaging and analysis platforms on the market have increased in number and capability in recent years (described below). Companies providing scanning and data analysis services have also emerged to capitalize on the growing field. Recent technological advances have significantly expanded the capabilities of HCA and helped establish its prevalence in the biopharmaceutical industry, while also pointing to areas to where improvements are still needed and possible future directions for the field.

In principle, HCA relies on the combination of fully automated microscopes and image analysis. For instance, screening systems need to possess the ability to quickly scan and assess cell populations at low magnifications, as well as to take high-resolution images of intracellular processes, without causing photobleaching of fluorescent labels or light-induced cellular damage (Bickle 2010). Most HCA platforms today have one of three types of instruments. Wide-field fluorescent microscopy systems are the most common, and they provide fast, adequate solutions for cellular imaging. Their main drawback, however, lies in a large image depth of field that results in insufficient probe colocalization accuracy (McCann 2010). On the other hand, true confocal HCA imaging systems are attractive alternatives in that they provide higher resolution and optical slices, as well as more precise probe colocalization. Unfortunately, these systems can be significantly more expensive than wide-field systems and are often significantly slower to operate. Finally, scanning laser beam imaging systems are specifically designed for examining live cells (Bickle 2010).

There are many systems on the market that offer combinations of the capabilities of these imaging platforms, such as the ability to perform both wide-field and confocal microscopy (Bickle 2010). The main companies supplying these systems to industries include BD Biosciences, GE Healthcare, Molecular Devices, Olympus, Perkin Elmer, Carl Zeiss, Yokogawa, and ThermoFisher Cellomics (Bickle 2010; Kornblau et al. 2011; Lang et al. 2006; McCann 2010; Rayment and Williams 2010) (see Table 11.1). Many of these same companies are also offering upgrades, so that systems can be improved without having to be replaced. For instance, Cellomics offers a confocal-like wide-field upgrade called the Zeiss Apotome that acts as a light image enhancement system (McCann 2010). Many users want to integrate image analysis algorithms with their imaging systems to create all-in-one screening solutions. While some of the hardware companies also provide software, there are a number of independent companies offering customizable software solutions for different applications, as well as outsourced image processing and analysis—and, in some cases, even assay development services (Liptrot 2001; Mack 2004; Walter et al. 2010) (see Table 11.3).

All of these tools for working with images share basic principles for examining cellular properties. First of all, most systems use fluorescent markers to label particular structures or components of interest (Lang et al. 2006; Walter et al. 2010; Zanella et al. 2010). Immunostaining techniques are used to visualize components of fixed cells, and

TABLE 11.3

Service and Software and Analysis Companies

Company	Description of Services
Definiens	Data mining services and software, accompanying quantitative image analysis. Can work with tissue slides, cell-based assays and fully body scans
Cellectis Bioresearch	Tools for the generation of stable cell lines for drug discovery (i.e., gene knockout or modification). Provides outsourced, customizable cell generation
Gene Network Sciences	Industrial-scale data analysis capabilities for the health care industry

fluorescent proteins (i.e., green fluorescent protein and red fluorescent protein) tag elements of live cells for spatiotemporal event analyses (Walter et al. 2010). Certain aspects of these labels, such as fluorescence intensity changes and fluorescence distribution—and the features that they highlight, like overall cell morphology or cell movement—can be quantified and used to define specific metrics of highlighted cellular features (Walter et al. 2010; Zanella et al. 2010). As before, common metrics include overall cell morphology, size, texture, spatial distribution, area, perimeter, circularity, number, localization, and dynamic movement (Rayment and Williams 2010; Stephens and Allan 2003; Walter et al. 2010; Zanella et al. 2010). Many users also like the ability to define their own metrics of interest; thus, many current software solutions are providing this flexibility along with integrated standard metrics (Bickle 2010).

11.3.3 Recent Advances in Technology

Improvements in both microscopes and image analysis programs have helped increase the effectiveness, and thus prevalence, of computational cellular phenotypic analyses in industry. Advances in charge-coupled diode (CCD) camera and chip technology, as well as light enhancement systems and laser-based autofocus methods, have vastly improved imaging speed, accuracy, flexibility, and resolution. New microscope modules for scanning, optical sectioning, and deconvolution have also improved imaging methods (Bickle 2010; McCann 2010). Along with these hardware upgrades, innovations in assay designs and components have helped improve the ability to observe and quantify cellular features and phenotypic behavior dynamics. For instance, efforts to develop improved fluorescent labeling technologies for live cell HCA assays have yielded promising advances over traditional stains and dyes. Two such advances include quantum dots and enzymatically activated fluorescent protein labeling. While work remains to minimize the potential drawbacks associated with these labels, including functional interference with the molecule of interest and ineffective delivery into cells, efforts in the area are continuing as the ability to image live cell behavior is crucial for the progression of HCA (Zanella et al. 2010).

The most apparent advancement in HCA technology, however, is the advent of automated and integrated imaging and analysis platform packages (Lang et al. 2006; Liptrot 2001; McCann 2010; Zanella et al. 2010) (Table 11.4). Specifically, many companies with high screening volumes and limited time and personnel resources want the ability to simply load samples into a hands-off machine that will later return results on specified metrics. To achieve this goal, many companies are incorporating robotic fluidics control, plate handling, and even incubation chambers into their systems that allow for live cell culturing and analysis in addition to fixed cell immunostaining assays. The time and resources required for live cell assays are often prohibitive for companies without automation. However, the

TABLE 11.4

HCA Imaging Systems

Company	Equipment Name	Detection Method
ThermoFisher Cellomics	ArrayScan VTI HCS	White light, single-CCD camera fluorescent microscope
Molecular Devices	ImageXpressMICRO	White light, single-CCD camera fluorescent microscope
	ImageXpressULTRA	Laser point scanning confocal microscope
GE Healthcare	IN Cell 1000	White light, single-CCD camera fluorescent microscope
	IN Cell 3000	3-CCD, slit laser line scanning confocal microscope
BD Biosciences	Pathway 855	White light, single-CCD camera confocal microscope
	Pathway 435	White light, single-CCD camera disc-based confocal microscope
Olympus	Scan^R	White light, single-CCD camera fluorescent microscope
Perkin Elmer	Opera	3-CCD, multi-beam laser illumination confocal microscope
	OperaLX	1-CCD, multi-beam laser illumination confocal microscope
Leica	TCS SP5	Laser point scanning confocal microscope
Yokogawa	CellVoyager	EMCCD camera; laser light confocal microscope

new integrated platforms allow live cell analyses, and the important dynamic behavioral information they yield, to become more widely used in industry. Finally, most systems also include some type of image processing and statistical analysis software to provide the user with tangible assay results. Options offering customizable tools and training methods, as well as links to storage databases or networks, make these platform components even more desirable (Zanella et al. 2010). In the aggregate, these advances in technology and automated platform packages help improve large-scale screening capabilities, but more importantly, they allow for the acquisition of data that are unbiased by human intervention. This is critical in industrial applications where the resulting statistically robust data are used to make decisions concerning the pursuit of a drug target or compound (Lang et al. 2006).

11.3.4 Current Limitations

Despite the major advancements in the area of computational phenotypic analyses in industry, the field has notable shortcomings that need to be addressed before continued growth can occur in the coming years. First of all, optimized protocols and stable, well-characterized cell lines need to be readily available for reliable and robust analyses across multiple assays and scales (Lang et al. 2006; McCann 2010; Zanella et al. 2010). As previously stated, advances in labeling probes are also imperative moving forward. New technology like DNA-based erasable molecular probes show potential for expanding the number of cellular components or structures that can be labeled and explored within the same cell population and indicate progress in the area (Duose et al. 2010, 2012; Schweller et al. 2012). However, there still exist other industrial needs, such as additional options for live cell labeling, as well as improvements that minimize fluorophore fading and photobleaching.

There are also significant hardware and software issues that must be addressed for HCA to grow. Both image acquisition and throughput speed must continue to increase to minimize fluorophore fading and maximize the number of cells and samples that can be visualized, respectively (Lang et al. 2006; McCann 2010). There may be no perfect solutions for other problems like inadequate autofocus methods, uneven culture plates, and poor assay designs, but efforts to improve these factors can significantly decrease associated poor image quality (McCann 2010). In the area of software, understanding how to standardize image parameters across populations, samples, and assays; define universal analysis metrics; and integrate metric data will help users detect meaningful patterns and exploit all of the available results to robustly quantify phenotypic behavior of cells (Lang et al. 2006; Walter et al. 2010; Zanella et al. 2010). Finally, data handling and storage methods will need to maintain pace with steadily increasing levels of data coming from higher-through-put screens. In addition to systems being able to save large data quantities (terabytes per month) for long periods (5 years or more), they should have data mining tools that allow for rapid, efficient queries during analyses and be amenable to the incorporation of new algorithms (Lang et al. 2006; McCann 2010). With improvements in all of these areas, HCA will continue to be a driving force in biopharmaceutical drug discovery processes and should provide increasingly accurate quantitative descriptions of cell populations and phenotypic behavior vital to target and compound identification and validation.

11.3.5 Case Study

Leveraging HCA techniques to identify drug targets against schistosomiasis, Paveley et al. (2012) describe screening for drug-induced effects on in vitro cultured schistosomula lar-vae by utilizing bright-field imaging. The team coupled automated, time-lapsed image analysis to Bayesian statistical methods to scan more than 10,000 compounds for morpho-logical damage and motility phenotyping, successfully detecting 99.8% of all leads. Such a cell-based methodology, not needing labels, can be readily adapted toward drug screens against a wide variety of organs and over a large swath of chemical libraries, speeding the development of clinically useful antiparasite therapeutics.

11.3.6 Summary

High content screening and analysis has proven itself to be a powerful resource in the bio-pharmaceutical industry by providing important information to users about detailed cel-lular behaviors and phenotypic responses to stimuli. HCA can analyze massive amounts of samples like traditional high-throughput screens but has additional tools for obtain-ing spatially and temporally relevant cellular data that is not possible with the fixed end point assays of HTS. With these highly detailed analyses, HCA is able to more thoroughly exploit the wealth of information available in cellular microscopy images by quantitatively describing the intricacies of biological processes and painting a physiologically relevant picture of cellular behavior (Bickle 2010).

Recent advances in HCA hardware and software have greatly increased its capabilities and its applicability in industry, specifically for detailed cellular imaging and analyses in biopharmaceutical drug development screens. The associated technology is still far from perfect, but small improvements in microscope hardware, analysis programs and algo-rithms, and storage methods will go a long way in helping HCA continue to grow and maintain its prevalence in industry. Ideally, companies hope that by providing detailed information about phenotypic behavior of cells, HCA will be able to integrate multiple steps of the drug discovery pipeline in a shorter period than traditional screens. Not only does this accelerated process have the potential to make a good candidate drug's jump to the clinic faster, it eliminates poor targets and compounds at an earlier stage, thus saving companies significant amounts of time, resources, and money. Finally, with similar quan-titative image analysis and cellular phenotyping methods being employed in the labora-tory and in the clinic, the biopharmaceutical industry's use of HCA technology provides opportunities for collaborative studies to improve their R&D methods and monitor and map their success rate in the clinic.

11.4 Cell Phenotyping in the Clinic

Despite being subjected to rigorous evaluations in both the lab and the pharmaceutical industry, any new drugs, compounds, or treatment methods that make it to the clinic must continue to be tested extensively for safety and efficacy. Physicians often assess these criteria at multiple scales: from the genomic level all the way to the tissue and whole-body level. Cellular actions and behaviors are of particular importance in a number of diseases and are thus monitored closely by expert pathologists. Traditionally, pathologists examine dyed tissue or cell samples and use them to both diagnose the presence or absence of a disease and grade its progression using a predetermined scale (Gurcan et al. 2009). However, this system has demonstrated low reproducibility and raises concerns regarding variability in interpretations between individuals (Furness et al. 2003). This problem has been extensively studied in the context of using the Gleason scale to grade prostate cancer (Allsbrook et al. 2001; King and Long 2000; Ruijter et al. 2000) and grading breast cancer (Gurcan et al. 2009). It was found to be the cause of significant variation in the grading of both conditions. To combat these potential sources of error and variability, the same quantitative cell phenotyping approaches employed in both the lab and industry have recently been pursued as the next generation of technology for the classically qualitative, subjective fields of histology and pathology.

Digital pathology is a new approach to this problem that allows for the automation or semi-automation of the diagnostic and grading processes. By digitally imaging and analyzing cell or tissue samples, a wealth of information about the subcellular components, morphology, and patterning of cells can be collected (Laurinavicius et al. 2012). These acquired metrics can be used to categorize a cell being studied for a range of diagnostic and screening purposes into a phenotype based on shared characteristics with other similar cells. For a semi-automated process, these data can be used to direct the pathologists' attention away from benign areas of tissue or cells and toward sections that contain information relevant to the diagnosis, reducing a work-intensive aspect of interpreting histological data. Additionally, the pathologist can use the quantitative data generated to guide or support their own diagnostic decisions (Isse et al. 2012). In a fully automated process, a program could use an algorithm based on criteria determined by a pathologist to directly interpret these data to make a diagnostic decision (Gurcan et al. 2009). Thus, by providing quantitative histological data for both diagnostic use and investigative clinical research, digital pathology allows for more consistent results between settings and deeper analysis of the patient samples.

11.4.1 Basics of Digital Pathology

Quantitative pathology began as a means of digitizing histopathology slides for easier collaboration between remote sites and to lessen dependence on slides, which can easily be lost or damaged (Isse et al. 2012). As image analysis and computational capabilities have improved, the utility of these digital images has also grown. Currently, digital pathology includes scanning entire tissue slides that have been appropriately dyed, processing resulting images to isolate components relevant to the specific sample, quantifying image components and characteristics, and potentially making a diagnosis or diagnostic suggestion (Gurcan et al. 2009).

More specifically, in tissue slide preparation, areas of interest can be dyed to reveal a range of cellular components and subcellular signals. Traditional dyes include hematoxylin and eosin, and variations on the Pap smear stain, which identify general cellular components and structures. Dyes that have been more recently developed are generally linked to a biomarker associated with a certain disease and utilize fluorescent tagging (Price et al. 2002). These labels provide more specific data about the tissue sample being studied and are easily distinguished by unique wavelengths, thus lending themselves nicely to digital interpretation (Price et al. 2002).

Once the tissue samples have been treated and stained, they undergo whole-slide imaging (WSI) to capture the entire sample into one image. This is achieved with specialized slide scanners, which adjust the z-plane focus as they navigate in the x–y plane to stitch together images to capture the entire slide. Although this process can be performed at any magnification, pathologists generally prefer a 40× magnification because a high level of detail is necessary to differentiate between many tissue characteristics important for diagnostic decisions (Isse et al. 2012).

Next, the first step in processing these images is normalizing the color and illumination so that samples taken in different conditions and created by a range of techniques can be analyzed equally (Gurcan et al. 2009). Using image analysis software, cells, glands, and other features of the tissue can be isolated for further investigation. Once these objects have been identified, a range of metrics relating to size, morphology, texture, and density can be measured. The spatial relationship between these objects can also be investigated using a graph-based approach. Finally, diagnosis or grading information is generated on the basis of these quantitative definitions of the objects.

The specific image features investigated will depend upon the type of tissue being studied, the dyes used to stain the components, and the purpose of the histopathological analysis. These metrics may be categorized by size and shape, radial and density, texture, and those related to chromatin (Gurcan et al. 2009). The choice of which of these to use will often be based off of how a pathologist approaches a tissue sample to make a diagnosis. For example, one study that applies digital pathology to grade follicular lymphoma quantitatively measured the same components of the cells, namely, morphology of the cytoplasm and nucleus, that a pathologist would qualitatively assess (Sertel et al. 2009). This approach is reflected in available pathology analysis software, which allows users to build their own pipeline to extract desired data and characteristics and emulate how a pathologist would analyze the images.

11.4.2 Recent Advances in Digital Pathology

Digital pathology has mostly emerged as a major trend in the clinic in the last 10 years, and in that short time, many significant advances have been made in the methods and analysis tools available. The most significant of these have been developments in cellular component labeling, tissue imaging, and segmentation and analysis of the captured images.

11.4.2.1 Biomarkers

Traditionally, histologists have dyed tissue samples with contrasting stains, such as hematoxylin and eosin, and visualized them using bright-field microscopy. More recently, immunofluorescent dyes have gained popularity because they can be used as molecular markers and can be more easily separated by their emission wavelengths. Because of chemical incompatibilities between stains and the fluorescent activity of traditional dyes, a newly developed method is to sequentially stain and image the same sample with different molecular biomarkers of interest (Can et al. 2008). While this method provides more data for subsequent cellular phenotyping and analysis, it also increases the time and labor necessary to image the sample for digital pathology (Gurcan et al. 2009).

11.4.2.2 Imaging Tissue Using Spectroscopy

The use of spectroscopy for imaging tissue can provide detailed information regarding the chemical composition of a tissue sample at both specific locations and as a whole. Although spectroscopy does not provide data regarding individual cells specifically, it can be used in conjunction with microscopy to phenotype cells and characterize tissue for diagnostic purposes (Gurcan et al. 2009).

11.4.2.3 Segmentation and Analysis

A number of image analysis tools exist on the market with a wide range of capabilities, many of which are identical to those used in the lab and in industry. One class includes programs that are not intended specifically for pathology but have image analysis tools that can be harnessed for different applications, such as MATLAB and ImageJ (Gurcan et al. 2009). There are also other types of software packages that integrate multiple analysis steps by automatically segmenting, analyzing, and quantifying characteristics from provided images (Tables 11.1 and 11.2). In many of these programs, the user can adjust the parameters used by the program and even teach it to identify characteristics like a pathologist.

Work in the use of digital pathology has demonstrated promising results. A study comparing the scoring from commercially available software for the analysis of estrogen receptor and human epidermal growth factor receptor-2 stains in tumor samples for the diagnosis of breast cancer found that all 33 of the automated image analysis scores fell within a satisfactory range of the pathologists' scores (Lloyd et al. 2010). Although the software implemented was not US Food and Drug Administration (FDA) approved, it was chosen for its adjustable parameters, such as segmentation, and intensity and curvature thresholds, which were used to train the software to match the pathologists' scoring of tissue samples. The study stressed the importance of these adjustments for the strong match between the automatic and pathologist-generated readings, as well as the necessity for pathologists to double check all software-generated scores.

Digital pathology may also be used in an exploratory capacity to correlate a disease prognosis or grade with cellular characteristics that pathologists would not be able to identify without computational aid. One study used this approach to investigate spatial differences in various types of pancreatic cancer tumors by utilizing their own image analysis tools to quantify differences in stromal area. The resulting correlation may have prognostic value, but without the use of computational phenotyping tools, this parameter would have been inaccessible to pathologists (Sims et al. 2003). The use of digital pathology allows researchers to harvest information from patient samples to quantitatively explore relationships between cell or tissue structures and disease states that would have been difficult or impossible to obtain using traditional histology methods.

11.4.3 Current Limitations

Although digital pathology promises to vastly improve the standardization and quantification of current histopathology practices, drawbacks remain. The first, which exists across many digitization processes, is how to handle the large quantity of data and images being produced. A single WSI on average ranges from 200 MB to 5 GB in size, depending upon the magnification and quality of the image (Price et al. 2002). Additionally, analyzing these images is a computationally intense process. Using quantitative pathology on the scale that would be necessary in a clinical or academic setting requires robust computing and storage capabilities (Gurcan et al. 2009).

The possibility of employing digital pathology as a diagnostic tool also raises the issue of ensuring accuracy, and not just precision, in the design systems. Further complicating this is the lack of a clear gold standard of comparison for results from an automated system; although the diagnosis by pathologists is the current standard of care, it still exhibits both intra- and interpersonal variability (Furness et al. 2003). Any viable solutions to this problem must demonstrate that digital pathology improves upon the accuracy of diagnoses being made, and not just the precision.

Finally, digital pathology must overcome the hurdle of being integrated into the workflow of clinical histopathology. Although most current research in digital pathology is working toward creating tools to assist pathologists rather than replace them, these innovations would still create significant differences in the way that histopathology has been used for many years. Current equipment and systems can be quite expensive, and it may be difficult to rationalize the additional expenses for improvements or overhauls in many smaller-scale settings and projects. Furthermore, no digital pathology software has yet been FDA approved for primary diagnostic use. Although many researchers believe that the use of digital pathology would create marked improvements in pathology in clinical settings, clinicians may still need to be convinced.

11.4.4 Case Study

In order to develop an automated method to quantitate immune infiltrates in colorectal cancer and determine their prognostic relationship with clinical outcome, Angell et al. (2013) combined immunohistochemistry with digital image analysis. Staining primary colorectal adenocarcinoma tissue with hematoxylin, along with antibodies against Foxp3, CD8, CD68, and CD31, and imaging the resultant slides with a digital scanner, Angell et al. used Genie pattern recognition software to visually segregate the tumor, immune infiltrate, and nonneoplastic regions. Results uncovered a possible metastasis-indicating immunosuppressive phenotype, demonstrating the clinical utility compared to qualitative histopathological investigation.

11.5 Conclusions

Evolving practices in research and design in the lab, plant, and clinic are necessitating the development of improvements on traditional assays and analysis tools in order to obtain enhanced biological understanding. Of particular interest in all three settings is the ability to capture dynamic cell behavior information from microscopy images and movies and use resulting data to make inferences about cellular behavior and response. As a result, the field of computational cell phenotyping has emerged to harness the wealth of descriptive, spatially resolved information present in detailed cellular microscopy images. Thus far, it has assisted researchers in making novel discoveries about cellular actions, allowed the biopharmaceutical industry to accelerate the drug development process, and provided assistance to pathologists in making clinical diagnosis and decisions. While the field is still continuing to evolve, it is clear that its impact is already widespread in biomedical sciences. With continued progress, computational cell phenotyping may revolutionize medicine by providing novel methods for therapeutic discovery and design, testing and production, and clinical implementation and assessment.

References

Agrawal, V, and Jamwal, S. 2012. "Top Ten Global Pharma." World Pharmaceutical Frontiers, pp. 10–11.

Allsbrook, W C, K A Mangold, M H Johnson, R B Lane, C G Lane, M B Amin, D G Bostwick et al. 2001. "Interobserver Reproducibility of Gleason Grading of Prostatic Carcinoma: Urologic Pathologists." *Human Pathology* 32: 74–80. doi:10.1053/hupa.2001.21134.

Amir-Aslani, A, and S Negassi. 2006. "Is Technology Integration the Solution to Biotechnology's Low Research and Development Productivity?" *Technovation* 26: 573–582. doi:10.1016/j.technovation .2005.06.001.

Angell, H K, N Gray, C Womack, D I Pritchard, R W Wilkinson, and M Cumberbatch. 2013. "Digital Pattern Recognition-based Image Analysis Quantifies Immune Infiltrates in Distinct Tissue Regions of Colorectal Cancer and Identifies a Metastatic Phenotype." *Br J Cancer* 109: 1618–1624.

Bass, G T, K A Ryall, A Katikapalli, B E Taylor, S T Dang, S T Acton, and J J Saucerman. 2011. "Automated Image Analysis Identifies Signaling Pathways Regulating Distinct Signatures of Cardiac Myocyte Hypertrophy." *Journal of Molecular and Cellular Cardiology* 52: 923–930. doi:10.1016/j.yjmcc.2011.11.009.

Bentley, K, H Gerhardt, and P A Bates. 2008. "Agent-based Simulation of Notch-mediated Tip Cell Selection in Angiogenic Sprout Initialisation." *Journal of Theoretical Biology* 250 (1): 25–36. doi:10.1016/j.jtbi.2007.09.015.

Bickle, M. 2010. "The Beautiful Cell: High-content Screening in Drug Discovery." *Analytical and Bioanalytical Chemistry* 398 (1): 219–226. doi:10.1007/s00216-010-3788-3.

Brugger, S D, C Baumberger, M Jost, W Jenni, U Brugger, and K Mühlemann. 2012. "Automated Counting of Bacterial Colony Forming Units on Agar Plates." *PLoS One* 7 (3): e33695. doi:10.1371/journal.pone.0033695.

Can, A, M Bello, H E Cline, X Tao, F Ginty, A Sood, M Gerdes, and M Montalto. 2008. "Multi-modal Imaging of Histological Tissue Sections." *Biomedical Imaging: From Nano to Macro, 2008. ISBI 2008. 5th IEEE International Symposium On.* doi:10.1109/ISBI.2008.4540989.

Chen, T-S, S-Q Zeng, Q-M Luo, Z-H Zhang, and W Zhou. 2002. "High-order Photobleaching of Green Fluorescent Protein Inside Live Cells in Two-photon Excitation Microscopy." *Biochemical and Biophysical Research Communications* 291 (5): 1272–1275. doi:10.1006/bbrc.2002.6587.

Chung, K, M M Crane, and H Lu. 2008. "Automated On-chip Rapid Microscopy, Phenotyping and Sorting of C. Elegans." *Nature Methods* 5 (7): 637–643.

Clemons, P A. 2004. "Complex Phenotypic Assays in High-throughput Screening." *Current Opinion in Chemical Biology* 8 (3): 334–338.

Contag, P R. 2002. "Whole-animal Cellular and Molecular Imaging to Accelerate Drug Development." *Drug Discovery Today* 7: 555–562.

Cottens, S, M Eaton, J Fuhr, S Geary, D S Johnson, G Li, L Raveglia, G M Robertson, and A Westwell. 2011. "Ask the Experts: Future of the Pharmaceutical Industry." *Future Medicinal Chemistry* 3 (15): 1863–1872.

Cox, J, and M Mann. 2007. "Is Proteomics the New Genomics?" *Cell* 130 (3): 395–398.

David, E, T Tramontin, and R Zemmel. 2009. "Pharmaceutical R&D: The Road to Positive Returns." *Nature Reviews. Drug Discovery* 8 (8): 609–610. doi:10.1038/nrd2948.

Deckers, R, B Quesson, J Arsaut, S Eimer, F Couillaud, and C T W Moonen. 2009. "Image-guided, Noninvasive, Spatiotemporal Control of Gene Expression." *Proceedings of the National Academy of Sciences of the United States of America* 106 (4): 1175–1180.

Dehmelt, L, and P I H Bastiaens. 2010. "Spatial Organization of Intracellular Communication: Insights from Imaging." *Nature Reviews Molecular Cell Biology* 11 (6): 440–452.

Duose, D Y, R M Schweller, W N Hittelman, and M R Diehl. 2010. "Multiplexed and Reiterative Fluorescence Labeling via DNA Circuitry." *Bioconjugate Chemistry* 21 (12): 2327–2331. doi:10.1021/bc100348q.

Duose, D Y, R M Schweller, J Zimak, A R Rogers, W N Hittelman, and M R Diehl. 2012. "Configuring Robust DNA Strand Displacement Reactions for in Situ Molecular Analyses." *Nucleic Acids Research* 40 (7): 3289–3298. doi:10.1093/nar/gkr1209.

Furness, P N, N Taub, K J Assmann, G Banfi, J P Cosyns, A M Dorman, C M Hill et al. 2003. "International Variation in Histologic Grading Is Large, and Persistent Feedback Does Not Improve Reproducibility." *The American Journal of Surgical Pathology* 27: 805–810.

Gerhardt, H. 2008. "VEGF and Endothelial Guidance in Angiogenic Sprouting." *Organogenesis* 4 (4): 241–246.

Gurcan, M N, L E Boucheron, A Can, A Madabhushi, N M Rajpoot, and B Yener. 2009. "Histopathological Image Analysis: A Review." *IEEE Rev Biomed Eng* 2: 147–171. doi:10.1109/RBME.2009.2034865.

Hoehme, S, M Brulport, A Bauer, E Bedawy, W Schormann, M Hermes, V Puppe et al. 2010. "Prediction and Validation of Cell Alignment Along Microvessels as Order Principle to Restore Tissue Architecture in Liver Regeneration." *Proceedings of the National Academy of Sciences of the United States of America* 107 (23): 10371–10376. doi:10.1073/pnas.0909374107.

Huth, J, M Buchholz, J M Kraus, K Mølhave, C Gradinaru, G v. Wichert, T M Gress, H Neumann, and H A Kestler. 2011. "TimeLapseAnalyzer: Multi-target Analysis for Live-cell Imaging and Time-lapse Microscopy." *Computer Methods and Programs in Biomedicine* 104 (2): 227–234. doi:10.1016/j.cmpb.2011.06.002.

Isse, K, A Lesniak, K Grama, B Roysam, M I Minervini, and A J Demetris. 2012. "Digital Transplantation Pathology: Combining Whole Slide Imaging, Multiplex Staining and Automated Image Analysis." *American Journal of Transplantation* 12: 27–37. doi:10.1111/j.1600-6143.2011.03797.x.

Jones, T R, A E Carpenter, M R Lamprecht, J Moffat, S J Silver, J K Grenier, A B Castoreno et al. 2009. "Scoring Diverse Cellular Morphologies in Image-based Screens with Iterative Feedback and Machine Learning." *Proceedings of the National Academy of Sciences of the United States of America* 106 (6): 1826–1831. doi:10.1073/pnas.0808843106.

Kandemir-Cavas, C, and E Nasibov. 2009. "Alternative Hierarchical Clustering Approach in Construction of Phylogenetic Trees." *2009 14th National Biomedical Engineering Meeting*. doi:10.1109/BIYOMUT.2009.5130304.

Karr, J R, J C Sanghvi, D N Macklin, M V Gutschow, J M Jacobs, B Bolival, N Assad-Garcia, J I Glass, and M W Covert. 2012. "A Whole-Cell Computational Model Predicts Phenotype from Genotype." *Cell* 150 (2): 389–401. doi:10.1016/j.cell.2012.05.044.

King, C R, and J P Long. 2000. "Prostate Biopsy Grading Errors: A Sampling Problem?" *International Journal of Cancer* 90: 326–330.

Kornblau, S M, Y H Qiu, N Zhang, N Singh, S Faderl, A Ferrajoli, H York, A A Qutub, K R Coombes, and D K Watson. 2011. "Abnormal Expression of Friend Leukemia Virus Integration 1 (FLI1) Protein Is an Adverse Prognostic Factor in Acute Myeloid Leukemia." *Blood* 118 (20): 5604–5612. doi:10.1182/blood-2011-04-348052.

Lang, P, K Yeow, A Nichols, and A Scheer. 2006. "Cellular Imaging in Drug Discovery." *Nature Reviews. Drug Discovery* 5 (4): 343–356. doi:10.1038/nrd2008.

Lange, T, V Roth, M L Braun, and J M Buhmann. 2004. "Stability-based Validation of Clustering Solutions." *Neural Computation* 16 (6): 1299–1323. doi:10.1162/089976604773717621.

Laurinavicius, A, A Laurinaviciene, D Dasevicius, N Elie, B Plancoulaine, C Bor, and P Herlin. 2012. "Digital Image Analysis in Pathology: Benefits and Obligation." *Anal Cell Pathol (Amst)* 35: 75–78. doi:10.3233/ACP-2011-0033.

Lee, I, and J Yang. 2009. "Common Clustering Algorithms." In *Comprehensive Chemometrics*, eds. S D Brown, R Tauler, and B Walczak, 577–618. Waltham, MA: Elsevier. doi:10.1016/B978-044452701-1.00064-8.

Lee, J, S Kotliarova, Y Kotliarov, A Li, Q Su, N M Donin, S Pastorino et al. 2006. "Tumor Stem Cells Derived from Glioblastomas Cultured in bFGF and EGF More Closely Mirror the Phenotype and Genotype of Primary Tumors Than Do Serum-cultured Cell Lines." *Cancer Cell* 9 (5): 391–403. doi:10.1016/j.ccr.2006.03.030.

Liptrot, C. 2001. "High Content Screening—From Cells to Data to Knowledge." *Drug Discovery Today* 6 (16): 832–834.

Liu, G, A A Qutub, P Vempati, F Mac Gabhann, and A S Popel. 2011. "Module-based Multiscale Simulation of Angiogenesis in Skeletal Muscle." *Theoretical Biology & Medical Modelling* 8 (1): 6. doi:10.1186/1742-4682-8-6.

Lloyd, M C, P Allam-Nandyala, C N Purohit, N Burke, D Coppola, and M M Bui. 2010. "Using Image Analysis as a Tool for Assessment of Prognostic and Predictive Biomarkers for Breast Cancer: How Reliable Is It?" *J Pathol Inform* 1: 29. doi:10.4103/2153-3539.74186.

Ludwig, J A, and J N Weinstein. 2005. "Biomarkers in Cancer Staging, Prognosis and Treatment Selection." *Nature Reviews Cancer* 5 (11): 845–856.

Mac Gabhann, F, A A Qutub, B H Annex, and A S Popel. 2010. "Systems Biology of Pro-angiogenic Therapies Targeting the VEGF System." *Wiley Interdiscip Rev Syst Biol Med* 2 (6): 694–707. doi:10.1002/wsbm.92.Systems.

Mack, G S. 2004. "Can Complexity Be Commercialized?" *Nature Biotechnology* 22 (10): 1223–1229. doi:10.1038/nbt1004-1223.

McCann, T. 2010. "Live Cell Imaging: An Industrial Perspective." In *Live Cell Imaging*, ed. D B Papkovsky, 47–66. New York: Springer.

Mioulane, M, G Foldes, N N Ali, M D Schneider, and S E Harding. 2012. "Development of High Content Imaging Methods for Cell Death Detection in Human Pluripotent Stem Cell-Derived Cardiomyocytes." *Journal of Cardiovascular Translational Research* 5 (5): 593–604. doi:10.1007/s12265-012-9396-1.

Möller, C, and M Slack. 2010. "Impact of New Technologies for Cellular Screening Along the Drug Value Chain." *Drug Discovery Today* 15 (9–10): 384–390. doi:10.1016/j.drudis.2010.02.010.

Murtagh, F, P Contreras, and W Place. 2011. "Methods of Hierarchical Clustering arXiv : 1105 . 0121v1 [Cs . IR] 30 Apr 2011." *Computer* 38 (2): 1–21. doi:10.1007/s00181-009-0254-1.

Narro, M L, F Yang, R Kraft, C Wenk, A Efrat, and L L Restifo. 2007. "NeuronMetrics: Software for Semi-automated Processing of Cultured Neuron Images." *Brain Research* 1138: 57–75. doi:10.1016/j.brainres.2006.10.094.

Noah, J W. 2010. "New Developments and Emerging Trends in High-throughput Screening Methods for Lead Compound Identification." *International Journal of High Throughput Screening* 2010: 1.

Ohya, Y, J Sese, M Yukawa, F Sano, Y Nakatani, T L Saito, A Saka et al. 2005. "High-dimensional and Large-scale Phenotyping of Yeast Mutants." *Proceedings of the National Academy of Sciences of the United States of America* 102 (52): 19015–19020.

Parsa, H, R Upadhyay, and S K Sia. 2011. "Uncovering the Behaviors of Individual Cells Within a Multicellular Microvascular Community." *Proceedings of the National Academy of Sciences of the United States of America* 108 (12): 5133–5138. doi:10.1073/pnas.1007508108.

Paveley, R A, N R Mansour, I Hallyburton, L S Bleicher, A E Benn, I Mikic, A Guidi, I H Gilbert, A L Hopkins, Q D Bickle. 2012. "Whole organism high-content screening by label-free, image-based Bayesian classification for parasitic diseases." *PLoS Negl Trop Dis.* 6 (7): e1762.

Petushi, S, F U Garcia, M M Haber, C Katsinis, and A Tozeren. 2006. "Large-scale Computations on Histology Images Reveal Grade-differentiating Parameters for Breast Cancer." *BMC Medical Imaging* 6: 14. doi:10.1186/1471-2342-6-14.

Price, J H, A Goodacre, K Hahn, L Hodgson, E A Hunter, S Krajewski, R F Murphy, A Rabinovich, J C Reed, and S Heynen. 2002. "Advances in Molecular Labeling, High Throughput Imaging and Machine Intelligence Portend Powerful Functional Cellular Biochemistry Tools." *Journal of Cellular Biochemistry. Supplement* 39: 194–210. doi:10.1002/jcb.10448.

Qutub, A A, and A S Popel. 2009. "Elongation, Proliferation & Migration Differentiate Endothelial Cell Phenotypes and Determine Capillary Sprouting." *BMC Systems Biology* 3: 13. doi:10.1186/1752-0509-3-13.

Qutub, A A, F Mac Gabhann, E D Karagiannis, P Vempati, and A S Popel. 2009. "Multiscale Models of Angiogenesis: Integration of Molecular Mechanisms with Cell- and Organ-Level Models." *IEEE Engineering in Medicine and Biology Magazine.* 28 (2): 14–31. doi:10.1109/MEMB.2009.931791 .Multiscale.

Qutub, A A, G Liu, P Vempati, and A S Popel. 2009. "Integration of Angiogenesis Modules at Multiple Scales: From Molecular to Tissue." *Pacific Symposium on Biocomputing* 1: 316–327.

Qutub, A A, D Ryan, B Long, J Hu, B Zaunbrecher, C W Hu, and J Slater. 2013. "An Automated Method for Measuring, Classifying and Matching the Dynamics and Information Passing of Single Objects Within an Image." Patent: 61/865,642, Rice University Office of Technology Transfer, Houston, TX.

Rayment, E A, and D J Williams. 2010. "Concise Review: Mind the Gap: Challenges in Characterizing and Quantifying Cell- and Tissue-based Therapies for Clinical Translation." *Stem Cells* 28: 996–1004. doi:10.1002/stem.416.

Ricci-Vitiani, L, R Pallini, M Biffoni, M Todaro, G Invernici, T Cenci, G Maira et al. 2010. "Tumour Vascularization via Endothelial Differentiation of Glioblastoma Stem-like Cells." *Nature* 468 (7325): 824–828. doi:10.1038/nature09557.

Rosenson, R S. 2010. "New Technologies Personalize Diagnostics and Therapeutics." *Current Atherosclerosis Reports* 12 (3): 184–186. doi:10.1007/s11883-010-0103-x.

Ruijter, E, G van Leenders, G Miller, F Debruyne, and C van de Kaa. 2000. "Errors in Histological Grading by Prostatic Needle Biopsy Specimens: Frequency and Predisposing Factors." *The Journal of Pathology* 192: 229–233.

Ryan, D R, J Hu, B L Long, and A A Qutub. 2013. "Predicting Endothelial Cell Phenotypes in Angiogenesis." *ASME 2nd Global Congress on NanoEngineering for Medicine and Biology.* Boston, Massachusetts: ASME.

Schweller, R, J Zimak, A A Qutub, W N Hittleman, and M R Diehl. 2012. "Multiplexed In Situ Immunofluorescence via Dynamic DNA Complexes." *Angewandte Chemie* 51: 9292–9296.

Sertel, O, J Kong, U V Catalyurek, G Lozanski, J H Saltz, and M N Gurcan. 2009. "Histopathological Image Analysis Using Model-based Intermediate Representations and Color Texture: Follicular Lymphoma Grading." *Journal of Signal Processing Systems* 55: 169–183.

Shillingford, C A, and C W Vose. 2001. "Effective Decision-making: Progressing Compounds Through Clinical Development." *Drug Discovery Today* 6: 941–946.

Sims, A J, M K Bennett, and A Murray. 2003. "Image Analysis Can Be Used to Detect Spatial Changes in the Histopathology of Pancreatic Tumours." *Physics in Medicine and Biology* 48: N183–N191.

Sozzani, R, and P N Benfey. 2011. "High-throughput Phenotyping of Multicellular Organisms: Finding the Link Between Genotype and Phenotype." *Genome Biology* 12 (3): 219. doi:10.1186 /gb-2011-12-3-219.

Stephens, D J, and V J Allan. 2003. "Light Microscopy Techniques for Live Cell Imaging." *Science Signalling* 300 (5616): 82–86. doi:10.1126/science.1082160.

Tan, Y, L H Schwartz, and B Zhao. 2013. "Segmentation of Lung Lesions on CT Scans Using Watershed, Active Contours, and Markov Random Field." *Medical Physics* 40 (4): 43502–43510.

Tibshirani, R, G Walther, and T Hastie. 2000. "Estimating the Number of Clusters in a Dataset via the Gap Statistic." *Journal of the Royal Statistical Society, Series B* 63: 411–423.

Tyers, M, and M Mann. 2003. "From Genomics to Proteomics." *Nature* 422 (6928): 193–197.

Walter, T, D W Shattuck, R Baldock, M E Bastin, A E Carpenter, S Duce, J Ellenberg et al. 2010. "Visualization of Image Data from Cells to Organisms." *Nature Methods Supplement* 7 (3): S26–S41. doi:10.1038/NmEtH.1431.

Wang, Y, J Y-J Shyy, and S Chien. 2008. "Fluorescence Proteins, Live-cell Imaging, and Mechanobiology: Seeing Is Believing." *Annual Review of Biomedical Engineering* 10 (1): 1–38.

Wilkin, G A, and X Huang. 2007. "K-Means Clustering Algorithms: Implementation and Comparison." *Second International MultiSymposiums on Computer and Computational Sciences IMSCCS 2007.* IEEE. doi:10.1109/IMSCCS.2007.51.

Wood, L B, A Das, R D Kamm, and H H Asada. 2008. "A Stochastic Control Framework for Regulating Collective Behaviors of an Angiogenesis Cell Population." *2008 2nd IEEE RAS & EMBS International Conference on Biomedical Robotics and Biomechatronics* (October): 390–396. doi:10.1109/BIOROB.2008.4762822.

Yoshigi, M, E B Clark, and H J Yost. 2003. "Quantification of Stretch-induced Cytoskeletal Remodeling in Vascular Endothelial Cells by Image Processing." *Cytometry. Part A: The Journal of the International Society for Analytical Cytology* 55 (2): 109–118. doi:10.1002/cyto.a.10076.

Yuan, Y, H Failmezger, O M Rueda, H R Ali, S Gräf, S-F Chin, R F Schwarz et al. 2012. "Quantitative Image Analysis of Cellular Heterogeneity in Breast Tumors Complements Genomic Profiling." *Science Translational Medicine* 4 (157): 157ra143.

Zanella, F, J B Lorens, and W Link. 2010. "High Content Screening: Seeing Is Believing." *Trends in Biotechnology* 28 (5): 237–245. doi:10.1016/j.tibtech.2010.02.005.

12

Molecular Simulation of Protein–Surface Interactions

Xianfeng Li and Robert A. Latour

CONTENTS

ABSTRACT Various computational methods used for the simulation of protein–surface interaction are reviewed in this work. Among these methods, molecular simulations based on empirical force fields are used extensively in modeling protein–surface adsorption since they are able to provide detailed structural information of a molecular system in reasonable computational time. However, force fields that have been specifically developed for modeling the behavior of proteins in aqueous solution or the bulk behavior of solid materials may not accurately represent protein adsorption behavior simply because the force field parameters were never tuned to represent interfacial interactions. In order to accurately represent these types of interactions, interfacial force field (IFF) parameters must be specifically developed, tested, and validated. For this purpose, the adsorption of host–guest peptides on self-assembled monolayer surfaces has been used as a model system in both experimental and simulation studies. Experimentally, adsorption free energies have been determined from adsorption isotherms, while the biased-energy replica-exchange molecular dynamics method has been used to calculate the adsorption free energy for various combinations of these adsorption systems. By matching the calculated adsorption free energies with the corresponding experimental results, IFF parameters can be developed that accurately represent peptide adsorption affinity to these types of surfaces. Once IFF parameters are determined, simulations can then be confidently extended to model protein adsorption behavior. Given the substantial increase in the size and complexity of the molecular systems involved, additional advanced sampling methods and coarse-graining techniques are required to increase the efficiency of simulations of protein–surface interactions, and these methods are also introduced.

12.1 Introduction

The adsorption of proteins to biomaterial surfaces plays a key role in many natural processes [1–6] and has therefore been a topic of widespread research over the past several decades. For example, when a medical implant is placed in vivo, the implant's surfaces are immediately coated with proteins that are adsorbed from blood and other body fluids, with this adsorbed layer of proteins mediating subsequent cellular responses. These processes are quite complex and still not well understood. The resulting structure and composition of the adsorbed layer of proteins on a surface can be expected to be significantly different from their structure and distribution in bulk solution, with the bioactivity of the adsorbed layer being determined by the proteins' conformations, orientations, packing states, and dynamical behavior on the surface. The highly complex nature of protein–surface interactions originates from a combination of the complexities of protein structure itself along with the diversity of the properties of a surface, which can be hydrophobic, like the surfaces of polyethylene, graphite, and carbon nanotubes, or hydrophilic, like the surfaces of mica, TiO_2, and Al_2O_3 bioceramics, or chemically heterogeneous with both hydrophilic and hydrophobic domains formed by the phase separation in synthetic polymers. In addition, other properties such as surface charge, wettability, shape, roughness, and compliance can also have considerable influence on protein adsorption behavior.

Over the past several decades, protein adsorption processes have been extensively studied by experimental methods [7–10]. However, experimental methods are very limited in terms of assessing the behavior of a system at molecular-level time and length scales. Therefore, protein adsorption behavior on surfaces is still not well understood, with surface design to influence protein–surface interactions and subsequent cellular responses being still largely relegated to trial-and-error approaches. For this reason, molecular simulation has become increasingly recognized as a valuable addition to research aimed at understanding and interpreting protein adsorption processes at various levels of time and length scales. Accordingly, various approaches for the simulation of protein–surface interaction have been developed over the past couple of decades with reviews of these efforts provided in a number of publications [11–27].

Early modeling methods for studies of protein–surface adsorption were developed largely based on phenomenological adsorption models aimed at extracting adsorption equilibria and kinetics using macroscopic rate equations [28–33]. On the basis of stochastic strategies, parameters for these models were generally obtained from bulk system properties, which were relatively easy to estimate or directly measurable, and then applied to given sets of experimental conditions. These types of models were able to include factors such as competitive adsorption [28], protein denaturation [29], adsorbate self-association [30], surface hydrophobicity [31], and pH and surface charge density [33] to describe the adsorption and desorption kinetics and surface diffusion mechanisms for protein adsorption. Some models were also able to provide useful structural information, such as the preferred orientation of a protein in the vicinity of the surface [33]. However, these phenomenological models still were not able to give detailed structural information of protein–surface interactions at a molecular level. The practical demand of exploring the microscopic causes for macroscopic observations of the adsorption behavior of proteins on material surfaces then naturally led to efforts to develop simulation methods that were able to predict protein–surface interactions at the atomistic levels of structure.

Presently, molecular simulation methods for studies of protein–surface interactions are being pursued along two directions of development: (i) quantum mechanical–based ab initio methods and (ii) empirical force field–based classical methods. Ab initio quantum mechanics (QM) methods, which treat electrons as the fundamental unit of the system through various approximations to the Schrödinger equation, have been applied to address aspects of protein–surface systems relatively recently [34–42]. These types of methods can accurately describe the interactions between functional groups of a protein and a surface by calculating the electronic structure of the atoms that are represented in the model without requiring the addition of any empirical fitting parameters to describe the behavior of the system. However, because of the complexities of the calculations involved, these methods are at this time primarily useful for understanding adsorption events that happen over very small time and length scales, such as the binding of an individual amino acid on model surfaces with different types of head-groups, often with the implicit representation of hydration effects [35,36]. Of the various types of QM methods available, density functional theory (DFT) has relatively low computational costs compared to conventional QM methods and therefore is most applicable for the simulation of larger molecular systems. In DFT simulations, the properties of an atom are determined by using a functional representation of the electron density of the molecular system. The DFT method has recently been applied to study microscopic wetting of self-assembled monolayer (SAM) surfaces [37], the adsorption of individual amino acids on carbon nanotube [38] and graphene surfaces [39,40], and the adsorption of small peptides on hydroxyapatite surfaces [41,42]. While ab initio methods are advantageous in terms of having the potential to achieve a very high level of accuracy without requiring the addition of empirical parameters to describe the behavior of a given molecular system, their usefulness for application for the simulation of protein adsorption behavior at this point in time is fairly limited because their high computational cost limits their application to systems typically composed of no more than a few hundred atoms over time frames of no more than a few hundred picoseconds.

While phenomenological adsorption models are very computationally efficient but provide little structural information of a system at the molecular level, and ab initio methods provide full atomic-level detail but are too computationally costly for application to whole proteins, empirical force field methods provide a happy medium between these two extremes by enabling atomic-level structural information of large molecular systems to be calculated with manageable levels of computation time. Because of these attributes, empirical force field methods, including a broad range of molecular mechanics (MM), molecular dynamics (MD), and Monte Carlo (MC) simulation techniques, have become the most widely used tools used for computer simulations to represent the atomistic structure and dynamics of protein–surface interactions. Table 12.1 outlines some of the recent publications [43–75] reporting on studies using empirical force field–based molecular modeling methods for the simulation of protein adsorption behavior. In addition, studies of the adsorption behavior of various single amino acids on Au surfaces [76] and the adsorption of amino acids or their analogues on quartz [77,78] and titania [79] surfaces are also representative efforts using empirical force field methods.

When compared to the ab initio methods, which treat the electronic structure of individual atoms, empirical force field schemes treat individual atoms or groups of atoms as the fundamental units of the system, with empirical force fields employed to represent the energetics of the interactions between individual atoms, from which thermodynamics and kinetic properties of the system can be calculated. The functional form of the force field equation and the values of the parameters used with it are optimized to reproduce a certain set of experimental or theoretical data (the latter being typically obtained from QM calculations), which are selected to represent the desired characteristics of the system that the simulation is intended to predict, such as protein folding behavior in aqueous solution or protein

TABLE 12.1

Examples of Publications Using MD and MC Techniques Using Empirical Force Field–Based Methods

Surface	Aβ	Albumin Subdomain	BMP-2	Cytochrome c	Fibrinogen	Fibronectin	Lysozyme
				Protein			
Carbon nanotube	43[a], 44[a]						22[a], 45[a]
Charged surface							46[b], 47[b], 48–50[a]
Graphite	51[a]	52[a], 53[b], 54[a]	55[a]			56[a]	22[a], 57[a]
Hydroxyapatite			58[a]			59[a]	
Mica							60[b], 61[a]
TiO₂ rutile		62[a]	63[a]			62[a], 64[a]	
SAM	65–67[a]			68[a,b], 69[a,b]	70[a]	71[a]	72[a]
Silica							73[a]
Polymer				74[a]			22[a], 75[a]

Note: Aβ, amyloid-β peptide; BMP-2, bone morphogenetic protein-2; SAM, self-assembly monolayer.

[a] Using MD technique.

[b] Using MC technique.

adsorption to a surface. Because of their empirical nature, the accuracy of an empirical force field method thus critically depends on the functional form of its force field potential and the values of the force field parameters that are used to represent the behavior of a given molecular system. Also, because these methods do not typically consider changes in the electronic structure of the system, they are generally not able to represent electron transfer–related events during a simulation such as covalent-bond breaking, functional group protonation/deprotonation, charge-transfer interactions, or environment-dependent polarization effects, which typically require QM methods. This being stated, newer, more advanced empirical force field–based methods are presently being developed to incorporate various aspects of these types of atomic interactions as well. Such methods include the reactive empirical bond-order (REBO) method [80–84], which allows for bond breaking and bond formation to occur; the adaptive intermolecular reactive empirical bond-order method, which is an improved REBO by modifying nonbonded interactions to fit bond properties [85–87]; the AMOEBA polarized force field (Atomic Multipole Optimized Energetics for Biomolecular Applications) method [88]; the AMOEBAPRO polarizable force field method [89–92]; the TIP4P/FQ water model incorporating fluctuating charges [93]; and the image-charge approximation developed for the calculation of the electrostatic effects in the simulations of protein adsorption on gold surfaces [94]. The possibilities also exist to develop new hybrid simulation schemes that combine either force field and phenomenological methods, force field and ab initio methods, or all three together in multilevel global–local-type approaches.

While there are currently no reports of using a hybrid force field/phenomenological scheme in the published literature, hybrid QM/MM (or QM/MD) methods have been reported that treat systems involving electronic structure changes, such as the adsorption of a peptide onto an ionized metal surface [34], and the effect of hydration on the configuration of polar head-groups of lipids [95–102]. These hybrid approaches typically use QM to treat a small part of the overall system, which is of particular interest, thus enabling electron transfer–type events to be accurately represented, and then MM or MD to treat the larger surrounding regions of the system, thus providing a relatively realistic representation of the overall molecular environment that the smaller region resides in. The challenges in building a hybrid scheme include how to partition the subsystems for the methods that are used at the different levels of complexity and how to treat the boundary between the subsystems. The Car–Parrinello molecular dynamics (CPMD) method, which combines DFT and MD in one algorithm [103], was recently implemented by Langel et al. in studying the adsorption of amino acids on hydroxylated rutile (100) and (110) surfaces [104,105], anatase titania (101) and (001) surfaces, and a rutile (110) surface [105], in explicit water. The CPMD method explicitly includes the electrons as effective dynamical variables. The ab initio electronic and ion potential energies contribute to the total potential energy in classical MD so that the quantum mechanical effect of the electrons is included in the calculation of energy and forces for the classical motion of the atoms in a system. The combined QM and MD methods (such as the hybrid QM/MD method and the unified CPMD method introduced above) have the potential to provide a much more comprehensive understanding of adsorption phenomena in the future by enabling the interfacial region of the system to be represented with a suitable ab initio method while representing the nonreactive parts of the system (e.g., atoms of the bulk aqueous solution and bulk surface) by an empirical force field method with low computational cost.

As described above, the molecular simulation of protein–surface interactions encompasses a very broad range of topics, all of which cannot be adequately addressed in a single chapter. This chapter is therefore focused on introducing empirical force field methods. In the following sections, we will provide general information on their application for the simulation of protein–surface interactions and highlight their primary limitations. We will then introduce some of the recent efforts that have been reported to overcome some of these limitations and address what we see as the future directions of this field for further development.

12.2 Classical Force Field Methods

Because of the size of the molecular systems involved, the simulation of protein adsorption behavior requires the use of empirical force field–based simulation methods. A force field is defined as an overall package including a list of atom types, functional forms for the components of the energy expression, and parameters for atoms (atomic mass and charge) and for the force field functional terms. A force field functional calculates the total potential energy of a molecular system by summing up contributions to the potential energy from the various types of atom–atom interactions in the system. The parameters in the functional are obtained by interpolating or extrapolating from the empirical data of a small set of model systems and then applied to a larger set of related models. In practice, the accuracy of a force field is limited to the set of element types and the specific molecular environment that the force field parameters are set up to represent. For biochemistry, a typical example is the CHemistry at HARvard Molecular Mechanics (CHARMM) force field [106,107]. The CHARMM force field functional is represented as

$$E = \sum_{bonds} k_b (b - b_o)^2 + \sum_{angle} k_\theta (\theta - \theta_o)^2 + \sum_{dihedrals} k_\phi [1 + \cos(n\phi - \delta)]$$

$$+ \sum_{vdW} \varepsilon_{ij} \left[\left(\frac{R_{ij}}{r_{ij}} \right)^{12} - 2 \left(\frac{R_{ij}}{r_{ij}} \right)^{6} \right] + \sum_{Coulomb} \frac{q_i q_j}{4 \pi \varepsilon_o r_{ij}},$$

(12.1)

where the first three terms on the right-hand side represent the potential energy contributions from the covalently bonded atoms in the system. The parameters b, θ, and ϕ represent the bond length, bond angle, and dihedral angle, respectively, of the molecular system being represented, while b_o and θ_o represent the zero-energy position of the bond length and bond angle, respectively, with $(b - b_o)$ and $(\theta - \theta_o)$ thus representing covalent bond stretching and bending, respectively. The parameters k_b, k_θ, and k_ϕ are force constants (or stiffnesses) constraining the bond geometries about their zero-energy positions. The contributions of the nonbonded interactions to the potential energy are represented by the last two terms of the force field functional. The first of these two terms is the Lennard-Jones (L-J) 12–6 potential (or van der Waals [vdW] interactions), considered as pairwise repulsive and attractive interactions for all nonbonded atoms (i.e., atoms separated by more than two covalent bonds), where ε_{ij} and R_{ij} represent the L-J well depth and the atomic separation distance between two nonbonded atoms, i and j, when they are in their minimum energy positions, respectively. The second term represents the energy contributions from the electrostatic interactions between pairs of atoms, which are represented by Coulomb's law, where q_i and q_j represent the assigned partial charges centered on atoms i and j, and ε_o is the relative permittivity of free space.

CHARMM belongs to the classical first-generation force field type, referred to as a Class I force field. It is capable of accurately representing a variety of systems, from isolated small molecules to solvated biological macromolecules. However, Class I force fields are generally not considered to be highly accurate for the representation of more highly strained condensed-phase polymer system, which generally present much more complex energy-surface topographies, with the molecular states typically being further removed from their minimum energy configurations. For these types of more complex systems, second-generation force fields (i.e., Class II force fields) may be required, which use higher-order terms to represent bonded interactions as well as additional cross-terms between the bonded interactions of the force field in order to accurately represent the energetics of the system. Thus, for systems such as a protein adsorbed onto a polymer surface, the use of two types of force fields should ideally be employed to accurately represent each phase of the simulation: a protein force field, such as CHARMM, to represent the protein and aqueous solution, and a polymer force field, such as the Polymer Consistent Force Field [108–111], to represent the polymer. However, the use of two separate force fields in the same simulation creates the additional challenge of how to represent interactions at the interfacial region where the two different phases of the system, each represented by their own respective force fields, meet and interact with each other.

Moreover, in order to simulate protein–surface interactions, the force field should not simply be borrowed from other force fields that were specifically tuned for the simulation of protein folding behavior in solution or molecular interactions within solid-phase materials. Rather, if a force field is expected to accurately represent the interactions between a protein and a material surface, it must be carefully and specifically developed and validated for that specific type of system. For example, force fields have been specifically developed for simulations of protein–metal surface interactions, such as the GoIP force field [112], which was developed by the Corni group to accurately represent protein interactions with a gold (111) surface, and the ProMetCS force field [94] developed by the Wade group for modeling protein interactions with other types of metal surfaces. Figure 12.1 depicts the requirements of these types of systems [113]. This figure illustrates a protein in aqueous solution (phase 1) over a solid-phase material surface (phase 2) with the protein color coded by amino acid residue type. The force field expression is shown above this molecular system. Compared to the force field functional (Equation 12.1), which applies to

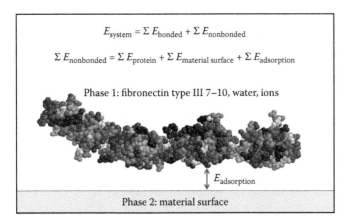

$$E_{system} = \Sigma\, E_{bonded} + \Sigma\, E_{nonbonded}$$

$$\Sigma\, E_{nonbonded} = \Sigma\, E_{protein} + \Sigma\, E_{material\ surface} + \Sigma\, E_{adsorption}$$

Phase 1: fibronectin type III 7–10, water, ions

$E_{adsorption}$

Phase 2: material surface

FIGURE 12.1
Illustration of a fibronectin protein fragment (PDB# 1FNF [114] color coded by amino acid residue type) inter-acting with a material surface. Because of the presence of the surface, the force field functional has an extra term, $E_{adsorption}$, when compared to the force field functional for each single phase. (Partially reprinted with permission from Latour, R.A. et al. Understanding protein–surface interactions at the atomistic level through the synergistic development of experimental and molecular simulation methods. In *Proteins at Interfaces III*, ed. T.A. Horbett, J. Brash, and W. Norde, ACS symposium series, Chapter 9, pp. 197–228. Copyright 2012 American Chemical Society.)

each individual phase shown in Figure 12.1, the force field functional form for the system shown in Figure 12.1 contains an extra term, which accounts for the potential energy of the nonbonded interactions between the two phases of the system. Thus, for the simulation of this type of multiphase system, force field parameters are necessary to describe how the atoms in the protein interact with each other, with the surrounding water and ions of the aqueous solution, and with the atoms from the material surface, and how the atoms contained within the material surface interact with each other. Fortunately, force field parameters have already been fairly well developed for individual phases (e.g., protein force fields for representing protein folding behavior in aqueous solution and material sci-ence force fields for representing atomic behavior in solid-phase materials). However, force fields have largely not yet been designed to represent the interfacial interactions between two different phases of a system, such as the interaction between a protein in aqueous solution and solid-phase material surfaces. Consequently, the adsorption energy term can-not be confidently represented with presently available force fields. To directly address this issue, Vellore and Latour evaluated the transferability of an existing empirical protein force field (CHARMM22/CMAP) for use with all-atom molecular simulations of protein adsorption behavior [115]. Using a biased-energy replica-exchange molecular dynamics (REMD) method (see Section 12.4), they evaluated the adsorption behavior of five model nine-amino-acid host–guest peptides over nine different functionalized alkanethiol SAM surfaces with explicitly represented solvent. Their simulation results revealed that the sim-ulations with this protein force field greatly underestimated peptide adsorption affinity on hydrophobic and positively charged amine surfaces, with calculated adsorption free energies deviating as much as 4 kcal/mol from corresponding experimental measure-ments for closely matched peptide–SAM–solvent systems. Their results clearly showed that improvements in force field methods and parameterization are necessary in order to accurately represent interactions between amino acid residues and functional groups of a surface.

In addition to the necessity of developing interfacial force field (IFF) parameters to simulate protein adsorption behavior, molecular modeling methods are also needed in order to provide simulation results that can be most directly compared to experimental data. The difficulty herein lies with the extremely large differences in time and length scale of data generated by a typical MD simulation compared to data generated by an experiment. An MD simulation generally consists of a series of incrementally time-sequenced numerical solutions of the classical equations of motion, which for a single atom may be written in Newton's notation as

$$\vec{F}_i = m_i \ddot{\vec{r}}_i, \quad \vec{F}_i = \frac{\partial E}{\partial \vec{r}_i}, \tag{12.2}$$

where m_i and $\vec{r}_i$ are mass and position of the ith atom, respectively, and $\vec{F}_i$ is the force vector acting on that atom, which directs the evolution of the conformation of a system over time. The force vector is usually derived from the derivative of the potential energy equation with respect to coordinate position, $dE(\vec{r}^N)/d\vec{r}^N$, with $E(\vec{r}^N)$ given by Equation 12.1 where $\vec{r}^N = \vec{r}_1, \vec{r}_2, \ldots, \vec{r}_N$ represents the whole set of $3N$ atomic coordinates of a system composed of N atoms (i.e., x, y, z coordinates for each atom). When performing a conventional MD simulation to represent protein adsorption behavior, the simulation represents the behavior of a single protein molecule over a time frame on the order of tens of nanoseconds. In distinct contrast to this, experimental measurements of protein adsorption/desorption processes typically represent the average behavior of billions of proteins over time frames ranging from seconds to hours. Because of this large disconnect between the physical and temporal conditions, direct comparisons between results obtained by a conventional MD simulation and experimental results can be very difficult to make with any degree of confidence. To overcome these types of problems, methods referred to as advanced or accelerated sampling have been developed and applied. For example, recently, the steered molecular dynamics (SMD) method has been applied in modeling protein adsorption behavior in an attempt to speed up the kinetics represented by the system [58,59,63]. In this method, artificial forces are used to pull the protein in designated directions to accelerate the adsorption/desorption processes. Although the SMD method can increase the speed of protein diffusion to or away from the surface, thus effectively increasing the time frame of the simulation, it still does not solve the kinetic trapping problem. Kinetic trapping causes protein conformations to stay in local energy minima for relatively long periods, impeding the ability to sufficiently sample all of the relevant protein conformational states in reasonable simulation time. To overcome this problem, advanced sampling methods that enable molecular simulations to rapidly construct thermodynamically equilibrated ensembles of states of the molecular system are required. Averages obtained from the resulting ensembles of states can then be confidently compared with experimental data on the basis of the ergodic hypothesis, which states that equilibrated conformational ensemble averages of a system are equal to equilibrated time averages of the same system [116]. Correspondingly, new experimental methods are needed to provide molecular-level information that can be used to evaluate, tune, and validate the methods developed for molecular simulation. For example, experimental data on the amount of protein adsorbed to a particular surface, which is the most commonly measured parameter in protein adsorption experiments, is of little use for comparison with molecular simulation results. Rather, experimental data are needed that quantitatively provide information regarding the specific interactions between individual amino acid residues of a protein and functional groups on a surface so that force field parameterization can be appropriately assessed and tuned to represent these types of interactions. In addition, there is also a need for experimental methods that provide quantitative information regarding the orientational and conformational state of proteins after they adsorb on a surface, with minimal influence of protein–protein effects, so that the accuracy of predictions made by simulations of protein adsorption behavior can be properly assessed.

12.3 Design of Model Peptide–Surface Interacting Systems

As noted at the end of Section 12.2, before force field parameters can be assessed and tuned to represent the interactions between amino acid residues of a protein and a surface, quantitative experimental data are first required for properties that characterize these types of interactions and that can be calculated by molecular simulation for direct comparison. In order to generate these kinds of data sets, our laboratory has designed a variety of experimental model peptide–surface systems over the past decade. Then, as a means of characterizing amino acid–surface interactions using these model systems, we have also developed and applied methods to determine the standard-state free energy of peptide–surface interactions (ΔG°_{ads}) using surface plasmon resonance (SPR) spectroscopy [117,118] and atomic force microscopy (AFM) methods [119,120].

12.3.1 Host–Guest Peptide Model

The host–guest model peptides that we designed (synthesized by Biomatik, Wilmington, Delaware; characterized by analytical high-performance liquid chromatography and mass spectral analysis with 98% purity) have the amino acid sequence of TGTG–X–GTGT (for SPR studies) and TGTG–X–GTCT (for AFM studies) with zwitterionic end groups, where G, T, and C are glycine (–H side chain), threonine (–CH(CH₃)OH side chain), and cysteine (–CH₂SH side chain), respectively. X represents a *guest* amino acid residue, which can be any of the 20 naturally occurring amino acid types. The guest amino acid residue is placed in the middle of the peptide to represent the characteristics of a mid-chain amino acid in a protein by positioning it relatively far from the zwitterionic end groups of the peptide. The threonine (T) residues and the zwitterionic end groups were selected to enhance aqueous solubility and to provide additional molecular weight (MW) for SPR detection while the nonchiral glycine residues were selected to inhibit the formation of secondary structure. The cysteine (C) residue was required for the AFM studies as the linker to connect our host–guest peptide sequences to the AFM probe tip. SPR studies were conducted using both of these peptide models to show that the TGTG–X–GTCT peptide can be used in AFM studies as an equivalent system for comparison with the TGTG–X–GTGT peptide model used by SPR [120,121].

12.3.2 SAM Surfaces

As model experimental surfaces for both SPR and AFM studies, Wei et al. synthesized alkanethiol SAM monolayers on gold with the structure of HS(CH₂)₁₁–Y, with Y representing functional groups contained in a wide range of organic polymers, such as Y = OH, CH₃, OC₆H₅, NH₂, COOH, NHCOCH₃, COOCH₃, and EG₃OH (EG: ethylene glycol segment,

TABLE 12.2

Values of $\Delta G°_{ads}$ (in Kilocalories per Mole) for Peptide–SAM Combinations

-X-	SAM-OH	SAM-COOH	SAM-EG$_3$OH	SAM-NH$_2$	SAM-NHCOCH$_3$	SAM-COOCH$_3$	SAM-OC$_6$H$_5$	SAM-OCH$_2$CF$_3$	SAM-CH$_3$
Nonpolar Guest Residues									
-L-	-0.003 (0.001)	-1.30 (0.43)	-0.40 (0.28)	-2.34 (0.80)	-1.04 (0.30)	-2.06 (0.31)	-2.68 (0.72)	-3.09 (0.31)	-3.87 (0.69)
-F-	a	a	-0.30 (0.13)	a	-2.44 (0.40)	a	a	-3.97 (0.24)	-4.16 (0.16)
-V-	-0.002 (0.001)	-1.11 (0.31)	-0.26 (0.06)	-3.90 (0.12)	-0.16 (0.10)	a	a	-3.99 (0.22)	-4.40 (0.31)
-A-	a	a	-0.97 (0.36)	a	a	a	a	a	a
-W-	-0.001 (0.001)	-1.14 (0.52)	-1.72 (0.33)	-2.71 (0.32)	-1.94 (0.45)	-0.92 (0.36)	-1.65 (0.60)	-3.42 (0.27)	-3.89 (0.34)
Polar Guest Residues									
-T-	-0.001 (0.001)	-0.87 (0.46)	-0.28 (0.15)	-3.15 (0.50)	-0.16 (0.09)	-0.40 (0.14)	-2.89 (0.75)	-2.81 (0.40)	-2.76 (0.28)
-G-	-0.001 (0.001)	-0.68 (0.36)	-0.30 (0.20)	-2.56 (0.32)	-1.86 (0.20)	-1.18 (0.30)	-3.51 (0.22)	-3.30 (0.37)	-3.40 (0.39)
-S-	-0.002 (0.001)	-1.10 (0.10)	-0.34 (0.11)	-2.09 (0.98)	-1.49 (0.47)	-1.55 (0.26)	-3.20 (0.28)	-3.22 (0.24)	-2.75 (0.23)
-N-	-0.004 (0.003)	-0.86 (0.38)	-0.59 (0.11)	-3.22 (0.41)	-1.64 (0.23)	-1.37 (0.68)	-3.02 (0.16)	-3.41 (0.32)	-4.33 (0.62)
Charged Guest Residues									
-R-	-0.002 (0.001)	-1.53 (0.19)	-0.20 (0.10)	-3.03 (0.31)	-1.60 (0.80)	-1.17 (0.35)	-2.26 (0.82)	-3.45 (0.31)	-4.15 (0.55)
-K-	-0.001 (0.001)	-1.71 (0.19)	-0.19 (0.07)	-3.14 (0.20)	-0.12 (0.07)	-1.77 (0.07)	-3.35 (0.25)	-3.54 (0.45)	-3.34 (0.39)
-D-	-0.003 (0.001)	-1.06 (0.09)	-0.44 (0.14)	-3.75 (0.20)	-1.93 (0.52)	-1.34 (0.50)	-3.89 (0.23)	-3.59 (0.37)	-3.54 (0.60)

Source: Reprinted with permission from Wei, Y. and R.A. Latour. Benchmark experimental data set and assessment of adsorption free energy for peptide–surface interactions. *Langmuir* 25: 5637–5646. Copyright 2009 American Chemical Society.

Note: The guest amino acids (X) are ranked by a standard hydrophobicity scale [10] from the most-to-least degree of hydrophobicity. Data are expressed as mean (±95% confidence interval) ($n = 6$).

a A condition in which peptide adsorption was so strong that it was determined to be irreversible, in which case $\Delta G°_{ads}$ could not be determined.

–(O–CH$_2$–CH$_2$)–) [117,122]. They have also investigated material surfaces that are not conducive for SPR, including fused silica glass (Chemglass Life Sciences, Vineland, New Jersey), high-density polyethylene (MW = 125,000 Da, Sigma Chemical Co., St. Louis, Missouri), and poly(methyl-methacrylate) (PMMA) (MW = 350,000 Da, Sigma Chemical Co.). All of the surfaces were characterized for quality assurance by x-ray photoelectron spectroscopy, static water contact angle, ellipsometry for thickness, and AFM for surface roughness.

The combination of the designed host–guest model peptides and SAM surfaces produced a large range of peptide–surface adsorption systems. For each of these systems, adsorption free energy, $\Delta G°_{ads}$, was determined by adsorption isotherm measurements by SPR spectroscopy or correlated desorption force measurements by AFM. Table 12.2 presents the adsorption free energies for various host–guest peptide/SAM combinations. The experimental methods in determining $\Delta G°_{ads}$ are discussed in detail in Refs. [10] and [123]. These methods thus provide a means to obtain adsorption free energies that are useful for the evaluation, modification, and validation of empirical force field parameters that should then be able to be used to enable peptide and protein adsorption behavior to be accurately represented by molecular simulation.

12.4 Peptide–Surface Adsorption Free Energy Calculation

Corresponding to the peptide–surface systems used in the SPR and AFM studies, molecular simulations were conducted to calculate adsorption free energies using the CHARMM22/CMAP force field for comparison to the experimental data sets. For these studies, molecular models were constructed for each of the nine different types of alkanethiol SAM and material surfaces, and eight TGTG–X–GTGT peptides, with X = V, F, T, W, G, N, D, and K (thus representing each class of amino acid: nonpolar aliphatic, aromatic, polar, negatively charged, and positively charged). The bottom sulfur atom of each alkanethiol chain composing the SAM surface was fixed in position to provide stability for the surface. Each system was then constructed by placing a water layer on top of the surface using the TIP3P water model [115]. The host–guest peptide was then placed in the top water layer and an additional 15-Å water layer with waters kept fixed was placed between the top water layer and adjacent (bottom) of the surface layer to prevent interaction of the peptide with the bottom of the surface layer when periodic boundary conditions are applied. A representative illustration of the model system for the X = V peptide over a CH$_3$–SAM surface is shown in Figure 12.2. Specific details about the setup of the adsorption model are provided in Ref. [115]. It should be noted that when performing MD simulations for a system with fixed atoms, traditional isobaric algorithms (e.g., NPT simulation; constant number of atoms [N], constant temperature [T], and constant pressure [P]) often cannot be used since the presence of fixed atoms prevents atom-coordinate rescaling, which is used to control the pressure of the system. Furthermore, for simulation programs that are able to avoid this rescaling issue and thus enable NPT conditions to be used, the presence of fixed atoms can cause the calculated pressure of the system to be substantially different from the actual pressure in the solution phase of the system owing to contributions from the nonphysical nature of the atomic constraints applied to the fixed atoms and their influence upon the surrounding atoms of the surface layer. To overcome these problems, Yancey et al. have proposed an accurate approach to calculate the internal pressure for systems with constraint components [124].

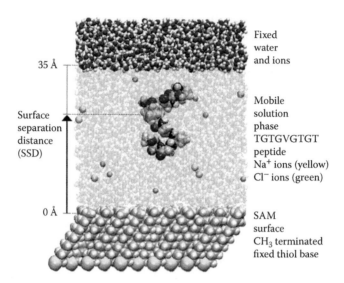

35 Å

Surface
separation
distance
(SSD)

0 Å

Fixed
water
and ions

Mobile
solution
phase
TGTGVGTGT
peptide
Na$^+$ ions (yellow)
Cl$^-$ ions (green)

SAM
surface
CH$_3$ terminated
fixed thiol base

FIGURE 12.2
Molecular model of a TGTG–V–GTGT peptide over a hydrophobic CH$_3$–SAM surface in TIP3P water. (Reprinted with permission from Vellore, N.A. et al. Assessment of the transferability of a protein force field for the simulation of peptide–surface interactions. *Langmuir* 26: 7396–7404. Copyright 2009 American Chemical Society.)

Molecular simulations were conducted for each of these systems using the CHARMM molecular simulation program and the CHARMM22/CMAP force field with advanced sampling methods applied in order to calculate the adsorption free energy for comparison with the experimental results. Adsorption free energy for each of these systems was determined by using the surface separation distance (SSD) as the reaction coordinate. SSD represents the z-coordinate distance (i.e., direction normal to the surface plane) from the center of mass of the peptide to the center of mass of all surface head atoms. To accurately calculate adsorption free energy, an effective molecular simulation method must (1) adequately sample the peptide's position over the entire range of SSD and (2) adequately sample the conformational state of the peptide at each SSD position. Once this degree of sampling of the system is achieved using an appropriate advanced sampling scheme (addressed below), the resulting sampled ensemble of states over the SSD-coordinate can be translated into a probability density profile representing the probability of the peptide being positioned in an adsorbed state over the surface relative to its probability to be in a nonadsorbed state in bulk solution above the surface. The ratio of these probabilities provides the ability to then calculate adsorption free energy from the simulation in a manner that is analogous to that used in the SPR experiments where adsorption free energy is determined at equilibrium by the concentration of the peptide when adsorbed to a surface compared to its concentration in solution [114].

For a peptide–surface adsorption process at room-temperature conditions, the potential of mean force (PMF) as a function of SSD (which is equivalent to a free energy vs. SSD profile) typically follows the relationship presented by Line A in Figure 12.3, which indicates strongest adsorption around about SSD = 6 Å. In a simulation using a conventional sampling method like straightforward MD, once the peptide is positioned within this range of SSD, it tends to become trapped within the deep part of the potential well for the entire simulation instead of sampling over the entire range of SSD, which is necessary for the proper calculation of adsorption free energy [14]. This situation is referred to as the SSD-sampling problem. To overcome this problem, Wang et al. [125] and O'Brien et al. [126] developed a sampling

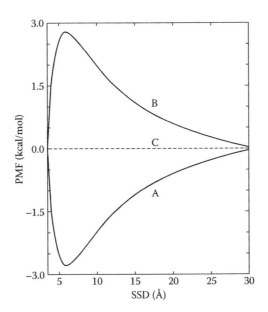

FIGURE 12.3
Schematic representations of the curve shape of (A) the PMF for peptide–surface adsorption without biasing, (B) the bias PMF, and (C) the flattened residual PMF.

method in which a biased energy function (Line B in Figure 12.3), which is derived as closely as possible to exactly mirror the free energy profile (Line A in Figure 12.3), is added to the force field functional form as a biasing energy term. This biasing term thus serves to effectively counter the presence of the low-energy well that was previously causing the peptide to be trapped at the surface, with the resulting PMF versus SSD profile becoming flat (Line C in Figure 12.3), thus eliminating the local energy well that was previously trapping the peptide close to the surface and thereby overcoming the SSD-sampling problem. For practical implementation, an estimate of the biasing function is first derived using the umbrella sampling method to obtain an estimate of the PMF versus SSD profile [127,128]. For this method, a series of parallel simulations is conducted with constraining potentials applied to force the peptide to sample overlapping, incrementally increasing regions of SSD positions over the full SSD-coordinate space (e.g., set to sample SSD values between 3 and 25 Å in 1-Å increments). The resulting sampled SSD trajectories from the umbrella sampling simulations are then analyzed using the statistical mechanics–based weighted histogram analysis method (WHAM) [129,130], which removes the effects of the applied biasing potentials to calculate an unbiased PMF profile as a function of SSD. The resulting PMF profile is then fitted to a modified Derjaguin, Landau, Verwey, and Overbeek (DLVO) potential [131,132] and the negative of this fitted function is added to the force field functional as a biasing potential in subsequent MD simulations. This procedure thus enables the peptide to escape from a strongly adsorbing surface during the simulation, which is needed to adequately sample the position of the peptide over the full SSD-coordinate space for the proper calculation of ΔG°_{ads}. After conducting a simulation with the biased potential, the resulting biased probability densities are corrected using statistical mechanics principles to remove the effects of the applied biased-energy function to give an unbiased probability distribution. This distribution is then used to calculate a final free energy of adsorption value using the probability-ratio method. Further details of these methods are provided elsewhere [125,126].

Although the use of this energy-biasing method can provide adequate sampling over the SSD-coordinate space, it is still not sufficient by itself to provide adequate sampling of the conformation states of the peptide at each SSD position. In order to generate a properly equilibrated ensemble of states from a simulation, Wang et al. [125] and O'Brien et al. [126] used a combined scheme of the biased-energy method along with the replica-exchange molecular dynamics (REMD) method (further addressed in Section 12.6.1) [133,134]. The REMD method uses elevated temperatures combined with statistical mechanics algorithms to greatly improve the sampling of the conformation space of the peptide. While the use of either of these advanced sampling methods alone does not provide adequate sampling for the accurate calculation of adsorption free energy, their combined use enables both sampling problems to be efficiently overcome in a single simulation, thus enabling adsorption free energy to be properly determined.

After performing a biased-energy REMD simulation and correcting the resulting ensemble of sampled conformational states, the adsorption free energy can be calculated based on the unbiased probability distribution [125,126]:

$$\Delta G^{\circ}_{ads} = -RT \ln \left\{ \frac{W}{\delta} \sum_{i=1}^{N} (P_i/P_b) \right\}, \qquad (12.3)$$

where N is the number of SSD bins over the full SSD-coordinate space, δ is the theoretical thickness of the adsorbed layer (approximately 12 Å for a nine-amino-acid residue peptide; see Refs. [10] and [123] for further details), and W is the SSD bin width used to produce the probability distribution. P_i and P_b are the probabilities of the peptide being at positions SSD_i, and SSD_b, respectively, with SSD_b defined to be the distance from the surface for which peptide–surface interactions become negligibly small, which is typically beyond 15 Å from the surface plane for these host–guest peptides. Once ΔG°_{ads} values are determined from the simulations, the accuracy of the force field used in the simulations can be evaluated by comparing the simulation results with the experimental results obtained from the SPR and AFM studies for corresponding systems. Differences between the calculated and experimental ΔG°_{ads} values are then used to identify situations where IFF parameters need to be adjusted to properly represent peptide adsorption behavior. However, as discussed below, before IFF parameters can be applied to correct identified problems in peptide adsorption behavior, additional modifications to the applied simulation methods are required.

12.5 IFF Method

The development and application of an IFF to predict peptide and protein adsorption behavior more accurately is a relatively new area of research in the biomaterials field. The use of IFF parameters in a simulation requires tuning the nonbonded parameters (i.e., electrostatic and vdW interactions) that control the interactions between atoms of the peptide/protein and water with the atoms of the surface. However, simply changing the CHARMM nonbonded parameters that control the interactions of the peptide, water, and ions with the atoms of a surface is ill-advised because these parameters were previously carefully optimized over the past several decades by the CHARMM development group to accurately represent protein folding behavior in aqueous solution. Therefore, modification of these parameters in order to correct peptide adsorption behavior will likely have the undesirable consequence of causing unknown errors in peptide folding behavior. Of course, in order to accurately represent protein adsorption interactions, both protein–surface interactions and protein folding behavior must accurately be represented. In order to overcome this problem, our laboratory developed what we refer to as the dual force field (Dual-FF) simulation method and implemented it in the CHARMM molecular simulation program [135]. The Dual-FF method uses two separate sets of nonbonded force field parameters within the same simulation: one set to represent intraphase interactions (i.e., the interactions between atoms of the solution phase or solid phase with other atoms of the same phase) and a separate set to independently represent interphase interactions (i.e., interactions between atoms of the solution phase with atoms of the solid phase). Using this approach, the interfacial parameters can thus be independently adjusted to correct errors in peptide adsorption free energy while maintaining the use of the regular CHARMM protein force field to properly control peptide conformational behavior in solution, as well as a material force field to properly control the conformational behavior of the atoms of the material surface.

The concept of the Dual-FF method is illustrated in Figure 12.4. To implement the Dual-FF capability into CHARMM, a phase-type identifier for each atom in the simulated system is set to a user-defined value for each phase present in the system. The CHARMM topology and parameter files and storage arrays are also updated to include an interfacial set of partial charges and vdW parameters. The potential energies from pairwise nonbonded interactions that are calculated during a simulation are then modified to be dictated by a comparison of the atom phase types for each specific interaction: if the two atoms being compared belong to the same phase (i.e., solution phase or solid phase in Figure 12.4), the standard intraphase parameters of the CHARMM force field are used, and if the two atoms

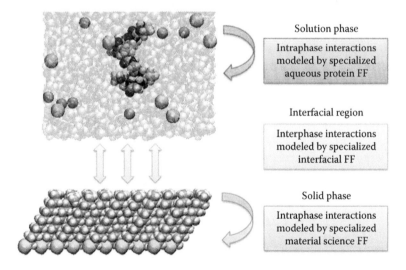

FIGURE 12.4
Schematic representation of the Dual-FF model applied to a peptide adsorption simulation. The solution and solid surface phases are modeled by specialized force fields that accurately represent intraphase interactions while all interactions between atoms of the solution phase and the solid phase are handled by a specialized IFF that is tuned to accurately represent peptide adsorption free energy. (Reprinted with permission from Latour, R.A. et al. Understanding protein–surface interactions at the atomistic level through the synergistic development of experimental and molecular simulation methods. In *Proteins at Interfaces III*, ed. T.A. Horbett, J. Brash, and W. Norde, ACS symposium series, Chapter 9, pp. 197–228. Copyright 2012 American Chemical Society.)

compared belong to different phases, the interfacial parameters are then used. The implementation of such a nonbonded scheme is relatively simple for cutoff-based nonbonded interactions; however, implementing Ewald summation [136] for the rigorous treatment of long-range electrostatic interactions is more involved and still under development. Despite this current limitation, preliminary studies comparing the handling of electrostatic effects using simple cutoffs versus Ewald summation have shown that differences in the use of these two methods for the calculation of adsorption free energies for peptide–surface interactions result in a difference of less than approximately 0.5 kcal/mol [114].

In Dual-FF parameterization, only the vdW and electrostatic interaction terms of the force field need to be considered. To determine which of these two factors have the greatest influence on peptide adsorption behavior, the contributions of electrostatic and vdW interactions can be separated by appropriate changes made in the Dual-FF parameterization. For example, electrostatic interactions can be eliminated by setting partial charges controlling the interactions between the solution-phase atoms and the surface-phase atoms to zero, while vdW interactions can be effectively eliminated by setting the well depth parameter (ε) of the Lennard-Jones potential to a very low value (e.g., 10^{-4}), which then makes vdW attraction negligibly small while maintaining atomic repulsion to prevent atom–atom overlap. By comparing PMF versus peptide SSD profiles obtained from simulations using these conditions in comparison to the behavior provided by the regular set of CHARMM force field parameters, assessment can be made regarding which set of parameters most strongly influences the adsorption behavior, thus indicating which parameters can be adjusted to most effectively correct identified errors in the adsorption free energy. Specific details in parameterizing the Dual-FF can be found in Refs. [115] and [135]. Figure 12.5 presents an example comparing experimentally determined adsorption

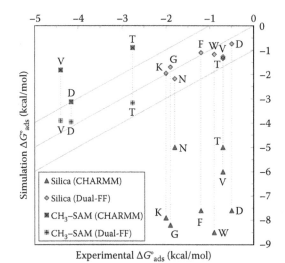

FIGURE 12.5

Comparison of the calculated ΔG°_{ads} values with corresponding experimental values. The values shown in dark gray are those obtained from a simulation with regular CHARMM parameters and the values shown in light gray are obtained from a Dual-FF simulation using optimized IFF parameters. Confidence intervals for both the experimental and simulation mean values are on the order of approximately 0.5 kcal/mol. (Reprinted with permission from Latour, R.A. et al. Understanding protein–surface interactions at the atomistic level through the synergistic development of experimental and molecular simulation methods. In *Proteins at Interfaces III*, ed. T.A. Horbett, J. Brash, and W. Norde, ACS symposium series, Chapter 9, pp. 197–228. Copyright 2012 American Chemical Society.)

free energies and calculated adsorption free energies using the regular CHARMM force field and Dual-FF parameters. These simulations were conducted for the adsorption of different TGTG–X–GTGT host–guest peptides over silica glass and CH_3–SAM surfaces. The results from these studies indicated that the adsorption free energies from simulations using the regular CHARMM force field are moderately underestimated for the CH_3–SAM surface and greatly overestimated for the silica glass. As indicated, IFF parameter modification using the Dual-FF approach enabled the calculated adsorption free energies to be brought into close agreement with the experimental data, thus indicating that a much more realistic balance has been achieved between the attraction of individual amino acids of these peptides and water molecules for the functional groups presented by each of these surfaces [114].

12.6 Advanced Sampling Methods

As introduced in Section 12.2, conventional MD methods are largely computationally insufficient for modeling protein–surface interactions, both because of the extremely large number of degrees of freedom that must be represented in a simulation and because of the inherent problem of very slow phase-space sampling that arises owing to the presence of relatively high-energy barriers separating the extremely numerous local energy minima contained within these types of systems. More efficient methods of searching the conformational phase space of a complex molecular system have been developed to address these issues. The most promising types of methods to overcome these problems include (i) the combination of statistical mechanics algorithms along with elevated temperature to accelerate the crossing of energy barriers in the system and (ii) the use of coarse graining combined with the implicit representation of solvation effects, which involves combining groups of atoms into single *bead* elements and incorporating solvation energy effects directly within the force field. The first type of approach accelerates the sampling of the system by speeding up the kinetics of energy-barrier crossing, while the second approach provides accelerated sampling by greatly reducing the number of degrees of freedom in the system. In this section, we provide an overview of our efforts to develop and implement both of these types of advanced sampling techniques for the efficient simulation of protein adsorption behavior.

12.6.1 Advanced Sampling Techniques

Among these types of methods, REMD has proven to be one of the most successful and extensively used for the simulation of biological molecules [133,134]. Figure 12.6 schematically compares a conventional MD simulation with an REMD simulation for a simple model system containing three potential energy wells. As shown in Figure 12.6, REMD conducts a number of parallel simulations at sequentially increasing temperature levels and periodically attempts to exchange configurations between adjacent levels following a Boltzmann-weighted process. By sampling and exchanging over the temperature space, the molecular system is able to overcome the kinetic trapping problem experienced in conventional MD simulations. Recently, the REMD method has been applied to study protein–surface interactions. These efforts include the work of Garcia's group studying the adsorption of proteins on a carbon nanotube surface [45], the work of Walsh's group

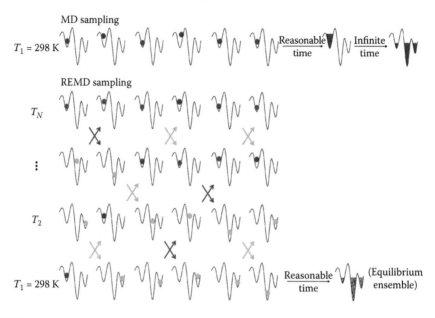

FIGURE 12.6
Schematic comparison of a conventional MD sampling with an REMD sampling for a model system containing three potential energy wells. Although the MD method can build an equilibrium ensemble at a very long (or infinite) simulation time, it is trapped in a local low-energy well during the reasonable simulation time, resulting in a poorly sampled system, whereas the REMD simulation uses thermal energy to enable the system to readily escape from the potential energy well. The Metropolis-type exchange procedure used to swap replicas at adjacent temperature levels enables the development of an equilibrium ensemble of states being sampled at the baseline temperature in reasonable time, thus representing a much more efficient sampling method.

studying quartz binding peptides [137], and the studies of adsorption of peptides on various surfaces conducted in our laboratory [115,124–126,135]. Still, practical difficulties remain in the application of REMD for large molecular systems [138,139]. In REMD, the size of the molecular system being simulated is dictated by the REMD algorithm, with large molecular systems requiring the use of a large number of replicas at closely spaced temperature levels to create sufficient overlap between the sampled potential energy states of adjacent replicas in order to obtain an acceptable degree of exchange. The implementation of REMD thus becomes increasingly computationally expensive as the size of the molecular system being simulated increases. In addition to the large computational cost, the use of a large number of replicas also results in the slow diffusion of replicas over the numerous temperature levels, thus resulting in poor sampling efficiency. Recently, some successful attempts aimed at improving the efficiency of the conventional REMD method have emerged. The efforts include the reservoir REMD method [140] developed by Roitberg et al. and the convective REMD method [141] developed by Spill et al. The reservoir REMD uses a fewer number of replicas by coupling replica exchange to a prebuilt, non-Boltzmann-populated reservoir as a source of additional conformational states at the highest temperature level to effectively seed the sampling with states that otherwise may not be readily sampled, and the convective REMD method eliminates the random travel of replicas in conventional REMD by forcing a replica to travel in one direction both up and down the temperature ladder.

To overcome the above problems of the conventional REMD method, we have developed a new empirical sampling method, which we call "temperature intervals with global exchange of replicas" (TIGER2) [139,142]. This advanced sampling method was specifically designed for systems that are deemed to be too large for REMD. Similar to REMD, a TIGER2 simulation involves the use of a number of replicas (N_r) running in parallel at different temperature levels. However, the number of replicas used in a TIGER2 simulation is independent on the size of the system; hence, it is able to use a much lower number of replicas when compared to REMD, thus allowing the user to set the computational cost of the simulation to match the available computational resources at hand. In a TIGER2 simulation, the sampling is composed of a series of cycles (shown in Figure 12.7) with each cycle containing four stages: (1) rapid heating from a baseline temperature (T_B) to the replica temperature (T_m) by rescaling the momenta of the atoms within the replica by a factor of $\sqrt{T_m/T_B}$ and thermally equilibrating, (2) MD sampling at constant temperature (T_m), (3) rapid quenching replicas sampled at elevated temperatures back down to T_B by rescaling the momenta by a factor of $\sqrt{T_B/T_m}$ followed by thermal equilibration, and (4) global replica reassignment. Stage 4 consists of two substeps: (i) one state from among the set of ($N_r - 1$) quenched states is randomly selected with a probability of $1/(N_r - 1)$, and the potential energy of this state is then compared with the potential energy from the production run of the baseline replica using the Metropolis criterion, and (ii) all replicas except the selected baseline replica are then reassigned to higher temperature levels according to their potential energies; that is, a higher potential energy state is assigned to a higher temperature level. This algorithm thus enables temperature to be used to accelerate the crossing of energy barriers in the system with much less computational cost than REMD. The validity of this new advanced sampling method has been demonstrated by comparison with REMD simulation results for the folding behavior of relatively small peptides and proteins that could be handled by both methods, including alanine dipeptide, $(AAQAA)_3$ [(Ala-Ala-Gln-Ala-Ala)$_3$], chignolin (Gly-Tyr-Asp-Pro-Glu-Thr-Gly-Thr-Trp-Gly) peptides [139], and protein G [142]. The TIGER2 results closely matched the REMD results for each of these model systems, thus demonstrating that the TIGER2 algorithm is able to closely approximate Boltzmann statistics, which is required for the accurate simulation of a

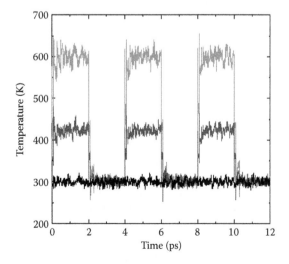

FIGURE 12.7

Three representative heating–sampling–quenching cycles generated by a TIGER2 simulation for alanine dipeptide in explicit solvent using three replicas at 300, 425, and 600 K temperature levels.

molecular system. Interested readers are referred to Ref. [139], which provides more detail regarding how this algorithm functions, and Ref. [142], which provides guidance regarding parameter set up for the proper implementation of the TIGER2 method.

The adsorption of proteins on the surface of amorphous polymers is another important area of research, which adds the additional challenge of accurately representing the complex behavior of the long-chain entangled molecules of the polymer surface as well as protein adsorption processes [22,74,105,143,144]. These types of simulations thus require the development of efficient algorithms to equilibrate condensed-phase polymers with high chain-packing density. Recently, a number of efficient sampling techniques have been developed for this purpose. For example, a method developed by Auhl et al. [145] is based on the prepacking of Gaussian chains and gradual introduction of the excluded volume. Alternatively, the pivot and bridging algorithms developed by Graessley et al. [146] and Kamio et al. [147] rapidly change the configuration of systems by forming new bonds across pairs of chains. In our efforts to develop algorithms for the efficient equilibration of amorphous polymer surfaces, we developed a new scheme termed "temperature intervals with global exchange of replicas and reduced radii" (TIGER3) [148]. The TIGER3 process is similar to that of TIGER2 in cycling. The only difference of TIGER3 from TIGER2 is that, in TIGER3, the sampling stage at elevated temperature levels is conducted with four substeps under constant volume conditions composed of (1) MC sampling with reduced vdW radii (we used zero vdW radii to turn off both attraction and repulsion terms), (2) energy minimization with the vdW radii recovered to their regular force field values, (3) relaxation using the MC method, and (4) MD sampling for further equilibration. Basically, The TIGER3 method allows chain segments to pass through one another at elevated temperature levels during the sampling stage by reducing the vdW radii of the atoms, thus eliminating chain entanglement problems. Atomic radii are then returned to their regular values and reequilibrated at elevated temperature before quenching to the baseline temperature (see Figure 12.8a). For its actual application, we use a mixed TIGER2/TIGER3 scheme with which the TIGER3 part enables the crossing of polymer chain segments while the TIGER2 part relaxes and equilibrates the system after chain passing and the return of the atomic radii to their normal sizes. The ratio of TIGER2 to TIGER3 cycles implemented in the mixed method is determined by the value of the exchange acceptance ratio that is obtained from pretest runs of the molecular system. A schematic illustrating the TIGER2/TIGER3 algorithm is schematically shown in Figure 12.8b. The TIGER3 method has been applied to generate bulk structures of a series of amorphous polymers such as PMMA, PBMA [148], and hydrated PDLLA [149] at their correct amorphous-phase densities. The equilibrium structure factors of all the calculated systems have been found to provide excellent agreement with the experimentally measured values, thus indicating that TIGER2/TIGER3 is a promising sampling method for building condensed-phase polymer surfaces.

12.6.2 Representation of Solvation Effect

The importance of properly representing solvation (water in most cases) effects in simulations of protein adsorption on material surfaces was addressed by Latour in Ref. [19]. As was pointed out, the contribution of water to the adsorption interaction includes water–water, water–protein, and water–surface interactions in the interfacial region of the molecular system. The most direct and most accurate way of representing aqueous solvation effects in an MD simulation is to explicitly include individual water molecules along with salt ions (e.g., 140 mM Na^+/Cl^- for representing the physiological environment) plus additional counter-ions for overall charge neutrality. Various explicit water models have been

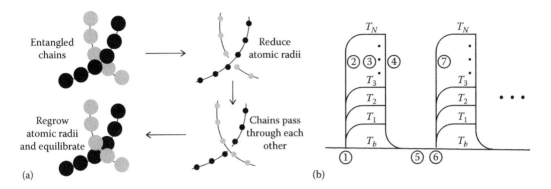

FIGURE 12.8

(a) A schematic representation of the TIGER3 scheme. (Reprinted with permission from Li, X., and R.A. Latour. Construction and validation of all-atom bulk-phase models of amorphous polymers using the TIGER2/TIGER3 empirical sampling method. *Macromolecules* 44: 5452–5464. Copyright 2009 American Chemical Society.) (b) A schematic representation of the TIGER2/TIGER3 algorithm. TIGER2: (1) A set of $N + 1$ replicas is assigned to temperatures ranging from T_b (baseline temperature of interest) to T_N with uniform separation between temperature levels. (2) Replicas assigned to elevated temperatures are rapidly heated by velocity rescaling. (3) Replicas are equilibrated at each assigned temperature. (4) Replicas are rapidly quenched by velocity rescaling to T_b and (5) equilibrated at T_b. (6) One quenched replica is randomly selected and its potential energy is compared with that of the baseline replica using the Metropolis criterion. If the Metropolis criterion is satisfied, the selected high-temperature replica is added to the sampled ensemble of states and reassigned to T_b. If not, the baseline replica is added to the ensemble and reassigned to T_b for the next cycle. Replicas not reassigned to T_b are then assigned to the elevated temperature levels on the basis of their potential energies, with the highest potential energy being assigned to T_N. A TIGER3 cycle is similar to TIGER2, except that the radii of the CG beads for the replicas assigned to the higher temperature are reduced to zero to allow chain segments to pass through one another. As part of step 3, the beads are then regrown in size and the systems are energy minimized and then reequilibrated to their designated elevated temperature level before quenching back down to T_b. (Reprinted with permission from Li, X. et al. Structure of hydrated poly(D,L-lactic acid) studied with x-ray diffraction and molecular simulation methods. *Macromolecules* 45: 4896–4906. Copyright 2009 American Chemical Society.)

developed over the years, the most popular of which include SPC [150,151], SPC/E [151], TIP3P [152], TIP4P [152–154], TIP4P/Ew [155,156], and TIP5P [157].

While the explicit representation of water provides the most accurate representation of protein–surface interactions, it greatly increases the number of degrees of freedom in a molecular system, thus greatly increasing the computational cost of the simulation. In order to reduce the computational cost of using explicit solvation, approximate methods have been developed to represent solvation effects without representing individual water molecules. The development of these approximate methods has been undertaken in two directions: (1) implicit solvation methods based on mean-field continuum approximations and (2) coarse-grained (CG) methods in which a number of water molecules are clustered together and represented by a single bead.

One of the simplest methods that have been applied in attempts to implicitly represent solvation effects is known as the distance-dependent dielectric method [158], in which a relative dielectric screening parameter is included in the denominator of the Coulomb's law expression in the force field (see Equation 12.1). This parameter is typically set to be equal to the radial distance between the interacting atoms, thus serving to increasingly screen electrostatic interactions as two charged species move apart from one another. While the use of this method is extremely attractive because it results in minimal additional computational cost, several comparative studies have shown this method to be highly inaccurate [159,160] and at best represents dampened vacuum-like environmental conditions as opposed to the representation of aqueous solution [158]. Thus, this method should never be used for the simulation of peptide/protein–surface interactions and results obtained from simulations using this implicit solvation method should not be taken seriously. More respectable and physically based numerical approaches to implicitly represent solvation effects are the Poisson–Boltzmann equation method and its much less computational expensive approximation, the generalized Born (GB) equation method [161–167]. However, as was pointed by Latour [19] and Sun et al. [168], the GB method alone is not able to properly describe protein–surface interaction because it substantially overestimates the strength of hydrogen bond interactions between functional groups that are explicitly represented in the system. Furthermore, it only addresses the electrostatic component of solvation effects, while completely neglecting hydrophobic interactions.

Over the past couple of decades, more sophisticated and accurate implicit solvation models have been developed, such as the Screened Coulomb Potentials Implicit Solvent Model (SCP-ISM) [169–172] and the GB models based on solvent-accessible surface area method (GB/SA) [167,173]. These models provide a more accurate representation of hydrogen bonding and hydrophobic effects and are able to offer excellent balance between efficiency and accuracy for protein folding in aqueous solution. Unfortunately, none of the currently available implicit solvation models have yet been validated to accurately represent the competitive interaction of water for protein adsorption behavior, which limits their use for this type of application at this time. The use of implicit solvation methods, however, is still highly desirable because of the reduction in computational requirements that they provide. Thus, there is a great need for the development of new implicit solvation methods that are specifically designed, tuned, and validated for use for the simulation of protein–surface interactions.

The use of CG water models provides another approach to accurately simulate protein–surface interactions in aqueous solution with improved computational efficiency. These methods have been recently reviewed by Riniker et al. [174]. In general, the CG water model represents more than one and up to five water molecules by a single CG bead with two oppositely charged interaction sites. The two charged sites, which are connected by an unconstrained bond, form a polarizable dipole, thus allowing explicit treatment of the electrostatic interactions but with reduced computational cost. CG water models are typically parameterized by reproducing the experimental density, surface tension, and static relative dielectric permittivity of water. As may be expected, the hydrogen bond pattern represented by the CG water model differs from that represented by individual water molecules. To correct this problem, Riniker et al. recently developed a hybrid scheme [175] in which a fine-grained (FG) water layer composed of individual water molecules was used locally around a protein, separating it from the surrounding CG water environment. This approach thus provides a more accurate representation of solvation effects immediately surrounding a protein while still providing a substantial reduction in the overall number of degrees of freedom in the overall system. Although not as computationally efficient as fully implicit solvation models, the CG or mixed CG/FG water schemes may have application for use in simulations of protein interactions with a material surface as an approach to reduce computational cost while maintaining reasonably high accuracy compared with fully explicit solvation methods.

12.6.3 CG Methods

Coarse graining of solute molecules is another effective way to reduce the computational cost and accelerate the equilibration of large molecular systems [176,177]. This method provides a means of greatly reducing the number of degrees of freedom in the system while keeping the description of microscopic properties at an acceptable level of accuracy and detail. To map an atomistic model onto a CG model, several atoms are grouped together into a relatively simple *super-atom assembly* (or CG bead) and the interaction energies between respective CG beads are obtained by the application of an optimization procedure that reproduces the structural distributions obtained from atomistic simulations. With a CG model, the bulk structure of a condensed phase can be equilibrated in a much reduced time frame. After equilibration, the atomistic bulk structures of the system can then be reconstructed from superpositions of atomistic counterparts on the corresponding CG beads.

CG models for protein modeling have been reviewed by Tozzini [177]. In our efforts to develop CG approaches for the simulation of protein adsorption on surfaces, we use a *Gō-like* CG model to represent the protein [178–181], in which each amino acid residue is treated as a single bead. Others have also used this CG model to represent protein adsorption behavior. For example, Thomas et al. [182] and Wei et al. [183,184] have represented proteins with the Gō-like model to theoretically study the change of protein conformation over unstructured flat surfaces. In our simulation dealing with structured polymer surfaces, the groups of polymer surface atoms are also combined into CG bead elements. On the basis of the Dual-FF method introduced above, for each type of surface, the IFF parameters of protein are tuned by mapping calculated adsorption free energies to available experimental data, as presented in Table 12.2, using our Dual-FF CHARMM program, which thus enables solvation effects to be directly incorporated into the CG parameters.

Using the tuned residue–surface interaction parameters and the CG model for both the protein and polymer surface, the adsorbed orientation and conformation of the protein with respect to the surface can be explored in a greatly accelerated time frame to obtain a molecular-level understanding of the factors influencing protein–surface interactions. Figure 12.9 presents an example of an adsorption system composed of a segment of the

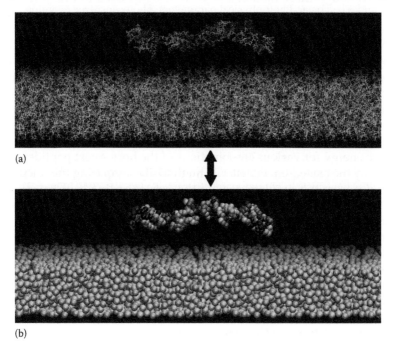

(a)

(b)

FIGURE 12.9
The adsorption of a segment of the protein fibronectin (7–10 type III domains) over a PMMA surface represented by all-atom (a) and CG (b) models.

protein fibronectin (7–10 type III domains) over an amorphous PMMA surface. The atomic and CG representations of the system are shown in the upper and lower panels, respectively. After system equilibration using an advanced sampling method such as TIGER2, the CG models are reverse-mapped back to all-atom models with explicit solvation added back into the system. The entire molecular system is then further equilibrated using TIGER2 to provide the final predicted ensemble of adsorbed protein states. The resulting equilibrated distribution of adsorbed protein states can then be analyzed to characterize the adsorbed orientation and conformational structure of the protein on the surface. Bioactivity assessment can also be conducted by evaluating the solvent accessibility and conformational state of designated bioactive sites within the protein. These results can then be compared with data from synergistically matched experimental studies for validation.

12.7 Conclusions and Future Perspective

Computer simulation studies on protein–surface interactions have become an increasingly active area of research and development in recent years. Currently, the most effective modeling methods for these types of systems are the force field–based method since they are able to provide structural information of the system at an atomic level in reasonable computational time. Presently, there are many force field parameter sets that have been developed and successfully applied in both the biophysics and material science communities. Although these methods work well when used to evaluate the properties of single-phase, relatively homogeneous systems, such as a protein in aqueous solution or a solid-phase bulk material, they generally cannot be directly borrowed and applied to simulate protein–surface adsorption simply because they have not been parameterized to accurately represent adsorption processes. In this chapter, we introduced the Dual-FF method developed in our laboratory at Clemson University, in which the energetic and force contributions of intraphase interactions and interphase interactions are processed separately. In order to tune the IFF parameters, the adsorption behavior of a wide range of host–guest peptides on a wide range of functionalized SAM surface systems have been designed and evaluated both experimentally and by simulation. In these simulations, the adsorption free energy for various combinations of the host–guest peptide–SAM systems was calculated by the biased-energy REMD method. By comparing the calculated adsorption free energies from the simulations with the corresponding experimental results, IFF parameters have been able to be evaluated and tuned to accurately represent peptide adsorption affinity to these types of surfaces.

We also introduced the current progress made in our laboratory, as well as others, toward the development of advanced sampling techniques with specific application for the simulation of protein–surface interactions. These include the development of the TIGER2 and TIGER3 advance sampling methods and CG techniques. These methods are able to greatly improve the efficiency of computer simulation and, thus, enable large, complex molecular systems to be readily equilibrated as is necessary for the comparison of results with experimentally determined values. Once fully developed, these methods have the potential to provide the ability to predict, understand, and control protein–surface interactions, thereby serving as a powerful tool to support a knowledge-based design approach for the optimization of biomaterial systems at the atomic level.

References

1. Castner, D. G., and B. D. Ratner, 2002. Biomedical surface science: Foundations to frontiers. *Surf Sci* 500: 28–60.
2. Hlady, V., and J. Buijs, 1996. Protein adsorption on solid surfaces. *Curr Opin Biotechnol* 7: 72–77.
3. Tsai, W. B., J. M. Grunkemeier, C. D. McFarland, and T. A. Horbett, 2002. Platelet adhesion to polystyrene-based surfaces preadsorbed with plasmas selectively depleted in fibrinogen, fibronectin, vitronectin, or von Willebrand's factor. *J Biomed Mater Res* 60: 348–359.
4. Blasi, P., S. Glovangnoli, A. Schoubben, M. Ricci, and C. Rossi, 2007. Solid lipid nanoparticles for targeted brain drug delivery. *Adv Drug Deliv Rev* 59: 454–477.
5. Dobrovolskaia, M. A., and S. E. Mcneil, 2007. Immunological properties of engineered nanomaterials. *Nat Nanotechnol* 2: 469–478.
6. Geelhood, S. J., T. A. Horbett, W. K. Ward, M. D. Wood, and M. J. Quinn, 2007. Passivating protein coatings for implantable glucose sensors: Evaluation of protein retention. *J Biomed Mater Res B: Appl Biomater* 81B: 251–260.
7. Ramsden, J. J., 1993. Experimental methods for investigating protein adsorption kinetics at surfaces. *Q Rev Biophys* 27: 41–105.
8. Hlady, V., J. Buijs, and H. P. Jennissen, 1999. Methods for studying protein adsorption. *Methods Enzymol* 309: 402–429.
9. Ostumi, E., B. A. Grzybowski, M. Mrksich, C. S. Roberts, and G. M. Whitesides, 2003. Adsorption of proteins to hydrophobic sites on mixed self-assembled monolayers. *Langmuir* 19: 1861–1872.
10. Wei, Y., and R. A. Latour, 2009. Benchmark experimental data set and assessment of adsorption free energy for peptide-surface interactions. *Langmuir* 25: 5637–5646.
11. Talbot, J., G. Tarjus, P. R. Van Tassel, and P. Viot, 2000. From car parking to protein adsorption: An overview of sequential adsorption processes. *Colloids Surf A* 165: 287–324.
12. Euston, S. R., 2004. Computer simulation of proteins: Adsorption, gelation and self-association. *Curr Opin Colloid Interface Sci* 9: 321–327.
13. Mantelli, M., A. Curtis, and P. Rolfe, 2005. Protein-surface interactions—An energy-based mathematical model. *Cell Biochem Biophys* 43: 407–417.
14. Raut, V. P., M. A. Agashe, S. J. Stuart, and R. A. Latour, 2005. Molecular simulation to characterize the adsorption behavior of a fibrinogen gamma-chain fragment. *Langmuir* 21: 1629–1639.
15. Latour, R. A., 2008. Biomaterials: Protein–surface interactions. In *Encyclopedia of Biomaterials and Biomaterials and Bioengineering*, 2nd edition, eds. G.E. Wnek and G.L. Bowlin, 1: 270–284. Informa Healthcare, New York.
16. Ganazzoli, F., and G. Raffaini, 2005. Computer simulation of polypeptide adsorption on model biomaterials. *Phys Chem Chem Phys* 7: 3651–3663.
17. Höök, F., B. Kasemo, M. Grunze, and S. Zauscher, 2008. Quantitative biological surface science: Challenges and recent advances. *ACS Nano* 2: 2428–2436.
18. Latour, R. A., 2008. Molecular dynamics simulation of protein-surface interactions: Benefits, problems, solutions, and future directions. *Biointerphases* 3: FC2–FC12.
19. Latour, R. A., 2009. Molecular simulation of protein-surface interactions. In *Biological Interactions on Materials Surfaces: Understanding and Controlling Protein, Cell, and Tissue Responses,* Chapter 4, eds. D. A. Puleo, and R. Bizios, 69–95. Springer Science & Business Media, LLC, New York.
20. Zhang, L., and Y. Sun, 2010. Molecular simulation of adsorption and its implications to protein chromatography: A review. *Biochem Eng J* 4: 408–415.
21. Wang, M. H., and J. P. Wang, 2010. Application of molecular simulation in biosensor development. *Prog Chem* 22: 845–851.
22. Raffaini, G., and F. Ganazzoli, 2010. Protein adsorption on biomaterial and nanomaterial surfaces: A molecular modeling approach to study non-covalent interactions. *J Appl Biomater Biomech* 8: 135–145.

23. Latour, R. A., 2011. Molecular simulation methods to study protein adsorption behavior at the atomic level. In *Comprehensive Biomaterials*, eds. P. Ducheyne, K. E. Healy, D. W. Hutmacher, D. W. Grainger, and C. J. Kirkpatrick, 3: 171–192. Elsevier, Oxford, UK.

24. Makarucha, A. J., N. Todorova, and I. Yarovsky, 2011. Nanomaterials in biological environment: A review of computer modelling studies. *Eur Biophys J* 40: 103–115.

25. Rabe, M., D. Verdes, and S. Seeger, 2011. Understanding protein adsorption phenomena at solid surfaces. *Adv Colloid Interface Sci* 162: 87–106.

26. Tanzi, M. C., P. Vena, S. Vesentini, S. Bozzini, G. Candiani, A. Cigada, L. DeNardo, S. Farè, F. Ganazzoli, D. Gastaldi, L. Levi, P. Metrangolo, F. Migliavacca, R. Osellame, P. Petrini, G. Raffaini, G. Resnati, and P. Zunino, 2011. Trends in biomedical engineering: Focus on smart bio-materials and drug delivery. *J Appl Biomater Biomech* 9: 87–97.

27. Gray, J. J., 2004. The interaction of proteins with solid surfaces. *Curr Opin Struct Biol* 14: 110–115.

28. Nadarajah, A., C. F. Lu, and K. K. Chittur, 1995. Modeling the dynamics of protein adsorption to surfaces. In *Proteins at Interfaces II: Fundamentals and Applications Book Series: ACS Symposium Series*, eds. T. A. Orbett, and J. L. Brash, 602: 181–194. American Chemical Society, Washington, DC.

29. Zhdanov, V. P., and B. Kasemo, 1998. Monte Carlo simulations of the kinetics of protein adsorption. *Surf Rev Lett* 5: 615–634.

30. Minton, A. P., 1999. Adsorption of globular proteins on locally planar surfaces. II. Models for the effect of multiple adsorbate conformations on adsorption equilibria and kinetics. *Biophys J* 76: 176–187.

31. Zhdanov, V. P., and B. Kasemo, 2010. Protein adsorption and desorption on lipid bilayers. *Biophys Chem* 146: 60–64.

32. Siegismund, D., T. F. Keller, K. D. Jandt, and M. Rettenmayr, 2010. Fibrinogen adsorption on biomaterials—A numerical study. *Macromol Biosci* 10: 1216–1223.

33. Hartving, R. A., M. van de Weert, J. Østergaard, L. Jorgensen, and H. Jensen, 2011. Protein adsorption at charged surfaces: The role of electrostatic interactions and interfacial charge regulation. *Langmuir* 27: 2634–2643.

34. Yang, Z. Y., and Y. P. Zhao, 2006. QM/MM and classical molecular dynamics simulation of histidine-tagged peptide immobilization on nickel surface. *Mat Sci Eng A-Struct* 423: 84–91.

35. Rimola, A., M. Corno, C. M. Zicovich-Wilson, and P. Ugliengo, 2008. Ab initio modeling of protein/biomaterial interactions: Glycine adsorption at hydroxyapatite surfaces. *J Am Chem Soc* 130: 16181–16183.

36. Rimola, A., M. Sodupe, and P. Ugliengo, 2009. Affinity scale for the interaction of amino acids with silica surfaces. *J Phys Chem C* 113: 5741–5750.

37. Xu, Z., K. Song, S. L. Yuan, and C. B. Liu, 2011. Microscopic wetting of self-assembled mono layers with different surfaces: A combined molecular dynamics and quantum mechanics study. *Langmuir* 27: 8611–8620.

38. Ganji, M. D., 2009. Density functional theory based treatment of amino acids adsorption on single-walled carbon nanotubes. *Diamond Relat Mater* 18: 662–668.

39. Qin, W., X. Li, W. W. Bian, X. J. Fan, and J. Y. Qi, 2010. Density functional theory calculations and molecular dynamics simulations of the adsorption of biomolecules on graphene surfaces. *Biomaterials* 31: 1007–1016.

40. Cazorla, C., 2010. Ab initio study of the binding of collagen amino acids to graphene and A-doped (A = H, Ca) grapheme. *Thin Solid Films* 518: 6951–6961.

41. Almora-Barrios, N., and N. H. de Leeuw, 2010. A density functional theory study of the interaction of collagen peptides with hydroxyapatite surfaces. *Langmuir* 26: 14535–14542.

42. Rimola, A., Y. Sakhno, L. Bertinetti, M. Lelli, G. Martra, and P. Ugliengo, 2011. Toward a surface science model for biology: Glycine adsorption on nanohydroxyapatite with well-defined surfaces. *J Phys Chem Lett* 2: 1390–1394.

43. Fu, Z. M., Y. Luo, P. Derreumaux, and G. H. Wei, 2009. Induced beta-barrel formation of the Alzheimer's A beta 25-35 oligomers on carbon nanotube surfaces: Implication for amyloid fibril inhibition. *Biophys J* 97: 1795–1803.

44. Jana, A. K., and N. Sengupta, 2012. Adsorption mechanism and collapse propensities of the full-length, monomeric A beta(1-42) on the surface of a single-walled carbon nanotube: A molecular dynamics simulation study. *Biophys J* 102: 1889–1896.

45. Vaitheeswaran, S., and A. E. Garcia, 2011. Protein stability at a carbon nanotube interface. *J Chem Phys* 134: Article Number 125101.

46. Carlsson, F., E. Hyltner, T. Arnebrant, M. Malmsten, and P. Linse, 2004. Lysozyme adsorption to charged surfaces. A Monte Carlo study. *J Phys Chem B* 108: 9871–9881.

47. Xie, Y., J. Zhou, and S. Y. Jiang, 2010. Parallel tempering Monte Carlo simulations of lysozyme orientation on charged surfaces. *J Chem Phys* 132: Article Number 065101.

48. Kubiak, K., and P. A. Mulheran, 2009. Molecular dynamics simulations of hen egg white lysozyme adsorption at a charged solid surface. *J Phys Chem B* 113: 12189–12200.

49. Freed, A. S., and S. M. Cramer, 2011. Protein-surface interaction maps for ion-exchange chromatography. *Langmuir* 27: 3561–3568.

50. Kubiak-Ossowska, K., and P. A. Mulheran, 2011. Multiprotein interactions during surface adsorption: A molecular dynamics study of lysozyme aggregation at a charged solid surface. *J Phys Chem B* 115: 8891–8900.

51. Yu, X., Q. M. Wang, Y. N. Lin, J. Zhao, C. Zhao, and J. Zheng, 2012. Structure, orientation, and surface interaction of Alzheimer amyloid-beta peptides on the graphite. *Langmuir* 28: 6595–6605.

52. Raffaini, G., and F. Ganazzoli, 2006. Adsorption of charged albumin subdomains on a graphite surface. *J Biomed Mater Res-A* 76A: 638–645.

53. Abdulhakeem, A. M., M. Mohammed, and N. Golam, 2009. Prediction of protein conformation in water and on surfaces by Monte Carlo simulations using united-atom method. *Mol Simulat* 35: 292–300.

54. Muecksch, C., and H. M. Urbassek, 2011. Molecular dynamics simulation of free and forced BSA adsorption on a hydrophobic graphite surface. *Langmuir* 27: 12938–12943.

55. Muecksch, C., and H. M. Urbassek, 2011. Adsorption of BMP-2 on a hydrophobic graphite surface: A molecular dynamics study. *Chem Phys Lett* 510: 252–256.

56. Raffaini, G., and F. Ganazzoli, 2004. Molecular dynamics simulation of the adsorption of a fibronectin module on a graphite surface. *Langmuir* 20: 3371–3378.

57. Raffaini, G., and F. Ganazzoli, 2010. Protein adsorption on a hydrophobic surface: A molecular dynamics study of lysozyme on graphite. *Langmuir* 26: 5679–5689.

58. Dong, X. L., W. Qi, W. Tao, L. Y. Ma, and C. X. Fu, 2011. The dynamic behaviours of protein BMP-2 on hydroxyapatite nanoparticles. *Mol Simulat* 37: 1097–1104.

59. Shen, J. W., T. Wu, Q. Wang, and H. H. Pan, 2008. Molecular simulation of protein adsorption and desorption on hydroxyapatite surfaces. *Biomaterials* 29: 513–532.

60. Mulheran, P. A., D. Pellenc, R. A. Bennett, R. J. Green, and M. Sperrin, 2008. Mechanisms and dynamics of protein clustering on a solid surface. *Phys Rev Lett* 100: Article Number 068102.

61. Mulheran P. A., and K. Kubiak, 2009. Protein adsorption mechanisms on solid surfaces: Lysozyme-on-mica. *Mol Simulat* 35: 561–566.

62. Raffaini, G., and F. Ganazzoli, 2012. Molecular modelling of protein adsorption on the surface of titanium dioxide polymorphs. *Philos Trans A Math Phys Eng Sci* 370: 1444–1462.

63. Utesch, T., G. Daminelli, and M. A. Mroginski, 2011. Molecular dynamics simulations of the adsorption of bone morphogenetic protein-2 on surfaces with medical relevance. *Langmuir* 27: 13144–13153.

64. Wu, C. Y., M. J. Chen, and C. Xing, 2010. Molecular understanding of conformational dynamics of a fibronectin module on rutile (110) surface. *Langmuir* 26: 15972–15981.

65. Wang, Q. M., C. Zhao, J. Zhao, J. D. Wang, J. C. Yang, X. Yu, and J. Zhen, 2010. Comparative molecular dynamics study of A beta adsorption on the self-assembled monolayers. *Langmuir* 26: 3308–3316.

66. Wang, Q. M., C. Zhao, J. Zhao, J. D. Wang, J. C. Yang, X. Yu, and J. Zhen, 2010. Alzheimer A beta(1-42) monomer adsorbed on the self-assembled monolayers. *Langmuir* 26: 12722–12732.

67. Zhao, J., Q. Wang, G. Liang, and J. Zheng, 2011. Molecular dynamics simulations of low-ordered Alzheimer beta-amyloid oligomers from dimer to hexamer on self-assembled monolayers. *Langmuir* 27: 14876–14887.

68. Zhou, J., J. Zheng, and S. Y. Jiang, 2004. Molecular simulation studies of the orientation and conformation of cytochrome c adsorbed on self-assembled monolayers. *J Phys Chem B* 108: 17418–17424.

69. Trzaskowski, B., F. Leonarski, A. Les, and L. Adamowicz, 2008. Altering the orientation of proteins on self-assembled monolayers: A computational study. *Biomacromolecules* 9: 3239–3245.

70. Agashe, M., V. Raut, S. J. Stuart, and R. A. Latour, 2005. Molecular simulation to characterize the adsorption behavior of a fibrinogen gamma-chain fragment. *Langmuir* 21: 1103–1117.

71. Wilson, K., S. J. Stuart, A. Garcia, and R. A. Latour, 2004. A molecular modeling study of the effect of surface chemistry on the adsorption of a fibronectin fragment spanning the 7–10th type-III repeats. *J Biomed Mater Res A* 69A: 686–698.

72. He, Y., S. Chen, J. C. Hower, M. T. Bernards, and S. Jiang, 2008. Molecular simulations of the interactions between a protein and phosphorylcholine self-assembled monolayers in the presence of water. *Langmuir* 24: 10358–10364.

73. Hanasaki, I., H. Takahashi, G. Sazaki, K. Nakajima, and S. Kawano, 2008. Single-molecule measurements and dynamical simulations of protein molecules near silicon substrates. *J Phys D Appl Phys* 41: Article Number 095301.

74. Gubskaya, A. V., V. Kholodovych, D. Knight, J. Kohn, and W. J. Welsh, 2007. Prediction of fibrinogen adsorption for biodegradable polymers: Integration of molecular dynamics and surrogate modeling. *Polymer* 48: 5788–5801.

75. Wei, T., M. A. Carignano, and I. Szleifer, 2011. Lysozyme adsorption on polyethylene surfaces: Why are long simulations needed? *Langmuir* 27: 12074–12081.

76. Feng, J., R. B. Pandey, R. J. Berry, B. L. Farmer, R. R. Naik, and H. Heinz, 2011. Adsorption mechanism of single amino acid and surfactant molecules to Au {111} surfaces in aqueous solution: Design rules for metal-binding molecules. *Soft Matter* 7: 2113–2120.

77. Notman, R., and T. R. Walsh, 2009. Molecular dynamics studies of the interactions of water and amino acid analogues with quartz surfaces. *Langmuir* 25: 1638–1644.

78. Wright, L. B., and T. R. Walsh, 2012. Facet selectivity of binding on quartz surfaces: Free energy calculations of amino-acid analogue adsorption. *J Phys Chem C* 116: 2933–2945.

79. Monti, S., and T. R. Walsh, 2010. Free energy calculations of the adsorption of amino-acid analogues at the aqueous titania interface. *J Phys Chem C* 114: 22197–22206.

80. Abell, G. C., 1985. Empirical chemical pseudopotential theory of molecular and metallic bonding. *Phys Rev B* 31: 6184–6196.

81. Tersoff, J., 1988. New empirical approach for the structure and energy of covalent systems. *Phys Rev B* 37: 6991–7000.

82. Brenner, D. W., 1990. Empirical potential for hydrocarbons for use in simulating the chemical vapor deposition of diamond films. *Phys Rev B* 42: 9458–9471.

83. Brenner, D. W., 1992. Erratum: Empirical potential for hydrocarbons for use in simulating the chemical vapor deposition of diamond films. *Phys Rev B* 46: 1948.

84. Brenner, D. W., O. A. Shenderova, J. A. Harrison, S. J. Stuart, and S. B. Sinnott, 2002. A second-generation reactive empirical bond order (REBO) potential energy expression for hydrocarbons. *J Phys Condens Matter* 14: 783–802.

85. Stuart, S. J., A. B. Tutein, and J. A. Harrison, 2000. A reactive potential for hydrocarbons with intermolecular interactions. *J Chem Phys* 112: 6472–6486.

86. Ni, B., S. B. Sinnott, P. T. Mikulski, and J. A. Harrison, 2002. Compression of carbon nanotubes filled with C60, CH4, or Ne: Predictions from molecular dynamics simulations. *Phys Rev Lett* 88: 205505.

87. Nikitin, A., H. Ogasawara, D. Mann, R. Denecke, Z. Zhang, H. Dai, K. Cho, and A. Nilsson, 2005. Hydrogenation of single-walled carbon nanotubes. *Phys Rev Lett* 95: 225507.

88. Ponder, J. W., C. J. Wu, P. Y. Ren, V. S. Pande, J. D. Chodera, M. J. Schnieders, I. Haque, D. L. Mobley, D. S. Lambrecht, R. A. DiStasio Jr., M. Head-Gordon, G. N. I. Clark, M. E. Johnson, and T. Head-Gordon, 2010. Current status of the AMOEBA polarizable force field. *J Phys Chem B* 114: 2549–2564.

89. Ren, P., and J. W. Ponder, 2002. A consistent treatment of inter- and intramolecular polarization in molecular mechanics calculations. *J Comput Chem* 23: 1497–1506.

90. Ren, P., and J. W. Ponder, 2003. Polarizable atomic multipole water model for molecular mechanics simulation. *J Phys Chem B* 107: 5933–5947.

91. Ponder, J. W., and D. A. Case, 2003. Force fields for protein simulation. *Adv Protein Chem* 66: 27–85.

92. Tomásio, S. D., and T. R. Walsh, 2007. Atomistic modelling of the interaction between peptides and carbon nanotubes. *Mol Phys* 105: 221–229.

93. Rick, S. W., S. J. Stuart, and B. J. Berne, 1994. Dynamical fluctuating charge force fields: Applications to liquid water. *J Chem Phys* 101: 6141–6156.

94. Kokh, D. B., S. Corni, P. J. Winn, M. Hoefling, K. E. Gottschalk, and R. C. Wade, 2010. An atomistic force field for modeling protein–Metal surface interactions in a continuum aqueous solvent. *J Chem Theory Comput* 6: 1753–1768.

95. Yin, J., and Y. P. Zhao, 2009. Hybrid QM/MM simulation of the hydration phenomena of dipalmitoylphosphatidylcholine headgroup. *J Colloid Interface Sci* 329: 410–415.

96. Landin, J., I. Pascher, and D. Cremer, 1995. Ab initio and semiempirical conformation potentials for phospholipid head groups. *J Phys Chem* 99: 4471–4485.

97. Li, W., and J. B. Lagowski, 1999. Ab initio study of phospholipid headgroups: GPE and GPC. *Chem Phys Lipids* 103: 137–160.

98. Pullman, B., and H. Berthod, 1974. Quantum-mechanical studies on the conformation of phospholipids. The conformational properties of the polar head. *FEBS Lett* 44: 266–269.

99. Pullman, B., H. Berthod, and N. Gresh, 1975. Quantum-mechanical studies on the conformation of phospholipids. The effect of water on the conformational properties of the polar head. *FEBS Lett* 53: 199–204.

100. Liang, C. X., C. S. Ewig, T. R. Stouch, and A. T. Hagler, 1993. Ab initio studies of lipid model species. 1. Dimethyl phosphate and methyl propyl phosphate anions. *J Am Chem Soc* 115: 1537–1545.

101. Landin, J., I. Pascher, and D. Cremer, 1997. Effect of a polar environment on the conformation of phospholipid head groups analyzed with the Onsager continuum solvation model. *J Phys Chem A* 101: 2996–3004.

102. Kubica, K., 2002. Computer simulation studies on significance of lipid polar head orientation. *Comput Chem* 26: 351–356.

103. Car, R., and M. Parrinello, 1985. Unified approach for molecular dynamics and density-functional theory. *Phys Rev Lett* 55: 2471–2474.

104. Langel, W., and L. Menken, 2003. Simulation of the interface between titanium oxide and amino acids in solution by first principles MD. *Surf Sci* 538: 1–9.

105. Koppen, S., O. Bronkalla, and W. Langel, 2008. Adsorption configurations and energies of amino acids on anatase and rutile surfaces. *J Phys Chem C* 112: 13600–13606.

106. Brooks, B. R., R. E. Bruccoleri, B. D. Olafson, D. J. States, S. Swaminathan, and M. Karplus, 1983. CHARMM: A program for macromolecular energy, minimization, and dynamics calculations. *J Comput Chem* 4: 187–217.

107. MacKerell, A. D., D. Bashford, M. Bellott, R. L. Dunbrack, J. D. Evanseck, M. J. Field, S. Fischer, J. Gao, H. Guo, S. Ha, D. Joseph-McCarthy, L. Kuchnir, K. Kuczera, F. T. K. Lau, C. Mattos, S. Michnick, T. Ngo, D. T. Nguyen, B. Prodhom, W. E. Reiher, B. Roux, M. Schlenkrich, J. C. Smith, R. Stote, J. Straub, M. Watanabe, J. Wiorkiewicz-Kuczera, D. Yin, and M. Karplus, 1998. All-atom empirical potential for molecular modeling and dynamics studies of proteins. *J Phys Chem B* 102: 3586–3616.

108. Hariharan, P. C., and J. A. Pople, 1973. Influence of polarization functions on MO hydrogenation energies. *Theor Chim Acta* 28: 213–222.

109. Francl, M. M., W. J. Pietro, W. J. Hehre, J. S. Binkley, M. S. Gordon, D. J. DeFrees, and J. A. Pople, 1982. Self-consistent molecular orbital methods. XXIII. A polarization-type basis set for second-row elements. *J Chem Phys* 77: 3654–3665.

110. Dinur, U., and A. T. Hagler, 1991. New approaches to empirical force fields. In *Reviews in Computational Chemistry*, eds. K. B. Lipkowitz, and D. B. Boyd, 2: 99–164. VCH Publishers, New York.

111. Maple, J. R., M. J. Hwang, T. P. Stockfisch, U. Dinur, M. Waldman, C. S. Ewig, and A. T. Hagler, 1994. Derivation of class II force fields. 1. Methodology and quantum force field for the alkyl functional group and alkane molecules. *J Comput Chem* 15: 162–182.

112. Iori, F., R. Di Felice, E. Molinari, and S. Cornij, 2009. GolP: An atomistic force-field to describe the interaction of proteins with Au(111) surfaces in water. *Comput Chem* 30: 1465–1476.

113. Latour, R. A., T. Abramyan, G. Collier, T. G. Kucukkal, X. Li, J. A. Snyder, A. A. Thyparambil, N. A. Vellore, Y. Wei, J. A. Yancey, and S. J. Stuart, 2012. Understanding protein-surface interactions at the atomistic level through the synergistic development of experimental and molecular simulation methods. In *Proteins at Interfaces III*, eds. T. A. Horbett, J. Brash, and W. Norde. ACS symposium series, Chapter 9, pp. 197–228. American Chemical Society, Washington, DC.

114. Leahy, D. J., I. Aukhil, and H. P. Erickson, 1996, 2.0 Å Crystal structure of a four-domain segment of human fibronectin encompassing the RGD loop and synergy region. *Cell* 84: 155–164.

115. Vellore, N. A., J. A. Yancey, G. Collier, R. A. Latour, and S. J. Stuart, 2010. Assessment of the transferability of a protein force field for the simulation of peptide-surface interactions. *Langmuir* 26: 7396–7404.

116. Allen, M. P., and D. J. Tildesley, 1989. *Computer Simulation of Liquids*. Oxford University Press, Oxford, UK.

117. Tamerler, C., E. E. Oren, M. Duman, E. Venkatasubramanian, and M. Sarikaya, 2006. Adsorption kinetics of an engineered gold binding peptide by surface plasmon resonance spectroscopy and a quartz crystal microbalance. *Langmuir* 22: 7712–7718.

118. Green, R. J., R. A. Frazier, K. M. Shakesheff, M. C. Davies, C. J. Roberts, and S. J. B. Tendler, 2000. Surface plasmon resonance analysis of dynamic biological interactions with biomaterials. *Biomaterials* 21: 1823–1835.

119. Wei, Y., and R. A. Latour, 2010. Correlation between desorption force measured by atomic force microscopy and adsorption free energy measured by surface plasmon resonance spectroscopy for peptide-surface interactions. *Langmuir* 26: 18852–18861.

120. Thyparambil, A. A., Y. Wei, and R. A. Latour, 2012. Determination of peptide-surface adsorption free energy for material surfaces not conducive to SPR or QCM using AFM. *Langmuir* 28: 5687–5694.

121. Wei, Y., A. A. Thyarambil, and R. A. Latour, 2012. Peptide-surface adsorption free energy comparing solution conditions ranging from low to medium salt concentrations. *Chem Phys Chem* 13: 3782–3785.

122. Silin, V. V., H. Weetall, and D. J. Vanderah, 1997. SPR studies of the nonspecific adsorption kinetics of human IgG and BSA on gold surfaces modified by Self-Assembled Monolayers (SAMs). *J Colloid Interface Sci* 185: 94–103.

123. Wei, Y., and R. A. Latour, 2008. Determination of adsorption free energy for peptide-surface interactions by SPR spectroscopy. *Langmuir* 24: 6721–6729.

124. Yancey, J. A., N. A. Vellore, G. Collier, S. J. Stuart, and R. A. Latour, 2010. Development of molecular simulation methods to accurately represent protein-surface interactions: The effect of pressure and its determination for a system with constrained atoms. *Biointerphases* 5: 85–95.

125. Wang, F., S. J. Stuart, and R. A. Latour, 2008. Calculation of adsorption free energy for solute-surface interactions using biased replica-exchange molecular dynamics. *Biointerphases* 3: 9–18.

126. O'Brien, C. P., S. J. Stuart, D. A. Bruce, and R. A. Latour, 2008. Modeling of peptide adsorption interactions with a poly(lactic acid) surface. *Langmuir* 24: 14115–14124.

127. Beutler, T. C., and W. F. van Gunsteren, 1994. The computation of a potential of mean force: Choice of the biasing potential in the umbrella sampling technique. *J Chem Phys* 100: 1492–1497.

128. Harvey, S. C., and M. Prabhakaran, 1987. Umbrella sampling: Avoiding possible artifacts and statistical biases. *J Chem Phys* 91: 4799–4801.

129. Kumar, S., J. M. Rosenberg, D. Bouzida, R. H. Swendsen, and P. A. Kollman, 1992. The weighted histogram analysis method for free-energy calculations on biomolecules. I. The method. *J Comput Chem* 13: 1011–1021.

130. Kumar, S., J. M. Rosenberg, D. Bouzida, R. H. Swendsen, and P. A. Kollman, 1995. Multidimensional free-energy calculations using the weighted histogram analysis method. *J Comput Chem* 16: 1339–1350.

131. Overbeek, J. T. G., 1977. Recent development in understanding of colloid stability. *J Colloid Interface Sci* 58: 408–422.

132. Israelachvili, J. N., 1992. *Intermolecular and Surface Forces.* Academic Press, New York.

133. Sugita, Y., and Y. Okamoto, 1999. Replica-exchange molecular dynamics method for protein folding. *Chem Phys Lett* 314: 141–151.

134. Garcia, A. E., and K. Y. Sanbonmatsu, 2006. Exploring the energy landscape of a β hairpin in explicit solvent. *Proteins* 42: 345–354.

135. Biswas, P. K., N. A. Vellore, J. A. Yancey, T. G. Kucukkal, G. Collier, B. R. Brooks, S. J. Stuart, and R. A. Latour, 2012. Simulation of multiphase systems utilizing independent force fields to control intra-phase and inter-phase behavior. *J Comput Chem* 33: 1458–1466.

136. Darden, T., D. York, and L. Pedersen, 1993. Particle Mesh Ewald-an N.Log(N) method for Ewald sums in large systems. *J Chem Phys* 98: 10089–10092.

137. Notman, R., E. E. Oren, C. Tamerler, M. Sarikaya, R. Samudrala, and T. R. Walsh, 2010. Solution study of engineered quartz binding peptides using replica exchange molecular dynamics. *Biomacromolecules* 11: 3266–3274.

138. Li, X., C. P. O'Brien, N. A. Vellore, F. Wang, D. A. Bruce, S. J. Stuart, and R. A. Latour, 2007. An improved replica-exchange sampling method: Temperature intervals with global energy reassignment (TIGER). *J Chem Phys* 127: Article number 164116.

139. Li, X., S. J. Stuart, and R. A. Latour, 2009. TIGER2: An improved algorithm for temperature intervals with global exchange of replicas. *J Chem Phys* 130: Article number 174106.

140. Roitberg, A. E., A. Okur, and C. Simmerling, 2007. Coupling of replica exchange simulations to a non-Boltzmann structure reservoir. *J Phys Chem B* 111: 2415–2418.

141. Spill, Y. D., G. Bouvier, and M. Nilges, 2012. A convective replica-exchange method for sampling new energy basins. *J Comput Chem* 34: 132–140.

142. Li, X. F., and R. A. Latour, 2011. The TIGER2 empirical accelerated sampling method: Parameter sensitivity and extension to a complex molecular system. *J Comput Chem* 32: 1091–1100.

143. Lu, D. R., and K. Park, 1991. Calculation of solvation interaction energies for protein adsorption on polymer surfaces. *J Biomater Sci Polym Ed* 1: 243–260.

144. Noinville, V., C. Vidal-Madjar, and B. Sebille, 1995. Modeling of protein adsorption on polymer surfaces. Computation of adsorption potential. *J Phys Chem* 99: 1516–1522.

145. Auhl, R., R. Everaers, G. S. Grest, K. Kremer, and S. J. Plimpton, 2003. Equilibration of long chain polymer melts in computer simulations. *J Chem Phys* 119: 12718–12729.

146. Graessley, W. W., R. C. Hayward, and G. S. Grest, 1999. Excluded volume effects in polymer solutions. Comparison of experimental results with numerical simulation data. *Macromolecules* 32: 3510–3517.

147. Kamio, K., K. Moorthi, and D. N. Theodorou, 2007. Coarse grained end bridging Monte Carlo simulations of poly(ethylene terephthalate) melt. *Macromolecules* 40: 710–722.

148. Li, X., and R. A. Latour, 2011. Construction and validation of all-atom bulk-phase models of amorphous polymers using the TIGER2/TIGER3 empirical sampling method. *Macromolecules* 44: 5452–5464.

149. Li, X., N. S. Murthy, and R. A. Latour, 2012. Structure of hydrated poly(D,L-lactic acid) studied with x-ray diffraction and molecular simulation methods. *Macromolecules* 45: 4896–4906.

150. Glättli, A., X. Daura, and W. F. van Gunsteren, 2002. Derivation of an improved simple point charge model for liquid water: SPC/A and SPC/L. *J Chem Phys* 116: 9811–9828.

151. Mark, P., and L. Nilsson, 2001. Structure and dynamics of the TIP3P, SPC, and SPC/E water models at 298 K. *J Phys Chem A* 105: 9954–9960.

152. Jorgensen, W. L., J. Chandrasekhar, J. D. Madura, R. W. Impey, and M. L. Klein, 1983. Comparison of simple potential functions for simulating liquid water. *J Chem Phys* 79: 926–935.

153. Jorgensen, W. L., and J. D. Madura, 1985. Temperature and size dependence for Monte Carlo simulations of TIP4P water. *Mol Phys* 56: 1381–1392.

154. Jorgensen, W. L., and C. Jenson, 1998. Temperature dependence of TIP3P, SPC, and TIP4P water from NPT Monte Carlo simulations: Seeking temperatures of maximum density. *J Comput Chem* 19: 1179–1186.

155. Horn, H. W., W. C. Swope, J. W. Pitera, J. D. Madura, T. J. Dick, G. L. Hura, and T. Head-Gordon, 2004. Development of an improved four-site water model for biomolecular simulations: TIP4P-Ew. *J Chem Phys* 120: 9665–9678.

156. Horn, H. W., W. C. Swope, and J. W. Pitera, 2005. Characterization of the TIP4P-Ew water model: Vapor pressure and boiling point. *J Chem Phys* 123: 194504.

157. Mahoney, M. W., and W. L. Jorgensen, 2001. Diffusion constant of the TIP5P model of liquid water. *J Chem Phys* 114: 363–366.

158. Schaefer, M., C. Bartels, and M. Karplus, 1999. Solution conformations of structured peptides: Continuum electrostatics versus distance-dependent dielectric functions. *Theor Chem Acc* 101: 194–204.

159. Yeh, I. C., M. S. Lee, and M. A. Olson, 2008. Calculation of protein heat capacity from replica-exchange molecular dynamics simulations with different implicit solvent models. *J Phys Chem B* 112: 15064–15073.

160. Sun, Y., and R. A. Latour, 2006. Comparison of implicit solvent models for the simulation of protein-surface interactions. *J Comput Chem* 27: 1908–1922.

161. Sharp, K. A., and B. Honig, 1990. Calculating total electrostatic energies with the nonlinear Poisson-Boltzmann equation. *J Phys Chem* 94: 7684–7692.

162. Bertonati, C., B. Honig, and E. Alexov, 2007. Poisson-Boltzmann calculations of nonspecific salt effects on protein-protein binding free energies. *Biophys J* 92: 1891–1899.

163. Still, W. C., A. Tempczyk, R. C. Hawley, and T. Hendrickson, 1990. Semianalytical treatment of solvation for molecular mechanics and dynamics. *J Am Chem Soc* 112: 6127–6129.

164. Dominy, B. N., and C. L. Brooks III, 1999. Development of a generalized Born model parameterization for proteins and nucleic acids. *J Phys Chem B* 103: 3765–3773.

165. Bashford, D., and D. A. Case, 2000. Generalized born models of macromolecular solvation effects. *Annu Rev Phys Chem* 51: 129–152.

166. Feig, M., and C. L. Brooks III, 2004. Recent advances in the development and application of implicit solvent models in biomolecule simulations. *Curr Opin Struct Biol* 14: 217–224.

167. Feig, M., A. Onufriev, M. S. Lee, W. Im, D. A. Case, and C. L. Brooks III, 2004. Performance comparison of generalized Born and Poisson methods in the calculation of electrostatic solvation energies for protein structures. *J Comput Chem* 25: 265–284.

168. Sun, Y., B. N. Dominy, and R. A. Latour, 2007. Comparison of solvation-effect methods for the simulation of peptide interactions with a hydrophobic surface. *J Comput Chem* 28: 1883–1892.

169. Hassan, S. A., E. L. Mehler, D. Zhang, and H. Weinstein, 2003. Molecular dynamics simulations of peptides and proteins with an implicit solvent model based on screened Coulomb potentials. *Proteins* 51: 109–125.

170. Hassan, S. A., F. Guarnieri, and E. L. Mehler, 2000. A general treatment of solvent effects based on screened Coulomb potentials. *J Phys Chem B* 104: 6478–6489.

171. Hassan, S. A., and E. L. Mehler, 2001. A general screened coulomb potential based implicit solvent model: Calculation of secondary structure of small peptides. *Int J Quant Chem* 83: 193–202.

172. Hassan, S. A., and E. L. Mehler, 2010. Modeling aqueous solvent effect through local properties of water. In *Modeling Solvent Environments: Applications to Simulations of Biomolecules*, ed. M. Feig. Wiley-VCH, Weinheim, Germany.

173. Chen, J. H., and C. L. Brooks III, 2008. Implicit modeling of nonpolar solvation for simulating protein folding and conformational transitions. *Phys Chem Chem Phys* 10: 471–481.

174. Riniker, S., and W. F. van Gunsteren, 2011. A simple, efficient polarizable coarse-grained water model for molecular dynamics simulations. *J Chem Phys* 134: Article Number 084110.
175. Riniker, S., A. P. Eichenberger, and W. F. van Gunsteren, 2012. Structural effects of an atomic-level layer of water molecules around proteins solvated in supra-molecular coarse-grained water. *J Phys Chem B* 116: 8873–8879.
176. Hess, B., S. León, N. van der Vegt, and K. Kremer, 2006. Long time atomistic polymer trajectories from coarse grained simulations: Bisphenol-A polycarbonate. *Soft Matter* 2: 409–414.
177. Tozzini, V., 2005. Coarse-grained models for proteins. *Curr Opin Struct Biol* 15: 144–150.
178. Ueeda, Y., H. Taketomi, and N. Gō, 1978. Studies on protein folding, unfolding, and fluctuations by computer simulation. II. A. Three-dimensional lattice model of lysozyme. *Biopolymers* 17: 1531–1548.
179. Karanicolas, J., and C. L. Brooks III, 2002. The origins of asymmetry in the folding transition states of protein L and protein G. *Prot Sci* 11: 2351–2361.
180. Karanicolas, J., and C. L. Brooks III, 2003. Improved Go-like models demonstrate the robustness of protein folding mechanisms towards non-native interactions. *J Mol Biol* 334: 309–325.
181. Karanicolas, J., and C. L. Brooks III, 2003. The structural basis for biphasic kinetics in the folding of the WW domain from a formin-binding protein: Lessons for protein design? *Proc Natl Acad Sci USA* 100: 3954–3959.
182. Thomas, A., I. V. Knotts, N. Rathore, and J. J. de Pablo, 2005. Structure and stability of a model three-helix-bundle protein on tailored surfaces. *Proteins* 61: 385–397.
183. Wei, S., A. Thomas, and I. V. Knotts, 2010. Predicting stability of alpha-helical, orthogonal-bundle proteins on surfaces. *J Chem Phys* 133: Article Number 115102.
184. Wei, S., A. Thomas, and I. V. Knotts, 2011. Effects of tethering a multistate folding protein to a surface. *J Chem Phys* 134: Article Number 185101.

13

Structure of the Electrical Double Layers: Insights from Continuum and Atomistic Simulations

Guang Feng, Guoqing Hu, Rui Qiao, and Narayana R. Aluru

CONTENTS

ABSTRACT   Electrical double layers (EDLs) are found ubiquitously in biomedical and engineering systems. While the critical dimension of EDLs rarely exceeds hundreds of nanometers, they often dictate the macroscopic behavior of systems in which they exist. In this chapter, we summarize the key features of EDLs and researches devoted to the thermodynamic aspects of EDLs. In particular, we will focus on theoretical and computational studies on the structure of EDLs. In theoretical studies, we focus on the Poisson–Boltzmann (PB) model and how physics such ion–ion correlations and dielectric saturation are incorporated in several generations of modified PB models and their effects on EDL structure. In simulation studies, we focus on molecular dynamics modeling of EDLs in aqueous systems and highlight how the discreteness and finite size of ion, solvent, and surface atoms affect EDL structures near open surfaces and in confined spaces. New directions for theoretical and computational studies of EDLs are discussed.

13.1 Introduction

An electrical double layer (EDL) is "a system, electrically neutral as a whole, in which a layer of positive charges opposes a layer of negative charges and in which, moreover, layers of oriented polar molecules and (or) polarized atoms are present" [1]. Though the

EDL can be commonly found at various interfaces and surfaces, in this chapter, we focus mainly on the EDL at the solid–liquid interface. For example, when a charged surface is in contact with an electrolyte solution, an EDL will appear near the surface. The study of EDL is of great importance to many surface and interfacial phenomena occurring in various physical, chemical, and biological systems. Here, we provide a few examples in which the behaviors or characteristics of the system depend critically upon the EDL structure.

- *Ion transport through charged channels of biological or physical membranes.* This transport is controlled in part by the charge distribution near the surface and the rate of transport is determined by the electrical potential distribution and the thickness of the EDL inside the channels [2,3].
- *Colloid stability.* The double layer interactions between the colloid particles in an electrolyte solution are responsible for the stability of the colloid. The classical DLVO theory of colloid stability, which accounts for the stability of colloid based on the competition of double layer interaction with van der Waals attraction between colloid particles, has successfully explained many experimental observations in colloid science [4,5].
- *Electrochemical reaction.* Since most of the interfacial electrochemical reactions occur within the formed double layer, the charge and electrical potential distributions in the EDL will have a strong influence on the kinetics of the reactions.
- *Electrokinetic phenomena.* These include mainly the electrophoresis, electroosmotic transport, sedimentation potential, and streaming potential. These phenomena have been widely used in the transport [6–9] and separation of bio-/chemical samples. For example, the electrophoresis and electroosmotic transport have become the standard separation and transport method used in the booming lab-on-a-chip technology [10].

13.1.1 A General Picture of EDLs

EDLs have been extensively studied since the early 1900s and various models have been proposed. Herein, we briefly summarize the characteristics of four major EDL models. The first model (see Figure 13.1a) for EDL, proposed by Helmholtz, states that a layer of counter-ions will bind to charged surface such that the surface charge is balanced exactly by this counter-ion layer [11]. In this model, the thickness (and the electrical field) of the EDL is limited to the thickness of a single molecular layer. While this simple model can explain some measurements of capacity of the EDL, it cannot explain most of the electrokinetic experiments. The second model (see Figure 13.1b), also referred to as a diffusive EDL model, was first proposed by Gouy [12] and Chapman [13]. In this model, the ions in the entire EDL are mobile, and the total charge, originating from counter-ions and co-ions in the liquid phase, balances the surface charge. They further proposed the Poisson–Boltzmann (PB) equation, which will be discussed in Section 13.2.1, for use in describing the potential and space charge distribution in the EDL.

Though the Gouy–Chapman model considers the diffusive nature of EDL, its treatment of ions as point charges can result in an unphysically high local concentration of counter-ions near highly charged surfaces. To address this issue, the concept of *Stern layer* (see Figure 13.1c) was introduced. Inside a Stern layer, the ion distribution depends mainly on the ion size and short-range interactions between ion, solvent, and the surface. Though very thin, the Stern layer is important, because, in many systems, a majority of the counter-ions balancing surface charges lie within the Stern layer.

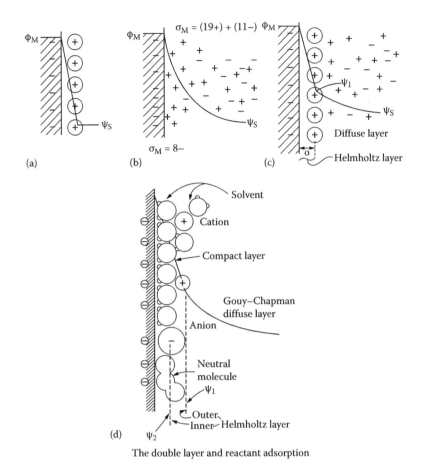

The double layer and reactant adsorption

FIGURE 13.1
Various models for EDL and the electric potential distribution across the EDL. (a) Helmholtz model, (b) Gouy–Chapman model, (c) Gouy–Stern model, and (d) a modern view of the EDL. (Reproduced from Conway, B.E. *Encyclopedia of Surface and Colloid Science*: Dekker Publishing Co., 2002.)

A more refined model for the EDL is shown in Figure 13.1d. In such a model, the diffusive part of the EDL begins at the outer Helmholtz plane (OHP). Some ions can be specifically adsorbed [1] on the surface and may be only partially hydrated. The plane of the specifically adsorbed ions is called the inner Helmholtz plane (IHP). Since the specifically adsorbed ions usually approach the surface more closely than other ions, there is usually no charge within the IHP. The region between the OHP and the surface is called an inner layer or compact layer. Note that the orientation of the water molecules within the inner layer may depend upon some extent on the surface charge, the polarity of solvent molecules, and adsorbed ions within the compact layer.

Most notably in the last two models, the EDL is split into certain distinct regions, in which the ion and potential distributions are dominated by different interactions. Such a split is rather artificial and a rigorous treatment of the EDL should model the entire transitions from the inner layer to the diffusive part of the EDL smoothly. Though the theoretical modeling of this transition is very complicated and has been rarely used in engineering practice [14], the splitting has been proven usefully especially in understanding various electrokinetic phenomena [5,14]. This is mainly because by splitting the EDL into an inner and a diffusive layer, one can encapsulate the complicated physics near the surface into the inner layer and rely on the experimental techniques to obtain quantitative information of the inner layer, while simple theories, for example, PB equation, may be concurrently used to analyze the diffusive layer quantitatively and thus provide useful information for engineering applications. With the advent of powerful computers and more reliable models for interactions between atoms in liquid phase developed over the last few decades, the EDL is now being studied via atomistic simulations. Consequently, molecular-level information of the EDL is now becoming available. This information, which can be valuable to the further refinement of the above models, can be useful in developing theoretical models applicable to engineering problems.

In this chapter, we shall focus on the ion distribution in the EDL, since once the ion distribution is known, other observables, for example electrical potential distributions, can be obtained without too much difficulty. This chapter is organized as follows: Section 13.2 shows the various theoretical models that have been developed to predict the ion distribution in EDLs, and Section 13.3 describes the atomistic simulations of the ion distribution in EDLs.

13.2 Continuum Modeling of EDLs

13.2.1 PB Equation

The PB equation was first proposed by Gouy [12] and Chapman [13] in the early 19th century. There are many ways to derive the PB equation, for example, from basic statistical mechanics principles [15], using the concept of electrochemical equilibrium [4], using the phenomenological free energy approach [16], or using the lattice gas model [16]. Here, we follow the original idea of Gouy and Chapman. That is, the distribution of electric potential ψ in the EDL can be described by the Poisson equation

$$\nabla^2 \psi = -\frac{\rho_e}{\varepsilon}, \tag{13.1}$$

where ρ_e and ε are the local ion charge density and the permittivity of the electrolyte solution, respectively. The Boltzmann distribution states that the number density of ion i at any position r can be expressed as

$$n_i(r) = n_{i,0} e^{\phi_{MF}(r)/k_B T}, \tag{13.2}$$

where $n_{i,0}$ is the number density of ion i at the reference point, k_B is the Boltzmann constant, and T is the absolute temperature. $\phi_{MF}(r)$ is the potential of mean force (PMF) of ion i at a position r, and it corresponds to the energy cost of moving an ion from the reference point to the position r. By approximating ϕ_{MF} to the electric potential, it is possible to obtain

$$n_i = n_{i,0} e^{-ez_i \psi / k_B T}, \tag{13.3}$$

where $n_{i,0}$ is the number density of ion i at the reference point where the potential ψ is zero, e is the electron charge, and z_i is the valence of ion species i. By expressing the local charge density in terms of the ion number density and combining Equations 13.1 and 13.3, the PB equation is obtained as

$$\nabla^2 \psi = -\frac{e}{\varepsilon} \sum_{i=1}^{N} z_i n_{i,0} e^{-\frac{z_i e \psi}{k_B T}}, \tag{13.4}$$

where N is the number of ion species in the solution. For symmetric, binary, single-charged ionic solution, the equation can be rewritten as

$$\nabla^2 \psi = \frac{2en_0}{\varepsilon} \sinh\left(\frac{e\psi}{k_B T}\right). \tag{13.5}$$

For small potential, that is, $|\psi| \ll k_B T/e$ (at room temperature, $k_B T/e \approx 25$ mV), the above equation can be linearized to obtain the linearized PB equation as

$$\nabla^2 \psi = \frac{2e^2 n_0}{\varepsilon k_B T} \psi. \tag{13.6}$$

By introducing the Debye length λ_D in the form of

$$\lambda_D = \left(\frac{\varepsilon k_B T}{2e^2 n_0}\right)^{\frac{1}{2}}, \tag{13.7}$$

the linearized PB equation can be written as

$$\nabla^2 \psi = \frac{1}{\lambda_D^2} \psi. \tag{13.8}$$

It is then possible to elucidate useful insights into the structure of EDLs from the PB equation by applying the PB equation to a simple problem. Here, a charged planar surface is in contact with a large electrolyte reservoir, and the interface between the planar surface and electrolyte is at $x = 0$. For this problem, the boundary conditions for the PB equation are given as

$$\psi\big|_{x=0} = \psi_0 \tag{13.9}$$

$$\psi\big|_{x\to\infty} = 0 \tag{13.10}$$

or

$$\frac{d\psi}{dx} = -\frac{\sigma}{\varepsilon} \tag{13.11}$$

$$\psi\big|_{x\to\infty} = 0 \tag{13.12}$$

depending on whether ψ_0 or σ (surface charge density) is known. Here, we assume that the surface potential is known ($\psi_0 = 20$ mV) and study the ion and potential distributions in the EDL for two different bulk electrolyte concentrations, that is, $c_0 = 0.1$ M and $c_0 = 1.0$ M. Using Equation 13.7 and taking the temperature and dielectric constant of the electrolyte solution to be 300 K and 80.0, respectively, the Debye length for the two cases is 0.98 and 0.31 nm, respectively. Figure 13.2a and b show the ion concentration and potential distribution near the charged surface for these two cases. We observe that as the bulk concentration increases (or as the Debye length decreases), the counter-ion concentration and the potential near the surface change more rapidly as it moves away from the surface, and the width of the EDL shrinks. This is because as the ion concentration increases, the screening of the surface charge becomes more effective, and thus the influence of the surface charge on ions and potential distributions in the solution penetrates less deeply into the electrolyte solution. These observations also suggest that the Debye length can serve as an indicator of the thickness of EDLs.

To date, the PB equation has been a major tool used to study various problems where electrostatic interactions between either the ions or the ion–surface are important. Its major advantage is its simplicity, which thus provided a solution for even complicated systems (e.g., biological membranes). Its major problem is that it is developed based on a mean field theory in which the correlation between ions and the nonelectrostatic interactions are totally neglected, and the solvents are treated as a dielectric medium. The success of the PB equation is quite impressive given the various assumptions made in its derivation. However, there are many situations where assumptions made in the PB equation become unrealistic, and the PB equation fails to render predictions that are even qualitatively consistent with experimental observations [17,18]. It is therefore very important to understand the limitation of the PB equation. Indeed, elucidating these limitations has been discussed ever since the first derivation of the PB equation. Though there have been several excellent

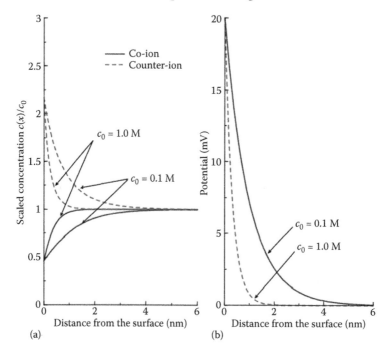

FIGURE 13.2

Ion (a) and potential (b) distribution near a charged surface with a surface potential of 20 mV for a bulk electrolyte concentration of 0.1 and 1.0 M.

reviews of this topic [4,14,19], we only list a few most widely scrutinized limitations of the PB equation.

- The finite size of the ions is neglected. This limitation is most problematic when the surface charge density is high because the PB equation can predict a counter-ion concentration far in excess of the concentration of counter-ions defined by the steric packing limit.

- The nonelectrostatic interactions between ion–ion are neglected and the nonelec-trostatic ion–surface interactions are considered using a hard-sphere model. These short-ranged interactions are responsible for the specific adsorption of ions on the surface.

- The correlations between ions are neglected. Because of the ion–ion correlations, the PMF of an ion at a position r is different from the average electric potential at that point even if only the electrostatic ion–ion interactions are considered.

- Water is taken as a structureless dielectric continuum, and its dielectric constant is usually taken as a constant in the entire EDL although more elaborate treatments do exist. Because of the strong electric field in the EDL, the dielectric constant of water can vary at different positions in the EDL [5,20]. In particular, dielectric saturation can occur at positions very close to a highly charged surface.

- The image forces between the ion and the surface are neglected.

Because of these limitations in the PB equation, a significant amount of work has been undertaken to develop better mathematical models for EDLs. Most of these models fall into two categories: (1) some are based on the PB equation or its thermodynamic extensions [21,22] and (2) some are based on the principles of basic statistical mechanics [23–26]. The first approach is usually easier to handle mathematically and is readily applicable to complicated systems. The second approach, usually much more involved mathematically, has not been widely used in the past. In this chapter, we will focus mainly on the first approach. For the second approach, the interested readers are referred to the excellent review by Lyklema [14] and the literature therein.

13.2.2 Modified PB Equation

It is difficult to cover all the work related to developing a modified PB (MPB) equation. Therefore, our discussion will focus on (1) an MPB equation that accounts for the finite ion-size effect [16,21], (2) an MPB equation that accounts for the effect of fluctuating poten-tial [27,28], (3) the work by Woelki and Kohler [29,30] where contributions of many effects to EDLs were compared, and (4) an MPB equation that accounts for solvent effects [22,31].

A major problem with the PB equation is that under a high surface charge density, it predicts unphysically high counter-ion concentrations at positions near the surface [14]. This is mainly caused by the fact that as ion concentration increases, the ion–ion distance decreases and the short-range ion–ion interactions become comparable to the electrostatic interactions, and thus can no longer be neglected. In particular, the ion concentration is bounded by a maximum value corresponding to the *close-packing* of counter-ions. Such an effect is especially prominent when the counter-ion size is large and has been incorporated into many MPB equations. A detailed history of such MPBs and their recent applications can be found in several recent reviews [32–34]. Here, we only introduce the MPB equation developed by Borukhov et al. [16,21]. Their MPB equation can be derived either by using a lattice gas formulation or by using a phenomenological free energy approach. For 1:z electrolytes, the MPB equation reads

$$\nabla^2\Psi = -\frac{zec_b}{\varepsilon}\frac{e^{zBe\Psi} - ze^{-Be\Psi}}{1-\phi_0 + \dfrac{\phi_0(e^{zBe\Psi} + ze^{-Be\Psi})}{z+1}}, \tag{13.13}$$

where c_b is the bulk concentration of the electrolyte. $\phi_0 = 2a^3c_b$, and a is the ion size. In either the low ion concentration limit ($\phi_0 \to 0$) or the low electrostatic potential ($|\beta e\Psi| \ll 1$), Equation 13.13 reduces to the classical PB equation (Equation 13.4). However, for large electrostatic potential ($|\beta e\Psi| \gg 1$), Equation 13.13 is significantly different from the classical PB equation. In particular, the ion concentration is always bounded by $1/a^3$ (close-packing) in the MPB equations.

Figure 13.3 shows the concentration profiles of the negative multivalent ion $c^-(x)$ near a positively charged surface, as obtained by solving Equation 13.13. Note that at positions close to the channel wall, the concentration saturation occurs, which deviates significantly from that obtained from the classical PB equation (especially when the counter-ion has a large size). Figure 13.4 shows the surface concentration of counter-ions as a function of the surface charge density for different ion sizes, a. The PB prediction is also shown for comparison. Clearly, for large ions, the surface concentration becomes saturated at a very low surface charge density. As the ion size decreases, the deviation between the MPB and PB equations becomes smaller.

Next, we introduce the MPB equations that consider the influence of the fluctuating potentials, an approach pioneered by Kirkwood [35], followed by Bell and Rangecroft [27], and refined by Outhwaite et al. [28,36–41]. The central idea of these MPB equations is that because of the ion–ion correlations, an ion with an opposite sign is more likely to be found near a given ion than one of the same sign, giving rise to the *self-atmosphere*. Therefore, the electrostatic potential at a point near an ion differs from the mean potential at the same

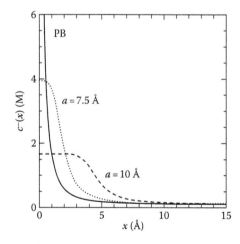

FIGURE 13.3

Concentration profiles of the negative multivalent ion $c^-(x)$ near a positively charged surface obtained by solving Equation 13.13 for two different ion sizes, $a = 7.5$ Å and $a = 10$ Å, respectively. The solid line represents the results obtained from the classical PB equation. The bulk concentration is $c_b = 0.1$ M for the 1:4 electrolyte. The surface charge density σ is taken as one electron charge per 50 Å^2. The temperature and dielectric constant of the aqueous solution are taken as 298 K and 80, respectively. (Reproduced from Borukhov, I. et al., *Phys. Rev. Lett.* 79 (3): 435–438, 1997.)

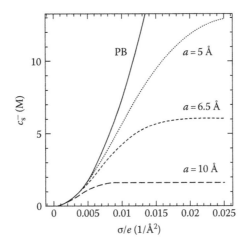

FIGURE 13.4
Concentration of the negative ion as a function of the surface charge density for different ion size, a. The bulk concentration is $c_b = 0.001$ M for the 1:4 electrolyte. The temperature and dielectric constant of the aqueous solution are taken as 298 K and 80, respectively. (Reproduced from Borukhov, I. et al., *Phys. Rev. Lett.* 79 (3): 435–438, 1997.)

point by the amount known as the fluctuating potential. Here, the fluctuating potential accounts mainly for the following three effects [27]:

1. The self-atmosphere of an ion is modified in the EDL by the image effects owing to the adjacent dielectric continuity.

2. The deviation of the local ionic concentrations from bulk values; if the diffuse region has a net charge, there is a *cavity effect* owing to the displacement of the charge by the ionic volume.

3. The *excluded volume* effect comes from the finite size of the ions and the difference between local ionic concentrations and their value in the bulk electrolyte.

Though many approaches have been suggested for incorporating the fluctuating potential into MPB equations, we refer interested readers to the work by Outhwaite and Bhuiyan [39]. Here, we only present some of the most important predictions of these equations. Figure 13.5 shows the comparison of singlet distribution $g_{0i}(X)$, that is, the ion distribution near surface, obtained from Monte Carlo (MC) simulation and from the MPB equation derived in Ref. [39]. It indicates that the prediction by the MPB equation agrees very well the MC results. Figure 13.6 shows the variation of the diffusive-layer potential drop $\phi\left(\dfrac{1}{2}\right)$ ($\phi = |e|\beta\psi$) with dimensionless surface charge density σ^* for a 1:1 electrolyte as predicted by both the MC simulation and the MPB equation. Again, very good agreement is evident.

Though the above MPB equations help take into account the effect of the fluctuating potential, they fail to account for other important effects such as the variation of the dielectric constant in the EDL. There exists very few work where various effects are accounted for in an MPB equation, and it seems that the work by Woelki and Kohler shows the most comprehensive model published so far [29,30]. Their derivation is based on the local thermodynamic equilibrium conditions of constant electrochemical potentials of the

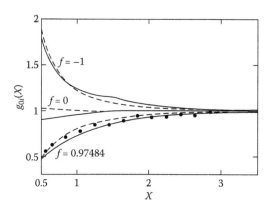

FIGURE 13.5

Singlet distribution function $g_{0i}(X)$ for a 1:1 electrolyte at $c_b = 0.1$ M and zero surface charge density, both with and without imaging. The solid points are the MC results of Croxton et al. [42]. The dotted dashed line denotes the results obtained using the MPB equation developed in Ref. [28]. (Reproduced from Outhwaite, C.W. and Bhuiyan, L.B., *J. Chem. Soc., Faraday Trans.* 2 79 (5): 707–718, 1983.)

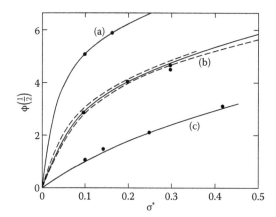

FIGURE 13.6

Variation of the diffuse-layer potential drop $\phi\left(\frac{1}{2}\right)$ ($\phi = |e|\beta\psi$) with a surface charge density of $\sigma^* = (\sigma a^2/|e|)$ for a 1:1 electrolyte: (a) $c_b = 0.01$ M, (b) $c_b = 0.1$ M and (c) $c_b = 1.0$ M. The solid points are from the MC results of Croxton et al. [42]. The curves marked (—), (–··–), and (- - -) are for no imaging, a metallic wall, and an insulating wall, respectively. (Reproduced from Outhwaite, C.W. and Bhuiyan, L.B., *J. Chem. Soc., Faraday Trans.* 2 79 (5): 707–718, 1983.)

components. They divided the EDL into a Stern layer and a diffusive layer and assumed that the thickness of the Stern layer is the radius of the smallest counter-ion and that only solvent molecules exist within the Stern layer. They developed a set of local-balance differential equations involving ϕ (the electrostatic potential), E (the electrical field in the normal direction of the surface), p (pressure), and c_i (the molar concentration of solute i). In their derivation, it was assumed that the compressibility of electrolyte solution was zero and the dielectric permittivity ε depended not upon the pressure but upon the composition and the field strength. In that their derivation is rather complicated, we only briefly summarize some of the most important features of their model.

- The size of ions are accounted for explicitly in the MPB by expressing the volume of the solution as

$$V = n_0^f \bar{V}_i + \sum_{i=1}^{K} n_i \bar{V}_i,$$ (13.14)

where $i = 0$ denotes the solvent, $i = 1 \cdots K$ denotes the K ionic species in the solution, and $\bar{V}_i (i = 0 \cdots K)$ denotes the partial molar volume of species i. Note that the water molecules in the solvation shell are assumed as an integral part of the ions and thus form part of their effective partial molar volume $\bar{V}_i$.

- The dielectric permittivity ε is a linear function of the solute concentration

$$\varepsilon = \sum_{i=0}^{K} \bar{\varepsilon}_i \bar{V}_i c_i,$$ (13.15)

where $\bar{\varepsilon}_i$ is a constant and $\bar{V}_i$ is the partial molar volume of species i. In their work, $\bar{\varepsilon}_i$ is taken as 1.0 for ions and the dielectric constant of water is taken as

$$\bar{\varepsilon}_0(E) = a + \frac{b}{cE} \arctan(cE),$$ (13.16)

where $a = 2.65 \times 10^{-11}$ C^2 J^{-1} m^{-1}, $b = 6.69 \times 10^{-10}$ C^2 J^{-1} m^{-1}, and $c = 3.46 \times 10^{-9}$ m V^{-1}. Figure 13.7 shows the variation of the dielectric constant of water with the electrical field strength.

- The effect of the self-atmosphere around the ion and the solvation of ion by water are taken into account by introducing the self-atmosphere energy into the chemical potential of the ion.

- The ion polarization effect is accounted for by introducing the electrical field dependence into the calculation of the electrochemical potential gradient across the EDL.

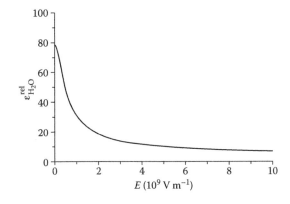

FIGURE 13.7
Relative dielectric constant of water $\varepsilon_{H_2O}^{rel} = \varepsilon_0 / \bar{\varepsilon}_0$, as a function of the electrical field strength according to Equation 13.16. (Reproduced from Woelki, S. and Kohler, H.-H., *Chem. Phys.* 261 (3): 411–419, 2000.)

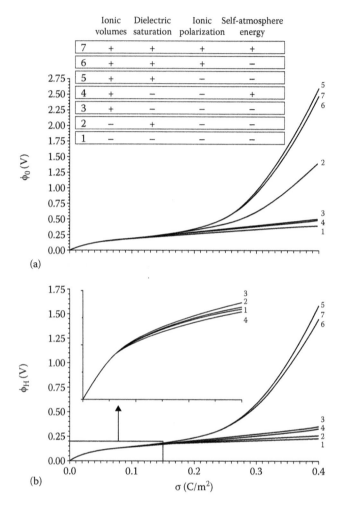

	Ionic volumes	Dielectric saturation	Ionic polarization	Self-atmosphere energy
7	+	+	+	+
6	+	+	+	−
5	+	+	−	−
4	+	−	−	+
3	+	−	−	−
2	−	+	−	−
1	−	−	−	−

FIGURE 13.8

Influence of several factors on the (a) surface potential ($\phi(0)$) and on the (b) Helmholtz potential (ϕ_H). In the table, the effects included in the individual curves are denoted with "+." Parameters: plane surface, $\varepsilon_p = 2\varepsilon_0$; electrolyte: KI, $c_{KI}^\infty = 0.01$ M, $\bar{V}_{I^-} = 37.1 \times 10^{-6}$ m^3 mol^{-1}, $\bar{V}_{K^+} = 44.2 \times 10^{-6}$ m^3 mol^{-1}; Stern layer: $\delta = \bar{r}_{I^-} = 2.45$ Å. (Reproduced from Woelki, S. and Kohler, H.-H., *Chem. Phys.* 261 (3): 411–419, 2000.)

Figure 13.8a and b show the influence of various factors upon the dependence of surface potential $\phi(0)$ and Helmholtz potential ϕ_H (potential at the Helmholtz plane) on the surface charge density. We observe that at low surface charge densities ($\sigma < 0.15$ C/m^2), the prediction of the MPB equation does not deviate greatly from that of the PB equation (curve 1). However, at higher surface charge densities, the deviation from the PB equation becomes significant as various effects are added to the MPB equations. Curve 2 indicates that $\phi(0)$ is much higher compared to the classical PB prediction if the dielectric saturation effect is included. This is because the saturation-induced decrease of the permittivity leads to an increase of the electrical field strength and hence an increase of potential at both the surface and the Helmholtz plane. Curves 3 and 4 indicate that for the case investigated in Ref. [29], the influence of ionic volume and self-atmosphere effects is not significant even at very high surface charge densities. Curve 5 indicates that when the ionic volume effect is considered, the effect of dielectric saturation becomes more significant. This is because the dielectric saturation strongly increases the pressure at the Helmholtz plane, thus repelling the ion from the surface (note that such a pressure increase does not repel ions from the channel wall if the ions are assumed at zero volume, as in curve 2). This saturation again impedes the screening of surface charge, resulting in an extremely high $\phi(0)$ value. Curves 6 and 7 indicate that contributions from ionic polarization and self-atmosphere are small for the case under study.

In the MPB equations discussed above, water is mainly modeled as a dielectric continuum; the solvent effect and the discrete nature of the water molecules are not explicitly included. Accounting for these factors in the MPB equation is very difficult, since the water–ion interaction and its influences on the ion–ion interaction are extremely complicated.

Burak and Andelman [22,31] proposed an MPB equation in which they introduced the solvent effect by adding an effective interaction potential to the electrostatic ion–ion interactions. Figure 13.9 shows the schematic description of the effective interaction potential approach. The key idea is that the system, consisting of discrete water molecules and ions, is replaced by ions in a continuum dielectric medium with a dielectric constant ε, with electrostatic and short-range interactions $u_{ij}(r) = u_{ij}(|r|)$. The short-range interaction u_{ij} can be characterized by an effective interaction potential and accounts mainly for the solvent effect on the ion–ion interactions. They also obtained u_{ij} by using the *reverse Monte Carlo* method [22,43]. Figure 13.10 shows the effective potential between Na+ ions. It was observed that because of the solvent effect, the Na+ ions experience an attractive interaction at close distance (e.g., at a separation of 3.8 Å). At a large separation, their interactions reduce to the pure electrostatic interactions. Burak and Andelman [22] also showed that, by considering these interactions, a new MPB formulation can be derived as

$$\ln \frac{c_i(r)}{\zeta_i} + \sum_j \int c_j(r')U_{ij}(r-r')\mathrm{d}^3r + \beta e_i \psi(r) = 0, \tag{13.17}$$

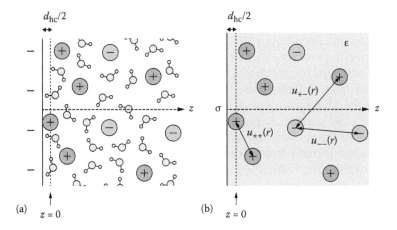

FIGURE 13.9
A schematic description of the aqueous pair potential model. An aqueous ionic solution in contact with a charged plate in (a) is replaced in (b) by ions in a continuum dielectric medium having a dielectric constant ε, with electrostatic and short-range interactions $u_{ij}(r) = u_{ij}(|r|)$. The z-coordinate designates the distance from the charged plate, with $z = 0$ corresponding to the distance of closest approach ($d_{hc}/2$) of the ions to the plane. (Reproduced from Burak, Y. and Andelman, D., *Phys. Rev. E* 62 (4): 5296–5312, 2000.)

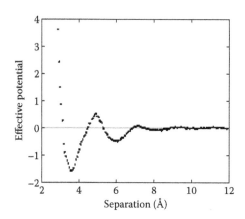

FIGURE 13.10

The short-range effective potential between Na^+ ion pairs using simulations in a bulk NaCl solution of concentration 0.55 M, at room temperature. The potential is shown in the unit of k_BT as a function of the distance between the ion centers. For ion separations smaller than 2.9 Å, a hardcore interaction was assumed. The Coulomb interaction is subtracted to show only the short-range hydration effect attributed to the water molecules. (Reproduced from Burak, Y. and Andelman, D., *Phys. Rev. E* 62 (4): 5296–5312, 2000.)

where c_i is the ion density and $\zeta_i = \exp(\beta\mu_i)/\lambda_T^3$ (μ_i is the chemical potential, λ_T is de Broglie thermal wavelength, and $\beta = 1/k_BT$). ψ is the electrostatic potential, and the weighted potential U_{ij} is defined as

$$U_{ij} = 1 - e^{-\beta u_{ij}(r-r')}, \tag{13.18}$$

where u_{ij} is the normal short-range interaction between ions of species i and j (see Figures 13.9 and 13.10). Note that this equation must be complemented by the Poisson equation.

Using the above MPB equation, Burak and Andelman studied the ion distribution near a charged planar surface in contact with an electrolyte solution of valence 1:1. Figure 13.11 shows the counter-ion density profile obtained from the MPB equation and the classical PB equation when the surface charge density is 0.333 C/m^2 and no salt is present in the solution. It indicates that the short-range attraction favors an increased concentration near the charged plate. Figure 13.12 shows the ratio c_+/c_+^{PB} between the positive ion densities obtained using the MPB and classical PB equations for three surface charge densities. It indicates that at a low surface charge density (e.g., $|\sigma| = 0.0333$ C/m^2), the effect of hydration is minor, but as the surface charge density increases, the deviation between MPB and PB equations becomes more and more significant. This is not surprising, because as the surface charge density increases, the counter-ion concentration near the surface increases (i.e., the distance between ions decreases), and thus the hydration effect, modeled by the short-range effective potential, becomes more important.

Even though this model captures some important aspects of the solvent effect, it has several limitations. For example, (1) the effective interaction potential for the ion–wall interaction, which is also influenced greatly by the solvent effect, is not considered; (2) it is assumed that the effective interaction potential between ions is independent of the ion position relative to the charged surface; and (3) the influence of the solvent structure on the ion–ion interaction is not included. Developing an MPB equation that accounts for all these missing effects is still an active research area and more rigorous models are emerging. For example, Lamperski and

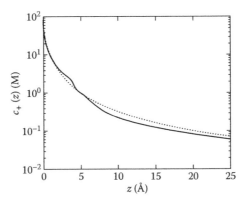

FIGURE 13.11
The counter-ion density profile (solid line) obtained from Equation 13.17, with the hydration interaction as in Figure 13.10. No slat is presented in the solution. The surface charge density is $|\sigma| = 0.333$ C/m². The dielectric constant is 78, and the temperature is 298 K. The dotted line shows the density profile predicted by the PB equation. (Reproduced from Burak, Y. and Andelman, D., *Phys. Rev. E* 62 (4): 5296–5312, 2000.)

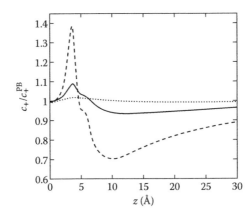

FIGURE 13.12
The ratio c_+ / c_+^{PB} between the positive ion density using the MPB and classical PB equation for surface charge densities $|\sigma| = 0.333$ C/m² (dashed line), 0.1 C/m² (solid line), and 0.0333 C/m² (dotted line). The bulk concentration c_b is 0.025 M. Other parameters are the same as in Figure 13.11. (Reproduced from Burak, Y. and Andelman, D., *Phys. Rev. E* 62 (4): 5296–5312, 2000.)

Outhwaite [44] developed an MPB equation where the water molecules are modeled as hard spheres with a dipole moment, and some interesting results are obtained to show how the density of solvent molecules can influence the ion distribution.

13.3 Atomistic Simulation of EDLs

The theoretical modeling approach discussed in Section 13.2 has provided valuable insights into the structure of EDLs. However, a major issue with such modeling is that it usually involves assumptions that are sometimes difficult to justify, which can compromise the accuracy of its predictions. Atomistic simulations offer a potential way to address this issue. In atomistic simulations, interactions between ion and ion, between ion and solvent, and between ion and surface are explicitly modeled and one obtains the ion distribution in EDLs without involving assumptions typically made in theoretical modeling. Atomistic simulations can provide quantitatively accurate results if accurate interaction parameters are used. In this section, we discuss the insights on ion distribution in EDLs obtained from atomistic simulations. The atomistic simulation of EDL can be broadly categorized into three groups [45]: (1) primitive model where solvent (i.e., water) is modeled as a dielectric continuum, (2) point dipole model where water is modeled as polarizable or nonpolarizable point dipole, and (3) molecular solvent model where the water is modeled as extended point charges; for example, in the SPC/E model, a water molecule is modeled as a three-atom molecule with each atom carrying a fixed partial charge. Atomistic simulations using primitive models are least demanding in terms of computational cost and have been extensively used [15,46–51]. Simulations of the second group are useful in studying the preferential adsorption of ions on surfaces and also have been used widely [43]. Compared to the first two groups, atomistic simulations of the last group provide the most complete description of the EDL, although their computational cost is the greatest. Enabled by the advent of fast electrostatic solvers (e.g., the Particle Mesh Ewald method [52] and the Particle–Particle Particle–Mesh method [53]) and improvement in computing hardware, simulations of the last group dominate present studies of EDLs and are the focus of discussion in this section.

Despite the fact that detailed atomistic simulations of EDLs near rigid surface have a relatively short history, much research has been undertaken in this realm. Here, we will focus on the insights on structure of EDLs revealed that cannot be easily captured using the classical PB or MPB equations, for example, the role of molecular nature of water and the ion specificity of EDLs. In particular, we will focus on how ion distribution in EDL is affected by interfacial water structure, ion size, molecular wall, and geometrical confinement. We note that because these effects are *closely* related (e.g., interfacial water structure effects are related to ion size effects), they should all be addressed simultaneously. However, for purposes of clarity, we will discuss them separately and comment on their relationships when appropriate.

13.3.1 Effects of Ion Hydration on EDLs

Water molecules play a dual role in determining the ion distribution within EDLs. First, they collectively serve as a dielectric medium that modulates the ion–ion and ion–wall interactions. Second, interactions between the ions and water molecules in their immediate vicinity can affect ion distributions within EDLs, which is known as the hydration effect. To appreciate this effect, we note that, in electrolyte solutions, water molecules near each ion are loosely bonded to the ion because of strong charge–dipole interactions between the ion and water molecules. These water molecules are usually referred to as the hydration water of the ion. Because the interactions between an ion and its hydration water molecules are highly attractive, it is energetically unfavorable (favorable) for an ion to lose (or increase) the number of its hydration water. Since the hydration of ion at different positions inside EDL can be different (e.g., the number of hydration water molecules of an ion will change as it moves from the electrolyte bulk to a solid surface owing to the simple geometrical confinement), ion hydration can affect the ion distribution. Since the strength of ion hydration depends on factors such as ion size and type, the proximity of ion to wall, and confinement, the effects of these factors on the ion distribution inside EDLs can often be traced to the ion hydration effects [54–56]. As such, we will not separately address the ion hydration effect but discuss their various manifestations through other effects.

13.3.2 Effects of Interfacial Water Structure on EDLs

Water layering occurs near solid–water interfaces, a phenomenon that has been observed in both atomistic simulations [57,58] and experimental studies [59]. Typically, the layering of water can extend a few water molecular diameters from the solid surface, and the density and orientation of water molecules within these layers are quite different from those in bulk [55,58]. Therefore, the hydration of ions near charged walls can be quite different from that in the bulk and significantly influence the ion distribution near the charged walls [55,57,58,60–65].

Figure 13.13 shows the water and K^+ ion concentration profiles near a solid wall with a surface charge density of $\sigma = -0.13$ C/m². The K^+ ion concentration computed from the PB equation (see Ref. [66] for details on the PB equation and its numerical solution) increases as ions approach the charged surface. However, for atomistic simulation results, in addition to the strong oscillation of water density near the wall, we observe that the K^+ ion concentration profile exhibits two peaks: the first peak at $z = 0.27$ nm corresponds to the closest approach of K^+ ions to the wall (i.e., contact adsorption) and the second peak at $z = 0.5$ nm originates from the ion hydration effect. Specifically, the significant accumulation of ions at the second peak is driven by the tendency of K^+ ions to appear at positions to maximize the number of their hydration water molecules. To see this quantitatively, we computed the hydration number of K^+ ions near the solid surface. An ion's hydration number is defined as the number of water molecules within the first hydration shell of this ion, and the radius of the first hydration shell (r_{min}) is usually defined as the location of the first minimum of the ion–water radial distribution function [67]. The radius of the hydration shell of a K^+ ion is found to be 0.365 nm (see Figure 13.14c). Figure 13.14a and b show the variation of K^+ ion concentration and K^+ ion's hydration number near the wall. The second K^+ ion concentration peak corresponds very well with the maximum of K^+ ion hydration number near wall, thus confirming that the accumulation of K^+ ion at the second peak is caused by the hydration effects.

We note that how significantly the interfacial water structure affects the ion distribution in EDL depends on both the physicochemical properties of the surface and the ion [45,58,60]. Such effects are most obvious for small ions (e.g., Na^+ ions) or near walls with low to moderate surface charge densities. For example, near a wall with $\sigma = -0.12$ C/m²,

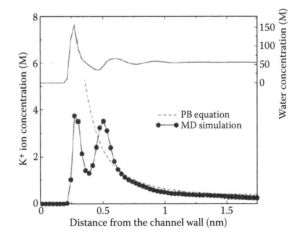

FIGURE 13.13
K^+ ion and water concentration profiles near a solid wall with a surface charge density of -0.13 C/m². (Reproduced from Qiao, R. and Aluru, N.R., *Colloids Surf. A* 267 (1–3): 103–109, 2005.)

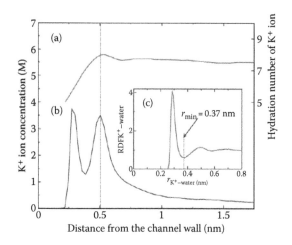

FIGURE 13.14

(a) Variation of the hydration number for K^+ ion near a solid wall with a surface charge density of -0.13 C/m². (b) The K^+ ion concentration profile near the solid wall. (c) The radial distribution function of K^+–water in bulk solution. (Reproduced from Qiao, R. and Aluru, N.R., *Colloids Surf. A* 267 (1–3): 103–109, 2005.)

driven by the tendency to maximize an ion's hydration number, the first Na^+ ion concentration peak is not located at the closet approach ($z \approx 0.15$ nm) but at $z = 0.5$ nm, where its hydration number is maximized [66]. However, near a wall with $\sigma = -0.285$ C/m², the ion hydration effects are overwhelmed by the ion–wall interactions and the first Na^+ ion concentration peak is shifted to $z \approx 0.15$ nm [68].

13.3.3 Molecular Wall Effects

In most theoretical studies of the ion distribution in EDL, the molecular ion–wall interactions are modeled by the hard-sphere interaction; that is, the ion can approach toward the surface up to a closest approach distance d_{ion}, and for wall–ion distance greater than d_{ion}, the molecular ion–wall interaction is neglected. Such a simplification, however, can be inaccurate when the ion approaches quite close to the surface, but not so close such that the ion–wall interaction is dominated by the molecular repulsion. In this case, because of van der Waals interactions, the wall atoms exert an attractive force on the ion, which helps increase the ion concentration near the surface. Figure 13.15a shows the Cl^- ion and water concentration profiles across a 3.49-nm-wide slit channel with a surface charge density of $+0.12$ C/m² as obtained from the atomistic simulation and from the PB equation solution. The Cl^- concentration peak predicted by atomistic simulation is approximately 88% higher compared to that predicted by the PB equation, and this deviation is mainly caused by the molecular wall–ion interactions. Figure 13.15b shows the potential energy of a Cl^- ion attributed to its molecular interactions (modeled by Lennard-Jones potential in the simulation) with the channel wall. It indicates that the potential energy attributed to the Cl^-–wall interaction is approximately $-1.8 k_BT$ ($T = 300$ K) at the position of 0.39 nm away from the channel wall (the location of the Cl^- ion concentration peak). Clearly, such a location with a negative potential energy is favorable for the Cl^- ions.

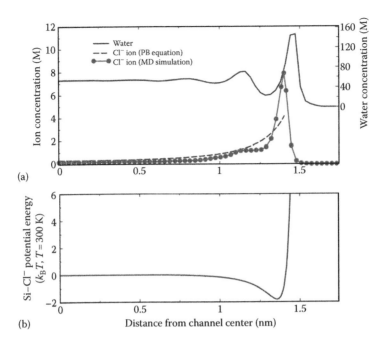

FIGURE 13.15

(a) Cl⁻ ion and water concentration across a 3.49-nm-wide silicon channel with a surface charge density of +0.120 C/m². The channel center is located at $z = 0$ nm. (b) The potential energy of the Cl⁻ ion over the channel wall computed using Lennard-Jones potential. It is assumed that the ion can access any position in the xy-plane with equal probability. (Reproduced from Qiao, R. and Aluru, N.R., *J. Chem. Phys.* 118 (10): 4692–4701, 2003.)

13.3.4 Ion Size Effects

In the classical PB equation, where the ions are assumed to be infinitesimal, the distribution of ions with the same valence but different size exhibits exactly the same behavior. However, the atomistic simulation results indicated that the distribution of ion in the EDL can be strongly influenced by its size [58,66,69].

In their systematic investigation of how the size of ions can influence their distribution in a 4.26-nm-wide slit pore, Crozier et al. [69] enclosed a slab of water molecules and ions between two rigid channel walls. The left channel wall had a surface charge density of +0.1 C/m², and the right channel wall had a surface charge density of −0.1 C/m². To model the ions with different sizes, they varied the Lennard-Jones parameter for different cases. The Lennard-Jones potential for the molecular interactions between molecules i and j can be written as $V_{LJ} = 4\varepsilon \left[\left(\dfrac{\sigma}{r_{ij}} \right)^{12} - \left(\dfrac{\sigma}{r_{ij}} \right)^{6} \right]$, where σ and ε are the interaction parameters. As σ increases, the closest distance molecules i and j can approach toward each other increases, and this corresponds to a large diameter of molecules i and j. Table 13.1 shows the various parameters used in their study.

Figure 13.16 shows the anion concentration profile across the channel for the various cases investigated. The upper panel shows the absolute value of the ion concentration and the lower panel shows the deviation of the ion concentration from the reference case (case 1). We observe that, in cases 3 and 4, the increased anion size produces a 20-fold increase in

TABLE 13.1

Anion and Cation Lennard-Jones Parameter for the Five Cases Studied in Ref. [69]

Case	Name	Cation–Cation		Anion–Anion		Cation–Anion		Cation–Oxygen		Anion–Oxygen	
		σ (Å)	ε/k_B (K)	σ (Å)	ε/k_B (K)	σ (Å)	ε/k_B (K)	σ (Å)	ε/k_B (K)	σ (Å)	ε/k_B (K)
1	Reference	3.169	78.2	3.169	78.2	3.169	78.2	3.169	78.2	3.169	78.2
2	Small cation	2.730	78.2	3.169	78.2	2.950	78.2	2.950	78.2	3.169	78.2
3	Large anion	3.169	78.2	4.860	78.2	4.015	78.2	3.169	78.2	4.015	78.2
4	Small cation–large anion	2.730	78.2	4.860	78.2	3.795	78.2	2.950	78.2	4.015	78.2
5	Reference	2.730	43.0	4.860	20.2	3.870	20.5	2.876	62.7	3.250	62.7

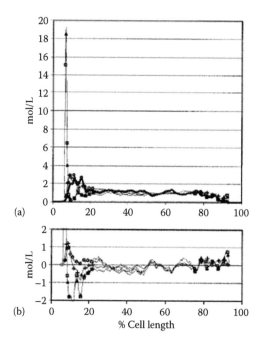

FIGURE 13.16

Anion concentration (a) and concentration deviation (b) from the reference case (case 1) as a function of distance from the left channel wall. The individual lines represent case 1 (thick line), case 2 (-o-o-), case 3 (-□-□-), case 4 (-Δ-Δ-), and case 5 (-+-+-). (Reproduced from Crozier, P.S. et al., *J. Chem. Phys.* 114 (17): 7513–7517, 2001.)

the local anion concentration near the left channel wall. Such a strong contact adsorption is mainly induced by the weaker Coulombic hydration of the larger anions and is accompanied by a replacement of adsorbed water molecules on the left channel wall as evidenced by the substantial decrease in the water peak shown in the bottom of Figure 13.17.

13.3.5 Microconfinement Effects

In the above discussions, the EDLs are either near isolated surfaces or in wide channels/ pores such that overlapping of EDLs is negligible. In many practical systems, however, the

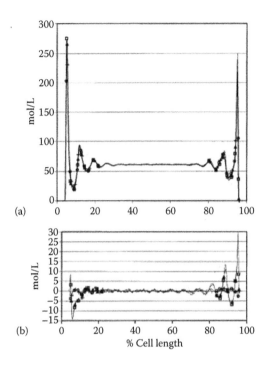

FIGURE 13.17

Oxygen atom concentration (a) and the concentration deviation (b) from the reference case (case 1) as a function of distance from the left channel wall. The individual lines represent case 1 (thick line), case 2 (-o-o-), case 3 (-□-□-), case 4 (-∆-∆-), and case 5 (-+-+-). (Reproduced from Crozier, P.S. et al., *J. Chem. Phys.* 114 (17): 7513–7517, 2001.)

distance between opposing walls is so small that a significant overlapping between the EDLs near these walls occurs. Such a situation has been extensively examined using the classical PB equation, which is applicable for dilute electrolytes and relatively wide pores. For example, the classical EDL theories predict that counter-ions would accumulate primarily in separate layers near each wall of a slit-shaped pore with fixed wall charge densities [4]. In very narrow pores (e.g., micropores, which are defined as pores with a width or diameter smaller than 2 nm [70]), the EDL structure can be conveniently studied using atomistic simulations. Studies in this regard, while scarce at present, have revealed interesting EDL phenomena in such situations [65,71].

Figure 13.18a shows the water and K^+ ion concentration profiles inside the slit-shaped pores with width W ranging from 9.36 to 14.7 Å [71]. Each wall carries a surface charge density of -0.055 C/m². The co-ions (i.e., the negatively charged ions [71]) are not included in the simulation, however, because the concentration of co-ions inside the pores is expected to be very low because of the strong electrostatic repulsion by charged pore walls. From Figure 13.18a, we observe that the water distribution inside the slit pore changes as pore width decreases: three layers of water molecules can be identified in slit pores with $W > 10.7$ Å while only two layers of water molecules develop in slit pores with $W \leq 10.7$ Å. In the widest slit pore studied ($W = 14.7$ Å), the K^+ ion distribution profile revealed that counter-ions accumulate in separate layers near *each* slit wall, in line with the expectation from the classical EDL theories to some extent. In contrast, K^+ ions, in slits between 10 and 14.7 Å, accumulate primarily in the central plane of each pore to form only one layer, which contradicts the prediction by classical PB equations. Interestingly, in slit pores with $W = 9.36$ Å, the K^+ ion concentration profile

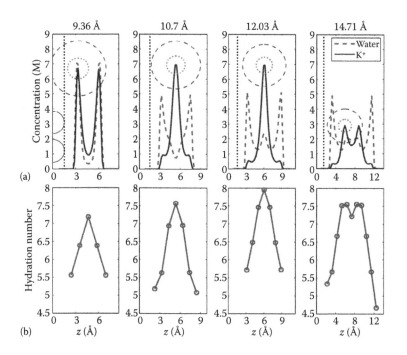

FIGURE 13.18

(a) Concentration profiles of water and K⁺ ions inside slit pores with various widths. For clarity, the water concentration has been scaled down by a factor of 30. The concentric circles denote the size of bare and hydrated K⁺ ions. The hemi-circle in the leftmost figure denotes the van der Waals radius of the wall atom and the dashed line denotes the effective boundary of the lower wall. (b) Hydration number of K⁺ ions across slit pores with various widths. All slit walls have the same surface charge density of −0.055 C/m². (Reproduced from Feng, G. et al., *ACS Nano* 4 (4): 2382–2390, 2010.)

again shows a distinct peak near *each* slit wall, in qualitative agreement with the classical PB equation. Different from those in the 14.7-Å-wide pore, K⁺ ions in each peak adjacent to the 9.36-Å-wide pore wall are contact-adsorbed as inferred from the size of the K⁺ ion (shown as circle in Figure 13.18a) and the water concentration profile in the slit pore.

To understand the origins of the evolution of K⁺ ion distribution in slit pores as the pore width varies, based on insights from the continuum and atomistic simulations of EDLs in Sections 13.2 and 13.3, we note that the distribution of counter-ions in electrified micropores free of co-ions is governed mainly by five factors: (1) the long-range electrostatic ion–ion repulsion, which always drives ions toward the slit walls; (2) the nonelectrostatic ion–wall attractions that consist of the van der Waals and steric interactions between the ion and slit wall atoms; (3) the hydration of ions, which drives ions toward positions where they can maximize interactions with their hydration water molecules; (4) the interactions between an ion's hydration water molecules and their surrounding water molecules; and (5) entropic effects that drive ions and water molecules inside pore toward a uniform distribution. These factors compete/cooperate with each other till the free energy of the entire system (ion and water) is minimized at equilibrium.

To clarify the role of ion hydration in determining the K⁺ ion distribution shown in Figure 13.18a, the hydration number, N_{hyd}, of K⁺ ions across various slit pores was computed (Figure 13.18b). In slit pores with $W = 14.7$ Å, as a K⁺ ion moves away from the slit wall, N_{hyd} increases sharply and reaches a maximum of 7.5 at a position 5.8 Å from the pore wall, exactly where the K⁺ ion concentration peak is located. In pores with $W = 10.7$

and 12.03 Å, N_{hyd} increases monotonically from the wall toward the pore center, and the K^+ peak again is located at a position where N_{hyd} is maximized. These results confirm that the ion hydration effects play a key role in determining the K^+ ion distribution in these pores, in line with observations for EDLs near open surfaces or in wide pores. However, it is clear that, in pores with a width between 10 and 14 Å, ion hydration plays a more decisive role in shaping the EDL structure in that it leads to a qualitative breakdown of the classical EDL picture; that is, it forces K^+ ions to form a single layer midway between two pore walls. As the pore width reduces to 9.36 Å, the K^+ ion distribution shows an abrupt transition; that is, they now form distinct layers near each slit wall, although the ion hydration effects should still drive them toward the pore center. Since the entropy effects do not favor the formation of distinct ion concentration peaks in any pore, the most straightforward reason for such a transition is that electrostatic ion–ion repulsions (factor 1 identified above) or nonelectrostatic ion–wall interactions (factor 2 identified above) overwhelm the hydration effects in this pore since these interactions strengthen with a decreasing pore width. A quantitative analysis, however, shows that neither the enhanced ion–ion repulsion nor the enhanced ion–wall attraction in the 9.36-Å-wide pore is the essential mechanism driving the transition observed here [71]. Instead, it was found that, in the 9.36-Å-wide pore, as a contact-adsorbed K^+ ion moves toward the pore center, while its interactions with hydration water molecules enhance as expected, the average coordination number of its hydration water molecules (defined as the water molecules within r_{min1} from the hydration water molecule being examined, where $r_{min1} = 3.30$ Å is the first local minimum of the water–water pair correlation function) reduces from 4.29 to 3.98, and the average interaction energy, between each of the ion's hydration water molecules and its primary coordination water molecules, increases by 5.5 kJ/mol. These results indicate that as the contact-adsorbed K^+ ion moves to the slit center, although it attracts more water molecules toward itself to improve hydration (thus lowering the system energy), it also causes its hydration water molecules to interact with fewer water molecules, therefore weakening these interactions (thus increasing the system energy). Such enthalpic effects associated with the interactions between the hydration water molecules and their coordinate water molecules dominate the ion hydration effects and play a critical role in causing the contact adsorption of K^+ ions on the pore wall, thus reducing the transition of the K^+ distribution profile as a pore width from 10.7 to 9.36 Å. The reduction of the coordination number of the hydration water of K^+ ions, as K^+ ion moves from the wall toward the pore center, is caused by the geometrical confinement posed by pore walls, and a thorough analysis of which is in Ref. [71].

From the above discussion, it is clear that in electrified pores with widths comparable to the size of hydrated ions, the ion distribution inside the pore is governed by the subtle interplay between ion–ion interactions, ion–water interactions, and water–water interactions, which are in turn controlled by the size of the pore, ion, and water molecules. While these insights elucidate a model of the EDL far more complex than those suggested by the classical PB equation or its various extensions, they open up new avenues for manipulating the structure of EDLs through rational design of micropores.

13.4 Future Perspective

As evident from the discussion in Sections 13.1 through 13.3, research on EDLs has a very long history, and much progress has been made in elucidating its structure and how physicochemical properties of ions and surfaces control the structure and other thermo-dynamic properties of EDLs. Despite extensive prior researches, there still exist much unexplored physics of EDLs that require new research on this topic, and the insights from these researches can positively affect the development of new biomedical and engineering technologies. Specifically, a majority of studies on EDLs have focused on the simplest situations; that is, the physicochemical properties (e.g., surface charge and atomic structure) of the surface are uniform and time invariant. While these situations resemble the EDLs encountered in some applications, most practical EDLs are much more complex. Some of the most interesting and technically relevant situations of EDL that remain little studied (as least compared to works devoted to traditional EDLs) include the following:

1. EDLs near heterogeneous surfaces. A key question for these EDLs is how atomistic-level heterogeneities of surface charge and topology regulate the structure of EDLs near these surfaces and interactions between opposing surfaces.

2. EDLs near soft surfaces. Soft surfaces are surfaces whose molecular structure can respond to external conditions and often exhibit significant thermal fluctuations. Cell membranes, lipid bilayers, and lipid vesicles are classical soft surfaces that can support significant surface charge. Unlike conventional EDLs near hard sur-face, the structure of EDLs near these soft surfaces can be coupled to the structure of soft surfaces themselves.

3. EDLs in complex environments, for example, EDLs near protein molecules con-fined in nanopores or nanochannels. Competition between the different effects governing EDL structure highlighted in Section 13.3 will likely introduce new features for such EDLs.

Research on EDLs in the above situations will benefit from the fast advance in compu-tational models and power and will also benefit from emerging experimental capabilities to probe the structure of EDLs in extreme scales. Work in these directions will open new chapters of EDL research.

References

1. Sparnaay, M. J. 1972. *The Electrical Double Layer*, Oxford: Pergamon Press.
2. Weetman, P., Goldman, S., and Gray, C. G. 1997. Use of the Poisson–Boltzmann equation to estimate the electrostatic free energy barrier for dielectric models of biological ion channels. *J. Phys. Chem. B* 101 (31): 6073–6078.
3. Jordan, P. C., Bacquet, R. J., McCammon, J. A., and Tran, P. 1989. How electrolyte shield-ing influences the electrical potential in transmembrane ion channels. *Biophys. J.* 55 (6): 1041–1052.
4. Israelachvili, J. N. 1992. *Intermolecular and Surface Forces*, New York: Academic Press.
5. Hunter, R. J. 1981. *Zeta Potential in Colloid Science: Principles and Applications*, London: Academic Press.
6. Probstein, R. F. 1994. *Physicochemical Hydrodynamics*, New York: John Wiley & Sons, Inc.
7. Harrison, D. J., Fluri, K., Seiler, K., Fan, Z. H., Effenhauser, C. S., and Manz, A. 1993. Micromachining a miniaturized capillary electrophoresis-based chemical analysis system on a chip. *Science* 261 (5123): 895–897.

8. Kemery, P. J., Steehler, J. K., and Bohn, P. W. 1998. Electric field mediated transport in nanometer diameter channels. *Langmuir* 14 (10): 2884–2889.

9. Kuo, T. C., Sloan, L. A., Sweedler, J. V., and Bohn, P. W. 2001. Manipulating molecular transport through nanoporous membranes by control of electrokinetic flow: Effect of surface charge density and debye length. *Langmuir* 17 (20): 6298–6303.

10. Reyes, D. R., Iossifidis, D., Auroux, P. A., and Manz, A. 2002. Micro total analysis systems. 1. Introduction, theory, and technology. *Anal. Chem.* 74 (12): 2623–2636.

11. Conway, B. E. 2002. *Encyclopedia of Surface and Colloid Science*, New York: Marcel Dekker.

12. Gouy, G. 1910. Constitution of the electric charge at the surface of an electrolyte. *J. Phys.* 9 (4): 457–468.

13. Chapman, D. L. 1913. Theory of electrocapillarity. *Philos. Mag.* 25 (148): 475–481.

14. Lyklema, J. 1995. *Fundamentals of Interface and Colloid Science*, San Diego, CA: Academic Press.

15. Joensson, B., Wennerstroem, H., and Halle, B. 1980. Ion distributions in lamellar liquid crystals. A comparison between results from Monte Carlo simulations and solutions of the Poisson-Boltzmann equation. *J. Phys. Chem.* 84 (17): 2179–2185.

16. Borukhov, I., Andelman, D., and Orland, H. 2000. Adsorption of large ions from an electrolyte solution: A modified Poisson–Boltzmann equation. *Electrochem. Acta* 46 (2–3): 221–229.

17. Otto, F., and Patey, G. N. 1999. Forces between like-charged plates in electrolyte solution: Ion-solvent packing versus electrostatic effects. *Phys. Rev. E* 60 (4): 4416–4422.

18. Terao, T., and Nakayama, T. 2001. Charge inversion of colloidal particles in an aqueous solution: Screening by multivalent ions. *Phys. Rev. E* 63 (4): 041401.

19. Onsager, L. 1933. Theories of concentrated electrolytes. *Chem. Rev.* 13 (1): 73–89.

20. Teschke, O., Ceotto, G., and de Souza, E. F. 2001. Interfacial water dielectric-permittivity-profile measurements using atomic force microscopy. *Phys. Rev. E* 64 (1): 011605.

21. Borukhov, I., Andelman, D., and Orland, H. 1997. Steric effects in electrolytes: A modified Poisson-Boltzmann equation. *Phys. Rev. Lett.* 79 (3): 435–438.

22. Burak, Y., and Andelman, D. 2000. Hydration interactions: Aqueous solvent effects in electric double layers. *Phys. Rev. E* 62 (4): 5296–5312.

23. Marcelja, S. 2000. Exact description of aqueous electrical double layers. *Langmuir* 16 (15): 6081–6083.

24. Carnie, S. L., and Chan, D. Y. C. 1981. The statistical mechanics of the electrical double layer: Stress tensor and contact conditions. *J. Chem. Phys.* 74 (2): 1293–1297.

25. Netz, R. R., and Orland, H. 1999. Field theory for charged fluids and colloids. *Europhys. Lett.* 45 (6): 726–732.

26. Lue, L., Zoeller, N., and Blankschtein, D. 1999. Incorporation of nonelectrostatic interactions in the Poisson–Boltzmann equation. *Langmuir* 15 (11): 3726–3730.

27. Bell, G. M., and Rangecroft, P. D. 1972. A linearized potential equation for the interfacial region in an unsymmetrical electrolyte. *Mol. Phys.* 24 (2): 255–267.

28. Outhwaite, C. W., Bhuiyan, L. B., and Levine, S. 1980. Theory of the electric double layer using a modified poisson-boltzman equation. *J. Chem. Soc., Faraday Trans. 2* 76: 1388–1408.

29. Woelki, S., and Kohler, H.-H. 2000. A modified Poisson–Boltzmann equation: I. Basic relations. *Chem. Phys.* 261 (3): 411–419.

30. Woelki, S., and Kohler, H.-H. 2000. A modified Poisson–Boltzmann equation: II. Models and solutions. *Chem. Phys.* 261 (3): 421–438.

31. Burak, Y., and Andelman, D. 2001. Discrete aqueous solvent effects and possible attractive forces. *J. Chem. Phys.* 114 (7): 3271–3283.

32. Bazant, M. Z., Kilic, M. S., Storey, B., and Ajdari, A. 2009. Towards an understanding of induced-charge electrokinetics at large applied voltages. *Adv. Colloid Interface Sci.* 152: 48–88.

33. Bazant, M. Z., and Squires, T. M. 2010. Induced-charge electrokinetic phenomena. *Curr. Opin. Colloid Interface Sci.* 15: 203–213.

34. Kilic, M. S., Bazant, M. Z., and Ajdari, A. 2007. Steric effects in the dynamics of electrolytes at large applied voltages. II. Modified Poisson-Nernst-Planck equations. *Phys. Rev. E* 75 (2): 021503.

35. Kirkwood, J. G. 1934. On the theory of strong electrolyte solutions. *J. Chem. Phys.* 2 (11): 767–781.
36. Outhwaite, C. W. 1970. A modified Poisson-Boltzmann equation in the double layer. *Chem. Phys. Lett.* 7 (6): 636–638.
37. Outhwaite, C. W., and Bhuiyan, L. B. 1982. A further treatment of the exclusion-volume term in the modified Poisson-Boltzmann theory of the electric double layer. *J. Chem. Soc., Faraday Trans. 2* 78 (5): 775–785.
38. Bhuiyan, L. B., Outhwaite, C. W., and Levine, S. 1981. Numerical solution of a modified Poisson-Boltzmann equation for 1 : 2 and 2 : 1 electrolytes in the diffuse layer. *Mol. Phys.* 42 (6): 1271–1290.
39. Outhwaite, C. W., and Bhuiyan, L. B. 1983. An improved modified Poisson-Boltzmann equation in electric-double-layer theory. *J. Chem. Soc., Faraday Trans. 2* 79 (5): 707–718.
40. Andreu, R., Molero, M., Calvente, J. J., Outhwaite, C. W., and Bhuiyan, L. B. 1996. Application of the MPB theory to the analysis of the ion-free layer thickness. *Electrochem. Acta* 41 (14): 2125–2130.
41. Das, T., Bratko, D., Bhuiyan, L. B., and Outhwaite, C. W. 1995. Modified Poisson-Boltzmann theory applied to linear polyelectrolyte solutions. *J. Phys. Chem.* 99 (1): 410–418.
42. Croxton, T., McQuarrie, D. A., Patey, G. N., Torrie, G. M., and Valleau, J. P. 1981. Ionic solution near an uncharged surface with image forces. *Can. J. Chem.* 59 (13): 1998–2003.
43. Lyubartsev, A. P., and Marčelja, S. 2002. Evaluation of effective ion-ion potentials in aqueous electrolytes. *Phys. Rev. E* 65 (4): 041202.
44. Lamperski, S., and Outhwaite, C. W. 1999. A non-primitive model for the electrode | electrolyte interface based on the Percus-Yevick theory. Analysis of the different molecular sizes, ion valences and electrolyte concentrations. *J. Electroanal. Chem.* 460 (1–2): 135–143.
45. Spohr, E. 2002. Molecular dynamics simulations of water and ion dynamics in the electrochemical double layer. *Solid State Ionics* 150 (1–2): 1–12.
46. Wennerstrom, H., Jonsson, B., and Linse, P. 1982. The cell model for polyelectrolyte systems. Exact statistical mechanical relations, Monte Carlo simulations, and the Poisson—Boltzmann approximation. *J. Chem. Phys.* 76 (9): 4665–4670.
47. Torrie, G. M., and Valleau, J. P. 1980. Electrical double layers. I. Monte Carlo study of a uniformly charged surface. *J. Chem. Phys.* 73 (11): 5807–5816.
48. Jamnik, B., and Vlachy, V. 1993. Monte Carlo and Poisson-Boltzmann study of electrolyte exclusion from charged cylindrical micropores. *J. Am. Chem. Soc.* 115 (2): 660–666.
49. Lo, W. Y., Chan, K. Y., Lee, M., and Mok, K. L. 1998. Molecular simulation of electrolytes in nanopores. *J. Electroanal. Chem.* 450 (2): 265–272.
50. Lee, M., Chan, K.-Y., Nicholson, D., and Zara, S. 1999. Deviation from electroneutrality in cylindrical pores. *Chem. Phys. Lett.* 307 (1–2): 89–94.
51. Corry, B., Kuyucak, S., and Chung, S. H. 2000. Invalidity of continuum theories of electrolytes in nanopores. *Chem. Phys. Lett.* 320 (1–2): 35–41.
52. Darden, T., York, D., and Pedersen, L. 1993. Particle mesh Ewald: An N•log(N) method for Ewald sums in large systems. *J. Chem. Phys.* 98 (12): 10089–10092.
53. Hockney, R. W., and Eastwood, J. W. 1988. *Computer Simulation Using Particles*, Bristol: Taylor & Francis Inc.
54. Rajamani, S., Ghosh, T., and Garde, S. 2004. Size dependent ion hydration, its asymmetry, and convergence to macroscopic behavior. *J. Chem. Phys.* 120 (9): 4457–4466.
55. Cui, S. T., and Cochran, H. D. 2002. Molecular dynamics simulation of interfacial electrolyte behaviors in nanoscale cylindrical pores. *J. Chem. Phys.* 117 (12): 5850–5854.
56. Qiao, R., and Aluru, N. R. 2005. Atomistic simulation of KCl transport in charged silicon nanochannels: Interfacial effects. *Colloids Surf. A* 267 (1–3): 103–109.
57. Rose, D. A., and Benjamin, I. 1991. Solvation of Na^+ and Cl^- at the water-platinum (100) interface. *J. Chem. Phys.* 95 (9): 6856–6865.
58. Spohr, E. 1998. Computer simulation of the structure of the electrochemical double layer. *J. Electroanal. Chem.* 450 (2): 327–334.

59. Cheng, L., Fenter, P., Nagy, K. L., Schlegel, M. L., and Sturchio, N. C. 2001. Molecular-scale density oscillations in water adjacent to a mica surface. *Phys. Rev. Lett.* 87 (15): 156103.
60. Spohr, E. 1999. Molecular simulation of the electrochemical double layer. *Electrochem. Acta* 44 (11): 1697–1705.
61. Rose, D. A., and Benjamin, I. 1993. Adsorption of Na^+ and Cl^- at the charged water-platinum interface. *J. Chem. Phys.* 98 (3): 2283–2290.
62. Dietter, J., and Morgner, H. 1997. Structure and dynamics at the surface of a concentrated aqueous solution of CsF. *Chem. Phys.* 220 (3): 261–278.
63. Leote de Carvalho, R. J. F., and Skipper, N. T. 2001. Atomistic computer simulation of the clay–fluid interface in colloidal laponite. *J. Chem. Phys.* 114 (8): 3727–3733.
64. Sachs, J. N., Petrache, H. I., Zuckerman, D. M., and Woolf, T. B. 2003. Molecular dynamics simulations of ionic concentration gradients across model bilayers. *J. Chem. Phys.* 118 (4): 1957–1969.
65. Yang, K.-L., Yiacoumi, S., and Tsouris, C. 2002. Monte Carlo simulations of electrical double-layer formation in nanopores. *J. Chem. Phys.* 117 (18): 8499–8507.
66. Qiao, R., and Aluru, N. R. 2003. Ion concentrations and velocity profiles in nanochannel electro-osmotic flows. *J. Chem. Phys.* 118 (10): 4692–4701.
67. Lee, S. H., and Rasaiah, J. C. 1996. Molecular dynamics simulation of ion mobility. 2. Alkali metal and halide ions using the SPC/E model for water at 25°C. *J. Phys. Chem.* 100 (4): 1420–1425.
68. Qiao, R., and Aluru, N. R. 2004. Charge inversion and flow reversal in a nanochannel electro-osmotic flow. *Phys. Rev. Lett.* 92 (19): 198301.
69. Crozier, P. S., Rowley, R. L., and Henderson, D. 2001. Molecular-dynamics simulations of ion size effects on the fluid structure of aqueous electrolyte systems between charged model electrodes. *J. Chem. Phys.* 114 (17): 7513–7517.
70. Sing, K. S. W., Everett, D. H., Haul, R. A. W., Moscou, L., Pierotti, R. A., Rouquerol, J., and Siemieniewska, T. 1985. Reporting physisorption data for gas/solid systems with special reference to the determination of surface area and porosity. *Pure Appl. Chem.* 57 (4): 603–619.
71. Feng, G., Qiao, R., Huang, J., Sumpter, B. G., and Meunier, V. 2010. Ion distribution in electrified micropores and its role in the anomalous enhancement of capacitance. *ACS Nano* 4 (4): 2382–2390.

14

A Solid-State Nanopore as Biosensor

Samuel Bearden and Guigen Zhang

CONTENTS

ABSTRACT Solid-state nanopores are important devices for future biosensing. They can be fabricated by using several different processing methods, such as selective etching, e-beam sculpting, and focused ion beam sculpting with a variety of materials. While the electrical and surface properties of the selected materials may affect the characteristics of nanopore behavior, different fabrication methods will also affect the shape of nanopores and sometimes even alter the electrical characteristics of the materials that make the nanopores. Because of such inherent complexity, analysis of the electrical and fluidic properties of a nanopore device requires the consideration of all relevant physics associated with the device. This may be accomplished by using either deterministic or probabilistic modeling techniques. Of particular importance to the modeling of the fluidics through a nanopore is the consideration of the electrical double layer. This chapter discusses the effects of various factors affecting the performance of a nanopore biosensor and presents a case study in which a nanopore consisting of a single-walled carbon nanotube is modeled.

14.1 Introduction

Biosensors are analytical devices that combine a biologically sensitive element with a physical transducer to selectively and quantitatively detect the presence of specific compounds in a given biological environment [1]. Like any conventional sensors, a biosensor is expected to be sensitive, responsive, and reliable over a long period. However, since a biosensor is often exposed to an environment containing many biological species that are similar in structures and binding behavior, it needs to be specific, that is, being responsive only to the specifically targeted analyte species. A biosensor may directly respond to a measurand of interest (as in the case of typical electrolytic pH sensors) or make indirect measurements that are related to the measurand of interest (as in the case of enzyme-mediated sensors). In any case, the key to designing and calibrating such biosensors is to know the underlying principle that describes how signal transduction occurs and how the output signal is related to the measurand. For example, in the case of the electrolytic pH meter, the input is the concentration of hydrogen ions and the output is an electric potential signal with the operations governed by the Nernst equation. In the case of an enzyme-mediated biosensor, the actual target is the enzyme substrate (e.g., glucose), but the measured signal is often an electrical current that occurs during the oxidation of the substrate [2–4].

For most biosensors, various physical and chemical methods are used for converting the biological events into electrical or optical signals, such as the mechanical, optical, electromagnetic, electrical, thermal, magnetic, and electrochemical methods, among others. The pH meter and enzyme-mediated biosensor mentioned earlier are of the electrochemical type. The performance of this type of biosensor relies not only on the kinetics of the underlying electrochemical reactions but also on the mass transport behavior near and around the electrodes. Since mass transport is a phenomenon affected by both temporal and spatial restrictions and limitations, predicting the performance of electrochemical-based biosensors has been difficult in certain cases, if not impossible, owing to the sophisticated fluidic designs of these biosensors.

Case in point: solid-state nanopores have been widely recognized as a promising sensor design, but their properties are inherently difficult to characterize. For example, in a typical case, a nanopore device is placed in a flow cell filled with an electrolytic solution. The device is often biased by an electric field across the pore while the resulting ionic through-pore current is measured (see Chapter 15 for more detailed discussion on this subject). Additional electric potentials may be applied near the nanopore surface to create a gating effect. By altering the geometric configurations or the materials comprising the nanopore, one may cause the nanopore to rectify the ionic current, creating a fluidic diode, or to increase the current, creating a fluidic amplifier [5–9]. Rectifying nanopores have been organized into fluidic logic gates, mimicking in a very simplified way the information processing logic found in neurophysiological structures [10]. Recently, there is a great deal of research into using a nanopore system as the basis of very fast and accurate DNA sequencers [11–20]. Chapter 15 discusses such an application. Several different transduction strategies have been implemented such as using ionic conductance through the nanopore and quantum tunneling across the two electrodes embedded in a nanopore [14,21–24].

The electro-driven fluidic transport through a nanopore is very complex and has been observed to exhibit unexpected behavior [6,25–27]. Therefore, a practical understanding of the processes governing the operations of a nanopore calls for elucidation of the interplay of electrochemistry, quantum mechanics, materials science, and fluid dynamics, among others. In situations like these, computational modeling provides an effective way for elucidating the mechanics of biosensor performance. In this chapter, we discuss the various aspects of computational modeling of electrofluidic transport through a nanopore. As a case study, we present in depth the study of electrofluidic flow through a nanopore made of a single-walled carbon nanotube (SWCNT).

14.2 The Making of a Solid-State Nanopore

A nanopore is often regarded as a single nanoscale opening through an otherwise impermeable material. Biological nanopores appearing in nature often serve as active or passive transporters through cell membranes. For example, in muscle and nerve tissues, sodium is transported across the cell membrane against an electrochemical gradient owing to active transport proteins [28]. Water is passively transported across cell membranes through aquaporins in response to osmotic and hydraulic pressure gradients [29]. Solid-state nanopores, on the other hand, are passive manmade structures. In this chapter, we limit our discussion to solid-state nanopores and ignore biological nanopores (discussions on biological nanopores can be found elsewhere [11,15,17]).

A solid-state nanopore can be fabricated using a wide variety of materials and can be shaped in various geometric configurations. For example, nanopores may be in a cylindrical shape when made using carbon nanotubes [5,26,30–32], in a conical shape [33], or in a bow-tie shape [34,35] as illustrated in Figure 14.1. The pore depth (sometimes it is also referred to as the pore channel length) may vary from a few angstroms (when made of graphene) [16,20,36,37] to several microns (when made of carbon nanotubes) [5,30,38] with a pore opening with sizes from a single to few tens of nanometers [34].

14.2.1 Materials for Fabricating Solid-State Nanopores

Because of the electrostatic nature of a nanopore and its electronic control in operations, the materials used to fabricate a nanopore will affect its performance. Nanopores are often

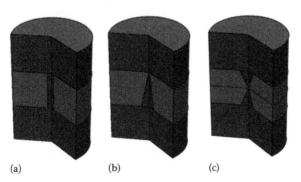

(a)   (b)   (c)

FIGURE 14.1
Typical solid-state pore geometries. (a) A cylindrical nanopore. Such nanopores may be formed by embedding a nanotube in a supporting material. (b) A conical nanopore. Conical nanopores may be created by depositing the pore material around an electrosharpened tip and then etching the tip. (c) A double conical nanopore. The double conical geometry occurs when a nanopore is formed by sputtering away material, as with a focused ion beam.

made using semiconductors and insulating materials such as Si_3N_4, SiO_2/Si, or various polymers [5,6,27,35]. They sometimes are constructed using composite materials in order to elicit specific effects [39].

The electrical permittivity, work function potential, and other properties of the materials used to make nanopores will dictate their performance. Because of the tiny dimensions of a nanopore, a slight change in the electric work potential and permittivity of its component materials could result in a large change in the electric field within the nanopore lumen, hence the overall sensing performance. For this reason, tuning of nanopore performance may be accomplished through careful selection of the component materials. Component materials are primarily chosen for their electronic and mechanical properties. For a nanopore with a very small pore depth, mechanical stability of the supporting material becomes extremely important [37] because the material must withstand the shearing forces associated with through-pore transport. Failure rates in some nanopore devices are found at 30% owing to mechanical failure of the supporting material alone.

Recently, graphene has emerged to become a popular material for nanopore fabrication [16,18,20,22,36,37,39] because of its atomically thin structure, allowing the creation of nanopores with extremely tiny pore depth. Graphene consists of a planar, hexagonal honeycomb of carbon atoms that exists in discrete layers. The layers may be mechanically cleaved using a process developed by Novoselov and integrated into freestanding membranes [40–43].

14.2.2 Fabrication Processes

The fabrication processes of nanopores depend highly on the desired geometry and chosen materials. While porous membranes can be made relatively easily through anodization or other lithographic techniques, fabrication of a single pore with desirable size, structure, and electrical properties requires greater controls. Here, we list three commonly used methods for nanopore fabrication.

14.2.2.1 Electron Beam/Focused Ion Beam

Electron beam (e-beam) sculpting is a commonly used top-down approach for silicon-based materials and is often used for nanopore drilling. Typically, a suspended membrane is prepared using silicon, silicon oxide, silicon nitride, or graphene and loaded into a tunneling electron microscope. Focusing the e-beam to a diameter of ~1 nm with energy of ~100 keV can drill (or burn) a small hole in the membrane [18,39,44]. E-beam sculpting offers fairly good control in the case of suspended graphene sheets [12,18,19,24,34,36,37,39,44–48]. Nanowires, nanogaps, nanoslits, and nanopores have all been produced in stable configuration using e-beam sculpting of graphene. For graphene, an e-beam may be used to add carbon to the lattice as well as to remove it, useful for shrinking the aperture in the lattice at low energy levels [36]. It has been shown that carbon present in the atmosphere will integrate into the honeycomb lattice graphene in a manner that may be controlled by temperature. This allows precise control over graphene structure and nanopores may be produced with very small diameters by sculpting an initial pore and gradually shrinking with a diffuse beam.

Focused ion beam (FIB) lithography is a technique that allows submicron patterning by controlling the energy level of the incident ions, the type of ions, and the exposure time. The technique consists of generating a stream of ions and focusing the stream at a location on a sample surface. The ions interact with the sample through sputtering, implanting, and heating the substrate [49]. FIB is a more versatile technique than e-beam sculpting in terms of the types and properties of the ion source. For example, a semiconductor sample may be selectively doped by implanting boron or arsenic, changing the electrical properties or the pore material. Formation of nanopores is possible by sputtering atoms off of the sample surface [50]. Sputtering occurs when ions are given low energy (typically in the 50–1000 eV range) while higher-energy ion beams tend to cause implantation. Treating a surface with a FIB will typically alter the crystalline structure of the sample, which will affect the electrical properties and chemical reactivity of the sample at the site of interaction. Nanopores have been fabricated in Al_2O_3, graphene, and Si_3N_4 membranes using FIB [39,51].

14.2.2.2 Swift Heavy Ion Tracks in Polymer

Conical nanopores in polymeric materials have been formed by a top–down track-etch process [6–9,33,52–55]. This process can create pores with a depth of ~10 μm and with a diameter as small as ~3 nm (up to 1–2 μm). In this process, polymer films of a desired thickness are irradiated by single swift heavy ions. A latent track is left in the polymer in the trail of the swift heavy ion, causing the alteration of the polymer structure along the track from semicrystalline to amorphous. This will help facilitate preferential etching along the latent track during an etching process. By etching the track from one side and monitoring the progress via ionic current, the opening of the pore can be controlled precisely.

14.2.2.3 Embedded SWCNTs in Insulation Material

Cylindrical nanopores with an extremely long depth can be produced through a bottom–up process of growing carbon nanotubes on an insulating substrate and covering the full-grown carbon nanotubes with another layer of the insulating material using e-beam evaporation [5,32,38]. This method has been employed to create highly efficient electrofluidic field effect transistors. SWCNTs with desirable dimension have been embedded in an insulating material (such as polymer or oxide materials) to form a sandwich structure, which is then selectively etched to reveal the ends of the nanotubes. The lumens at the two ends are subsequently opened by exposing the ends to oxygen plasma. This method has been used to create nanopores with diameters of 1 to 2 nm and lengths of up to 20 to 30 μm.

14.2.3 Electrolytic Solutions

Another important component of an electrofluidic nanopore system is the electrolyte fluid. The electrolyte fluid flows though the nanopore, responding dynamically to the electronic structure of the nanopore and the applied electric field. A typical electrolyte fluid is aqueous potassium chloride (KCl) of various concentrations, though other electrolytes (such as NaCl or KF) are also commonly used [9,34,54–56]. In a nanopore with a radius on the order of the Debye length, the relationship between the conductance of the device and the solution concentration is more complex than is typically observed in other systems. The electrical double layer (EDL) at the pore wall will typically overlap in the diffuse region owing to the radial symmetry of the nanopore structure, giving rise to ion selectivity, causing the intraluminal fluid to differ drastically from the bulk solution [57–63]. Additionally, the surface properties of the pore wall influenced by the presence of adsorbed charged species or distributed charge will affect the intraluminal fluid transport [9,24,31,63,64].

Electrolyte solutions often consist of various ionic compounds dissolved in water. In the case where the compounds are strong electrolytes, the ionic components of the compounds (e.g., K^+ and Cl^- from KCl) will dissociate completely and the conductivity of the solution will be a function of the limiting molar conductivities of the individual ionic components. Here, the limiting molar conductivity refers to the conductivity of an electrolyte as the solution approaches infinite dilution and is given as λ_0. It can be determined by linear superposition, $\lambda_0 = n_1\lambda_1 + n_2\lambda_2 + \ldots$, where λ_1, λ_2, and so on, are the limiting molar conductivity for each component, and n_1, n_2, and so on, are the number of moles of the corresponding individual electrolytes.

For a strong electrolytic solution, its conductivity (σ) can be estimated as $\sigma = \lambda_0 c$, where c is the concentration of the electrolyte. The conductance of this solution through a narrow channel can be estimated by using the conductance equation $G = \sigma \dfrac{A}{l}$, where G is conductance and A and l are geometric terms representing the minimum cross-section area and length of the channel, respectively. This equation, though often used to provide a baseline reference, is usually a poor predictor for the nanopore's conductance behavior. As examined by Kowalczyk et al., this equation predicted conductance well for small, double conical nanopores (<10 nm minimum diameter) but deviated from observed conductance by more than a factor of 2 for larger double conical pores [34]. In double conical nanopores larger than 10 nm, the resistance of the pore becomes comparable to the resistance of the fluid surrounding the pore (the access resistance), meaning that the access resistance is no longer negligible. A correction factor was proposed, which made prediction much more accurate for double conical nanopores with diameters between 10 and 100 nm by accounting for access resistance: $\left(G = \sigma \left[\dfrac{4l}{\pi d^2} + \dfrac{1}{d} \right]^{-1} \right)$. However, for other types of nanopores, this relationship may not apply. For instance, the conductance of a nanopore with a high aspect ratio made of SWCNTs was found to be two to three orders of magnitude larger than that predicted by this equation, despite the fact that the nanopore diameter was less than 10 nm [5,26,32].

14.3 Influence of the Electrode–Fluid Interface

In addition to solution conductivity, it is important to consider the interaction between the electrolytic fluid and the nanopore at their interface. EDL is a molecular structure that spontaneously forms at a solid/fluid interface because of the drive of thermodynamic equilibrium. The EDL structure is well studied in the context of electrochemistry, in light of the seminal theoretical and experimental works of Grahame and others in the middle of the 20th century [65,66], which is also discussed in detail in Chapter 13. For the sake of the discussion that follows, we describe it here in brief. EDL consists of a compact layer and a diffuse layer [57,65–67] made of ions and solvent molecules that are accumulated in solution near a solid/liquid interface. Unlike the compact layer, the ions in the diffuse later are not bound to the surface and may move freely in response to applied forces and potentials. Typically, the thickness of the diffuse later is given by the Debye length, where the Debye length is calculated as $\lambda_D = \sqrt{\dfrac{\varepsilon_0 \varepsilon_r RT}{2F_c^2 c_0}}$, where ε_0 and ε_r are the vacuum and relative permittivity, R is the gas constant, T is temperature, F_c is the Faraday constant, and c_0 is the electrolyte concentration. When the radius of a nanopore is less than or equal to the Debye length, the diffuse layer around the nanopore will overlap, making transport through the nanopore ion selective. In conical nanopore, this ion selectivity can lead to current rectification through the creation of depletion regions [7,54].

In both the compact and diffuse layers, the ions and solvent arrange themselves in response to an electrical field generated from the differential potential of the work functions of the nanopore materials and from any charge buildup at the pore wall. The work function of a material is defined as the energy needed to move an electron from the Fermi level to the vacuum energy level. The Fermi level can be thought of as the average energy level of carriers in a material. When a material has a bandgap in its electronic structure owing to quantum restrictions, the Fermi level often falls within the bandgap. The Fermi level may be altered by doping the material with hole or electron donors or by bringing the material in contact with another material possessing a different work function. This is the basis for the design of most diodes, bipolar junction transistors, and field effect transistors. The result is a potential drop at the surface of the nanopore structure relative to the solution that causes preferential accumulation of ions near the material interface. This accumulation and occlusion are important because the properties of the solution and the volume available for transport within the pore govern the function of the entire device.

14.4 Choosing a Modeling Platform

In modeling nanoscale systems, it is important to select an appropriate modeling platform for the system of interest. In general, there are four main types of mathematical modeling platforms, and they are (1) analytical, (2) numerical continuum, (3) molecular dynamics, and (4) Monte Carlo simulation. Analytical models typically offer the most complete solutions. But since solving an analytical model often requires knowing well-defined physics and boundary conditions, it is sometimes impossible to develop an analytical model or find a solution for it. Numerical continuum models may be used with much relaxed a priori conditions. Numerical methods (finite element modeling as an example) are used to solve weak forms of differential equations over a given domain. This is done by meshing the domain with many small elements over which the approximate solutions to the differential equations are computed. Typically, the size of the elements is gradually decreased, or the number of elements is increased, until the numerical error within the model is decreased to an acceptable level.

In molecular dynamics models, the continuum approach is abandoned in favor of modeling the motion and forces of individual particles. A system is designed as a group of molecules, with each atom and bond defined. The molecules themselves are defined in terms of atomic radius, bond lengths, mass, and charge. The interactions between the molecules are defined by thermodynamic potential energy fields or by force fields between particles (where the forces are typically attributed to electrostatics or physical interaction). One may also account for quantum mechanical phenomena in a molecular dynamics simulation. Solutions are often arrived at iteratively. Given an initial starting point for all species in the simulation, the spatially varying interactions between molecules are calculated. The time component of the simulation is then incremented in some small step and the molecules are moved in response to local forces according to Newtonian mechanics. Movement may be estimated by Newtonian mechanics or other more complicated methods. The process is repeated for as long as necessary or achievable.

Monte Carlo simulation is to molecular dynamics what finite element analysis is to analytical solutions. Monte Carlo simulation relies on probabilistic properties of complex systems to generate meaningful outcomes. This type of simulation is useful for systems dominated by Brownian motion or some other randomly varying mechanic. The method was developed at Los Alamos Scientific Laboratory as a way to model neutron scattering in nuclear experiments [68]. There is no standard system that describes Monte Carlo modeling, as methods may vary wildly between physical systems. For example, in optics, a photon may have some finite probability of being absorbed by a surface and some finite probability of being reflected, with a distribution of probabilities as to the direction of reflection. A famous Monte Carlo problem consists of calculating pi (π) by dropping needles on a striped surface (the Buffon's needle problem). Defining a system in terms of these interactions and repeating the experiment many times will produce a result that models reality. When performed computationally, a source of random numbers with known distribution is used to produce an outcome to each probabilistic event. Practically, the kind of probabilistic information needed to set up a Monte Carlo simulation is very different from the physical information used in other modeling methods. The advantage is that nondeterministic systems may be evaluated with reasonable computational resources. The disadvantage is that Monte Carlo simulations are *black box* and tend not to provide as much mechanistic information as physics-driven simulations. In one case, a Monte Carlo simulation was performed to investigate the conformation of DNA in a nanopore [69]. The pore geometry was defined and a model of a DNA chain was created. The DNA chain consisted of 10 basepairs in a freely jointed chain capable of random rotation and stretching. Starting with a random chain orientation, the model DNA was electrostatically driven into the pore. The results provided information about conformation and stretching of DNA in a nanopore (illustrated in Figure 14.2) that would be difficult or impossible to acquire from other simulation methods and provided insight into the meaning of several experimental nanopore current measurements.

To choose from these different methods of modeling, a decision is necessary in terms of whether to consider the system as composed of discrete particles (molecular dynamics or Monte Carlo) or as a structure of the continuum (analytical or finite element). To decide on this, a key factor to consider is whether the physical dimensions of the system permit the

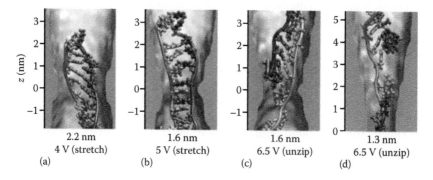

FIGURE 14.2

A Monte Carlo method was used to determine the conformation of DNA in a double conical nanopore. The possible configurations of hairpin DNA were investigated in a 2.2 nm (a) and a 1.6 nm nanopore (b). The conformation of the unzipped DNA was explored in a 1.6 nm (c) and a 1.3 nm nanopore (d). (From Comer J et al., *Biophys. J.* 96, 593–608, 2009.)

use of a continuum approach. This typically can be decided by examining the dimensionless Knudsen number. A Knudsen number less than 1 often justifies the use of a continuum model while other methods should be used for larger numbers, though to be convincing, the Knudsen number should be much smaller than 1. The Knudsen number is originally derived for use in rarefied gases in the upper atmosphere and is defined as the ratio of the mean free path of particles to some characteristic system length $\left(Kn = \dfrac{\lambda}{L} \right)$. The use of the Knudsen number in condensed fluid systems is not rigorously supported, yet it is often used as a rule of thumb in nanoscale fluidics [70]. The number is commonly used in studies of micro- and nanofluidics with good outcomes [5,32,70,71]. The mean free path length in aqueous solutions is often regarded to be the molecular diameter of water (0.3 nm) and the characteristic length will vary depending on the geometry of the system. A Knudsen value in the range from 0.1 down to 0.001 is in a transitional region between probabilistic and continuum approaches that is inherently difficult to model, and both approaches have been used [5,32,70]. A more accurate Knudsen number may be calculated by finding the mean free path of a solvent particle modeled as a sphere (with a radius of 0.15 nm, half the molecular diameter of water). The mean free path length is then defined by the formula $\lambda = \dfrac{MW}{4\pi r^2 N_{avogadro}\rho_v}$, where λ is the mean free path length, MW is the molecular weight of a solvent molecule, r is the molecular radius (0.15 nm in this case), and ρ_v is the mass density of the fluid. The mean free path length for water produced by this method is 0.105 nm, which decreases the Knudsen number by approximately a factor of 3. A small, transitional Knudsen number allows for the continuum model to be utilized, but it does not rule out the added value a probabilistic model may provide. However, the computational cost of a probabilistic model of the same scale as the continuum model may tend to be prohibitively high [70].

14.5 Considering the EDL

In continuum models, where the finite size of solute and solvent molecules is typically ignored, care must be taken to properly model the EDL. The difficulty in modeling the EDL is the fact that the compact layer forms owing to surface adsorption of species with a finite size. The finite size of the adsorbed particles creates a plane of closest approach (the outer Helmholtz plane) that defines the boundary between the compact and diffuse layers. The outer Helmholtz plane will become the practical boundary not only for fluidic flow but also for electron transfer, if any. Continuum modeling of the complete EDL has been extensively studied in the realm of electrochemical nanoelectrodes with investigation of various parameters such as electrode size, electrode spacing, compact layer thickness, reaction rate, and presence of supporting electrolyte.

Numerical continuum models of axisymmetric nanoscale electrodes have been produced investigating the effects of the EDL [57,67]. The operating principle of larger-scale electrodes is that the current response is limited only by diffusion of the reactant species near the electrodes; however, this model breaks down at nanoscale. Attempts to correct this failed to account for the nonelectroneutrality that occurs within the diffuse layer of the EDL. A nanoscale model, however, is able to account for most of the phenomena near the electrode that become prominent at nanoscale.

One of these computation models consisted of axisymmetric setting with a spherical electrode having a radius of r_0 and a compact layer thickness of μ (Figure 14.3a). The compact layer was divided into inner and outer Helmholtz planes where the inner plane consists of adsorbed ions or solvent molecules and the outer plane represents the plane of closest approach for nonadsorbed solution. In electrochemical experiments, the outer Helmholtz plane also serves as the position of electron transfer. The electrical permittivity within the compact layer was defined as smoothly varying between the permittivity of the electrode material and the electrolyte. The smoothly varying permittivity has been defined using segmented cosine and hyperbolic cosine equations or a single sigmoidal equation with good effect. The use of a smoothly varying permittivity within the compact layer produces more accurate models than assuming either a single uniform permittivity or a stepped permittivity where the compact layer is divided into two regions of different permittivity values. Moreover, it allows for the permittivity within the compact layer to be defined for electrodes constructed of any material and for any compact layer thickness.

For a continuum system, the steady-state electrostatic distribution of potential is governed by the Poisson equation and the transport and distribution of charged species are governed by the Nernst–Planck equation. The compact layer is considered to be composed of adsorbed solvent molecules and therefore containing no net charge. Thus, the Poisson equation for the compact layer region can be simplified to a Laplace equation. The presence of electroactive species undergoing redox reactions at the position of electron transfer may be dealt with by Bulter–Volmer kinetics equations. In the model, the Poisson equation is applied over the entire geometry, while the Nernst–Planck equation is only considered in the domain of the electrolytic solution, bound by a distant boundary held at constant concentration and the outer Helmholtz plane. At the outer Helmholtz plane, the concentration of electroactive species is defined by the flux of redox species governed by the Bulter–Volmer equation.

The modeling results were compared against the result of a large-scale diffusion-limited situation. For a single electrode, the limiting current deviates more as the electrode radius decreases, owing to differences in the potential drop across the compact layer that has a size-dependent effect. As a result, the diffuse layer is shorter in a relative sense for larger

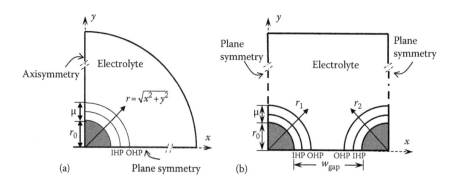

FIGURE 14.3
(a) The EDL occurs at the interface of an electrode (gray) and solution (white). The compact layer consists of immobilized ions and solvent molecules electrostatically held at the electrode surface. The finite size of these molecules creates a plane of closest approach to the electrode (the outer Helmholtz layer, OHM) with a thickness μ. (b) When electrodes are placed in proximity, the EDL overlaps itself. In a nanopore, EDL overlap is attributed to the small inner dimensions and is responsible for some of the unusual properties of nanopores.

electrodes than for smaller electrodes (100 nm vs. 1 nm). The diffuse layer consists of the region outside the compact layer where electroneutrality is not kept because of unequal concentrations of charged species of differing valence. This nonelectroneutrality is attributed to two causes: (1) the depletion of electroactive species at the position of electron transfer owing to electrochemical reaction, and (2) the electromigration of charged species in the electric field near the electrode surface. The concentration gradient of any species is dependent on the concentration of co-solutes owing to the screening of electric potential within the solution. The depletion gradient of the reactant species was found to increase in the presence of supporting electrolyte, altering the cyclic voltammetric current response of the electrode.

In the case of interdigitated electrodes, where collector and generator electrodes (see Figure 14.3b) are placed in proximity, the electrochemical properties are influenced by the overlapping of the diffuse layers of the two electrodes. The result is fast redox cycling between the two electrodes. Similar to the case of a single electrode, the influence of the EDL decreases as the size of the electrodes increases. Decreasing the space between the electrodes leads to an increased electrical field between the electrodes, contributing to enhanced electromigration between the collector and generator. Because of the screening effects of the electrolyte solution, the electrical fields of the two electrodes do not overlap when the gap spacing between them is large (>16 nm), but they strongly overlap when the gap spacing is small (4 nm). It is noted in the case of a single nanoscale electrode that when a supporting electrolyte is not included, the thickness of the diffusion layer will increase. When interdigitated electrodes are considered without a supporting electrolyte, the increased diffusion layer will overlap between the electrodes, creating a peak-shaped cyclic voltammogram. Increasing the thickness of the compact layer will lead to a greater potential drop within the compact layer, resulting in a smaller diffusion layer. These models of the EDL discussed here illustrate how a continuum approach can be used in a transitional domain where the benefits of a probabilistic mechanics approach may provide similar validity but with greater complexity.

14.6 Mass Transport

Mass transport through a nanopore is typically electrokinetically driven. Because of the small cross-sectional area and relative fragility of the supporting membranes comprising such a device, any significant pressure across the nanopore may lead to structural failure. Furthermore, because of the extremely small size of the lumen of the nanopore, fluid flow will likely be laminar and the Reynolds number will be low. Given laminar flow in a low-pressure gradient environment, the fluidic flow will likely be driven predominately by electrokinetics. The two mechanisms chiefly responsible for mass transport are electrophoresis and electroosmosis, where electrophoresis is the movement of ions owing to an electric field and electroosmosis is the movement of the supporting fluid. Diffusion exists as a balancing influence that is reactionary to the concentration gradients imposed on the system by the active mechanisms but does not significantly contribute to mass flux.

14.6.1 Electrophoresis

Electrophoresis is the transport of charged particles in fluid under an electric field. A subtlety of this definition is that the fluid may or may not be stationary. A moving fluid will increase the drag force on ions moving against the flow by increasing the velocity of the particles relative to the fluid, and vice versa, thus decreasing the drag force on ions moving with the fluid. Conceptually, one can separate the two mechanisms by considering ionic flux through the fluid (electrophoresis) and ionic flux with the fluid (electroosmosis). When an electrical field is applied across an electrolyte solution, each individual ion is subjected to a force proportional to the local electric field and the charge on the particle. Additionally, each ionic particle experiences a drag force in the direction opposite the electrical force in proportion to the velocity of the particle relative to the supporting fluid. The balance of these forces causes the particle to attain a final velocity dependent on the particle mass, charge, volume, and electrical field. The electrophoretic current flux can be determined as $\sum_j z_j \mu_j F_c \nabla V$ according to the Nernst–Planck equation, where z_j and μ_j are the valence charge and mobility of a jth species, respectively, F_c is the Faraday constant, and ∇V is the differential of the electric potential. Electronic mobility of a particular ionic species is often determined by the Stokes–Einstein relationship, $\mu_m = \dfrac{D_j}{k_B T}$, where D_j is the diffusion coefficient of j, k_B is the Boltzmann constant, and T is the temperature.

14.6.2 Electroosmosis

Just as the solvent exerts a drag force on mobile ions, mobile ions exert an equal and opposite drag force on the solvent. The force on the solvent can be expressed as a force per unit volume using the term $\vec{F} = F_c \sum_j (z_j c_j) E$, where $\vec{F}$ is the force per unit volume, c_j is the concentration of the jth species, and E is the electric field. In a free body diagram, this force would be balanced by friction at the channel wall and viscous interaction at the mouths of the pore. However, these boundary conditions are often difficult or impossible to obtain for a model of nanopore fluidics. For this reason, most studies of electrofluidic nanopores are solved numerically. Solving for electroosmosis gives a fluid velocity profile that is typically uniform (plug-like flow). The product of electroosmotic velocity and the concentration gradient in the diffuse layer of the EDL gives a mass flux, which may be converted to an ionic current if geometry and species charge terms are known.

14.7 Modeling a Nanopore Biosensor

14.7.1 Governing Differential Equations

Creating functional models for nanopores is an important part of designing nanopore-based biosensors. Having a good understanding of the underlying governing principles will help select better sensor design parameters. For complicated biosensors like nanopores, modeling can provide insight into the interplay of multiphysics phenomena as well as noise levels.

Numerical modeling of a nanopore is essentially the process of applying numerical techniques to solve differential equations that govern the nanopore system. These governing differential equations typically include the Poisson equation, the Nernst–Planck equation, and the Navier–Stokes equation. The Poisson equation takes the form $\nabla^2 V = -\dfrac{\rho_c}{\varepsilon_0 \varepsilon_r}$, where V is the spatial distribution of electric potential, ρ_c is the spatial distribution of charged species, and ε_0 and ε_r represent the vacuum and relative permittivity values, respectively. The charge term ρ_c allows for interaction between all charged species and electric fields, where charged species can be solvated ions or surface charges. The Nernst–Planck equation is given as $\nabla \cdot (-D_j \nabla c_j - z_j \mu_{m,j} F_c c_j \nabla V) + u \cdot \nabla c_j = R_j$, where D_j is the diffusion coefficient, c_j is the ion concentration, z_j is the ion valence, $\mu_{m,j}$ is the ion mobility, F_c is the Faraday constant, V is electric potential, u is fluid velocity, and R_j is the source term. When solved, the Nernst–Planck equation provides a concentration distribution (as well as other information) for the species of interest. In the case of an aqueous solution of a strong electrolyte, the species of interest are typically the dissociated ions. Coupling between the Poisson and Nernst–Planck equation occurs by feeding the ionic concentration profile into the charge distribution term of the Poisson equation and using the electric fields of the Poisson equation in the electrokinetic terms of the Nernst–Planck equation. Such coupling must be solved iteratively and self-consistently in order to produce a stable solution.

Additional physics (such as electroosmosis or chemical reactions) must also be considered with appropriate differential equations. In the case of electroosmosis, fluid velocity may be defined using a Stokes equation, which is appropriate for low Reynolds number flow. The Stokes equations $\rho_m (u \cdot \nabla) u = \nabla \cdot \left[-PI + \gamma \left(\nabla u + (\nabla u)^\tau \right) - \dfrac{2}{3} \gamma (\nabla \cdot u) I \right] + \vec{F}_V$ and $\nabla \cdot (\rho_m u) = 0$ account for all fluidic flow parameters, where ρ_m represents the fluid density (not to be confused with ρ_c, the distribution of charges in the Poisson equation), u is the fluid velocity, P is pressure, I is an identity matrix useful for numerical solutions, γ is viscosity, τ is the viscous stress tensor, and $\vec{F}_V$ is a volume force that may be calculated as $\left(\vec{F}_V = F_c \sum^i (z_j c_j) \cdot \nabla V \right)$.

Fluid flow through nanopores is not usually pressure driven (hindered by the inherent mechanical instability of most nanopore membranes), and electrokinetic terms usually dominate because of the interactions between moving charged particles (from the Poisson/Nernst–Planck equations) and a polar solvent (typically water). When a nanopore is composed of an embedded SWCNT, one should also consider the large fluidic slip length at the nanopore wall, which induces nearly frictionless flow through the carbon nanotube [5,26,31,32].

14.7.2 Setting Boundary Conditions

Setting boundary conditions for a nanopore system can be a complex process, particularly the conditions at the nanopore wall. Issues to consider include the following: (1) the wall has either free or trapped charges distributed on it, (2) differential potentials owing to material work function mismatches, (3) EDL structure, and (4) fluidic conditions, among others. Charge may become trapped in the wall when energetic particles are used to ablate the pore volume, as in e-beam and FIB sculpting. The presence of such trapped charge can alter the electric field within the nanopore, leading to anomalous flow effects. In some cases, pH-sensitive molecules may be purposely bonded to the pore surface, allowing the operator to control the distribution and charge present on the pore wall [9,33]. In cases where the nanopore is constructed out of conductor/insulator composites (such as SWCNT nanochannels), it has been theorized that charges trapped between the conductor and insulator can induce mobile charge on the conductor [5]. The resulting mobile charge distribution would have to be solved for in a manner consistent with the rest of the model.

In all of these situations, the actual amount of charge will generally need to be found iteratively by comparing the model output to external references.

EDL is a construct that arises naturally at material interfaces. In models that account for difference in material work functions or consider charges on the pore wall, the diffuse layer forms in the solution following the Poisson/Nernst–Planck equations. However, a continuum model inherently neglects the finite size of the solvated ions, so if the compact layer is to be considered, it must be included explicitly. The question remains as to what the physical thickness of the compact layer should be. The compact layer thickness is typically regarded in the literature to exhibit some variability around a typical value of 0.44–0.46 nm. However, within the interior of a nanopore, this value may be better solved for by comparing the model output to external references through iteratively altering the value.

Any chemical reactions or fluidic slip planes must be considered at the wall of the nanopore. Species in the fluid may undergo surface-catalyzed reactions, which will change the distribution of species in the EDL. The presence of redox species in the solution should be noted, especially if any portion of the nanopore is electrically biased. Chemical or electrochemical interactions will change the structure of the EDL, which will likely have an effect on the conductance and transport properties of the nanopore [57,67]. Additionally, the fluidic slip length at the nanopore wall should be considered. Some materials (notably SWCNTs) have been noted to have very long slip lengths resulting in essentially frictionless flow [26,32]. Correctly determining these conditions will help ensure accurate modeling of nanopore transport characteristics.

14.7.3 A Case Study: Effect of EDL on Electrofluidic Transport in an SWCNT Nanopore

As mentioned earlier, the ionic conductance through SWCNTs has been observed to be two to three orders of magnitude larger than expected based on the geometry of the channel and the conductivity of the solution. In this section, a nanopore system consisting of SWCNTs embedded in a variety of materials is investigated. The nanopore itself is formed in the lumen of the SWCNT with the embedding material forming an impermeable barrier around the nanopore. Several aqueous electrolyte solutions are examined, and the effects of the concentration of electrolyte on the EDL and transport properties of the pore are noted.

In SWCNTs with radii of 1–2 nm, the dimensions of the EDL are not negligible. The finite thickness of the compact layer of the EDL would effectively reduce the diameter of the carbon nanotube from a fluidics perspective, and changes in nanochannel diameter are known to alter the ionic conductance of a nanopore. The Knudsen number for this system was calculated to be 0.05 based on a mean free path length (λ) given by $\lambda = \dfrac{MW}{4\pi r^2 N_{\text{avogadro}} \rho_m}$ (where MW is the molecular weight of a solvent molecule, r is the molecular radius—0.15 nm for a water molecule, and ρ_m is the mass density of the fluid) and a characteristic length of 2 nm (the diameter chosen for a representative SWCNT). Based on the small, but transitional Knudsen number, a continuum approach is considered as appropriate to use for modeling this system.

The geometry of the system is defined in an axisymmetric way, to take advantage of the symmetry of the system about a longitudinal axis running through the length at the center of the carbon nanotube. The model consists of cylindrical fluid reservoirs continuous with the interior volume of the nanotube. The nanotube itself is considered as an infinitesimal layer at the boundary of the bulk insulating material and the nanochannel. A compact layer is explicitly modeled as a cylindrical shell at the junction of the infinitesimal carbon nanotube and the electrolyte fluid. Choosing a thickness for the compact layer presents a complication for the design of the model and is handled in a unique way. In the beginning, the thickness of the compact layer is given a parameterized variable thickness. Once the model is constructed, the thickness of the compact layer is allowed to vary and the model output is used along with a decision rule to identify allowable thicknesses.

Since the model in question is in the continuum regime, the model physics are defined by the Poisson, Nernst–Planck, and Stokes equations as discussed earlier. The Poisson equation is bounded by applied electric potentials at the far ends of the model reservoirs, which set up an electric field to drive ions through the nanopore formed by the carbon nanotube. Additionally, the model accounts for a potential at the surface of the carbon nanotube owing to differences in the work function of the insulating materials and the carbon nanotube. The only charged species considered in the model is the solvated ionic species. The transport of electrolytes is governed by the Nernst–Planck equation with a boundary of a constant concentration condition at the far ends of the fluid reservoirs.

A special property of SWCNTs is that they have a very long fluidic slip length for fluid transported through the interior nanochannel. The result is practically frictionless flow, which, when electrically driven, is called electroosmosis. Small-scale fluid flow may be modeled with the Stokes equation, but because of the slip condition at the wall of the carbon nanotube, the boundary conditions are not well defined (this is actually the reason that an analytical model has not yet been created for this system). The fluid is driven by a volume force attributed to electrostatic interaction with solvated ions, and this force is balanced by viscous interactions within the fluid.

With the physics of the model defined, a numerical mesh is constructed. A mesh with rectangular elements is implemented in order to reduce the computational load of the model. In order to obtain numerically converged results, the element size is iteratively reduced while monitoring the model output current at three different locations along the length of the carbon nanotube. Because mass will be conserved, it should be expected that the current at different positions along the length of the nanotube will be the same. An iterative approach is taken in which a mesh is first generated, the model solved, and the current measurements at these three locations compared. The number of elements is increased and the process is repeated until the three measurements are close within three significant digits.

Once the mesh is set, the thickness of the compact layer and other parameters of interest are evaluated. Here, we are interested in quantifying the thickness of the compact layer when the insulating material and the concentration of the electrolyte solution changes. To do that, we analyze the model under 12 conditions, where each conditional model is given one of three insulating materials and one of four possible solution concentrations. Care is taken in each conditional model: only the parameters of interest are changed and all other conditions and settings are kept identical between models. Each conditional model is solved with a parameterized sweep of 11 values for the compact layer thickness variable.

These conditional models are solved and ionic conductance is determined for each case. Since there are 11 solved conditional models (12 original conditional models minus 1 that could not be solved in a reasonable time) and 11 compact layer thicknesses evaluated in each conditional model, 121 output conductance values are collected. Of the selected compact layer thickness values, some are invalid. Thus, a filtering method is developed to eliminate the compact layer thickness values that seem unreasonable. From a survey of the literature, it is known that the ionic conductance of SWCNT devices is related to the concentration of the solution by a power law ($G = Ac^b$), where G is conductance, A is a fitting factor, c is the solution concentration, and b is a characteristic exponent. In functional carbon nanotube devices, the exponent (b) is found to be less than 1. Hence, the 11 conditional models were divided up into three separate groups by insulating material to be evaluated separately. Within each subgroup, the concentration and compact layer thickness parameters are iterated into every possible four-member ordered list, where each ordered list contains all four solution concentrations. Each ordered list is then fit to a power relationship using a least squares method and a power law exponent and goodness-of-fit statistic is produced in each case. The ordered lists are then filtered to find lists with exponents meeting the experimental criterion (b less than 1) from a good fit to the power relationship. The sorting and filtering of data are automated with custom scripting software, which greatly simplified and organized the process. The scripting approach is necessary because of the large amount of data produced by the 11 models. Since there are three insulating materials investigated at four concentrations with 11 parametric values for the compact layer thickness, a total of $11^3 + 11^4 + 11^4 = 30{,}613$ outputs are evaluated.

As shown in Figure 14.4, the conductance values from those models that deemed having a proper compact layer thickness are found to be in the range of one to three orders of magnitude greater than that predicted by the bulk conductance theory (Bulk theory). Empirical checks of electrophoresis and electroosmosis are possible because the numerical computation package used allows for such mechanistic separation. Electrophoresis may be approximated by the geometric conductance equation $G = \sigma \dfrac{A}{L}$, where G is the conductance, σ is the solution conductivity (a function of concentration as discussed earlier), A is the nanochannel cross-sectional area, and L is the nanochannel length. When the electrophoretic conductance is calculated in this way using concentration information from the output of the Nernst–Planck equation, good agreement is seen between the empirical relationship and the numerical model, as seen in Figure 14.5.

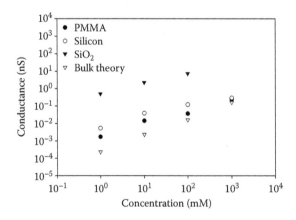

FIGURE 14.4
The conductance of the SWCNT nanopore is dependent on the work function of the embedding material. Higher work functions and electrolyte concentrations increase the overall conductance of the nanopore.

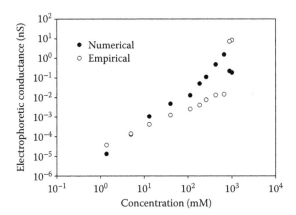

FIGURE 14.5
The numerical calculation of electrophoretic conductance and the empirically calculated electrophoretic conductance share similar values and relationships with the electrolyte concentration.

A similar test of electroosmosis can be made using the empirical electroosmotic equation $G = \dfrac{v_{eo}q}{LV}$ and the net charge within the nanotube from the Poisson–Nernst–Planck equations. The electroosmotic velocity in this empirical equation is calculated from $v_{eo} = \mu_{eo}E$, where μ_{eo} is the electroosmotic velocity and E is the applied electric field. μ_{eo} may be calculated from $\mu_{eo} = \dfrac{\varepsilon_0\varepsilon_r\xi}{\eta}$, where ξ is the zeta potential, η is the fluid viscosity, and ε_0 and ε_r are the vacuum and relative permittivity, respectively. The empirical relationship reasonably approximates the numerically derived electroosmotic conductance, as seen in Figure 14.6. It should be emphasized that the empirical results presented here were calculated using the concentration and net charge within the nanopore as derived from the numerical model. Thus, the good agreement between numerical and empirical methods suggests that the enhanced current conductance can be attributed to the increases in the electrolytic concentration and net change inside the nanopore.

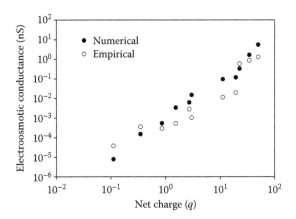

FIGURE 14.6
The numerical calculation of electroosmotic conductance and the empirically calculated electroosmotic conductance share similar values and relationships with the net charge of the fluid contained within the nanopore.

14.8 Summary and Future Perspectives

The design and analysis of the performance of a nanopore sensor is a complex and exciting subject. The properties of a nanopore may be tuned by carefully choosing proper materials and fabrication methods. Careful selection of materials allows the adjustment of the electrical and fluidic properties of the nanopore, and different fabrication methods may decide the shape of a nanopore device, which in turn may influence the nanopore behavior. While the materials and fabrication methods listed in this chapter are by no means comprehensive, they nevertheless bring our attention to the interdependence of the actual nanopore devices upon these selections.

The various modeling techniques discussed in this chapter provide an overview of common methods of deriving the physical basis of observed behavior in nanopores. The effect of the EDL and its dependence on the material properties are of particular importance when modeling pores with truly nanoscale dimensions. The case study presented in this chapter highlights the usefulness of multiphysics computational modeling. With careful execution and iterative investigation, it is capable of shining crucial insights into the operations of a complex nanopore device. While nanopores may become an important class of biosensors, the complex behavior and performance of each new design need to be fully investigated.

References

1. Zhang G. 2009. Nanotechnology-based biosensors in drug delivery. In *Nanotechnology in Drug Delivery*, eds. M M de Villiers, P Aramwit and G S Kwon (New York: Springer) pp. 163–89.
2. Gangadharan R, Anandan V, Zhang A, Drwiega J C and Zhang G. 2011. Enhancing the performance of a fluidic glucose biosensor with 3D electrodes. *Sens. Actuators B Chem.* **160**: 991–8.
3. Gangadharan R, Anandan V and Zhang G. 2008. Optimizing the functionalization process for nanopillar enhanced electrodes with GOx/PPY for glucose detection. *Nanotechnology* **19**: 395501.
4. Anandan V, Gangadharan R and Zhang G. 2009. Role of SAM chain length in enhancing the sensitivity of nanopillar modified electrodes for glucose detection. *Sensors (Basel)* **9**: 1295–305.
5. Pang P, He J, Park J H, Krstić P S and Lindsay S. 2011. Origin of giant ionic currents in carbon nanotube channels. *ACS Nano* **5**: 7277–83.
6. Kalman E B, Sudre O, Vlassiouk I and Siwy Z S. 2009. Control of ionic transport through gated single conical nanopores. *Anal. Bioanal. Chem.* **394**: 413–9.
7. Vlassiouk I, Smirnov S and Siwy Z. 2008. Ionic selectivity of single nanochannels. *Nano Lett.* **8**: 1978–85.
8. Siwy Z and Fuliński A. 2002. Fabrication of a synthetic nanopore ion pump. *Phys. Rev. Lett.* **89**: 4–7.
9. Siwy Z, Heins E, Harrell C C, Kohli P and Martin C R. 2004. Conical-nanotube ion-current rectifiers: The role of surface charge. *J. Am. Chem. Soc.* **126**: 10850–1.
10. Ali M, Mafe S, Ramirez P, Neumann R and Ensinger W. 2009. Logic gates using nanofluidic diodes based on conical nanopores functionalized with polyprotic acid chains. *Langmuir* **25**: 11993–7.
11. De Zoysa R S S, Krishantha D M M, Zhao Q, Gupta J and Guan X. 2011. Translocation of single-stranded DNA through the α-hemolysin protein nanopore in acidic solutions. *Electrophoresis* **32**: 3034–41.

12. Chang H, Kosari F, Andreadakis G, Alam M A, Vasmatzis G and Bashir R. 2004. DNA-mediated fluctuations in ionic current through silicon oxide nanopore channels. *Nano Lett.* **4**: 1551–6.

13. Gracheva M E, Xiong A, Aksimentiev A, Schulten K, Timp G and Leburton J-P. 2006. Simulation of the electric response of DNA translocation through a semiconductor nanopore–capacitor. *Nanotechnology* **17**: 622–33.

14. Ivanov A P, Instuli E, McGilvery C M, Baldwin G, McComb D W, Albrecht T and Edel J B. 2011. DNA tunneling detector embedded in a nanopore. *Nano Lett.* **11**: 279–85.

15. Timp W, Mirsaidov U M, Wang D, Comer J, Aksimentiev A and Timp G. 2010. Nanopore sequencing: Electrical measurements of the code of life. *IEEE Trans. Nanotechnol.* **9**: 281–94.

16. Min S K, Kim W Y, Cho Y and Kim K S. 2011. Fast DNA sequencing with a graphene-based nanochannel device. *Nat. Nanotechnol.* **6**: 162–5.

17. Deamer D W and Branton D. 2002. Characterization of nucleic acids by nanopore analysis. *Acc. Chem. Res.* **35**: 817–25.

18. Schneider G F, Kowalczyk S W, Calado V E, Pandraud G, Zandbergen H W, Vandersypen L M K and Dekker C. 2010. DNA translocation through graphene nanopores. *Nano Lett.* **10**: 3163–7.

19. Branton D, Deamer D W, Marziali A, Bayley H, Benner S A, Butler T, Di Ventra M, Garaj S, Hibbs A, Jovanovich S B, Krstic P S, Lindsay S, Sean X, Riehn R, Soni G V, Tabard-Cossa V, Wanunu M, Huang X, Ling X S, Mastrangelo C H, Meller A, Oliver J S, Pershin Y V, Ramsey J M, Wiggin M and Schloss J A. 2008. The potential and challenges of nanopore sequencing. *Genome Res.* **26**: 1146–53.

20. Nelson T, Zhang B and Prezhdo O V. 2010. Detection of nucleic acids with graphene nanopores: Ab initio characterization of a novel sequencing device. *Nano Lett.* **10**: 3237–42.

21. Ohshiro T and Umezawa Y. 2006. Complementary base-pair-facilitated electron tunneling for electrically pinpointing complementary nucleobases. *Proc. Natl. Acad. Sci. U. S. A.* **103**: 10–4.

22. Saha K K, Drndić M and Nikolić B K. 2011. DNA Base-specific modulation of microampere transverse edge currents through a metallic graphene nanoribbon with a nanopore. *Nano Lett.* **12**: 50–5.

23. Lee C Y, Choi W, Han J-H and Strano M S. 2010. Coherence resonance in a single-walled carbon nanotube ion channel. *Science* **329**: 1320–4.

24. Smeets R M M, Keyser U F, Krapf D, Wu M-Y, Dekker N H and Dekker C. 2006. Salt dependence of ion transport and DNA translocation through solid-state nanopores. *Nano Lett.* **6**: 89–95.

25. Yan Y, Wang L, Xue J and Chang H-C. 2013. Ion current rectification inversion in conic nanopores: Nonequilibrium ion transport biased by ion selectivity and spatial asymmetry. *J. Chem. Phys.* **138**: 044706.

26. Majumder M, Chopra N, Andrews R and Hinds B J. 2005. Enhanced flow in carbon nanotubes. *Nature* **438**: 43–4.

27. Bearden S and Zhang G. 2013. The effects of the electrical double layer on giant ionic currents through single-walled carbon nanotubes. *Nanotechnology* **24**: 125204.

28. Skou J C. 1965. Enzymatic basis for active transport of Na^+ and K^+ across cell membrane. *Physiol. Rev.* **45**: 596–617.

29. Scha A R. 1998. Review Aquaporin function, structure, and expression: Are there more surprises to surface in water relations? *Planta* **204**: 131–9.

30. Pang P, He J, Park J H, Krstić P S, Lindsay S and Page S. 2011. Supporting information for "Origin of giant ionic currents in carbon nanotube channels." *ACS Nano* **5**: 1–40.

31. Wu J, Gerstandt K, Majumder M, Zhan X and Hinds B J. 2011. Highly efficient electroosmotic flow through functionalized carbon nanotube membranes. *Nanoscale* **3**: 3321–8.

32. Holt J K, Park H G, Wang Y, Stadermann M, Artyukhin A B, Grigoropoulos C P, Noy A and Bakajin O. 2006. Fast mass transport through sub-2-nanometer carbon nanotubes. *Science* **312**: 1034–7.

33. Apel P Y, Korchev Y, Siwy Z, Spohr R and Yoshida M. 2001. Diode-like single-ion track membrane prepared by electro-stopping. *Nucl. Instrum. Methods Phys. Res. Sect. B Beam Interact. Mater. Atoms* **184**: 337–46.

34. Kowalczyk S W, Grosberg A Y, Rabin Y and Dekker C. 2011. Modeling the conductance and DNA blockade of solid-state nanopores. *Nanotechnology* **22**: 315101.
35. Firnkes M, Pedone D, Knezevic J, Döblinger M and Rant U. 2010. Electrically facilitated translocations of proteins through silicon nitride nanopores: Conjoint and competitive action of diffusion, electrophoresis, and electroosmosis. *Nano Lett.* **10**: 2162–7.
36. Lu N, Wang J, Floresca H C and Kim M J. 2012. In situ studies on the shrinkage and expansion of graphene nanopores under electron beam irradiation at temperatures in the range of 400–1200°C. *Carbon N. Y.* **50**: 2961–5.
37. Merchant C A, Healy K, Wanunu M, Ray V, Peterman N, Bartel J, Fischbein M D, Venta K, Luo Z, Johnson A T C and Drndić M. 2010. DNA translocation through graphene nanopores. *Nano Lett.* **10**: 2915–21.
38. Liu H, He J, Tang J, Liu H, Pang P, Cao D, Krstic P, Joseph S, Lindsay S and Nuckolls C. 2010. Translocation of single-stranded DNA through single-walled carbon nanotubes. *Science* **327**: 64–7.
39. Venkatesan B M, Estrada D, Banerjee S, Jin X, Dorgan V E, Bae M-H, Aluru N R, Pop E and Bashir R. 2012. Stacked graphene-Al2O3 nanopore sensors for sensitive detection of DNA and DNA-protein complexes. *ACS Nano* **6**: 441–50.
40. Novoselov K S, Geim A K, Morozov S V, Jiang D, Katsnelson M I, Grigorieva I V, Dubonos S V and Firsov A A. 2005. Two-dimensional gas of massless Dirac fermions in graphene. *Nature* **438**: 197–200.
41. Lecture N, Novoselov K S, Abbott E A and Romance F A. 2010. Graphene: Materials in the flatland. *Rev. Mod. Phys.* **83**: 106–31.
42. Novoselov K S, Jiang D, Schedin F, Booth T J, Khotkevich V V, Morozov S V and Geim A K. 2005. Two-dimensional atomic crystals. *Proc. Natl. Acad. Sci. U. S. A.* **102**: 10451–3.
43. Novoselov K S, Geim A K, Morozov S V, Jiang D, Zhang Y, Dubonos S V, Grigorieva I V and Firsov A A. 2004. Electric field effect in atomically thin carbon films. *Science* **306**: 666–9.
44. Nam S-W, Rooks M J, Kim K-B and Rossnagel S M. 2009. Ionic field effect transistors with sub-10 nm multiple nanopores. *Nano Lett.* **9**: 2044–8.
45. Allen M J, Tung V C and Kaner R B. 2010. Honeycomb carbon: A review of graphene. *Chem. Rev.* **110**: 132–45.
46. Krapf D, Wu M-Y, Smeets R M M, Zandbergen H W, Dekker C and Lemay S G. 2006. Fabrication and characterization of nanopore-based electrodes with radii down to 2 nm. *Nano Lett.* **6**: 105–9.
47. Wanunu M, Morrison W, Rabin Y, Grosberg A Y and Meller A. 2010. Electrostatic focusing of unlabelled DNA into nanoscale pores using a salt gradient. *Nat. Nanotechnol.* **5**: 160–5.
48. Heng J B, Aksimentiev A, Ho C, Marks P, Grinkova Y V, Sligar S, Schulten K and Timp G. 2005. Stretching DNA using the electric field in a synthetic nanopore. *Nano Lett.* **5**: 1883–8.
49. Melngailis J. 1987. Focused ion beam technology and applications. *J. Vac. Sci. Technol. B Microelectron. Nanom. Struct.* **5**: 469.
50. Matsunami N, Yamamura Y, Ltikawa Y, Itoh N, Kazumata Y, Miyagawa S, Morita K, Shimizu R and Tawara H. 1984. Energy dependence of sputtering yields of monatomic solids. *At. Data Nucl. Data Tables* **31**: 1–80.
51. Bacri L, Oukhaled A G, Schiedt B, Patriarche G, Bourhis E, Gierak J, Pelta J and Auvray L. 2011. Dynamics of colloids in single solid-state nanopores. *J. Phys. Chem. B* **115**: 2890–8.
52. Powell M R, Cleary L, Davenport M, Shea K J and Siwy Z S. 2011. Electric-field-induced wetting and dewetting in single hydrophobic nanopores. *Nat. Nanotechnol.* **6**: 798–802.
53. Siwy Z, Ausloos M and Ivanova K. 2002. Correlation studies of open and closed state fluctuations in an ion channel: Analysis of ion current through a large-conductance locust potassium channel. *Phys. Rev. E* **65**: 1–6.
54. Siwy Z S. 2006. Ion-current rectification in nanopores and nanotubes with broken symmetry. *Adv. Funct. Mater.* **16**: 735–46.
55. Cervera J, Schiedt B and Ramírez P. 2005. A Poisson/Nernst-Planck model for ionic transport through synthetic conical nanopores. *Europhys. Lett.* **71**: 35–41.

56. Nishizawa M, Menon V P and Martin C R. 1995. Metal nanotubule membranes with electrochemically switchable ion-transport selectivity. *Science* **268**: 700–2.

57. Yang X and Zhang G. 2008. The effect of an electrical double layer on the voltammetric performance of nanoscale interdigitated electrodes: A simulation study. *Nanotechnology* **19**: 465504.

58. Kovarik M L, Zhou K and Jacobson S C. 2009. Effect of conical nanopore diameter on ion current rectification. *J. Phys. Chem. B* **113**: 15960–6.

59. Pham P, Howorth M, Planat-Chrétien A and Tardu S. 2007. Numerical simulation of the electrical double layer based on the Poisson-Boltzmann models for AC electroosmosis flows. Excerpt from the Proceedings of the COMSOL Users Conference 2007 Grenoble.

60. Keh H J and Wu Y Y. 2011. Electroosmotic velocity and electric conductivity in a fibrous porous medium in the transverse direction. *J. Phys. Chem. B* **115**: 9168–78.

61. Smith C P. 1991. Theory of the voltammetric response of electrodes of submicron dimensions. Violation of electroneutrality in the presence of excess supporting electrolyte. *Anal. Chem.* **65**: 3343–53.

62. Berg P and Findlay J. 2011. Analytical solution of the Poisson-Nernst-Planck-Stokes equations in a cylindrical channel. *Proc. R. Soc. A Math. Phys. Eng. Sci.* **467**: 3157–69.

63. Movahed S and Li D. 2011. Electrokinetic transport through nanochannels. *Electrophoresis* **32**: 1259–67.

64. Karnik R, Duan C, Castelino K, Daiguji H and Majumdar A. 2007. Rectification of ionic current in a nanofluidic diode. *Nano Lett.* **7**: 547–51.

65. Grahame D C. 1947. The electrical double layer and the theory of electrocapillarity. *Chem. Rev.* **41**: 441–501.

66. Macdonald J R. 1954. Theory of the differential capacitance of the double layer in unadsorbed electrolytes. *J. Chem. Phys.* **22**: 1857.

67. Yang X and Zhang G. 2007. Simulating the structure and effect of the electrical double layer at nanometre electrodes. *Nanotechnology* **18**: 335201.

68. Ulam S M. 1990. Statistical Methods in Neutron Diffusion: With J. von Neumann and R. D. Richtmyer (LAMS-551, April 9, 1947) Analogies Between Analogies: The Mathematical Reports of S. M. Ulam and His Los Alamos Collaborators, eds. A R Bednarek and F Ulam (Oxford, UK: University of California Press), pp. 18–37.

69. Comer J, Dimitrov V, Zhao Q, Timp G and Aksimentiev A. 2009. Microscopic mechanics of hairpin DNA translocation through synthetic nanopores. *Biophys. J.* **96**: 593–608.

70. Gad-El-Hak M. 2005. Differences between liquid and gas transport at the microscale. *Bull. Polish Acad. Sci.* **53**: 301–16.

71. Hammack A, Chen Y-L and Pearce J. 2011. Role of dissolved salts in thermophoresis of DNA: Lattice-Boltzmann-based simulations. *Phys. Rev. E* **83**: 1–7.

15

DNA Electrokinetic Translocation through a Nanopore

Shizhi Qian and Li-Hsien Yeh

CONTENTS

ABSTRACT In the next-generation nanopore-based DNA sequencing technique, DNA nanoparticles are electrophoretically driven through a single nanopore by an externally imposed dc electric field, and the DNA sequence is determined based on the change in the recorded ionic current flowing through the nanopore as the DNA molecule passes through the nanopore. The DNA translocation process has been modeled by using a continuum-based model, composed of the coupled Poisson–Nernst–Planck (PNP) equations for the ionic mass transport and the modified Stokes equations for the hydrodynamic field. The DNA is modeled as a rigid cylindrical nanoparticle. The DNA translocation process in three types of nanopores, including ungated solid-state nanopores, gated solid-state nanopores by field effect transistor (FET), and soft nanopores comprising functionalized polyelectrolyte brushes engrafted to the solid-state nanopore wall, has been theoretically analyzed. The predictions of the developed model agree with the experimental data obtained from the literature. The developed model successfully captures the essential physics underlying the DNA translocation process and provides both necessary theoretical background and reasonable interpretations for the experimental observations on DNA translocation through a nanopore. In both solid-state and soft nanopores, current blockade occurs for thin electric double layer at high bulk salt concentration, while both current blockade and elevation occur at low bulk salt concentration. Two effects arising from the FET control, electroosmotic flow inside the nanopore and DNA nanoparticle–nanopore electrostatic interaction, could be used to actively regulate the DNA translocation process. The soft nanopore has the features of simultaneously enhancing the DNA capture rate before funneling the nanopore and slowing down DNA translocation velocity inside the nanopore.

15.1 Introduction

A single nanopore embedded in a thin synthetic or biological membrane has emerged as a promising platform for next-generation DNA sequencing technology [1–15]. In the nanopore-based DNA sequencing device, a voltage bias is externally applied across a single, short nanopore immerged in an aqueous electrolyte solution, as schematically shown in Figure 15.1. The imposed electric field generates an ionic current flowing through the nanopore [16]. The imposed electric field directed from the *trans* reservoir to the *cis* reservoir also drives negatively charged DNA molecules from the *cis* reservoir through the nanopore toward the *trans* reservoir by electrophoresis. In addition, electric double layer (EDL) forms in the vicinity of the charged nanopore wall with enriched (depleted) counterions (coions) within the EDL, and the interaction between the imposed electric field and the net charges within the EDL of the nanopore induces electroosmotic flow (EOF). The direction of the induced EOF is opposite to (the same as) the DNA electrophoretic motion, and the EOF retards (enhances) the DNA translocation if the nanopore wall is negatively (positively) charged. Therefore, the DNA nanoparticle experiences both hydrodynamic force arising from the induced EOF and electrostatic force during the translocation process. The resulting ionic current flowing through the nanopore is very sensitive to the properties of both the nanopore and the translocating DNA molecules, such as surface charges, sizes, and shapes of the nanopore and the DNA molecules, and salt concentration. The translocating DNA inside the nanopore displaces electrolyte solution out of the nanopore, resulting in a decrease in the ionic current flowing through the nanopore [17]. In addition, the enriched counterions within the EDL of the charged DNA molecule inside the nanopore enhance the nanopore conductance and accordingly ionic current flowing through

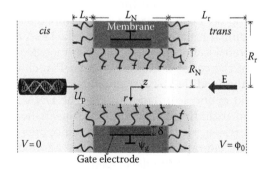

FIGURE 15.1

Schematics of a dsDNA translocation through a single nanopore embedded in a membrane under a negative axial electric field. A gate electrode is patterned on the outer surface of the dielectric nanopore for regulating the surface potential of the nanopore's inner surface next to the gate electrode. The inner surface of the solid-state nanopore is coated with a functionalized layer made of polyelectrolyte brushes.

the nanopore [18,19]. Therefore, single bases or strands of DNA electrophoretically passing through the nanopore will induce a change in the ionic current flowing through the nanopore [16,20,21]. Since the A, C, G, and T nucleotides on the DNA molecule carry different surface charges, each of them may tune the nanopore conductance to a different characteristic degree, resulting in different magnitudes of ionic current. Thus, the magnitude of the ionic current indicates which of the four nucleotides passing through the short nanopore and the sequence of bases in DNA can then be probed by monitoring the current modulations during the translocation of a whole DNA molecule through the nanopore [10,22]. The nanopore-based DNA sequencing technique examines the electronic signals in contrast to the existing paradigms based on chemical techniques and, therefore, does not require sample amplification. Because of the use of short nanopore, the sequencing time of nucleic acids is within a microsecond. In addition, the estimated cost of the nanopore-based sequencing of a human genome would be in the order of $1000, which meets the goals set by the National Institutes of Health in 2004 [23]. All these encouraging advantages of the nanopore-based DNA sequencing stimulated a fast-growing research area associated with nanopore analysis [1,2,4–15,24–30].

Since the fluid reservoirs are typically much larger than the nanopore, whose diameter is typically less than 10 nm, the local electric field within the nanopore is significantly higher than that in the fluid reservoirs [3]. The mismatch of the cross-sectional areas of the reservoir and nanopore results in very slow particle motion within the fluid reservoirs and very high translocation velocity inside the nanopore. Slow particle motion in the fluid reservoir leads to low throughput, while fast translocation inside the nanopore reduces the single base read-out accuracy [26,31–33]. Therefore, there are two major challenges in the nanopore-based DNA sequencing devices: (i) increase DNA capture rate into the nanopore and (ii) slow down DNA translocation within the nanopore. In addition, diverse ionic current signatures including current blockade and current enhancement during the translocation process have been observed in various experiments [6,18,34].

In order to better understand the diverse ionic current signatures underlying the translocation process and develop new methods to resolve the aforementioned challenges in the nanopore-based DNA sequencing devices, a continuum-based mathematical model, composed of the Poisson–Nernst–Planck (PNP) equations for the ionic mass transport and the modified Stokes equations for the hydrodynamic field, is developed to theoretically study DNA translocation process under various conditions. The model is verified by comparing its predictions to some experimental data obtained from the literature. The model provides a useful tool to design the next-generation DNA sequencing devices, to optimize the experimental conditions, and to interpret experimental data. The rest of this chapter is organized as follows. Section 15.2 details the mathematical model for the electric field–induced DNA translocation process. Section 15.3 describes the numerical procedures and code validation. Section 15.4 provides the typical results of DNA translocation in three types of nanopores: (i) ungated solid-state nanopore, (ii) solid-state nanopore gated by field effect transistor (FET), and (iii) ungated soft nanopore composed of a solid-state nanopore with polyelectrolyte (PE) brushes engrafted to the nanopore inner wall surface. This chapter concludes with Section 15.5.

15.2 Mathematical Model

Figure 15.1 schematically depicts an uncoiled dsDNA nanoparticle electrophoretically translocating from the *cis* reservoir along the axis of a cylindrical nanopore of length L_N

and radius R_N, toward the *trans* fluid reservoir under an applied negative axial electric field, **E**. The dsDNA is simulated by a long, rigid nanorod of radius $a = 1$ nm and length L_p bearing a constant surface charge density, σ_p [35,36]. The length of the DNA depends on its base pairs. The nanopore wall bears a fixed uniform surface charge density, σ_w. The nanopore and the *cis* and *trans* reservoirs are filled with an incompressible, binary KCl electrolyte solution of dynamic viscosity μ and permittivity ε. A gate electrode is coated on the outer surface of the dielectric nanopore of thickness δ in the middle region of the nanopore. A gate potential, ψ_g, is applied to the gate electrode for regulating the surface potential of the nanopore's inner surface next to the gate electrode, which in turn modulates the EOF and, accordingly, DNA translocation inside the nanopore. In addition, a functionalized soft layer made of PE brushes is coated on the inner wall surface of the entire solid membrane. For simplicity, we assume that the PE layer is ion penetrable, homogeneously structured, and bears dissociable function groups bearing a uniform fixed charge density ρ_{fix} [37]. In addition, the possible morphology deformation of the PE layer [38] is neglected. The fixed charge density of the PE layer is evaluated by $\rho_{fix} \cong (eZ\sigma_s/L_s)\beta$, where e, Z, σ_s, L_s, and β represent, respectively, the elementary charge, the valence of the dissociable groups per molecular chain, the molecular chain surface density grafted to the solid-state nanopore, the thickness of the PE layer, and the dissociated degree of functional groups in the PE layer. For illustration, we assume that $Z = -1$ and $\sigma_s = 0.6$ nm^{-2}, which correspond to a typical lipid bilayer [39]. The axial length L_r and the radius R_r of the *cis* and *trans* reservoirs are large enough so that bulk ionic concentration, C_0, is maintained far away from the nanopore.

To further simplify the problem, an axisymmetric model is used in the present study. Therefore, all the variables are defined in a cylindrical coordinate system (r, z) with the origin fixed at the center of the nanopore. In other words, we only considered DNA nanoparticle translating along the axis of the nanopore without rotation. In the present study, we consider three types of nanopores: (1) classical ungated solid-state nanopore without the PE brushes and the gate electrode, (2) solid-state nanopore gated by FET in the absence of the PE brushes, and (3) ungated solid-state nanopore coated with the PE brushes. We refer to the third type of nanopore as the soft nanopore. This study adopted a continuum-based model that includes the coupled PNP equations for the ionic mass transport, the modified Stokes equations for the flow field in the region outside of the PE layer, and the modified Brinkman equations for the hydrodynamic field inside the PE layer. The continuum model has been validated by Vlassiouk et al. [40] for the ion transport in a single nanochannel, by Liu et al. [41] for the electrophoresis of a spherical nanoparticle along the axis of a long cylindrical nanotube, by Yeh et al. [42] for the electrophoresis of a soft nanoparticle in an infinite electrolyte solution, and will be further validated by four benchmark problems described in Section 15.3.

15.2.1 Mathematical Model for the Ionic Mass Transport

The ionic mass transport within the binary electrolyte solution is described by the verified PNP equations

$$-\varepsilon\nabla^2 V = h\rho_{fix} + \rho_e = h\rho_{fix} + F(z_1c_1 + z_2c_2) \tag{15.1}$$

and

$$\nabla \cdot \mathbf{N}_j = \nabla \cdot \left(\mathbf{u}c_j - D_j\nabla c_j - z_j \frac{D_j}{RT}Fc_j\nabla V \right) = 0, \; j = 1 \text{ and } 2. \tag{15.2}$$

In the above, V is the electric potential; $\mathbf{u}$ is the fluid velocity; $\rho_e = F(z_1c_1 + z_2c_2)$ is the space charge density of the mobile ions; and $\mathbf{N}_j$, c_j, D_j, and z_j are the ionic flux density, the concentration, the diffusivity, and the valence of the jth ionic species, respectively ($j = 1$ for cations K^+ and $j = 2$ for anions Cl^-). F, R, and T are the Faraday constant, universal gas constant, and the absolute temperature, respectively. h is a unit region function with $h = 0$ in the region outside the PE layer and $h = 1$ inside the PE layer of the nanopore. The EDL thickness is characterized by the Debye length, $\lambda_D = \kappa^{-1} = \sqrt{\varepsilon RT \Big/ \sum_{j=1}^{2} F^2 z_j^2 C_0}$, based on the bulk salt concentration, C_0.

The axial symmetric boundary conditions for all the physical fields are applied on the axis of the nanopore. The following boundary conditions for the potential, V, are imposed: (1) At the ends of the two reservoirs, $V(r, - (L_r + L_N/2)) = 0$ and $V(r, (L_r + L_N/2)) = \phi_0$ with ϕ_0 being the imposed potential bias. (2) On the DNA nanoparticle surface, the Neumann boundary condition is applied for the surface charge density of the nanoparticle, $-\varepsilon \mathbf{n} \cdot \nabla V = \sigma_p$. (3) The Neumann boundary condition of a zero normal electric field is applied on other boundaries in contact with the fluid except the interface between the nanopore's inner wall and the fluid. (4) In the presence of the PE layer, electric potential and field are continuous at the PE layer/fluid interface. (5) Along the nanopore inner wall, surface charge density boundary condition, $-\varepsilon \mathbf{n} \cdot \nabla V = \sigma_w$, is imposed in the absence of the FET control. (6) In the presence of the FET control in the second type of nanopore, the following boundary condition is imposed on the nanopore's inner wall:

$$V = \psi \text{ and } -\varepsilon \mathbf{n} \cdot \nabla V + \varepsilon_d \mathbf{n} \cdot \nabla \psi = \sigma_w, \tag{15.3}$$

where ψ represents the potential inside the dielectric nanopore wall sandwiched between the gate electrode and the fluid, ε_d is the permittivity of the dielectric nanopore material, and $\mathbf{n}$ is the unit normal vector directed from the entity (i.e., nanopore or DNA nanoparticle) wall into the fluid. The potential inside the dielectric nanopore wall is governed by the Laplace equation:

$$\nabla^2 \psi = 0. \tag{15.4}$$

Gate potential $\psi = \psi_g$ is applied on the gate electrode, and electric insulation is applied on other boundaries for the electric potential ψ. Axial symmetric boundary condition for the ionic concentrations is also applied on the axis of the nanopore. The Dirichlet boundary condition is used for the ionic concentrations at the ends of the two big reservoirs, c_j (r, $\pm(L_r + L_N/2)) = C_0$, $j = 1$ and 2. Along the ion-impenetrable surface of the DNA nanoparticle, the normal ionic flux only includes the convective flux arising from the particle translation velocity, $\mathbf{n} \cdot \mathbf{N}_j = \mathbf{n} \cdot (\mathbf{u}c_j)$, $j = 1$ and 2 [43]. In the presence of the PE layer in the soft nanopore, ionic concentration and normal flux are continuous at the PE layer/liquid interface [37]. The normal ionic fluxes on all other ion-impenetrable boundaries are set to be zero.

15.2.2 Mathematical Model for the Hydrodynamic Field

The Reynolds numbers of the electrokinetic flows in the nanopore-based nanofluidic devices are extremely low. Therefore, it is appropriate to model the hydrodynamic flow field using the modified Stokes equations by neglecting the inertial terms in the Navier–Stokes equations

$$-\nabla p + \mu \nabla^2 \mathbf{u} - F(z_1 c_1 + z_2 c_2)\, \nabla V - h\gamma \mathbf{u} = 0 \tag{15.5}$$

and

$$\nabla \cdot \mathbf{u} = 0. \tag{15.6}$$

In the above, p is the hydrodynamic pressure and γ is the hydrodynamic frictional coefficient of the PE layer. The softness degree of the PE layer is characterized by $\lambda^{-1} = \sqrt{\mu/\gamma}$. Nonslip boundary condition is imposed on the surface of the DNA nanoparticle (i.e., $\mathbf{u} = U_p \mathbf{e_z}$) and that of the rigid part of the membrane surface (i.e., $\mathbf{u} = 0$). U_p and $\mathbf{e_z}$ represent, respectively, the DNA nanoparticle translation velocity along the axis of the nanopore and the axial unit vector. A normal flow without external pressure gradient is assumed at the ends of the two big reservoirs. Slip boundary condition is applied at the side boundaries of the two reservoirs, which are far away from the nanopore. In addition, the flow field is continuous on the PE layer/liquid interface in the third type of soft nanopore.

The DNA nanoparticle translational velocity, U_p, is determined based on the balance of the z-component forces acting on the particle using the quasi-static method [44]:

$$F_E + F_H = 0, \tag{15.7}$$

where

$$F_E = \int \varepsilon \left[\frac{\partial V}{\partial z} \frac{\partial V}{\partial r} n_r + \frac{1}{2}\left(\frac{\partial V}{\partial z}\right)^2 n_z - \frac{1}{2}\left(\frac{\partial V}{\partial r}\right)^2 n_z \right] d\Gamma \tag{15.8}$$

is the axial electrical force based on the integration of the Maxwell stress tensor over the particle surface and

$$F_H = \int \left[-p n_z + 2\mu \frac{\partial u_z}{\partial z} n_z + \mu\left(\frac{\partial u_r}{\partial z} + \frac{\partial u_z}{\partial r}\right) n_r \right] d\Gamma \tag{15.9}$$

is the axial hydrodynamic force acting on the DNA nanoparticle. Here, u_r and u_z are, respectively, the r- and z-components of the fluid velocity; n_r and n_z are, respectively, the r- and z-components of the unit vector, $\mathbf{n}$; Γ denotes the surface of the DNA nanoparticle.

The ionic current flowing through the nanopore is

$$I = \int_S F(z_1 \mathbf{N}_1 + z_2 \mathbf{N}_2) \cdot \mathbf{n}\, dS, \tag{15.10}$$

where S denotes either end of the two reservoirs owing to the current conservation. The nanopore conductance, G, can be evaluated by

$$G = I/\phi_0. \tag{15.11}$$

The performance of the DNA translocation process can be measured on the basis of the ionic current deviation,

$$\chi = \frac{I - I_\infty}{I_\infty},$$ (15.12)

with I and I_∞ being the ionic current when the DNA particle's center of mass is located at an arbitrary location z_p and that when the DNA is located far away from the nanopore. During the DNA translocation process (i.e., $-L_N/2 \le z_p \le L_N/2$), a negative (positive) value of χ represents a current blockade (enhancement) [45]. χ_0 represents the current deviation when the DNA nanoparticle's center of mass is located at the center of the nanopore (i.e., $z_p = 0$).

15.3 Numerical Implementation and Code Validation

In the ungated solid-state nanopore, one needs to solve Equations 15.1, 15.2, and 15.5 through 15.7 with $\rho_{fix} = \gamma = 0$. In the solid-state nanopore gated by FET, one needs to solve Equations 15.1, 15.2, and 15.4 through 15.7 with $\rho_{fix} = \gamma = 0$. In the third ungated soft nanopore, one needs to solve Equations 15.1, 15.2, and 15.5 through 15.7 with the appropriate values for the parameters ρ_{fix} and γ. The nonlinear coupled system is numerically solved by a commercial finite-element package COMSOL (version 3.5a; http://www.comsol.com/) operating in a high-performance cluster. The computational domain, as shown in Figure 15.1, is discretized into quadratic triangular elements. Nonuniform elements are employed with larger number of elements assigned locally as necessary. Finer mesh is used near the charged DNA nanoparticle and solid-state nanopore wall as well as inside the region of the PE brushes if they are present. The ionic current through the nanopore is obtained by using the weak constraint in COMSOL specially developed for an accurate calculation of the ionic flux. Rigorous mesh-refinement tests have been performed to ensure that the solutions obtained are convergent and mesh independent. Typically, the number of elements is 2×10^5. A maximum tolerance of 0.01% is imposed on the relative difference $|I_a - I_c|/I_a$, where I_a and I_c are, respectively, the current entering (anode) and leaving (cathode) the nanopore. Several benchmark tests were carried out to ensure the validity and accuracy of the numerical model. The following dimensional parameter values are used in the present study: $T = 300$ K, $D_1(K^+) = 1.95 \times 10^{-9}$ m²/s, $D_2(Cl^-) = 2.03 \times 10^{-9}$ m²/s, $\varepsilon = 7.08 \times 10^{-10}$ F/m, $\mu = 1 \times 10^{-3}$ Pa·s, and $F = 96,490$ C/mol.

15.3.1 Code Validation 1

In the absence of the DNA nanoparticle, gate electrode, and PE brushes, we used the aforementioned model to simulate EOF in a long charged solid-state nanotube filled with 10 mM KCl electrolyte. The surface charge density and radius of the nanotube are, respectively, $\sigma_w = -1$ mC/m² and $R_N = 50$ nm, and the negative axial electric field is $E = 50$ kV/m. The analytical solution of the fully developed axial EOF velocity is given by [46,47]

$$u_z(r) = -\frac{\lambda_D \sigma_w E}{\mu I_1(R_N/\lambda_D)}[I_0(R_N/\lambda_D) - I_0(r/\lambda_D)],$$ (15.13)

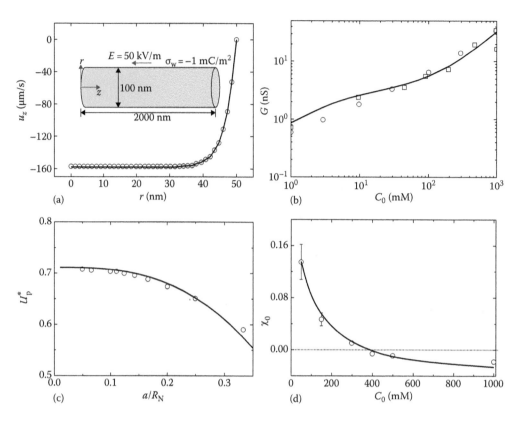

FIGURE 15.2

Axial EOF velocity in a long cylindrical nanotube. The inset shows the schematic view of the problem under consideration (a). Conductance in a solid-state nanopore as a function of bulk salt concentration C_0 (b). Electrophoretic velocity of a sphere of radius a translating along the axis of an uncharged cylindrical tube of radius R_N as a function of the ratio a/R_N (c). Current deviation change $\chi_0 = (I_0 - I_\infty)/I_\infty$ attributed to the presence of a dsDNA located at the center of a solid-state nanopore as a function of the bulk salt concentration C_0 (d). (Adapted from (a) Ai, Y. et al., *Journal of Physical Chemistry C* 114 (9):3883–3890, 2010; (b) Yeh, L.H. et al., *Nanoscale* 4 (16):5169–5177, 2012; (c) Ai, Y., and S.Z. Qian, *Physical Chemistry Chemical Physics* 13 (9):4060–4071, 2011; (d) Yeh, L.H. et al., *Nanoscale* 4 (8):2685–2693, 2012. With permission.)

where I_i is the modified Bessel functions of the first kind of order i. Figure 15.2a shows the radial distribution of the fully developed axial EOF velocity, and our numerical results (circles) are in good agreement with the analytical solution (solid line) [48].

15.3.2 Code Validation 2

In the absence of the DNA particle, gate electrode, and PE brushes, we used the afore-mentioned model to simulate electrokinetic ion and fluid transport in a silica solid-state nanopore of length $L_N = 34$ nm and radius $R_N = 5.5$ nm at the potential bias $\phi_0 = 200$ mV. The surface charge density of the silica nanopore wall is $\sigma_w = -60$ mC/m^2 [49], $L_r = 250$ nm, and $R_r = 250$ nm. Figure 15.2b depicts the nanopore conductance, G, as a function of the bulk concentration, C_0, of KCl electrolyte solution [50]. Our number results (solid line) agree well with the experimental data (circles with error bars) obtained by Smeets et al. [19].

15.3.3 Code Validation 3

In the absence of the gate electrode and the PE brushes, we simulated electrophoretic motion of a charged spherical particle of radius a translating along the axis of an infinitely long, uncharged cylindrical nanopore of radius R_N. Based on the Poisson–Boltzmann model (PBM), the approximation solution for the electrophoretic velocity has been derived when the EDL is not overlapped and the zeta potential of the particle, ζ_p, is relatively small ($\zeta_p/(RT/F) < 1$) [51]. Figure 15.2c shows the steady particle electrophoretic velocity normalized by $\varepsilon\zeta_p E/\mu$ as a function of the ratio of the particle radius to the nanopore radius, a/R_N, when $a = 1$ nm, $\kappa a = 2.05$, $\zeta_p = 1$ mV, and $E = 50$ kV/m [52]. The numerical results (circles) are in good agreement with the approximation solution (solid line) when the pore size is much larger than the particle size. However, the approximation solution underestimates the particle velocity as a/R_N increases since the PBM used to derive the approximation solution becomes inappropriate.

15.3.4 Code Validation 4

In the absence of the gate electrode and the PE brushes, we simulated the influence of a DNA nanoparticle located in the center of a solid-state silica nanopore on the ionic current flowing through the nanopore. The surface charge density of the silica nanopore wall is $\sigma_w = -60$ mC/m^2 [49]. The length and radius of the nanopore are, respectively, $L_N = 34$ nm and $R_N = 5.1$ nm [19]. The voltage bias is $V_0 = 0.35$ V, the reservoir dimensions are $L_r = 200$ nm and $R_r = 200$ nm, and $\sigma_p = \lambda_{DNA}/2\pi a$ (ca. -35.7 mC/m^2). Here, $a = 1$ nm, and $\lambda_{DNA} = \lambda_{bare}/\beta_M$ is the effective line charge density of the DNA estimated by dividing the bare line charge density of the DNA $\lambda_{bare} = 5.9$ e/nm by the Manning factor $\beta_M = 4.2$ [53]. Figure 15.2d depicts the relative ionic current change when a 147-bp DNA (ca. 14 helical pitches) is located at the center of the nanopore, χ_0, as a function of the bulk concentration of KCl electrolyte solution, C_0 [54]. The solid line in Figure 15.2d represents our numerical results, while circles with error bars represent the experimental data obtained by Smeets et al. [19]. Our model successfully captured the dependence of the ionic current on the bulk salt concentration, and its predictions agree with the experimental results. It predicts that current blockade occurs when C_0 exceeds a critical salt concentration (ca. 390 mM), and current enhancement occurs when C_0 is lower than that critical concentration. As pointed out by Smeets et al. [19], the current enhancement and blockade arise from two competing effects: (1) the ionic current decreases because of the displacement of ions out of the nanopore by the volume of the dielectric DNA strand present inside the nanopore, and (2) the screened counterions accompanied with the charged DNA strand increases the ionic concentration inside the nanopore and accordingly increases the ionic current.

15.4. Results and Discussion

15.4.1 DNA Translocation through an Ungated Solid-State Nanopore

Liu et al. [41] modeled DNA nanoparticle translocation in a solid-state nanopore without FET control and PE layer using three different models: the multi-ion model (MIM) described in Section 15.2, its simplified model based on the Poisson–Boltzmann model (PBM), and the Smoluchowski slip velocity model (SVM). The MIM takes into account the EDL polarization stemming from the strong electric field imposed and the generated hydrodynamic flow and is valid for all EDL thicknesses, while the PBM neglects the EDL polarization because of the imposed electric field and the induced fluid convection, and assumes that the ionic concentrations satisfy the Boltzmann distribution and the EDL is under its equilibrium state. The PBM does not require solving the Nernst–Planck equations (Equation 15.2) for the ionic concentration fields, and the PB equation derived from Equation 15.1 and the governing equations for the hydrodynamic field are then decoupled. Consequently, the computational complexity is significantly reduced. One would expect that the PBM would provide reasonable predictions when the external electric field is relatively small compared to the equilibrium electric field arising from the charge surfaces of the DNA nanoparticle and the nanopore wall. Both the MIM and PBM require one to determine the EDL. When the EDL thickness is very thin ($\lambda_D \ll a$ and R_N), it is not practical to resolve the EDL in the numerical simulations. Instead, the motion of the liquid at the *edge* of the EDL of the charged particle and solid boundaries is approximated by the Smoluchowski electroosmotic slip velocity in the SVM. Since the SVM does not need to determine the field within the EDL, it provides great simplification in the computational effort. The SVM has been widely used to model electrokinetic fluid and particle transport in microfluidics in which the EDL thickness is much smaller than the characteristic length of microfluidic devices [55].

When the EDL is thin at high bulk salt concentration, the predictions from the three models are in good agreement, and only current blockade is predicted. The magnitude of the current blockade is roughly proportional to the cross-sectional area of the DNA nanoparticle present inside the nanopore because the induced current blockade mainly arises from the displacement of ions out of the nanopore. The duration of the blockade is proportional to the length of the DNA nanoparticle. The blockade's amplitude is independent of the DNA nanoparticle's length as long as the DNA nanoparticle is longer than the nanopore. When the nanopore wall's surface charge is of the same sign and same magnitude (or larger) as the particle's surface charge, the opposite EOF will prevent the DNA nanoparticle from translocating and the particle will not go through the nanopore. Figure 15.3a depicts the ionic current change for a 3-kbp dsDNA translocating through a solid-state nanopore of 1.5 nm in radius and 5 nm in length when $\phi_0 = 120$ mV, $L_r = 0.3$ mm, and $R_r = 1.5$ mm, and the experimental result was obtained by Li et al. [9]. In the experiments, 1 M KCl and 10 mM TRIS–HCl buffer at pH = 8.0 was used, and the corresponding ratio $\lambda_D/(R_N - a)$ is approximately 0.08, implying that the EDL is very thin. In the experiments, the base current was 1430 ± 20 pA, the blockade current was 1310 ± 15 pA, $\chi_{min} = -0.084 \pm 0.02$, and the average translocation velocity was 0.85–1.13 cm/s. Figure 15.3b shows the predicted ionic current obtained by Liu et al. [41] using reduced fluid reservoirs of 0.6 μm in length and 0.3 μm in radius. The predicted base current, I_∞, is 1730 pA; the blockade current is 1100 pA; the corresponding current deviation, χ, is −0.36; and the average particle velocity is 0.81 cm/s. The experimental ionic current as a function of time (Figure 15.3a) is qualitatively similar to the prediction shown in Figure 15.3b. Figure 15.3c quantitatively compares the predictions and experimental results. The computational results are of the same order of magnitude as the experimental ones. The deviations between the experimental and theoretical results can be attributed, in part, to the complexity of the DNA molecule, which was not captured in the numerical simulations and, in part, to underestimation of the pore's size [56]. The reported nanopore geometry is interpreted from transmission electron microscope images. These images are, however, two-dimensional projections of the nanopore and capture the smallest dimensions of the nanopore along its length. In fact, the nanopores are often elliptical in cross section rather than circular and typically

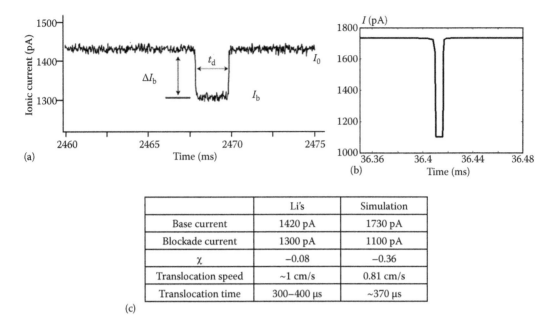

	Li's	Simulation
Base current	1420 pA	1730 pA
Blockade current	1300 pA	1100 pA
χ	−0.08	−0.36
Translocation speed	~1 cm/s	0.81 cm/s
Translocation time	300–400 μs	~370 μs

(c)

FIGURE 15.3
Measured (a) and predicted (b) ionic current change for a 3-kbp dsDNA translocating through an ungated solid-state nanopore, and comparisons between the experimental and numerical results (c). ((a) Adapted from Li, J. L. et al., *Nature Materials* 2 (9):611–615, 2003. With permission.)

have a conical shape along their length. Hence, the reported nanopore dimensions are an underestimate of the nanopore's true dimensions, and therefore the experimental $|\chi|$ is smaller than the computed one. The fact that the measured translocation velocity is nearly the same as the predicted one indicates that the translocation process is governed by a balance between the electrostatic and viscous forces and that, in this case, the entropic effects associated with the coiling of the molecule do not play a significant effect.

When the EDL is relatively thick, the excess ion concentration inside the EDL of the DNA nanoparticle and the EDL polarization contribute significantly to the ionic current. As a result, one may observe either both current blockade and elevation or current enhancement alone during the translocation process. Because of the neglect of the EDL in the SVM and the assumption of equilibrium EDL without considering the EDL polarization in the PBM, both SVM and PBM only predict current blockade and fail to predict the current enhancement phenomenon, which has been observed in many experiments [19,34,57,58]. Therefore, the SVM and PBM are not appropriate for simulating a DNA nanoparticle's translocation under the conditions of a thick EDL. In contrast, the MIM predicts current blockade along most of the particle's path, but current enhancement when the particle exits from the nanopore. Figure 15.4a shows the ionic current during the translocation of a 200-bp dsDNA through a silicon oxide nanopore with a radius of 2.2 nm and a length of 50 nm, and the experimental results were obtained by Chang et al. [34]. In the experiments, the imposed potential bias is 200 mV and the buffer solution is 0.1 M KCl solution with 2 mM Tris buffer at pH ~8.5. Under these conditions, the silicon oxide nanopore is expected to carry a negative surface charge density of approximately $\sigma_w = -9.5$ mC/m² and the surface charge density of the dsDNA is estimated as $\sigma_p = -150$ mC/m². The ratio $\lambda_D/(R_N - a) \approx 0.88$ suggests that the EDLs of the DNA nanoparticle and the nanopore wall are

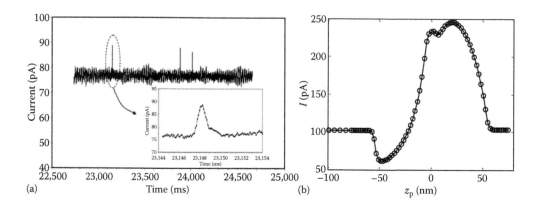

FIGURE 15.4

Measured (a) and predicted (b) ionic current change for a 220-bp dsDNA translocating through a solid-state nanopore of 2.2 nm in radius. ((a) Adapted from Chang, H. et al., *Nano Letters* 4 (8):1551–1556, 2004. With permission.)

overlapped when the DNA is inside the nanopore. Figure 15.4a, the experimental result from Chang et al. [34], shows that throughout most of the translocation process, the ionic current is above the base value. Figure 15.4b depicts the predicted ionic current during the translocation process. Although the simulation results are in qualitative agreement with the experimental data, there are significant differences in the current's magnitude. In the simulations, the ionic current changed from the base current of 100 pA to the maximum value of 240 pA while the corresponding values in the experiment were, respectively, 75 and 90 pA. The difference between the predicted and measured base currents may be attributed to differences between the modeled and the actual nanopore's dimensions (see earlier discussion in Figure 15.3).

15.4.2 DNA Translocation through a Solid-State Nanopore Gated by FET

Under the conditions of thin EDL, low surface potential, and weak electric field imposed, the electrophoretic velocity of a charged spherical particle of radius a along the axis of a cylindrical tube of radius R_N can be approximated by [59]

$$U_p = \frac{\varepsilon E}{\mu}\left[1 - 1.28987\left(\frac{a}{R_N}\right)^3 + 1.89632\left(\frac{a}{R_N}\right)^5 \right.$$
$$\left. -1.0278\left(\frac{a}{R_N}\right)^6 + O\left(\frac{a}{R_N}\right)^8\right](\zeta_p - \zeta_w), \tag{15.14}$$

where ζ_p and ζ_w are, respectively, the zeta potentials of the particle and the tube wall, and E represents the strength of the imposed electric field in the absence of the particle. Obviously, the particle velocity inside the tube depends on the zeta potential difference between the particle and the tube wall. The EOF arising from the charged tube wall retards (enhances) the particle electrophoretic motion when the polarities of ζ_p and ζ_w are the same (opposite). Therefore, one can tune the EOF by modulating ζ_w, which in turn tunes the particle motion. The potential at the solid/liquid interface can be tuned by an ionic FET. In the field effect control of the surface potential, a gate potential, ψ_g, is applied to the gate electrode patterned along the outer surface of the dielectric channel wall [43,60–63]. Figure 15.5 depicts the zeta potential at the SiO_2/fluid interface as a function of the imposed gate potential ψ_g in a SiO_2-based nanochannel embedded with a nanofluidic FET. The solid line represents the theoretical prediction from a model recently developed by Yeh et al. [63], and circles represent the experimental data obtained by Oh et al. [64]. The surface potential becomes more negative when a negative gate potential is applied and becomes positive if a sufficient positive gate potential is imposed. The field effect has also been used to actively control nanoparticle motion in a nanofluidic device [43,64–69].

Recently, Ai et al. [43] theoretically analyzed regulation of DNA particle translocation through a solid-state nanopore by a nanofluidic FET using the model described in Section 15.2 with $\rho_{fix} = 0$ and $\gamma = 0$. When a negative gate potential is applied to the gate electrode, more cations are accumulated in the vicinity of the inner wall of the nanopore next to the gate electrode. The induced EOF is opposite to the particle electrophoretic motion and thus retards the DNA translocation. When a positive gate potential is applied on the gate electrode, anions are predominantly occupied in the EDL region where the gate electrode is located, and the generated EOF is in the same direction of the DNA translocation, leading to the enhancement of the DNA translocation through the nanopore. Figure 15.6 shows the variation of the particle velocity along the axis of the nanopore under two different applied electric fields, $E = 10$ kV/m (a) and $E = 1000$ kV/m (b) at $C_0 = 100$ mM ($a/\lambda_D = 1.03$) and $\varepsilon_d = 3.45 \times 10^{-11}$ F/m (the corresponding dielectric nanopore material is silicon dioxide). The thickness of the dielectric nanopore wall is $\delta = 5$ nm, $L_N = 40$ nm, $R_N = 4$ nm, $\sigma_p = -10$ mC/m², $L_r = 40$ nm, $R_r = 40$ nm, $\sigma_w = 0$, the length of the DNA nanoparticle is $L_p = 10$ nm, and the FET covering half of the nanopore is located in the center region of the nanopore. In an ungated solid-state nanopore (circles in Figure 15.6), DNA is electrophoretically driven from the *cis* reservoir into the nanopore. Since the electric field inside the nanopore is higher than that in the reservoir, the particle velocity in the former is significantly higher than that in the latter. The particle phoretic velocity inside the nanopore is

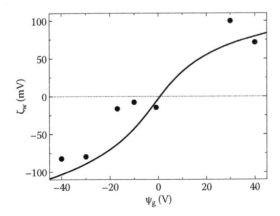

FIGURE 15.5
Zeta potential versus the gate potential in a SiO_2-based nanochannel gated by a nanofluidic FET. Circles represent the experimental data of Oh et al. [64] and the solid line represents the theoretical prediction based on the model developed by Yeh et al. [63]. (Adapted from Yeh, L.H. et al., *Journal of Physical Chemistry C* 116 (6):4209–4216, 2012. With permission.)

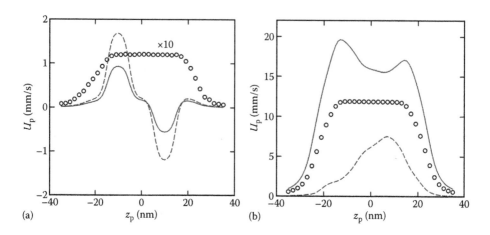

FIGURE 15.6
Particle velocity along the axis of the nanopore under $E = 10$ kV/m (a) and $E = 1000$ kV/m (b). Circles and solid lines represent, respectively, ψ_g = floating and 0.52 V. Dashed lines represent, respectively, $\psi_g = 1.03$ V (a) and -0.52 V (b). (Adapted from Ai, Y. et al., *Analytical Chemistry* 82 (19):8217–8225, 2010. With permission.)

nearly a constant. The particle velocity decreases after the particle exits the nanopore into the *trans* reservoir owing to the decrease in the local axial electric field.

For $E = 10$ kV/m, the particle velocity in an ungated nanopore is multiplied by a factor of 10 for comparison with the results in a FET-gated solid-state nanopore. Since the applied electric field is relatively low, to increase throughput, a positive gate potential is applied to generate an EOF in the same direction of the DNA translocation. The solid and dashed lines in Figure 15.6a represent, respectively, the particle velocities for $\psi_g = 0.52$ and 1.03 V. The induced EOF facilitates the DNA threading the nanopore, and a higher gate potential leads to a more significant EOF and, accordingly, a faster attraction of the DNA into the nanopore. The particle velocity attains its maximum at nearly $z_p = -10$ nm (the edge of gated nanopore) and subsequently decreases as the DNA translates further into the nanopore. When the DNA passes through the center of the nanopore ($z_p = 0$), the particle velocity becomes negative, implying that the DNA is unable to move further and is trapped inside the nanopore. The asymmetric particle velocity and particle trapping shown in Figure 15.6a are attributed to the electrostatic interaction between the negatively charged DNA and the induced positive surface potential of the nanopore next to the gate electrode. The particle–nanopore interaction induces an attractive force acting on the DNA particle, which drags the DNA into the nanopore in the region of $z_p < 0$. However, the attractive force becomes opposite to the particle phoretic motion in the region of $z_p > 0$, and, accordingly, retards the DNA translocation. Under low electric field imposed and thick EDL, the attractive particle–nanopore electrostatic interaction force dominates over the electrophoretic driving force and the hydrodynamic force arising from the EOF; the DNA is trapped inside the nanopore after passing through $z_p = 0$.

For a relatively high electric field such as $E = 1000$ kV/m (Figure 15.6b), a positive gate potential generates an EOF in the same direction of the particle electrophoretic motion, facilitating the DNA translocation. Therefore, the particle velocity for $\psi_g = 0.52$ V (solid line) is higher than that in the ungated nanopore (circles). In contrast to the case of $E = 10$ kV/m, particle trapping inside the nanopore is not observed for $E = 1000$ kV/m, implying that the electric driving force arising from the external electric field dominates over the particle–nanopore electrostatic interaction force. The asymmetric particle velocity profile with respect to the center of the nanopore, $z_p = 0$, is attributed to the particle–nanopore wall interaction. One can slow down DNA translocation speed inside the nanopore by imposing a negative gate potential. The particle velocity inside the nanopore for $\psi_g = -0.52$ V (dashed line) is lower than that in the ungated nanopore (circles). The particle velocity is also asymmetric with respect to the center of the nanopore owing to the spatially dependent particle–nanopore wall interaction. The surface potential of the FET-gated nanopore wall becomes negative for $\psi_g < 0$, resulting in an EOF opposite to the particle phoretic motion and accordingly slows down the particle motion inside the nanopore. In addition, the particle–nanopore wall electrostatic interaction induces repulsive force acting on the particle. When the particle is located in the region of $z_p < 0$, the electrostatic repulsive force further slows down the particle motion. However, the electrostatic repulsive force enhances the particle motion in the region of $z_p > 0$.

The systematic study by Ai et al. [43] concluded that there were two effects arising from the field effect, the EOF and the particle–nanopore electrostatic interaction. The EOF globally affects the DNA translocation in a consistent direction, while the particle–nanopore electrostatic interaction highly depends on the location of the DNA nanoparticle, acting as a local effect. The particle–nanopore electrostatic interaction dominates over the EOF effect only when the EDLs of the DNA nanoparticle and the nanopore wall are overlapped and the applied electric field is relatively low. By dynamically tuning the gate potential, one can slow down and even trap a DNA nanoparticle inside the nanopore. For example, a feedback FET nanofluidic control system was proposed by He et al. [68,69] to regulate the DNA translocation through a gated nanopore. In contrast to the symmetric particle velocity profile in the ungated nanopore, the particle velocity profile is asymmetric with respect to the center of the FET-gated nanopore owing to the particle–nanopore wall electrostatic interaction.

15.4.3 DNA Translocation through a Solid-State Nanopore Functionalized by PE Brushes

Recently, Yeh et al. [54] proposed and numerically demonstrated simultaneous increase in the DNA capture rate before funneling a nanopore and decrease in the DNA translocation velocity inside the nanopore by using a soft nanopore comprising a solid-state nanopore with functionalized PE brushes engrafted to the entire solid membrane wall. Figure 15.7a schematically illustrates a dsDNA translocating through a soft nanopore, and Figure 15.7b shows the mechanisms involved in the process.

Because of the imposed axial electric field **E**, an EOF is induced within the charged soft nanopore. The porous PE layer yields an extra friction force $\mathbf{F}_{friction}$ acting on the liquid flowing through it. Because of the extra friction force, the fluid flow inside the PE layer is slower than that in the central region outside the PE layer. In addition, the mobile charges accumulated inside the soft nanopore are higher than those in the corresponding solid-state nanopores. Figure 15.8a and b show, respectively, the spatial distributions of the normalized net ionic concentration difference, $(c_1 - c_2)/C_0$, in a soft nanopore and the corresponding solid-state nanopore. For comparison, the net amounts of charge in the soft and solid-state nanopores are assumed to be the same, that is, $\rho_{fix} \times \Phi_{soft\,layer} = \sigma_w \times \Delta_{membrane}$ with $\Phi_{soft\,layer}$ and $\Delta_{membrane}$ being the volume of the PE layer and the surface area of the membrane, respectively. The nanopore length and radius are, respectively, $L_N = 60$ nm and $R_N = 8$ nm. The thickness of the PE layer in the soft nanopore is $L_s = 5$ nm, and the size

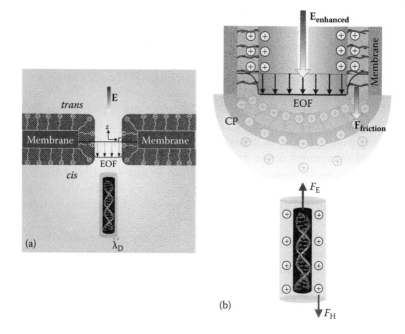

FIGURE 15.7
Schematics (a) and mechanism (b) of a dsDNA translocating through a soft nanopore. (Adapted from Yeh, L.H. et al., *Nanoscale* 4 (8):2685–2693, 2012. With permission.)

of the reservoirs is $L_r = 200$ nm and $R_r = 200$ nm. The imposed potential bias is $\phi_0 = 1.12$ V. Comparisons between Figure 15.8a and b reveal that the concentration of counterions is high in the vicinity of the rigid surface of the solid-state nanopore but remains high outside the PE layer in the soft nanopore. Because of the very strong electric field inside the nanopore and the ion selectivity of the charged nanopore, ion concentration polarization (CP) with enriched (depleted) ions occurs at the *cis* (*trans*) side of the nanopore [50,54]. Because of the induced ion CP, the concentrations of both ions at the cross section of $z = -L_N/2$ are higher than those at the cross section of $z = L_N/2$, resulting in a concentration gradient across the nanopore. In addition, the induced ion CP in a soft nanopore is more significant than that in the corresponding solid-state nanopore. Figure 15.8c and d show, respectively, the axial variations of $(c_1 - c_2)/C_0$ and the normalized axial electric field, $-E_z/E_0$, with $E_0 = RT/aF$. As can be seen in Figure 15.8c, the concentration of counterions near the entrance of the soft nanopore (dashed line) is significantly higher than that in the corresponding solid-state nanopore (solid line), implying that a significant counterion-rich CP occurs at the mouth of the soft nanopore, as schematically shown in Figure 15.7b. The electrostatic interaction between the enriched counterions at the nanopore mouth and the negatively charged DNA nanoparticle induces an attractive force, resulting in an increase in the DNA capture velocity inside the *cis* reservoir. The induced ion CP generates a concentration gradient, which in turn generates an axial electric field, the direction of which is opposite to the externally applied one. Figure 15.8d shows the axial variation of the net electric field in the soft nanopore and its corresponding solid-state nanopores. As expected, the electric field inside the nanopore is significantly higher than that inside the reservoirs because of the difference in their cross-sectional areas. $\mathbf{E}_{enhanced}$ in Figure 15.7b represents the enhanced local electric field inside the nanopore. In addition, the axial net

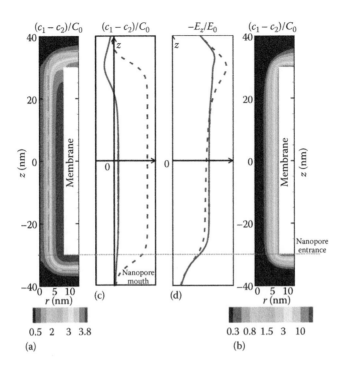

FIGURE 15.8
Spatial distribution of the normalized net ionic concentration difference, $(c_1 - c_2)/C_0$, for a soft nanopore with fixed charge density $\rho_{fix} = -9.1 \times 10^6$ C/m^3, softness degree $\lambda^{-1} = 1$ nm, and $\sigma_w = 0$ (a), and a solid-state nanopore with surface charge density σ_w (b), at bulk salt concentration $C_0 = 24$ nM. Axial variation of $(c_1 - c_2)/C_0$ (c) and $-E_z/E_0$ (d), with $E_0 = RT/aF$ (not to scale). The dashed curve in (a) denotes the outer boundary of the soft layer and the dashed and solid curves in (c) and (d) denote the results of the soft and solid-state nanopores, respectively. (Adapted from Yeh, L.H. et al., *Nanoscale* 4 (8):2685–2693, 2012. With permission.)

electric field inside the solid-state nanopore is nearly uniform, while that inside the soft nanopore becomes spatially dependent. Except near the nanopore exit where the local electric field in the soft nanopore is higher than that in the solid-state nanopore, which is attributed to more significant depletion of ions in that region of the soft nanopore, the local electric field within most region of the soft nanopore is lower than that in the solid-state nanopore. Because the ion CP in the soft nanopore is more significant than that in the solid-state nanopore, the induced electric field opposite to the externally imposed one in the soft nanopore is also higher than that in the solid-state nanopore, yielding a lower net electric field inside most region of the soft nanopore. The significant ion CP in the soft nanopore results in a spatially nonuniform electric field inside the soft nanopore. In summary, the presence of the PE layer induces the following effects on DNA nanoparticle translocation: (1) enhanced EOF in the central region outside the PE layer resulting in higher hydrodynamic force acting on the DNA particle and, accordingly, lower translocation velocity; (2) significantly enriched counterions (cations) at the nanopore mouth attracting DNA nanoparticle from the *cis* reservoir toward the nanopore entrance resulting in an increase in the DNA capture rate; and (3) decreased net electric field inside most region of the soft nanopore (owing to significant ion CP) leading to lower electrophoretic driving force, F_E, and accordingly lower translocation velocity. One can also tune the above effects by adjusting the bulk salt concentration, C_0, and the properties of the PE layer including the molecular chain surface density, σ_s, thickness of the PE layer, L_s, and softness degree of the PE layer, λ^{-1}.

Figure 15.9 depicts the particle velocity as a function of the particle's position for various values of ρ_{fix} at $C_0 = 100$ mM (a) and various bulk salt concentrations C_0 at $\rho_{fix} = -9.1 \times 10^6$ C/m³ (b). The solid line with circles in Figure 15.9a represents the results in the corresponding solid-state nanopore with $\rho_{fix} = \gamma = 0$. In the soft nanopore, the surface charge density of the membrane wall is assumed to be $\sigma_w = 0$. Figure 15.9a shows that the DNA translocation velocity inside the solid-state nanopore (-30 nm $\leq z_p \leq 30$ nm) is faster than that in the soft nanopore. As $|\rho_{fix}|$ increases, more counterions are accumulated inside the nanopore, resulting in an increase in the EOF inside the nanopore and, accordingly, slower particle translocation velocity. When ρ_{fix} is sufficiently large, the particle velocity becomes negative in the front of the nanopore, implying that the DNA is trapped there by the strong EOF opposite to the particle translocation motion. Figure 15.9b shows that the particle velocity decreases as the bulk salt concentration increases, which is mainly attributed to the decrease in the electrophoretic driving force with an increase in the bulk salt concentration [70]. The DNA could not enter the nanopore if the salt concentration exceeds a certain threshold value. In addition, the DNA velocity before threading the nanopore entrance, defined as the DNA capture velocity, significantly increases as it approaches the nanopore entrance (-70 nm $< z_p < -60$ nm) and then starts to decrease at $z_p \cong -55$ nm, as shown in Figure 15.9b. The enhancement in the capture velocity in the soft nanopore is attributed to the significant counterion-rich CP occurring at the nanopore mouth, as discussed before. Since the induced ion CP becomes more significant at higher ρ_{fix} and lower bulk salt concentration (thicker EDL), the enhancement in the capture velocity increases at higher fixed charge density of the PE layer and lower salt concentration, as can be seen in Figure 15.9.

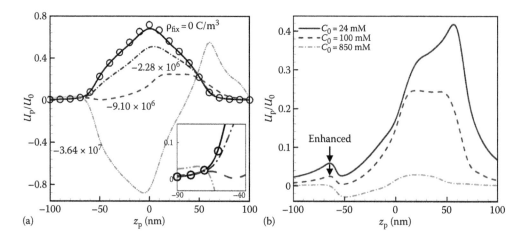

FIGURE 15.9
Variation of the DNA translational velocity (normalized with the reference Smoluchowski velocity $U_0 = \varepsilon R^2 T^2 / \mu a F^2$) as a function of the particle position z_p at various fixed charge density ρ_{fix} (a) and the bulk salt concentration C_0 (b) for $R_N = 8$ nm, $L_N = 60$ nm, $L_s = 5$ nm, the length of the dsDNA is $L_p = 49$ nm, $\sigma_p = -35.7$ mC/m², and $\phi_0 = 1.12$ V. (a) $\lambda^{-1} = 1$ nm, $C_0 = 100$ mM, and open circles denote the corresponding results for the corresponding solid-state nanopore (i.e., $\rho_{fix} = \lambda = 0$). (b) $\rho_{fix} = -9.1 \times 10^6$ C/m³ and $\lambda^{-1} = 1$ nm. The inset in (a) is the enlarged region for -90 nm $\leq z_p \leq -40$ nm; the arrows in (a) and (b) highlight that the capture velocity (DNA velocity before funneling the nanopore) is enhanced. (Adapted from Yeh, L.H. et al., *Nanoscale* 4 (8):2685–2693, 2012. With permission.)

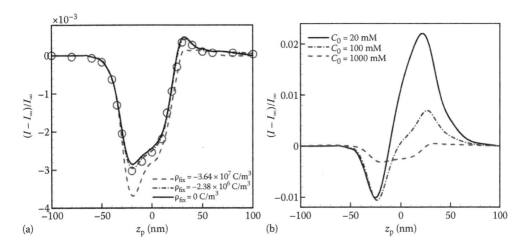

FIGURE 15.10

Ionic current deviation, $(I - I_\infty)/I_\infty$, as a function of the particle location z_p for various combinations of the fixed charge density ρ_{fix} and the softness degree λ^{-1} at bulk salt concentration $C_0 = 1000$ mM (a) and for various C_0 at $\rho_{fix} = -1.16 \times 10^7$ C/m^3 and $\lambda^{-1} = 0.3$ nm (b). The values of the parameters are chosen from those in the experiment [71] nanopore radius $R_N = 14$ nm, pore length $L_N = 12$ nm, thickness of soft layer $L_s = 3.4$ nm, and electric bias $\phi_0 = 0.5$ V. Curves in (a): $\lambda^{-1} = 0.3$ nm; open circles: $\lambda^{-1} = 0.5$ nm and $\rho_{fix} = -2.38 \times 10^6$ C/m^3. (Adapted from Yeh, L.H. et al., *Nanoscale* 4 (8):2685–2693, 2012. With permission.)

Figure 15.10 depicts the ionic current deviation as a function of the particle location for various soft layer properties (ρ_{fix} and λ^{-1}) and bulk salt concentration C_0. Under the conditions considered, DNA can translocate through the nanopore. Figure 15.10a shows that current blockade occurs in both solid-state and soft nanopores owing to higher salt concentration involved [45]. At fixed λ^{-1}, the magnitude of the current blockade increases as the fixed charge density of the PE layer increases. At fixed ρ_{fix}, the effect of λ^{-1} on the current signature is negligible. The same as solid-state nanopores, in the soft nanopore, current blockade occurs for thin EDL at high bulk salt concentration, and both current blockade and enhancement occur when the salt concentration is relatively low, as shown in Figure 15.10b.

15.5 Conclusions and Future Perspective

Electrokinetic translocation of DNA nanoparticle through ungated and FET-gated solid-state nanopores and soft nanopores has been modeled and verified using a continuum-based model, consisting of the PNP equations for the ionic mass transport, the modified Stokes equations for the flow field outside the PE layer, and the modified Brinkman equations for the hydrodynamic field within the PE layer. The fully coupled model takes into account the EDL polarization arising from the induced EOF and the externally imposed electric field. The theoretical predictions agree with experimental data obtained from the literature. Therefore, the model successfully captures the underlying physics of the DNA nanoparticle translocation process in the nanopore-based DNA sequencing technology. In both solid-state and soft nanopores, current blockade occurs for thin EDL at high salt concentration, and both current blockade and enhancement occur for thick EDL at low salt concentration.

Because of the mismatch of the cross-sectional areas of the fluid reservoirs and the nanopore, the local electric field inside the nanopore is significantly enhanced, resulting in very fast translocation. The feasibilities of slowing down DNA translocation inside the nanopore by using a nanofluidic FET and a soft nanopore have been numerically demonstrated. The FET control leads to two effects, EOF and particle–nanopore electrostatic interaction, which can effectively regulate the DNA translocation through a nanopore. The EOF globally affects the DNA translocation in a consistent direction, while the particle–nanopore electrostatic interaction highly depends on the location of the DNA nanoparticle, acting as a local effect. The particle–nanopore electrostatic interaction dominates over the EOF effect only when the EDLs are overlapped and the imposed electric field is relatively low. One can actively slow down DNA translocation by imposing a negative gate potential to the gate electrode. Comparing to the solid-state nanopore, three main effects arise from the PE layer engrafted to the solid-state nanopore wall: (1) enhanced EOF slows down particle translocation; (2) enhanced ion CP increases the capture rate at the nanopore entrance; and (3) enhanced ion CP reduces the net electric field inside the soft nanopore resulting in lower particle translocation velocity. These effects simultaneously yield an increase in the DNA capture velocity at the nanopore mouth and a decrease in its translocation velocity within the nanopore. If the bulk salt concentration is high (thin EDL) and the soft nanopore is short, regardless of the levels of the fixed charge density and the softness degree of the PE layer, current blockade always occurs. Therefore, soft nanopore can be applied to simultaneously increase the capture rate and slow down DNA translocation without changing the ionic current signature.

References

1. Akeson, M., D. Branton, J. J. Kasianowicz, E. Brandin, and D. W. Deamer. 1999. Microsecond time-scale discrimination among polycytidylic acid, polyadenylic acid, and polyuridylic acid as homopolymers or as segments within single RNA molecules. *Biophysical Journal* 77 (6):3227–3233.
2. Chen, P., J. J. Gu, E. Brandin, Y. R. Kim, Q. Wang, and D. Branton. 2004. Probing single DNA molecule transport using fabricated nanopores. *Nano Letters* 4 (11):2293–2298.
3. Cheng, L. J., and L. J. Guo. 2010. Nanofluidic diodes. *Chemical Society Reviews* 39 (3):923–938.
4. Fologea, D., M. Gershow, B. Ledden, D. S. McNabb, J. A. Golovchenko, and J. L. Li. 2005. Detecting single stranded DNA with a solid state nanopore. *Nano Letters* 5 (10):1905–1909.
5. Howorka, S., S. Cheley, and H. Bayley. 2001. Sequence-specific detection of individual DNA strands using engineered nanopores. *Nature Biotechnology* 19 (7):636–639.
6. Iqbal, S. M., D. Akin, and R. Bashir. 2007. Solid-state nanopore channels with DNA selectivity. *Nature Nanotechnology* 2 (4):243–248.
7. Kasianowicz, J. J., E. Brandin, D. Branton, and D. W. Deamer. 1996. Characterization of individual polynucleotide molecules using a membrane channel. *Proceedings of the National Academy of Sciences of the United States of America* 93 (24):13770–13773.
8. Kohli, P., C. C. Harrell, Z. H. Cao, R. Gasparac, W. H. Tan, and C. R. Martin. 2004. DNA-functionalized nanotube membranes with single-base mismatch selectivity. *Science* 305 (5686):984–986.

9. Li, J. L., M. Gershow, D. Stein, E. Brandin, and J. A. Golovchenko. 2003. DNA molecules and configurations in a solid-state nanopore microscope. *Nature Materials* 2 (9):611–615.

10. Meller, A., L. Nivon, E. Brandin, J. Golovchenko, and D. Branton. 2000. Rapid nanopore discrimination between single polynucleotide molecules. *Proceedings of the National Academy of Sciences of the United States of America* 97 (3):1079–1084.

11. Merchant, C. A., K. Healy, M. Wanunu, V. Ray, N. Peterman, J. Bartel, M. D. Fischbein, K. Venta, Z. T. Luo, A. T. C. Johnson, and M. Drndic. 2010. DNA translocation through graphene nanopores. *Nano Letters* 10 (8):2915–2921.

12. Schneider, G. F., S. W. Kowalczyk, V. E. Calado, G. Pandraud, H. W. Zandbergen, L. M. K. Vandersypen, and C. Dekker. 2010. DNA translocation through graphene nanopores. *Nano Letters* 10 (8):3163–3167.

13. Storm, A. J., J. H. Chen, H. W. Zandbergen, and C. Dekker. 2005. Translocation of double-strand DNA through a silicon oxide nanopore. *Physical Review E* 71 (5):051903.

14. Storm, A. J., C. Storm, J. H. Chen, H. Zandbergen, J. F. Joanny, and C. Dekker. 2005. Fast DNA translocation through a solid-state nanopore. *Nano Letters* 5 (7):1193–1197.

15. Venkatesan, B. M., A. B. Shah, J. M. Zuo, and R. Bashir. 2010. DNA sensing using nanocrystalline surface-enhanced Al_2O_3 nanopore sensors. *Advanced Functional Materials* 20 (8):1266–1275.

16. Dekker, C. 2007. Solid-state nanopores. *Nature Nanotechnology* 2 (4):209–215.

17. Meller, A., L. Nivon, and D. Branton. 2001. Voltage-driven DNA translocations through a nanopore. *Physical Review Letters* 86 (15):3435–3438.

18. Chang, H., B. M. Venkatesan, S. M. Iqbal, G. Andreadakis, F. Kosari, G. Vasmatzis, D. Peroulis, and R. Bashir. 2006. DNA counterion current and saturation examined by a MEMS-based solid state nanopore sensor. *Biomedical Microdevices* 8 (3):263–269.

19. Smeets, R. M. M., U. F. Keyser, D. Krapf, M. Y. Wu, N. H. Dekker, and C. Dekker. 2006. Salt dependence of ion transport and DNA translocation through solid-state nanopores. *Nano Letters* 6 (1):89–95.

20. Howorka, S., and Z. Siwy. 2009. Nanopore analytics: Sensing of single molecules. *Chemical Society Reviews* 38 (8):2360–2384.

21. Venkatesan, B. M., and R. Bashir. 2011. Nanopore sensors for nucleic acid analysis. *Nature Nanotechnology* 6 (10):615–624.

22. Clarke, J., H. C. Wu, L. Jayasinghe, A. Patel, S. Reid, and H. Bayley. 2009. Continuous base identification for single-molecule nanopore DNA sequencing. *Nature Nanotechnology* 4 (4):265–270.

23. Branton, D., D. W. Deamer, A. Marziali, H. Bayley, S. A. Benner, T. Butler, M. Di Ventra, S. Garaj, A. Hibbs, X. H. Huang, S. B. Jovanovich, P. S. Krstic, S. Lindsay, X. S. S. Ling, C. H. Mastrangelo, A. Meller, J. S. Oliver, Y. V. Pershin, J. M. Ramsey, R. Riehn, G. V. Soni, V. Tabard-Cossa, M. Wanunu, M. Wiggin, and J. A. Schloss. 2008. The potential and challenges of nanopore sequencing. *Nature Biotechnology* 26 (10):1146–1153.

24. Venkatesan, B. M., D. Estrada, S. Banerjee, X. Z. Jin, V. E. Dorgan, M. H. Bae, N. R. Aluru, E. Pop, and R. Bashir. 2012. Stacked graphene-Al_2O_3 nanopore sensors for sensitive detection of DNA and DNA-protein complexes. *ACS Nano* 6 (1):441–450.

25. Kowalczyk, S. W., M. W. Tuijtel, S. P. Donkers, and C. Dekker. 2010. Unraveling single-stranded DNA in a solid-state nanopore. *Nano Letters* 10 (4):1414–1420.

26. Kowalczyk, S. W., D. B. Wells, A. Aksimentiev, and C. Dekker. 2012. Slowing down DNA translocation through a nanopore in lithium chloride. *Nano Letters* 12 (2):1038–1044.

27. Tsutsui, M., M. Taniguchi, K. Yokota, and T. Kawai. 2010. Identifying single nucleotides by tunnelling current. *Nature Nanotechnology* 5 (4):286–290.

28. Mussi, V., P. Fanzio, L. Repetto, G. Firpo, S. Stigliani, G. P. Tonini, and U. Valbusa. 2011. "DNA-Dressed Nanopore" for complementary sequence detection. *Biosensors & Bioelectronics* 29 (1):125–131.

29. Min, S. K., W. Y. Kim, Y. Cho, and K. S. Kim. 2011. Fast DNA sequencing with a graphene-based nanochannel device. *Nature Nanotechnology* 6 (3):162–165.

30. Saha, K. K., M. Drndic, and B. K. Nikolic. 2012. DNA base-specific modulation of microampere transverse edge currents through a metallic graphene nanoribbon with a nanopore. *Nano Letters* 12 (1):50–55.
31. Fologea, D., J. Uplinger, B. Thomas, D. S. McNabb, and J. L. Li. 2005. Slowing DNA translocation in a solid-state nanopore. *Nano Letters* 5 (9):1734–1737.
32. de Zoysa, R. S. S., D. A. Jayawardhana, Q. T. Zhao, D. Q. Wang, D. W. Armstrong, and X. Y. Guan. 2009. Slowing DNA translocation through nanopores using a solution containing organic salts. *Journal of Physical Chemistry B* 113 (40):13332–13336.
33. Luan, B., G. Stolovitzky, and G. Martyna. 2012. Slowing and controlling the translocation of DNA in a solid-state nanopore. *Nanoscale* 4 (4):1068–1077.
34. Chang, H., F. Kosari, G. Andreadakis, M. A. Alam, G. Vasmatzis, and R. Bashir. 2004. DNA-mediated fluctuations in ionic current through silicon oxide nanopore channels. *Nano Letters* 4 (8):1551–1556.
35. van Dorp, S., U. F. Keyser, N. H. Dekker, C. Dekker, and S. G. Lemay. 2009. Origin of the electrophoretic force on DNA in solid-state nanopores. *Nature Physics* 5 (5):347–351.
36. Keyser, U. F., S. van Dorp, and S. G. Lemay. 2010. Tether forces in DNA electrophoresis. *Chemical Society Reviews* 39 (3):939–947.
37. Ohshima, H. 1995. Electrophoresis of soft particles. *Advances in Colloid and Interface Science* 62 (2–3):189–235.
38. Peleg, O., M. Tagliazucchi, M. Kroger, Y. Rabin, and I. Szleifer. 2011. Morphology control of hairy nanopores. *ACS Nano* 5 (6):4737–4747.
39. Marsh, D., R. Bartucci, and L. Sportelli. 2003. Lipid membranes with grafted polymers: Physicochemical aspects. *Biochimica Et Biophysica Acta-Biomembranes* 1615 (1–2):33–59.
40. Vlassiouk, I., S. Smirnov, and Z. Siwy. 2008. Ionic selectivity of single nanochannels. *Nano Letters* 8 (7):1978–1985.
41. Liu, H., S. Z. Qian, and H. H. Bau. 2007. The effect of translocating cylindrical particles on the ionic current through a nanopore. *Biophysical Journal* 92 (4):1164–1177.
42. Yeh, L. H., K. L. Liu, and J. P. Hsu. 2012. Importance of ionic polarization effect on the electrophoretic behavior of polyelectrolyte nanoparticles in aqueous electrolyte solutions. *Journal of Physical Chemistry C* 116 (1):367–373.
43. Ai, Y., J. Liu, B. K. Zhang, and S. Qian. 2010. Field effect regulation of DNA translocation through a nanopore. *Analytical Chemistry* 82 (19):8217–8225.
44. Qian, S. Z., A. H. Wang, and J. K. Afonien. 2006. Electrophoretic motion of a spherical particle in a converging-diverging nanotube. *Journal of Colloid and Interface Science* 303 (2):579–592.
45. Aksimentiev, A. 2010. Deciphering ionic current signatures of DNA transport through a nanopore. *Nanoscale* 2 (4):468–483.
46. Newman, J., and K. E. Thomas-Alyae. 2004. *Electrochemical Systems*, 3rd ed. John Wiley & Sons: Hoboken, NJ.
47. White, H. S., and A. Bund. 2008. Ion current rectification at nanopores in glass membranes. *Langmuir* 24 (5):2212–2218.
48. Ai, Y., M. K. Zhang, S. W. Joo, M. A. Cheney, and S. Z. Qian. 2010. Effects of electroosmotic flow on ionic current rectification in conical nanopores. *Journal of Physical Chemistry C* 114 (9):3883–3890.
49. Stein, D., M. Kruithof, and C. Dekker. 2004. Surface-charge-governed ion transport in nanofluidic channels. *Physical Review Letters* 93 (3):035901.
50. Yeh, L. H., M. Zhang, N. Hu, S. W. Joo, S. Qian, and J. P. Hsu. 2012. Electrokinetic ion and fluid transport in nanopores functionalized by polyelectrolyte brushes. *Nanoscale* 4 (16):5169–5177.
51. Ennis, J., and J. L. Anderson. 1997. Boundary effects on electrophoretic motion of spherical particles for thick double layers and low zeta potential. *Journal of Colloid and Interface Science* 185 (2):497–514.
52. Ai, Y., and S. Z. Qian. 2011. Electrokinetic particle translocation through a nanopore. *Physical Chemistry Chemical Physics* 13 (9):4060–4071.

53. Manning, G. S. 1969. Limiting laws and counterion condensation in polyelectrolyte solutions. I. Colligative properties. *Journal of Chemical Physics* 51 (3):924–933.
54. Yeh, L. H., M. K. Zhang, S. Z. Qian, and J. P. Hsu. 2012. Regulating DNA translocation through functionalized soft nanopores. *Nanoscale* 4 (8):2685–2693.
55. Qian, S., and Y. Ai. 2012. *Electrokinetic Particle Transport in Micro-/Nanofluidics: Direct Numerical Simulation Analysis.* CRC Press Taylor & Francis: Boca Raton, FL.
56. Ho, C., R. Qiao, J. B. Heng, A. Chatterjee, R. J. Timp, N. R. Aluru, and G. Timp. 2005. Electrolytic transport through a synthetic nanometer-diameter pore. *Proceedings of the National Academy of Sciences of the United States of America* 102 (30):10445–10450.
57. Heng, J. B., C. Ho, T. Kim, R. Timp, A. Aksimentiev, Y. V. Grinkova, S. Sligar, K. Schulten, and G. Timp. 2004. Sizing DNA using a nanometer-diameter pore. *Biophysical Journal* 87 (4):2905–2911.
58. Fan, R., R. Karnik, M. Yue, D. Y. Li, A. Majumdar, and P. D. Yang. 2005. DNA translocation in inorganic nanotubes. *Nano Letters* 5 (9):1633–1637.
59. Keh, H. J., and J. L. Anderson. 1985. Boundary effects on electrophoretic motion of colloidal spheres. *Journal of Fluid Mechanics* 153 (APR):417–439.
60. Ai, Y., J. Liu, B. K. Zhang, and S. Z. Qian. 2011. Ionic current rectification in a conical nanofluidic field effect transistor. *Sensors and Actuators B-Chemical* 157 (2):742–751.
61. Hu, N., Y. Ai, and S. Z. Qian. 2012. Field effect control of electrokinetic transport in micro/nanofluidics. *Sensors and Actuators B-Chemical* 161 (1):1150–1167.
62. Xue, S., N. Hu, and S. Z. Qian. 2012. Tuning surface charge property by floating gate field effect transistor. *Journal of Colloid and Interface Science* 365 (1):326–328.
63. Yeh, L. H., S. Xue, S. W. Joo, S. Qian, and J. P. Hsu. 2012. Field effect control of surface charge property and electroosmotic flow in nanofluidics. *Journal of Physical Chemistry C* 116 (6):4209–4216.
64. Oh, Y. J., A. L. Garcia, D. N. Petsev, G. P. Lopez, S. R. J. Brueck, C. F. Ivory, and S. M. Han. 2009. Effect of wall-molecule interactions on electrokinetic transport of charged molecules in nanofluidic channels during FET flow control. *Lab on a Chip* 9 (11):1601–1608.
65. Karnik, R., R. Fan, M. Yue, D. Y. Li, P. D. Yang, and A. Majumdar. 2005. Electrostatic control of ions and molecules in nanofluidic transistors. *Nano Letters* 5 (5):943–948.
66. Karnik, R., K. Castelino, and A. Majumdar. 2006. Field-effect control of protein transport in a nanofluidic transistor circuit. *Applied Physics Letters* 88 (12):123114.
67. Oh, Y. J., T. C. Gamble, D. Leonhardt, C. H. Chung, S. R. J. Brueck, C. F. Ivory, G. P. Lopez, D. N. Petsev, and S. M. Han. 2008. Monitoring FET flow control and wall adsorption of charged fluorescent dye molecules in nanochannels integrated into a multiple internal reflection infrared waveguide. *Lab on a Chip* 8 (2):251–258.
68. He, Y. H., M. Tsutsui, C. Fan, M. Taniguchi, and T. Kawai. 2011. Controlling DNA translocation through gate modulation of nanopore wall surface charges. *ACS Nano* 5 (7):5509–5518.
69. He, Y. H., M. Tsutsui, C. Fan, M. Taniguchi, and T. Kawai. 2011. Gate manipulation of DNA capture into nanopores. *ACS Nano* 5 (10):8391–8397.
70. Yeh, L. H., J. P. Hsu, and S. Tseng. 2010. Electrophoresis of a membrane-coated cylindrical particle positioned eccentrically along the axis of a narrow cylindrical pore. *Journal of Physical Chemistry C* 114 (39):16576–16587.
71. Yusko, E. C., J. M. Johnson, S. Majd, P. Prangkio, R. C. Rollings, J. L. Li, J. Yang, and M. Mayer. 2011. Controlling protein translocation through nanopores with bio-inspired fluid walls. *Nature Nanotechnology* 6 (4):253–260.

16

Dielectrophoresis for Bioengineering Applications and Some Associated Issues

Yu Zhao, Vandana Pandian, Johnie Hodge, Jozef Brcka,
Jacques Faguet, and Guigen Zhang

CONTENTS

ABSTRACT Dielectrophoresis (DEP) is a phenomenon that occurs when a dielectric particle is placed in a nonuniform electric field. The force generated by the DEP phenomenon has been exploited for various micro- and nanofluidics applications like positioning, sorting and separation of particles involved in medical diagnostics, drug discovery, cell therapeutics, biosensors, microfluidics, nanoassembly, particle filtration, and so on. This chapter aims to identify some of the problems associated with evaluating the DEP forces experienced by particles. Specifically, we will illustrate the consequences of ignoring some of the crucial factors. In addition, we will demonstrate the advantages of a new volumetric method we have developed for quantifying the DEP forces in investigating the alignment and movement of multiple particles under DEP.

16.1 Introduction

Dielectrophoresis (DEP) is a phenomenon occurring when a dielectric particle is placed in a nonuniform electric field. Although the DEP phenomenon was first observed in the early part of the 20th century, it was largely ignored until the 1950s when Herbert A. Pohl applied it to separate particles in a polymer solution [1]. In the past decades, DEP has attracted a lot of attention because of the advent and widespread use of micro- and nanofluidic systems in sensing, processing, and transporting applications, among others [2]. The main advantages of using DEP for these applications include user-friendliness, ease of implementation in micro- and nanofluidic systems, low cost, high throughput, operational at low electrical potentials, and providing motions without any physical contacts or moving parts, to name just a few [3–6]. DEP technology has been constantly evolving and branching out over the years. For example, instead of using metallic electrodes, it sometimes uses the strong local electric field generated by an insulation material such that the required potential can be greatly reduced, and it also uses a photo-conductive technique and material to form electrodes such that the geometry of electrodes can be altered instantly with optical patterns [7–9].

DEP has been commonly used in lab-on-a-chip systems for processing, sensing, and manipulation of synthetic particles as well as biological particles including cells and viruses, among others. Based on the fact that different particles and suspension media may have different dielectric permittivity and conductivity (either frequency dependent or independent), DEP has been used for trapping and separating cells [10–14], sorting particles and cells [15–18], and even studying cellular reactions to drugs [10,19]. Using DEP to separate live cells from dead ones offers a direct and less invasive way over other methods such as using chromogens and fluorophores. For example, since dead cells have significantly lower dielectrophoretic mobility than live cells, they will experience DEP forces with different polarity [20,21]. DEP has also been used to manipulate DNA [22,23] and separate viruses such as the tobacco mosaic virus (TMV) and herpes simplex virus (HSV) [24]. The two viruses are believed to experience DEP forces of different polarity: HSV is trapped under negative DEP (nDEP) forces at the field minimum while TMV experiences positive DEP (pDEP) and collects at the field maximum. Arranging cells into desired patterns is another attractive area of EDP application, especially for constructing bioactive scaffolds and tissue constructs [25–31]. Ho et al. [25] demonstrated the patterning of multiple lines of cells to mimic functioning organs using pDEP in which they aligned heterogeneous cells including hepatic cells and endothelial cells into pearl chains to mimic the lobular morphology of a real liver tissue.

An analytical expression (see Equation 16.1) for the force generated by DEP is commonly used to determine the magnitude and direction of DEP forces despite the force magnitude calculated using this equation often being found to deviate significantly from the actual values [32,33]. In close inspection, it is clear that this force expression assumes that the electrical field, E, will remain unchanged no matter whether particles are present or not. Since the generation of the DEP phenomenon is caused by the disparity in polarization between a particle and its surrounding medium, the presence of such a particle will surely affect the distribution of the electrical field. Additionally, it has been reported that the size of a particle also affects the conductivity of the particle [34–36]. Thus, particle size will have a concomitant effect on DEP forces. Moreover, in most cases, a particle is considered as homogeneous. This may not be the case for biological particles like cells, bacteria, and viruses. Unlike synthetic particles, biological particles (e.g., cells) generally have a complex heterogeneous structure containing multiple components [37]. For example, cells have different permittivity and conductivity from the cytoplasm [38] and even the nucleus. Thus, their structures are better described as a composite body and their dielectric properties may be determined from a combination of the properties of all components [39,40].

In view of these issues, Equation 16.1 may provide a good qualitative guide in predicting the DEP forces in situations like trapping and sorting applications. But for using DEP forces for patterning and alignment purposes, as well as for potential sensing applications, a more precise and quantitative evaluation of the DEP seems necessary. In this chapter, we will use a computational approach to assess some of the associated issues in using DEP for bioengineering applications and illustrate their corresponding consequences.

16.2 Current DEP Theory and Its Limitations

As defined by Pohl, the DEP phenomenon describes the relative motion of particles and suspension medium resulting from polarization forces produced by an inhomogeneous electrical field [1]. As illustrated in Figure 16.1, when a dielectric particle is placed in a medium having different dielectric permittivity, polarization in the particle will occur, leading to an induced dipole moment in the particle. When the induced dipole moment is placed in a nonuniform electrical field, one end of the dipole is in a weaker field than the other and the resulting electrostatic pull will cause the particle to move. When the particle is more polarizable than the suspension medium as shown in Figure 16.1a, the particle will experience a leftward net force, moving it in the direction of increasing electrical field strength. This behavior is referred to as pDEP. When the particle is less polarizable than the suspension medium as shown in Figure 16.1b, the particle will experience a rightward net force, moving it in the direction of decreasing electrical field strength. This behavior is referred to as nDEP.

For a homogeneous particle with a radius of r suspended in a medium, the DEP force can be calculated as follows:

$$F_{DEP} = 2\pi r^2 \varepsilon_m Re(f_{CM}) \nabla |E|^2 \tag{16.1}$$

where $Re(f_{CM})$ denotes the real part of the Clausius–Mossotti (CM) factor f_{CM}, r is the radius of the particle, ε_m is the permittivity of the suspension medium, and E is the electrical field. The CM factor is defined as

$$f_{CM} = \left(\varepsilon_p^* - \varepsilon_m^*\right) / \left(\varepsilon_p^* + 2\varepsilon_m^*\right), \tag{16.2}$$

where ε_p^* and ε_m^* are the complex permittivity of the particle and the suspension medium, respectively. It is worth noting that a modified CM factor has been proposed to deal with nonspherical particles [41]. Here, the complex permittivity $\left(\varepsilon_x^*\right)$ is determined by using $\varepsilon_x^* = \varepsilon_x - i(\sigma_x/\omega)$, in which the subscript x represents either the particle or the medium; thus, ε_x and σ_x are the permittivity and conductivity, respectively, of either the particle (when subscript x refers to the particle: x = p) or the medium (when subscript x refers to the medium: x = m), i is the imaginary symbol ($i = \sqrt{-1}$), and ω is the angular frequency of an

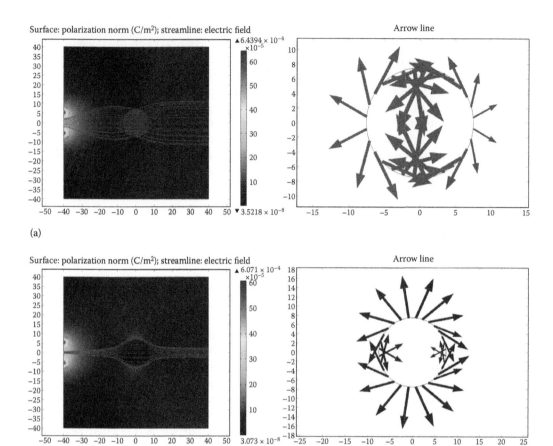

FIGURE 16.1

Illustration of DEP phenomena when a particle is suspended in a medium and subjected to a nonuniform electrical field generated by a small electrode on the left and a large electrode on the right. (a) Positive DEP: the particle is more polarizable than the suspension medium, and the resulting net force will point left, moving the particle in the direction of increasing electrical field strength. (b) Negative DEP: the particle is less polarizable than the suspension medium and the resulting net force will point right, moving the particle in the direction of decreasing electrical field strength.

alternating electrical field. Clearly, the DEP force varies with the properties and size of the particle (ε_p, σ_p, and r) and the suspension media (ε_m and σ_m), as well as the gradient of the field magnitude square ($\nabla|E|^2$). For this reason, DEP can be generated under either a direct current or alternating current (ac) electrical field. In the case of ac DEP, the alternating field can be used to minimize the interference of conventional electrophoresis and adds an extra control to the DEP force through the CM factor by adjusting the frequency (ω) of the alternating electrical field. To counter for the influence of the particle's size, Equation 16.1 scales the DEP force with the particle's volumetric size ($\sim r^3$) no matter what shape the particle takes or what a concomitant effect it might have. The only part in Equation 16.1 that considers the properties of the particle is the CM factor. As one can see from Equation 16.2, the CM factor is often determined by assuming a particle of homogeneous property. This assumption is valid for many synthetic particles, but it may not be for cells, bacteria, and viruses.

To date, Equation 16.1 is still the expression commonly used to determine the magnitude and direction of DEP forces. Although the DEP phenomenon is caused by the disparity in polarization between particles and the suspension medium, Equation 16.1 does not provide any information on how the polarization of particles will affect the distribution of the electrical field. To overcome this drawback, two methods have been developed. In the first one, multipolar moments are represented by a dyadic tensor to account for the higher-order terms, and this method seems to provide a more precise analytical solution [42,43]. The problem with this method, however, is that it treats particles as point dipoles and it is only applicable to particles with axisymmetrical geometrical shapes. The second method uses surface integration of Maxwell stress tensor to calculate the forces on particles. It has been used to simulate the interaction between particles [32,44–46] and the movement of particles [32,47]. This method, although powerful, is not without its limitation: it is based on the boundary element method. With the consideration of the outer shell (i.e., boundary) of a particle, it is difficult to deal with the discontinuty in electrical field across the boundary [44,46]. Furthermore, since DEP force is a volumetric force in essence, torques exerted by the electric field cannot be correctly determined with a boundary-based method. This indicates that the second method will have some problems in dealing with rotational movement of particles. This may explain why the predicted configuration of particle alignment from modeling differs from that of experimental observation [32,33]. Another limitation of the second method is that it is unable to model particles of nonhomogeneous property like cells. Therefore, in addition to assessing the consequences of ignoring some of the important factors, we will also demonstrate a new volumetric method we have developed recently for quantifying the DEP forces and use this method to investigate the alignment and movement of multiple particles.

16.3 Model Setup and Parameters

With a computational approach based on COMSOL Multiphysics, we first set out to build relevant models, investigate the influences of some commonly ignored factors and main issues on the DEP forces through parametric studies, and illustrate the potential consequences of ignoring these factors. After that, we will demonstrate our new volumetric method for quantifying the DEP forces, investigating the particle–particle interaction, and explaining particle alignment patterns.

16.3.1 Model Geometry, Parameters, and Variables

To induce DEP, it is necessary to create nonuniform electrical fields. A nonuniform electrical field can be generated with different methods including the use of electrodes of different sizes, and unique spatial arrangements of electrodes, among others [48–50]. In this work, we use a three-dimensional (3D) spatial arrangement of electrodes for this purpose. Figure 16.2 depicts a section of a setup that consists of a chamber filled with suspension medium with parallel electrodes lined at the bottom of the chamber. A cover layer is used to prevent the electrodes from directly contacting the medium. The parallel electrodes are biased in an alternating positive and ground manner with insulation gaps in between.

Figure 16.3 shows a 3D view of one of the developed COMSOL models. In this model, the width of electrodes is set at 100 μm, and the gap between electrodes is defined by assigning

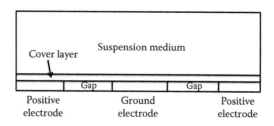

FIGURE 16.2
A schematic view of the physical setup of the models.

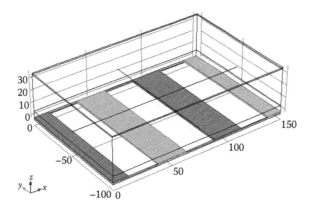

FIGURE 16.3
A 3D view of the actual computational model with electrodes at the bottom of the chamber electrically biased in an alternating +V and –V (or ground) seting.

a value that definines the ratio of electrode-to-gap width. Other parameters used are given in Table 16.1. Spherical polystyrene (PS) particles with various radii are considered and deionized water is used as the suspension medium. The values for the permittivity and conductivity of both the PS particles and water are given in Table 16.2. The electrodes are considered made of gold and the cover layer of silicon oxides.

TABLE 16.1

Parameters Defined for the Parametric Models

Parameters		
Name	**Expression**	**Description**
w_e	100 μm	Width of electrode
ratio	0.1 to 10	Ratio of w_e to w_g
w_g	ratio × w_e	Width of gap
pot	16 V	Electric potential
f	1 Hz to 1 MHz	Frequency
t_c	1 μm	Thickness of cover region

TABLE 16.2

Constants Used in the Models

	Variables	
Name	**Expression**	**Description**
ε_m	6.9×10^{-10} F/m	Permittivity of the medium
ε_p	2.21×10^{-11} F/m	Permittivity of the particle
σ_m	1×10^{-4} S/m	Conductivity of the medium
σ_p	4.8×10^{-4} S/m	Conductivity of the particle (size effect not considered)
r	1, 2.25, 5 µm	Radius of particle

16.3.2 Physics of Electrostatics

For the electrostatics problem, its governing equation follows Gauss's law as

$$\nabla \cdot D = \rho_v, \tag{16.3}$$

where D is the electric displacement and ρ_v is the free volume charge density. The electric displacement is related to the eletrical field by the following relationship: $D = \varepsilon_o E + P$, where E is the external electric field, P is the polarization, and ε_o and ε_r are the vacuum and relative permittivity, respectively. The electrical field can be determined by the negative gradient of the electrical potential as $E = -\nabla V$. Parametric sweeps are performed to analyze the different factors affecting the DEP forces acting on the particles. In these parametric studies, the electric potential is set to vary from 1 to 40 V, the electrode-to-gap ratio is set to vary from 0.1 to 10, and the frequency is set to vary from 1 Hz to 1 MHz.

16.4 Model Validation

To assure the validity and correctness of our modeling approach and results, we first performed an integrated study in which modeling results are compared with experimental results. In this study, we built a 3D model (Figure 16.4) with a unit cell containing two sawtooth-shaped electrodes separated by a gap. In the model, the lower electrode is electrically biased (+V) and the upper electrode is grounded (GND). From the modeling results, we found that on top of the biased electrode, the DEP forces point to an accumulation zone marked by several lines in Figure 16.4a and the forces are strong at the edges of the electrode and diminishes to almost zero near the edge of the accumulation zone. In corner regions of the gap space, the DEP force points from the ground electrode to the biased electrode in a symmetric manner with respect to an oblique angle marked by a diagonal line (see inset in Figure 16.4a). This kind of force distribution suggests that particles on top of the biased electrode will accumulate in a diamond-shaped zone with thin tails at the four vertices extending out along the electrodes and particles in the corners of the gap space will form oblique chains. A particle tracing study confirms this prediction. As shown in Figure 16.4b, particles (represented by the dots) accumulate on top of the biased electrode and align along an oblique line in corners of the gap space. Experimentally, we found that

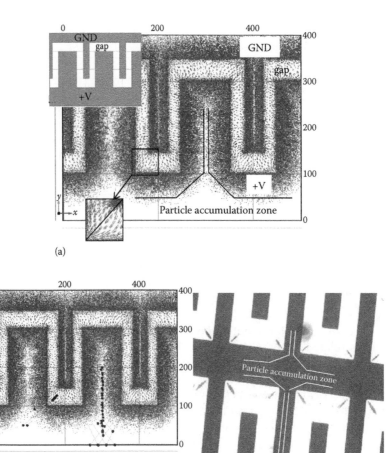

FIGURE 16.4
Results from an integrated modeling and experimental study. (a) Vector distribution of the DEP forces on top of the electrodes and in the gap space. (b) Particle alignment pattern on top of the biased (+V) electrode and in a corner of the gap space. (c) Experimental observation of the resulting particle accumulation and alignment.

particles indeed gathered on top of the large electrode in a diamond-shaped zone with thin-line extensions. Also in the corners of the gap space, particles form a chain aligning in an oblique angle in exactly the same way as the model predicted.

On close examination, we found that these particles actually rest at different height positions in different locations. As shown in Figure 16.5a, the particles aligning in oblique chains rest at the bottom, and the particles accumulating on top of the biased electrode rest at an elevated position. To confirm these modeling predictions experimentally, we used the focal-plane adjusting function of an optical microscope to discern the height locations of the particles. As shown in Figure 16.5b, when the focal plane is close to the electrode plane, the particles in an oblique chain are in focus, indicating that these particles are resting at the bottom of the liquid chamber. When the focal plane is moved upward, the particles on top of the electrode come into focus (Figure 16.5c), pointing to the fact that these particles are at an elevated position. These experimental observations agree very well with the predictions by our model, thus assuring the validity of our modeling approach.

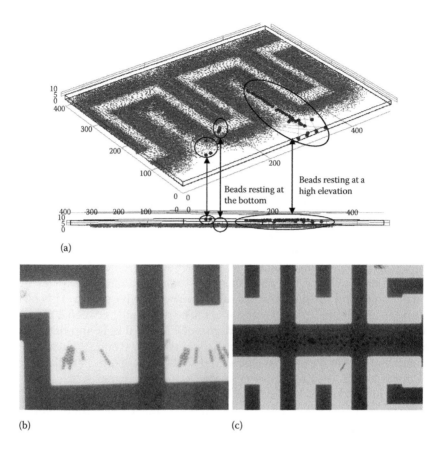

(a)

(b)   (c)

FIGURE 16.5
Examination of particle heights. (a) Modeling result: particles rest at different heights at different locations: particles in the corners of the gap space are at the bottom and those on top of the +V electrode are at an elevated position. Optical images confirm the modeling predictions: when the focal plane of the microscope is close to the plane of electrodes (b) and when the focal plane is at a high position (c).

16.5 Some Commonly Ignored Factors

With our modeling approach and results validated by experimental observations, we then move to assess the influences of ignoring some crucial factors in quantifying the DEP forces. To illustrate the consequences, in this chapter, we will just focus on a few selected factors including the effects of particle size on conductivity, particle nonhomogeneity, and the electrical double layer (EDL).

16.5.1 Effect of Particle Size on Its Conductivity

According to Markx et al. [36], the size of a particle affects its conductivity through the following relationship:

$$\sigma_p = \sigma_b + \frac{2\lambda}{r},$$ (16.4)

where σ_p is the effective particle conductivity, σ_b is the bulk conductivity of the material the particle is made of, λ is the surface conductivity, and r is the radius of the particle. To examine the effect of changing conductivity upon varying the particle size, we analyzed two cases. For the first case, the model considers the relationship defined by Equation 16.4, and for the second one, it treats the situation conventionally; that is, the effect of radius on conductivity is ignored.

To put this in a practical perspective, we examined this size effect using PS spherical particles of two different sizes—2 and 4.5 μm in diameter. For these small particles, the bulk conductivity can be ignored, while the surface conductivity of PS particles [51] is assumed to be $\lambda = 1.2$ nS. With the constants given in Table 16.2, we found the conductivity for the 2-μm ($r = 1$ μm) and 4.5-μm ($r = 2.25$ μm) PS particles as $\sigma_p = 2.410^{-3}$ S/m and 1.0710^{-3} S/m, respectively. With these modified particle conductivity values, we determined the CM factor for both types of particles. As shown in Figure 16.6, the real part of the CM factor goes through a positive-to-negative crossover [52] at a frequency around 400 kHz for the 2-μm particles and around 180 kHz for the 4.5-μm particles. Figure 16.7 shows the results of two particle tracing studies demonstrating this crossover behavior. For the smaller (2 μm) particles, they experience pDEP at 200 kHz and nDEP at 600 kHz, and the pDEP attracts the particles to the bottom of the well and the nDEP pushed them upward. This fact suggests that the particles indeed go through a crossover at a frequency between 200 and 600 kHz. For the larger (4.5 μm) particles, they experience pDEP at 100 kHz and nDEP at 200 kHz, suggesting the existence of a crossover frequency between 100 and 200 kHz.

Experimentally (see Figure 16.8), we observed that for the 2-μm particles, they experience pDEP forces and form line patterns in the gaps at a frequency below 400 kHz. But when the frequency increases beyond 400 kHz, particles start to experience nDEP forces and move away from the bottom of the gaps. At 600 kHz, no bead alignment is even visible. For the 4.5-μm particles, they experience pDEP forces at a frequency below 180 kHz and nDEP forces at a frequency above 200 kHz.

In addition to this change in crossover frequency, this size effect will also affect the force magnitude. Figure 16.9 shows the variation of DEP forces with particle radius for these two cases. Clearly, when Equation 16.4 is not incorporated in the model, the DEP force (dashed line) follows a trend that is proportional to r^3 as predicted by Equation 16.1. However, when

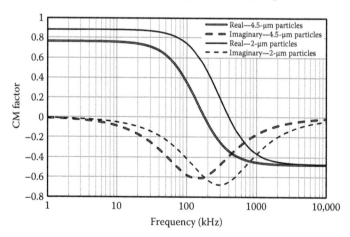

FIGURE 16.6
CM factors obtained for PS particles with different sizes when the effect of particle size on their conductivity is considered.

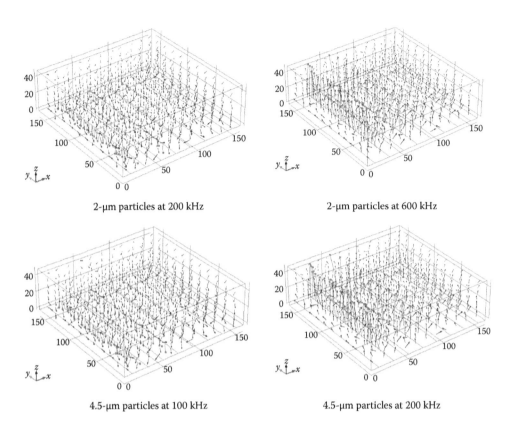

2-µm particles at 200 kHz

2-µm particles at 600 kHz

4.5-µm particles at 100 kHz

4.5-µm particles at 200 kHz

FIGURE 16.7
Results from particle tracing studies show the crossover behavior occurring between 200 and 600 kHz for the 2-µm particles and between 100 and 200 kHz for the 4.5-µm particles.

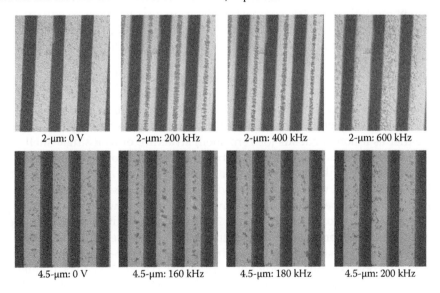

2-µm: 0 V

2-µm: 200 kHz

2-µm: 400 kHz

2-µm: 600 kHz

4.5-µm: 0 V

4.5-µm: 160 kHz

4.5-µm: 180 kHz

4.5-µm: 200 kHz

FIGURE 16.8
Optical images obtained for 2- and 4.5-µm PS particles under DEP forces. The alignments of these particles at different frequencies confirm the modeling predictions of the crossover behavior.

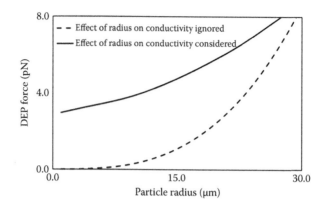

FIGURE 16.9
Difference in the DEP forces when the effect of particle size on conductivity is considered and when it is ignored.

this radius effect on the conductivity is incorporated in the model, the curve for the DEP force is found to deviate from the cubic trend with a left–upward shift, indicating that the force magnitude increases drastically as compared with the other case. This result suggests that ignoring the effects of radius on conductivity could lead to an underestimate for the magnitude of the DEP forces. Since separation of particles using DEP is often done for particles with different sizes, this outcome could have some practical implication when precise magnitudes of DEP forces are of great importance. In such a case, the particle's conductivity dependence upon its radius may not be ignored.

16.5.2 Effect of Particle Nonhomogeneity

When particles are not homogeneous, their structures are better described by a composite body made of multiple dielectric compartments. In many cases, these compartments are represented by layers of shell structures. For example, the structure of a yeast cell is often considered to consist of multiple shells of vacuole, vacuole membrane, cytoplasm, plasma membrane, and cell wall.

To illustrate the differences in considering a biological cell either as a homogeneous particle or as a composite particle with one-layer outer shell (or single shell), we considered the DEP force experienced by an *Escherichia coli* cell. Figure 16.10 shows the variation of DEP force with the frequency of the electrical potential experienced by the cell when it is modeled either as a homogeneous (or zero shell) structure or as a single-shell structure. When the cell is treated as a homogeneous structure, the DEP force it experiences shows a decreasing trend and exhibits a positive-to-negative crossover at a frequency of approximately 23 kHz. However, when the cell is modeled as a composite structure with a single shell, the DEP force it experiences exhibits an increasing trend with a negative-to-positive crossover at a frequency of approximately 4.2 kHz. Hence, on the basis of the single-shell model results, the cell is predicted to experience nDEP at low frequency and pDEP at high frequency. This, rather than the other way around, seems more reasonable judging from the experimental observations reported by Pethig et al. [11]. It needs to be pointed out that while the shell model has been used to denote cells in almost all cell-related DEP works, it only takes the nonhomogeneity of the membrane into consideration while neglecting that of other cellular structures such as the nucleus. A better way to deal with this nonhomogeneity is necessary.

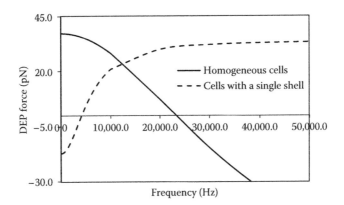

FIGURE 16.10
Variation of DEP forces with frequency experienced by a cell when it is modeled as a homogeneous body or as a nonhomogeneous body with a single shell.

16.5.3 Effect of Electric Double Layer on Crossover Frequency

In a similar way to the size of a particle affecting its conductivity, the presence of an EDL structure surrounding the particle also affects its conductivity [53–56]. In a simplified way of counting for this EDL effect, the following relationship can be used [57]:

$$\sigma_p = \sigma_b + \frac{2(k_s + k_d)}{r}, \tag{16.5}$$

where σ_p and σ_b are the effective particle and bulk conductivity, and k_s and k_d are the conductivity of the stern layer and diffuse layer, respectively. Figure 16.11 compares the DEP forces when the EDL effect on the particle's conductivity is considered and when it is ignored for latex particles suspended in deionized water.

It is seen that there is a considerable amount of shift in both the force magnitude and the crossover frequency when the EDL effect on the particle's conductivity is considered.

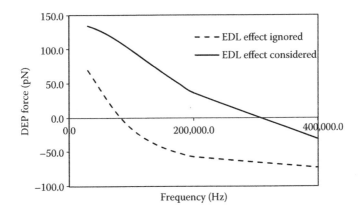

FIGURE 16.11
Variation of DEP forces with frequency experienced by a latex particle when the EDL effect is considered or not considered.

The upward shift will likely result in the particle experiencing a pDEP force under a wide range of frequency. This seems consistent with the argument made by Basuray and Chang [55] that the presence of EDL increases the nanocolloid conductivity to produce pDEP.

16.6 A Look into DEP-Induced Particle–Particle Interactions and Pearl-Chain Formation

Experimentally it is often observed that increasing the applied potential at a fixed frequency can induce a secondary particle alignment—the so-called pearl-chain alignment, which can be seen in some of the images in Figure 16.8. This pearl-chain alignment of particles is believed to be the result of particle realignment under the interaction between dipoles and the electrical field. Frustrated with the inability of using the conventional DEP equation to explain many of the experimentally observed phenomena, we developed 3D computational models to reevaluate the DEP forces exerted on particles. We hypothesized that the presence of the volumetric domain of a particle, which has different dielectric properties from the surrounding medium, will distort the electrical field, thus altering the DEP forces. Under this hypothesis, the size and location of a particle and the distance between neighboring particles will all play some roles in determining the resulting DEP forces.

16.6.1 Electrical Field Distortion Owing to the Presence of Particles

By going back to the fundamentals of physics, we treat a particle as a group of point dipoles and calculate the force density on a point dipole using the following relationship:

$$f = (P \cdot \nabla) E, \tag{16.6}$$

where P is the polarization of the particle. With the use of an effective real permittivity defined as $\varepsilon' = \sqrt{\varepsilon^2 + \left(\dfrac{\sigma}{\omega}\right)^2}$, we integrate this force density over the volumetric domain of the particle to obtain the DEP force as follows:

$$F = \frac{\varepsilon'_p - \varepsilon'_m}{\varepsilon'_p + 2\varepsilon'_m} \varepsilon_0 \int (P \cdot \nabla) E \, dV. \tag{16.7}$$

Since this DEP force is determined by integration over the entire volume of the particle, the effects of the particle size, shape, and its location are all inherently considered. This is not the case when using the conventional DEP force formula. Thus, with this new way of determining the DEP forces, we are able to consider the effects of the size, shape, and location of the particle on the induced electrical field and subsequently the DEP forces.

To evaluate the DEP force using Equation 16.7, it is necessary to use a computational approach, especially for many complex situations. For that, we use COMSOL Multiphysics to develop models to closely represent actual situations including the geometry and the underlying physics. Figure 16.12a shows a 3D model in which a spherical particle ($r = 5$ μm)

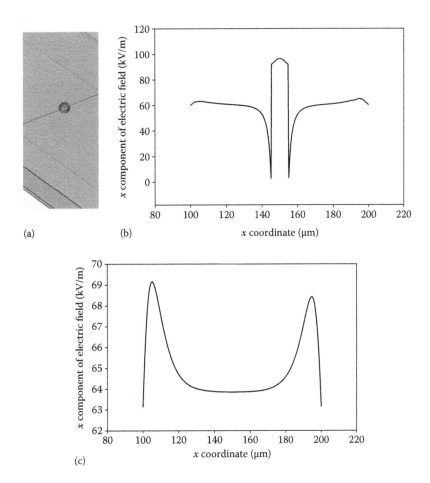

(a)

(b)

x coordinate (μm)

(c)

x coordinate (μm)

FIGURE 16.12
COMSOL model (a) and line plots (b and c) obtained for a 10-μm particle to demonstrate the influence of particle volumetric domain on the distortion of electrical field. In (b), the influence of the particle presence on the electrical field distortion is drastic as compared with (c) when the influence is ignored.

is placed in a nonuniform electrical field suspended in deionized water. Figure 16.12b shows the *x*-component of the induced electrical field along a line that goes through the center of the particle and Figure 16.12c shows the same electrical field distribution when the presence of the particle is ignored. Clearly, the electrical field surrounding the particle is distorted drastically when the presence of the particle is considered. This electrical field distortion is the result of differential conductivity and permittivity between the particle and the suspension medium. When the values for the particle conductivity and permittivity are replaced by those for the suspension medium (i.e., water), respectively, this electrical field distortion will vanish. This electrical field distortion suggests that ignoring it could lead to inaccurate quantification of the actual DEP forces.

Now, by considering a physical domain that has different conductivity and permittivity properties from the surrounding medium, we are able to determine an electrical field that represents the real situation more closely. To get a quantitative sense, we list here in Table 16.3 some quantitative values for the DEP forces evaluated for a particle placed at various locations using our new integration method (Equation 16.7) and the conventional equation

TABLE 16.3

DEP Force Comparison

Distance from Electrode Edge (μm)	New Integration Method		Conventional DEP Formula	
	DEP-X (N)	DEP-Z (N)	DEP-X (N)	DEP-Z (N)
10	2.03×10^{-13}	1.87×10^{-12}	1.05×10^{-11}	5.27×10^{-11}
20	5.26×10^{-14}	1.41×10^{-12}	3.83×10^{-12}	2.84×10^{-12}
30	1.17×10^{-14}	1.34×10^{-12}	1.24×10^{-12}	1.27×10^{-12}
40	1.94×10^{-15}	1.33×10^{-12}	1.21×10^{-13}	1.49×10^{-13}
50 (center of the gap)	-2.69×10^{-16}	1.32×10^{-12}	1.31×10^{-15}	1.10×10^{-13}

(Equation 16.1). We can see that while these force values are within a similar range, they differ slightly. From Table 16.3, it is clear that the vertical component of the DEP force, that is, the DEP-Z force, is much higher for the 10-μm case than that for the 50-μm case. Judging from the estimated particle liftoff force (gravitational force minus the buoyancy force), these force values indicate that the DEP-Z force at 10 μm is way higher and the DEP-Z force at 50 μm is way lower than the liftoff force. This seems unreasonable based on our experimental observation in which particle liftoff seems more uniform. Thus, we believe that the values obtained from the integration method are more reasonable and that our new method represents the real situation more closely.

16.6.2 Particle–Particle Interaction

When multiple particles are placed close to one another, the dipoles induced by the electrical field of one particle will interact with those of others [33,56–60]. Whether the interaction will result in an attractive or repelling force depends on the orientations of the dipoles. To show the interaction effect, we consider a case in which two particles are introduced in the gap region aligning in either the x or y direction (Figure 16.13a and b). When the two particles are placed along the x direction, which is perpendicular to the electrode orientation, we found (Figure 16.14a) that as the distance between the particles (center-to-center

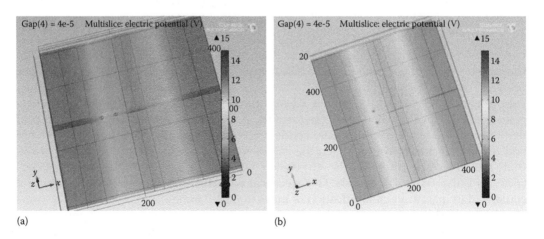

(a)   (b)

FIGURE 16.13
COMSOL models for elucidating particle–particle interaction: (a) two particles align in the x direction; (b) two particles align in the y direction.

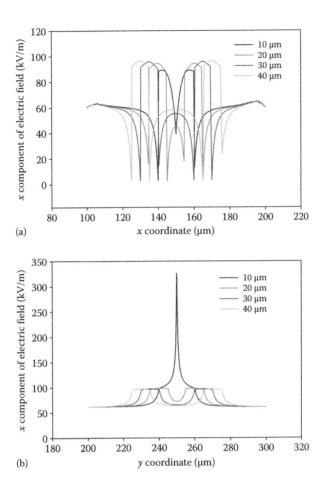

(a)

(b)

FIGURE 16.14
Influence of changing distance between the two particles on distorting the electrical field: (a) two particles align in the x direction; (b) two particles align in the y direction.

distance) increases from 10 to 40 μm, the x-component electrical field exhibits a transition from having overlapped peaks to having two distinct peaks, indicating a diminishing interaction between the two dipoles as the particle-to-particle distance increases. When the two particles are placed along the y direction, which is parallel to the electrode orientation, we found that (see Figure 16.14b) as the distance between the particles increases from 10 to 40 μm, the x-component electrical field at the center transits from having one large peak to two smaller plateaus. This transition indicates that particle–particle interaction will diminish as the distance between particles increases in the y direction as well.

We also investigated the interaction between particles by considering one particle at the center of the gap and another at a distance along the x axis (in the direction perpendicular to the electrodes). As shown in Figure 16.15a, in this case, the two particles experience an attractive DEP force and the force decreases as the neighboring particle moves away from it, an indication of weakening particle–particle interaction. When the second particle is placed along the y axis (a direction parallel to the electrodes), we found that the two particles experience a repelling force and the force decreases as the distance between the two particles increases as shown in Figure 16.15b. The repelling force becomes negligible when

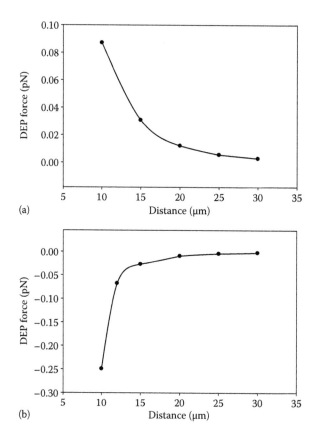

(a)

(b)

FIGURE 16.15
Particles experience an attractive DEP force when placed along the *x* direction (a) and repulsive force when placed along the *y* direction (b). (a) Attractive DEP force decreases as the particle distance increases. (b) Repulsive DEP force decreases as the particle distance increases.

the two-particle distance reaches a certain value (e.g., ~30 μm in this case), suggesting that particles along the *y* axis will repel one another until a certain distance is reached. This fact supports the experimental observation in which the chains formed by particles in secondary alignment (see Figure 16.8) are located at a certain distance apart. The predicted distance value (~30 μm; three times the particle size) based on our model is consistent with our experimental observation where particle chains are separated from each other by a distance of approximately two to three times the particle size.

16.6.3 Pearl-Chain Formation

With this new integration method for quantifying the DEP forces, we further investigated the formation of pearl chains. To simplify matters, we performed a two-dimensional investigation by implementing a moving mesh study. Figure 16.16a shows the positions of the two particles at the beginning of the simulation and Figure 16.16b shows their position after 12 s. These results show that the particle located closer to the electrode is pushed toward the center (the white circle). Please note that the particle on the right also moves, but in comparison with the one on the left, it moves much less because of its position closer to the center of the gap. This result provides a reasonable explanation for the formation of

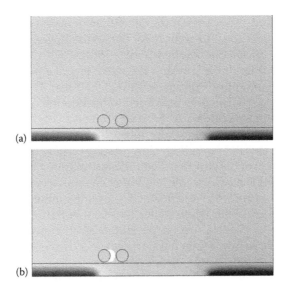

FIGURE 16.16

Modeling results show the movement of 10-μm particles favoring the formation of a pearl chain. The figure shows the positions of the particles (a) at the beginning of the simulation and (b) after 12 s.

pearl chains of beads near the center of the gap between electrodes in a direction perpendicular to the electrode orientation: the DEP forces along with the distortion of the electrical field by the neighboring particles actually generate a drive force to move the particle closer together in a line that is parallel to the overall electrical field or perpendicular to the electrode orientation. This result provides for the first time a quantitative estimate for the level of the driving forces for such pearl-chain formation, and it may present a direct way to quantify the changes in bioparticles by monitoring the change in their relative positions in a fixed period.

16.7 Conclusions and Future Outlook

DEP serves as a rapid technique that can be exploited for various biomedical applications such as processing, sensing, and manipulation of synthetic particles as well as biological particles including cells and viruses, among others. This chapter provides a short review of the field of DEP and identifies some common problems. Some of the problems are highlighted and their influences on the DEP force are illustrated through computational modeling. To assure the validity of our modeling approach and results, experiments are also performed and results are compared with the modeling predictions.

Evidently, it is important to recognize the problems identified, especially the discrepancy in the predicted DEP magnitudes and the actual ones. For instance, treating a nonhomogeneous particle such as a cell as a homogeneous one may lead to a shift in its crossover frequency. Since crossover frequency of cells serves as the basis for cell manipulations in many cases, a change in the actual frequency value may lead to wrong interpretation. While the commonly used shell models for dealing with the nonhomogeneity of biological cells offer some improved prediction of the cell behavior, it can only account for the non-homogeneity of cell membranes. To account for the nonhomogeneity in other cellular components including the nucleus, a volumetric way to deal with the cell body's composite structures is necessary. Moreover, ignoring the size effect of a particle on its conductivity may underestimate the magnitude of the resulting DEP force. The influence of the ubiquitous EDL surrounding a particle may also need to be accounted for in some situations in order to obtain more precise evaluation of the DEP forces.

This chapter also pinpoints another major problem in the commonly used DEP force equation (Equation 16.1)—it does not provide any information on how the polarization of particles will affect the distribution of the electrical field. Because of this, it cannot be used to quantify particle–particle interaction as well as the alignment and movement of particles, among others. To address this major problem, we developed a new integration-based numerical method to reevaluate the DEP forces by accounting for the effect of particle presence on the electrical field, and the effects of particle size, shape, and its location on the DEP forces. With this new method, we are able to investigate the electrical field distortion caused by the presence of particles with different polarization properties from the suspension medium and study particle–particle interactions as well as particle alignments and movements. The modeling results obtained from this new method compare favorably with experimental observations.

We expect that this new method of quantifying the DEP forces and its results will be subjected to more tests and validations through experimental means. We are hopeful that a closed-form analytical expression may be derived based on this new method to make it more accessible for scrutiny and validation, and subsequently for a more widespread use in quantifying the actual DEP forces. We believe that all these efforts may someday help realize the many desired features as well as other potential capabilities in using the DEP phenomenon for many important bioengineering applications including biosensing, drug screen and discovery, tissue engineering, and regenerative medicine.

References

1. Pohl, H., The motion and precipitation of suspensoids in divergent electric fields. *J. Appl. Phys.* 1951. 22: pp. 869–871.
2. Pethig, R., Dielectrophoresis-status of the theory, technology and applications. *Biomicrofluidics* 2010. 4: pp. 022811–022820.
3. Rodrigo, M., Microfabrication technologies in dielectrophoresis applications—A review. *Electrophoresis* 2012. 33: pp. 3110–3132.
4. Pohl, H., *Dielectrophoresis.* Cambridge University Press: Cambridge, 1978.
5. Crane, J., and Pohl, H. J., A study of living and dead yeast cells using dielectrophoresis. *Electrochem. Soc.* 1968. 115(6): pp. 584–586.
6. Germishuizen, W. A., Walti, C., Wirtz, R., Johnston, M. B., Pepper, M., Giles, A., and Middelberg, A., Selective dielectrophoretic manipulation of surface-immobilized DNA molecules. *Nanotechnology* 2003. 14: pp. 896–902.
7. Zellner, P., Shake, T., Sahari, A., Behkam, B., and Agah, M., Off-chip passivated-electrode, insulator-based dielectrophoresis (OπDEP). *Anal. Bioanal. Chem.* 2013. 405(21): pp. 6657–6666. doi:10.1007/s00216-013-7123-7.
8. Chau, L., Ouyang, M., and Liang, W., Inducing self-rotation of Melan-a cells by ODEP. Nano/Micro Engineered and Molecular Systems (NEMS). *2012 7th IEEE International Conference*, 2012, pp. 195–199.

9. Kale, A., Patel, S., Hu, G., and Xuan, X., Numerical modeling of Joule heating effects in insulator-based dielectrophoresis microdevices. *Electrophoresis* 2013. 34(5): pp. 674–683. doi:10.1002/elps .201200501.

10. Gossett, D., Weaver, W., Mach, A., Hur, S. C., Lee, W., Amini, H., and Carlo, D. D., Label-free cell separation and sorting in microfluidic systems. *Anal. Bioanal. Chem.* 2010. 397(8): pp. 3249–3267.

11. Pethig, R., Huang, Y., Wang, X. B., and Burt, J. P. H., Positive and negative dielectrophoretic collection of colloidal particles using interdigitated castellated microelectrodes. *J. Phys. D: Appl. Phys.* 1992. 24: pp. 881–888.

12. Morgan, H., Hughes, M. P., and Green, N. G., Separation of submicron bioparticles by dielectrophoresis. *Biophys. J.* 1999. 77: pp. 516–525.

13. Gascoyne, P., Huang, R. C. Y., Pethig, R., Vykoukal, J., and Becker, F. F., Dielectrophoretic separation of mammalian cells studied by computerized image analysis. *Meas. Sci. Technol.* 1992. 3: pp. 439–445.

14. Jen, C. P., and Chen, T. W., Selective trapping of live and dead mammalian cells using insulator-based dielectrophoresis within open-top microstructures. *Biomed. Microdevices* 2009. 11: pp. 597–607.

15. Fiedler, S., Shirley, S. G., Schnelle, T., and Fuhr, G., Dielectrophoretic sorting of particles and cells in a microsystem. *Anal. Chem.* 1998. 70: pp. 1909–1915.

16. Voldman, J., Gray, M. L., Toner, M., and Schmidt, M. A., A microfabrication-based dynamic array cytometer. *Anal. Chem.* 2002. 74: pp. 3984–3990.

17. Voldman, J., Toner, M., Gray, M. L., and Schmidt, M. A., Design and analysis of extruded quadrupolar dielectrophoretic traps. *J. Electrostat.* 2003. 57: pp. 69–90.

18. Ling, S. H., Lam, Y. C., and Chian, K. S., Continuous cell separation using dielectrophoresis through asymmetric and periodic microelectrode array. *Anal. Chem.* 2012. 84: pp. 6463–6470.

19. Duncan, L., Shelmerdine, H., Coley, H. M., and Labeed, F. H., Assessment of the dielectric properties of drug sensitive and resistant leukaemic cells before and after ion channel blockers using dielectrophoresis. *NSTI-Nanotech*, 2006, p. 2. ISBN 0-9767985-7-3.

20. Markx, G., and Davey, C., The dielectric properties of biological cells at radiofrequencies: Applications in biotechnology. *Enzyme Microb. Technol.* 1999. 25: pp. 161–171.

21. Markx, G. H., and Pethig, R., Dielectrophoretic separation of cells: Continuous separation. *Biotechnol. Bioeng.* 1995. 45: pp. 337–343.

22. Asbury, C., and Engh, G., Trapping of DNA in nonuniform oscillating electric fields. *Biophys. J.* 1998. 74: pp. 1024–1030.

23. Washizu, M., Kurosawa, O., Arai, I., Suzuki, S., and Shimamoto, N., Applications of electrostatic stretch-and-positioning of DNA. *IEEE Trans. Ind. Appl.* 1995. 31: pp. 447–456.

24. Hu, X., Bessette, P. H., Qian, J., Meinhart, C. D., Daugherty, P. S., and Soh, H. T., Marker-specific sorting of rare cells using dielectrophoresis. *Proc. Natl. Acad. Sci. U. S. A.* 2005. 102(44): pp. 15757–15761. ISSN 0027-8424.

25. Ho, C. T., Lin, R. Z., Chang, H. Y., Chang, W. Y., and Liu, C. H., Rapid heterogeneous liver-cell on-chip patterning via the enhanced field-induced dielectrophoresis trap. *Lab Chip* 2006. 6: pp. 724–734.

26. Lin, R. Z., Ho, C. T., Liu, C. H., and Chang, H. Y., Dielectrophoresis based-cell patterning for tissue engineering. *Biotechnol. J.* 2006. 1: pp. 949–957.

27. Verduzco-Luque, C., Alp, B., Stephens, G. M., and Markx, G. H., Construction of biofilms with defined internal architecture using dielectrophoresis and flocculation. *Biotechnol. Bioeng.* 2003. 83(1): pp. 39–44.

28. Mason, V. P., Markx, G. H., Thompson, I. P., Andrews, J. S., and Manefield, M., Colonial architecture in mixed species assemblages affects AHL mediated gene expression. *FEMS Microbiol. Lett.* 2005. 244(1): pp. 121–127.

29. Andrews, J. S., Mason, V. P., Thompson, I. P., Stephens, G. M., and Markx, G. H., Construction of artificially structured microbial consortia (ASMC) using dielectrophoresis: Examining bacterial interactions via metabolic intermediates within environmental biofilms. *J. Microbiol. Methods* 2006. 64(1): pp. 96–106.

30. Gagnon, Z. R., Cellular dielectrophoresis: Applications to the characterization, manipulation, separation and patterning of cells. *Electrophoresis* 2011. 32: pp. 2466–2487.

31. Tsutsui, H., Yu, E., Marquina, S., Valamehr, B., Wong, I., Wu, H., and Ho, C. M., Efficient dielectrophoretic patterning of embryonic stem cells in energy landscapes defined by hydrogel geometries. *Ann. Biomed. Eng.* 2010. 38: pp. 3777–3788.

32. House, D. L., Luo, H., and Chang, S., Numerical study on dielectrophoretic chaining of two ellipsoidal particles. *J. Colloid Interface Sci.* 2012. 374(1): pp. 141–149. doi:10.1016/j.jcis.2012.01.039.

33. Singh, J., Lele, P., Nettesheim, F., Wagner, N., and Furst, E., One- and two-dimensional assembly of colloidal ellipsoids in ac electric fields. *Phys. Rev. E* 2009. 79(5): p. 050401. doi:10.1103/PhysRevE.79.050401.

34. Kirby, B. J., *Micro- and Nanoscale Fluid Mechanics: Transport in Microfluidic Devices*. Cambridge University Press: New York, 2010. ISBN 978-0-521-11903-0.

35. O'Konski, C., Electric properties of macromolecules. V. Theory of ionic polarization in polyelectrolytes. *J. Phys. D: Appl. Phys.* 1997. 30: pp. 2470–2477.

36. Markx, G., Pethig, R., and Rousselet, J., The dielectrophoretic levitation of latex beads, with reference to field-flow fractionation. *J. Phys. D: Appl. Phys.* 1997. 30: pp. 2470–2477.

37. Pauly, H., and Schwan, H., Impedance of a suspension of ball-shaped particles with a shell: A model for the dielectric behaviour of cell suspensions and protein solutions. *Chem. Biochem.* 1959. 14(2): pp. 125–131.

38. Fuhr, G., Hagedorn, R., and Müller, T., Simulation of the rotational behavior of single cells by macroscopic spheres. *Stud. Biophys.* 1985. 107: pp. 109–116.

39. Arnold, W. M., and Zimmermann, U., Electro-rotation development of a technique for dielectric measurements on individual cells and particles. *J. Electrostat.* 1998. 21: pp. 151–191.

40. Schnelle, T., Müller, T., Fiedler, S., and Fuhr, G., The influence of higher moments on particle behaviour in dielectrophoretic field cages. *J. Electrostat.* 1999. 46: pp. 13–28.

41. Yang, C. Y., and Lei, U., Quasistatic force and torque on ellipsoidal particles under generalized dielectrophoresis force. *Biomicrofluidics* 2009. 3(1): p. 012003.

42. Liang, E., Smith, R., and Clague, D., Dielectrophoretic manipulation of finite sized species and the importance of the quadrupolar contribution. *Phys. Rev. E* 2004. 70(6): p. 066617. doi:10.1103/PhysRevE.70.066617.

43. Washizu, M., and Jones, T. B., Dielectrophoretic interaction of two spherical particles calculated by equivalent multipole-moment method. *IEEE Trans. Ind. Appl.* 1996. 32(2): pp. 233–242. doi:10.1109/28.491470.

44. Kurgan, E., Stress calculation in two-dimensional DC dielectrophoresis. *Przeglad Elektrotechniczny* 2011. 69(12): pp. 111–116.

45. Rosales, C., and Lim, K. M., Numerical comparison between Maxwell stress method and equivalent multipole approach for calculation of the dielectrophoretic force in single-cell traps. *Electrophoresis* 2005. 26(11): pp. 2057–2065. doi:10.1002/elps.200410298.

46. Wang, X., Wang, X.-B., and Gascoyne, P. R. C., General expressions for dielectrophoretic force and electrorotational torque derived using the Maxwell stress tensor method. *J. Electrostat.* 1997. 39(4): pp. 277–295. doi:10.1016/S0304-3886(97)00126-5.

47. Li, H., Ye, T., and Lam, K. Y., Numerical modeling of motion trajectory and deformation behavior of a cell in a nonuniform electric field. *Biomicrofluidics* 2011. 5(2): p. 21101. doi:10.1063/1.3574449.

48. Washizu, M., and Kurosawa, O., Electrostatic manipulation of DNA in microfabricated structures. *IEEE Trans. Ind. Appl.* 1990. 26: pp. 1165–1172.

49. Cummings, E. B., and Singh, A. K., Dielectrophoresis in microchips containing arrays of insulating posts: Theoretical and experimental results. *Anal. Chem.* 2003. 75: pp. 4724–4731.

50. Hernandez, H. M., Cardiel, B., Gonalez, P., and Encinas, L., Insulator-based dielectrophoresis of microorganisms: Theoretical and experimental results. *Electrophoresis* 2011. 32(18): pp. 2502–2511.

51. Sun, T., Holmes, D., Gawad, S., Green, N. G., and Morgan, H., High speed multi-frequency impedance analysis of single particles in a microfluidic cytometer using maximum length sequences. *Lab Chip* 2007. 7(8): pp. 1034–1040.

52. White, C. M., Holland, L. A., and Famouri, P., Application of capillary electrophoresis to predict crossover frequency of polystyrene particles in dielectrophoresis. *Electrophoresis* 2010. 31: pp. 2664–2671.

53. Stern, O., Theory of a double-electric layer with the consideration of the adsorption processes. *Z. Electrochem.* 1924. 30: pp. 508–516.

54. Arnold, W. M., Jäger, A. H., and Zimmermann, U., The influence of yeast strain and of growth medium composition on the electro-rotation of yeast cells and of isolated walls. *Dechema Biotechnology Conferences*, 1989. 3: pp. 653–656.

55. Basuray, S., and Chang, H., Designing a sensitive and quantifiable nanocolloid assay with dielectrophoretic crossover frequencies. *Biomicrofluidics* 2010. 4: pp. 013205 (1–11).

56. Shilov, V. N., Dielectrophoresis of nanosized particle. *Colloid J.* 2008. 70(4): pp. 515–528.

57. Castellanos, A., Ramos, A., Green, N. G., and Morgan, H., Electrohydrodynamics and dielectrophoresis in microsystems: Scaling laws. *J. Phys. D: Appl. Phys.* 2003. 36: pp. 2584–2597.

58. Ai, Y., and Qian, S., DC dielectrophoretic particle-particle interactions and their relative motions. *J. Colloid Interface Sci.* 2010. 346(2): pp. 448–454. doi:10.1016/j.jcis.2010.03.003.

59. Aubry, N., and Singh, P., Influence of particle-particle interactions and particles rotational motion in traveling wave dielectrophoresis. *Electrophoresis* 2006. 27(3): pp. 703–715. doi:10.1002/elps.200500606.

60. Sancho, M., Martínez, G., Muñoz, S., Sebastián, J. L., and Pethig, R., Interaction between cells in dielectrophoresis and electrorotation experiments. *Biomicrofluidics* 2010. 4(2): pp. 1–12. doi:10.1063/1.3454129.

17

Image-Based Modeling for Bioengineering Problems

Adrienne M. Madison and Mark A. Haidekker

CONTENTS

ABSTRACT   Computational modeling uses a numerical approach to simulate material behavior under defined spatial constraints and load conditions. For this purpose, a system is decomposed into a large number of interacting volume elements (called finite elements), which can be described by a set of partial differential equations. Numerical methods are then employed to solve the equation system for the unknown quantities, such as deformation and stress. Finite-element models have been employed to observe the mechanical response behavior of biological tissue as well as implant materials. Unlike in mechanical systems, where a relatively simple geometrical description is available, patient-specific models of organs or implants are often obtained from volumetric images. Image-based finite-element models have a highly complex geometry, and the assignment of material properties to individual elements from image information is difficult. In this chapter, the four steps to obtain an image-based finite element–based material simulation (segmentation, meshing, simulation, and postprocessing) are described in detail, and strategies to overcome the specific challenges of image-based computational modeling are discussed. A focus of this chapter lies on available software to perform the four steps with aspects of the practical realization of a finite-element modeling chain.

17.1 Overview

Finite-element analysis (FEA, or finite-element modeling [FEM]) is a numerical modeling technique used to solve engineering problems by obtaining approximate solutions from a large system of algebraic equations. The underlying principle requires the entire geometry of interest to be subdivided into a large number of small regions or *elements* that are considered homogeneous. These small elements have a variety of possible shape patterns (e.g., triangular, rectangular, tetrahedral, hexagonal, and cubic), depending on the number of geometric dimensions present, and they share their edges and vertices with neighboring elements. The vertices (referred to as *nodes*) are rigidly connected; therefore, each element has boundary conditions imposed upon it by its neighbors (internal boundary conditions) and by the environment (external boundary conditions). Internal boundary conditions are obtained from the balance of forces and from the equal displacement of a node that is common to multiple elements. External boundary conditions, such as pressure, forces, or spatial constraints, can be prescribed to the model as a whole. The actual finite-element *model* is represented by a series of partial differential equations that describe material properties, conservation of mass and energy, the laws of motion, and deformation of an element by forces acting upon its nodes. Ultimately, solutions are found for each region by the calculation of unknowns within the volume by only taking into account the regions located next to them.

Originally developed to analyze the twisting behavior of cylindrical objects in the early 1940s [1], FEM has been intensely used in biomedical contexts to examine, simulate, and predict the material behavior and nonlinear biomechanical properties of soft tissues [2,3], organs [4,5], bone [6,7], and joints [8,9]. It is also highly useful in applications of modeling, testing, and verification of medical device designs, such as vascular implants and stents [10–12], dental implants [13], and most recently in accident analysis and prevention [14]. The number of reported studies that utilize FEM and related computational numerical methods in the advancement of biomedical and clinical research, development, diagnosis, and treatment applications has constantly increased since 1980 and currently surpasses 10,000 [15].

Classical finite-element models are based on geometric descriptions of the object under examination: A motor, for example, can be composed of cylinders, pistons, rods, the crank shaft, and other interacting parts that can be represented by their exact geometrical description. In biomedical applications, two challenges appear. First, a tissue or organ can have a fairly complex geometry that necessitates an equally complex analytical description, sometimes with approximations made to simplify the model. Second, to obtain a patient-specific description, the geometry is often extracted from volumetric images, such as computed tomography (CT) or magnetic resonance (MR) images. FEM of biomedical structures involves four main steps (Figure 17.1) and begins with a volumetric image. In the first step, the object of interest is *segmented*, that is, separated from image elements not related to the object of interest. At this point, the object is still represented by individual voxels. The *meshing* step follows, in which the volumetric arrangement of voxels is parametrized (i.e., approximated by an analytical description of the surface with straight-line or curved segments), and during which boundary conditions and material properties are applied. The third step involves the actual finite-element simulation of the time-variable behavior of the created model under the established parameters. Once this step is completed, the output of the simulation process is visualized or postprocessed in the final step.

The objective of this chapter is twofold: (i) to explore the basic principles, theories, and techniques behind the execution of each component within this modeling chain, and (ii) to introduce the reader to software options along with trends and developments in which these methods and approaches could be better used in biomedical applications.

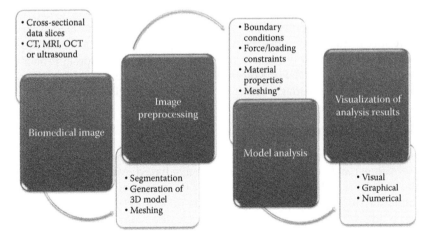

FIGURE 17.1
Flow process diagram for FEM of anatomical geometry extracted from medical imaging data. With a volumetric image as starting point, the first crucial step is the extraction of the geometry of the object of interest. For this purpose, a segmentation step is followed by the meshing step, in which an analytical description of the geometry is obtained. For this geometry, the constituent mechanical partial differential equations are then solved (i.e., the actual modeling step). The (*) symbol in the analysis step indicates that meshing can take place either during the preprocessing step or during the actual model analysis step. Lastly, the modeling results are visualized or further examined with respect to the property of interest, such as deformation, stress, or failure.

17.2 Segmentation

The preprocessing phase, which consists of the segmentation and meshing steps, is the most crucial and challenging component within the biomedical modeling chain. The segmentation process divides an image into meaningful regions in an attempt to delineate and extract objects or regions of interest (these are often referred to as *features* in the image). No uniform solution exists for the segmentation problem. The segmentation strategy strongly depends on the imaging modality, the object itself, and the varying image interpretations among different modalities. For example, CT allows for a relatively easy intensity-based segmentation of bone or the lungs because of the excellent bone-tissue and air-tissue contrast. Conversely, MR imaging can provide excellent contrast between tissues but is not usually used for imaging bone because of the low water content [16]. Frequently, image voxels are classified according to visual characteristics (e.g., intensity, texture, or color). Prerequisite is a form of contrast between healthy and abnormal tissue, or between the tissue of interest and adjoining regions—the latter are often referred to as *background* in a generalized sense.

A second goal of the segmentation process is the assignment of tissue properties, most often in inhomogeneous tissue regions. An assumed relationship between image intensities and material types is frequently the guiding standard in medical imaging segmentation application [5,17–21]. For example, the CT number of a bone voxel is related to its mineral content, and it can be argued that mineral content and stiffness are related [22,23]. Therefore, some empirical material properties are assigned to the voxel based on its CT number.

The segmentation step can be performed manually, with limited manual assistance, or in an automated fashion. In a manual segmentation step, a trained observer (such as the radiologist) delineates the boundary of the object. This process is often performed in two dimensions on a slice-by-slice basis. Manual segmentation suffers from variability owing to subjective influences. Computer-aided segmentation or fully automated segmentation is desirable to reduce intra- or interobserver variability [24,25] and to accelerate the segmentation process. A brief overview of some commonly used segmentation approaches is given in Sections 17.2.1 through 17.2.3. For a more comprehensive overview or for the underlying mathematical theories, the reader is referred to the pertinent literature [24,26–29].

17.2.1 First-Generation Processes

First-generation processes solely rely on information available within an individual image (i.e., its voxel values) and therefore are purely image based. Manual segmentation largely relies on the same contrast properties that enable these first-generation methods.

Automatic multistep segmentation approaches (discussed later) usually incorporate a combination of these first-generation methods or use them as a foundation for higher-level steps. First-generation processes can be partitioned into the following categories:

- *Intensity thresholding* (Figure 17.2b)
  - Intensity-based segmentation method that uses contrasting intensity levels to identify distinctive regions.
  - Each image pixel is compared to a threshold value such that all values
    - Above this range are labeled as *feature*
    - Equal to or below the indicated value are classified as *background*

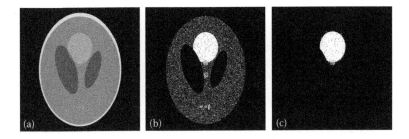

FIGURE 17.2
Intensity-based segmentation in a noisy variant of the Shepp–Logan head phantom. The additive noise causes major overlap of the image values between the *gray matter* and the large central *tumor* (a). Pure intensity-based thresholding (white pixels are those from (a) which lie above the threshold) cannot separate the tumor region from the gray matter region (b). When connectivity is considered, for example, with the region-growing algorithm, the segmented pixels are constrained to a connected region, and unconnected pixels within the thresholded intensity range are excluded (c).

- The ideal image case would contain pixels with nonoverlapping intensity values between feature and background.
- Often, a suitable transformation (e.g., local texture filters) can provide additional contrast.
- Multidimensional thresholding is an alternative option when a voxel is described by multiple criteria, such as intensity and one or more local neighborhood properties (e.g., smoothness or proximity to a gradient). When a voxel is associated with multiple orthogonal criteria, these are referred to as *feature vector*.

- *Region-based methods* (Figure 17.2c)
  - Extension of the intensity-based thresholding method under the assumption that the object forms a contiguous region.
  - Assumption of connectivity allows the separation of disjoint image features even if these have similar intensity.
- *Edge/boundary based* (Figure 17.3)
  - Relies on the identification of intensity gradients or sharp transitions of intensity levels.

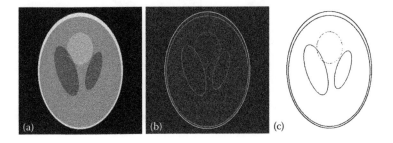

FIGURE 17.3
Edge-based segmentation. The source image is the head phantom with additive noise used in Figure 17.2 (a). The application of an edge enhancement filter (Sobel operator) converts gradients into higher-intensity pixels (b). As a side effect, the noise component is amplified. After thresholding and removal of isolated noise pixels, the edges remain; however, low-contrast features do not necessarily have a closed boundary, and the features with the lowest contrast have disappeared altogether (c).

- The anticipated result is that all of the pixels located near the gradient boundaries have higher intensity values than those lying outside or inside the object.

- The resulting image highlights the object surface rather than the volume; intensity-based thresholding is possible (Figure 17.3c).

17.2.2 Second-Generation Processes

Second-generation processes rely on the same intensity or contrast information that first-generation processes use but attempt to describe the image feature at a higher level of abstraction. Often, some form of numerical optimization or minimization is involved (purely discrete algorithms), or a physical model is approximated by numerical methods. Second-generation methods are purely image-based derivations of first-generation methods that occasionally use information gathered directly from initial first-generation segmentation results. The need for second-generation methods can be illustrated with the edge-based segmentation in Figure 17.3c, where it is desirable to obtain a closed contour for the large *tumor* in the same fashion as for the skull and the ventricles. Second-generation processes can be subdivided as follows:

- *Continuous Model Discretizations*: Based on a physical model, such as elastic contraction or viscous flow, but with an external, image-based driving force that lets the model converge on an image feature.

  - *Snakes*—Snakes are models of elastic rubber bands that are subjected to a stretching and a bending force. The external force is the negative image gradient. In the snake concept, a closed path contracts until an equilibrium is reached between the curvature-based internal force responsible for the contour's smoothness and the external force of the intensity gradient [30]. Figure 17.4 highlights the iterative progression of this process.

  - *Level Set Active Contours*—Level set active contours are implicit methods (in contrast to the explicit numerical formulations underlying the snakes). Level set–based active contours are derived from a numerical method designed to track an evolving contour deforming at a rate of speed based on curvature and gradient [31]. The model ceases deformation once the speed reaches an

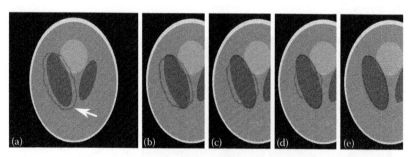

FIGURE 17.4
Semisupervised segmentation with active contours (snakes). A hand-drawn region (arrow) near one of the *ventricles* of a noisy Shepp–Logan head phantom serves as the starting point for the snake (a). The snake algorithm causes the snake to contract, but vertices are attracted by edges. Beginning contraction after five iterations (b); some convergence can be seen after 10 iterations (c); most of the snake has locked onto the edges after 20 iterations (d); final convergence of the snake (e). The vertices of the snake coincide with the edge of the ventricle, and the curve defined by the vertices serves as parametrization of the contour.

artificial preset speed assigned to desired boundary areas. Their main benefit over snakes is their ability to change the topology [32].

- *Live Wire*—The live wire formulation is a semiassisted method where a cost function is established from representative boundary points identified by the user. The live wire algorithm then connects those points along a minimum-cost path [33].

- *Purely Discrete Algorithms*:
  - *Clustering*—Automatic assignment of pixels to one of several classes (e.g., feature and background) based on minimum-distance criteria for a vector of descriptive metrics
    - *k*-means—A pixel belongs to exactly one class, with which it has the smallest distance to the class centroid [34].
    - Fuzzy *c*-means—A pixel initially belongs to a fuzzy extent to multiple classes, and final class membership is decided after the optimization process [35].
  - *Graph Based* (see below)
    - Watershed segmentation
    - Fuzzy connectedness

In graph-based methods [28,36], the nodes of the graph correspond to the voxels. The graph itself is the set of all paths that connect a voxel inside the feature with a background voxel. Some criteria can be found where a path traverses a discontinuity (such as an edge) that defines the object boundary. At this point, the graph is cut. The remaining connected regions show a higher voxel homogeneity with respect to the segmentation criteria than the uncut graph. It is possible to express the links of the graph as a cost function similar to the one that drives the live wire, and training of the cost function is performed with some user-selected seed points.

The watershed and fuzzy-connectedness algorithms are based on the graph-cut principle. Watershed segmentation demarcates the boundaries of regions on a topological surface using *watershed* lines [37]. The topological surface is built on the interpretation of pixel intensity as elevation. The object of interest is assumed to be the set of pixels that becomes flooded, and the low-elevation regions that become flooded first serve to cut disjunct features. Thus, watershed segmentation is used to separate overlapping features that are connected in a first-generation segmented image. Fuzzy connectedness [38] assigns a continuous voxel similarity to pairs of voxels, and the graph (in the sense introduced above) is cut at a certain level of dissimilarity.

Statistical pattern recognition and neural networks are related image-based segmentation methods that are often collaborative [39]. In statistical pattern recognition, a model is used to assign image pixels to a known set of classes. Neural networks can be trained to segment images based on pixel values manually designated to classes. Neural networks in particular rely on high-order feature vectors that include the voxel intensity and a number of neighborhood criteria that can be generated through texture description methods (e.g., Laws' texture energy [40]).

17.2.3 Third-Generation Processes

Third-generation methods of geometry extraction are model-based recognition procedures that require extensive a priori information. A simplified explanation to third-generation processes can be given when we consider Figure 17.3. The edge contours are known to be elliptical (this is the a priori knowledge). The image can now be searched for voxels that belong to an ellipse, for example, with the Hough transform [41]. In this fashion, the fragments of the central ellipse in Figure 17.3c would be recognized as belonging to one ellipse, and the segmentation would yield the completed ellipse rather than the fragments.

More generally, third-generation processes are based on the construction of a spatial statistical model for the object of interest that consists of prominent shape details and any potential variations from a set of training images. During analysis, image data are scanned to locate regions that resemble the model. *Active shape models* identify objects within an image set that are recognized as members of the same class by using landmark points [42]. Image patches, such as object intensity or texture, are incorporated to add region-based features in *active appearance models* [43]. In *atlas-based segmentation*, a composite image is constructed from segmented images of many subjects. Descriptive information besides the geometry and shape, such as intensity properties, object labeling, and relationship definitions, is also stored with the atlas. An image set is first matched to the atlas template via three-dimensional (3D) mapping, followed by the atlas using the accompanying descriptive properties for statistical pattern recognition.

Hybrid segmentation methods merge the complementary strengths of separate methods with an aim to create more complex methods that increase accuracy and precision while simultaneously overcoming some of the individual limitations. Many of the recent advances in segmentation have contributed to the varying combinations of the aforementioned techniques. Some comprehensive surveys and reviews are based on method type [44], medical application [45,46], image type and method [47], medical application and image type [48,49], or, more specifically, medical application, image, type, and method [50].

Almost all of the above segmentation methods are supervised, and some level of user interaction is required throughout the process. Hybrid methods incorporating unsupervised processes can significantly reduce the level of operator assistance. Rule-based systems attempt to achieve effective, unsupervised segmentations. In this multistep process, first- and second-generation methods extract desired image features, which are interpreted and labeled by third-generation knowledge-based approaches. The segmentation is carried out according to an explicit predefined set of rules [51]. Neural networks and fuzzy-connected filters are commonly implemented in rule-based systems and have been used in brain tumor extraction from MR images [52–54], breast cancer lumps [55], and skin cancer lesions [56].

At the end of the segmentation process, the image has been subdivided into the background and one or more features (objects) that will be analyzed in the finite-element simulation. At this point, the voxels are merely labeled as belonging to the background or to the image feature (or features if multiple materials are present). In the next step, the shape of the objects formed by those voxels needs to be described analytically such that the proper set of governing equations can be set up.

17.3 Meshing

In conventional engineering FEM applications, the meshing step is relatively straightforward, because an analytical description of the object usually exists. Notably, solid modeling software often allows automatic subdivision of a 3D model into nodes and elements and assigning material properties to the elements. The resulting finite-element shapes in these 3D models can be extensions of either a quadrilateral in the form of a *hexahedron* (8 vertices, 12 edges, 6 faces) or a triangle evolved into a *tetrahedron* (4 vertices, 6 edges, 4 faces).* The mesh is of fundamental importance, because it directly gives rise to the set of partial differential equations that are used in the FEM solver (i.e., the simulation step) to determine the unknown quantities of the simulation. The process of discretizing a known geometrical shape can be seen as a *top–down approach* to generating a finite-element model.

Conversely, the irregular shape of biomedical objects—especially when obtained from volumetric images—requires a piecewise analytical approximation of the shape. Usually, a large number of points on the surface is determined, and these points are connected with high-order curves, such as splines. The process of approximating a shape with discrete nodes can be seen as a *bottom–up approach*. The element shape, mesh arrangement, and algorithm selections to generate the most accurate mesh for evaluating biomechanical behavior are widely dependent on the analysis emphasis, material type, complexity of geometry, method of FEA, and other application characteristics. Adjustment or modification of one application parameter could potentially require the use of an entirely different meshing approach.

Moreover, in biomedical applications, the material properties are often unknown or uncertain, and a rigorous match between elements and their associated material properties cannot be obtained in a straightforward manner. For these reasons, *the overall meshing process based on patient-specific medical image data remains the most crucial bottleneck in the entire FEA chain.* However, a large body of literature has emerged in recent years where improvements and modifications are presented for tailored and application-specific mesh generation, and this section provides an overview of some of the most relevant approaches.

Image-based mesh generation begins with the segmented object, which is the outcome of any of the processes described in Section 17.2. To provide the necessary input for FEA, three steps are taken:

- *Surface mesh construction*: The shape of the object is discretized by a large number of nodes that are placed as close as possible to the surface of the segmented object. Ideally, these nodes are either evenly spaced or become denser in regions of higher curvature.

- *Volume mesh construction*: The areas between the surface boundaries can be meshed in a manner similar to the analytical top-down approach; that is, the object's volume is subdivided into a large number of small hexahedral or tetrahedral elements. Volume meshing usually begins at the nodes of the meshed surface. Similar to conventional mesh generation of computer-aided design (CAD)–based models, the elements are rigidly connected at the nodes and provide the boundary conditions for neighboring elements.

- *Application of material properties and external boundary conditions*: Material properties must be defined for all volume elements. External forces or spatial constraints can be applied to some of the nodes.

---

* In FEM terminology, the reference is the number of facets. A hexahedral element has six sides, and a cuboid would be a hexahedral element. A *hexagonal* prism, in FEM terminology, would count as octahedral.

17.3.1 Surface Mesh Construction

A 3D image volume is the yield, or end product, of the segmentation process. Each voxel within this volumetric scalar field is assigned a value to represent pixels that are a part of either the background or any of one or more segmented objects (including their associated material types) within the identified geometry. Two general mechanisms have been implemented to fit surfaces to data [57]: isosurface extraction and adaptive contours. Not coincidentally are these related to the first- and second-order processes in the segmentation step.

Isosurface extraction uses piecewise linear interpolation algorithms such as the marching cubes algorithm [58] or level sets, to subdivide (tessellate) the surface into triangular surface facets. For the isosurface extraction, the volume of interest is embedded into a regular, cuboid mesh. The assumption is that the object has higher voxel values than the background. Each node of the mesh is now checked whether it is above the isosurface value (i.e., lies within the object) or below the isosurface value (i.e., is part of the background). Edges that connect nodes inside and outside the object intersect the surface, and the intersection point is determined by linear interpolation. The intersection points then form the nodes of the surface mesh. Edges are shared by multiple cubes, and consequently, surface facets are connected. Whenever the intersection of any cuboid with the isosurface renders quadrilaterals or higher-order polygons, these are further subdivided into triangles, because triangles are always planar, and thus have a defined surface normal. Figure 17.5 demonstrates how the algorithm constructs triangular elements.

The alternative approach to surface reconstruction of a segmented volume is a 3D adaptation of the local energy-minimizing snake algorithm [59]. A net wraps around, and conforms to, a specific volumetric feature based on internal energy and image force calculation between the binary surface and the parametric surface in an iterative manner. The points on the surface and other parameters, for example the number of nodes, must be preassigned to determine the net's initial geometry. The definition of such parameters

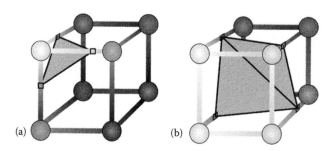

FIGURE 17.5

Two examples of an isosurface intersecting a cube. In both cases, the image value of the voxel centers (spheres) is known, and the image values between voxel centers are obtained by linear interpolation (thick lines with gradients). Interpolation provides the location of the desired isosurface value between two adjoining pixels, and this location serves as one vertex of the tessellated surface (small squares). (a) Only three edges cross the isosurface value, and all other edges lie below the isosurface value. The resulting element is a triangle. (b) The four front voxels have values above the isosurface value; the four back pixels lie below. Consequently, the vertices lie on the diagonal edges and form a quadrilateral. Since tessellation requires planar (triangular) elements, the quadrilateral is subdivided once.

contributes to the model's smoothness. A smoothed approximation of the surface by the model nodes is the output from this process, and nodes are connected to form triangles.

17.3.2 Volume Mesh Construction

The surface mesh can now be transformed into a FEM *volume mesh* by filling the interior region with the preferred element shape and arrangement. Mesh types can be broadly classified into *structured* or *unstructured* meshes according to their geometrical pattern. *Structured* mesh arrangements consist of an evenly spaced, fixed, uniform amount of nodes and elements and are composed entirely of hexahedral elements that are a result of grid-based surface construction algorithms. This template-based connectivity pattern was the initial attempt at meshing automation, and it produces meshes that approximate curved surfaces in a stair-step fashion. The disadvantage of a structured mesh is the inability to adapt to the shape curvature: the node density is the same in regular regions, where fewer nodes would yield an adequate discretization, and in irregular regions, where the node density may not be sufficient to describe the surface with adequate detail.

Unstructured meshes contain either all tetrahedral elements or a combination of hexahedral, tetrahedral, and wedge-shaped elements generated automatically in arbitrary configurations. The relationship between the number of vertices, edges, faces, and regions is unknown beforehand. Unstructured meshes are better capable of adhering to curved boundaries while being adaptable to general complex shapes with less user intervention. Figure 17.6 demonstrates the difference between structured and unstructured meshes.

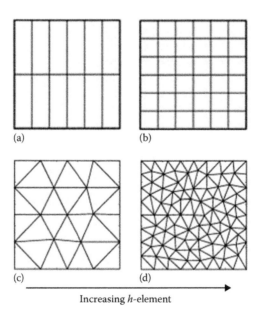

Increasing *h*-element

FIGURE 17.6
Comparison of mesh types. (a and b) Structured mesh with quadrilateral elements (corresponding to hexahedral elements in 3D); (c and d) unstructured mesh with triangular elements (corresponding to tetrahedral elements in 3D). The effects of increasing the *h*-element constraint can also be observed. The finer mesh patterns in (b) and (d) with smaller element size and increased element quantities are derived from the original patterns in (a) and (c) by subdivision of the original elements.

The following algorithms have been established for the generation of unstructured mesh types:

Tetrahedral-based mesh

- *Octree* [60,61]: Recursively partitions a cube containing the geometry into eight octants until a preferred resolution is reached. Nonuniform tetrahedral elements can be formed between the intersections of these cubes.
- *Advancing Front* [62,63]: Begins at a boundary and then progresses toward empty space within a region.
- *Delaunay* [64]: Creates nearly equilateral triangles (which are the faces of tetrahedrons) based on satisfaction of an *empty circle* criterion. For this method, each edge of a triangle lies near the edge of a circle, and vertices are prevented from being located within the circle's circumference. This approach minimizes the occurrence of *skinny* triangles that have very small angles or form sharp, jagged edges (see Figure 17.7).

Hexahedral-based mesh

- *Plastering* [65] is a hexahedral adaptation of *advancing front* mechanism. It begins with an all-quadrilateral mesh that projects faces into a volume, thereby creating hexahedral elements in an iterative manner.
- *Medial Surface* [66]: Decomposes a volume into hexahedral elements.
- *Grid Based* [67]: Imposes a 3D grid of hexahedral elements within volume interiors.
- *Whisker-Weaving* [68]: Builds a dual or spatial twist continuum with bisecting intersecting surfaces that fit hexagonal elements derived from quads into the volume based on connectivity followed by the subsequent determination of nodal locations.

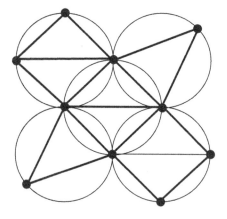

FIGURE 17.7

Triangular/tetrahedral mesh construction based on Delaunay algorithm. All points or vertices of each triangle lie near the edge of a circle, because the *empty circle* criterion prevents vertices from being placed within the circle or sphere's circumference.

17.3.3 Mesh Quality, Optimization, and Adaptive Refinement

Meshes must be feature preserving in the sense that they must be as close as possible to the original surfaces and be capable of handling complex topology [69,70]. Ideally, they also possess the adaptivity to increase node density in areas of high interest (e.g., areas of concentrated stress or high curvature) to limit the surface discretization error, while balancing the number of mesh elements. A mesh composed of nearly equilateral triangles is desirable, and vertices need to be seamlessly aligned with neighboring vertices.

A frequently employed strategy is to generate an initial mesh that is then refined until convergence is reached, that is, until further mesh refinement changes the simulation results by less than a predefined margin. The method to generate the initial mesh is referred to as *primal contouring method*, and the marching cubes algorithm is one example for a primal contouring method. The resulting initial mesh approximates the implicit geometry but generally has undesirable features that need to be suppressed. Common observations in meshed objects from biomedical images include the following [71,72]:

- A uniform stair-step surface appearance that does not fully align with the natural surface curvature
- Badly shaped triangles (e.g., triangles with very large and small angles that cause sharp, jagged edges)
- Excessive amounts of irrelevant nodal and faceted data
- The nonpreservation of sharp features within the data

Methods for subsequent refinement are referred to as *dual contouring methods* [73]. Dual contouring methods were derived to improve the quality of meshes with respect to the accurate reproduction of sharp features [70]. In the basic dual contouring algorithm, the region to be meshed is divided into overlapping cubic grids. The surface is then analyzed at vertices of the grids and classified as either being inside or outside the mesh. Cubes consisting of inside and outside combinations of vertices are denoted as containing surface portions. The dual contouring process creates a vertex pair per cube that straddles the surface, and the connection of each to the neighboring vertex pair shapes the final mesh.

Additional refinement is based either on local remeshing through swapping of edges or faces or on local refinement through insertion or deletion of vertices [74]. In fact, the methods described in Section 17.3.2 for the generation of unstructured meshes can be used for mesh refinement as well. The criteria that the octree, Delaunay, and advancing front algorithms act upon are responsible for the swapping of edges/faces and insertion or deletion of vertex points that lead to the final positions and number of the vertices of the mesh. It is at these locations at which the error is minimal between the planes and normals at the edge intersections [75–77].

In addition to dual methods, mesh smoothing can be applied. Smoothing occurs when vertices are relocated following some regularity criterion, but relocation does not affect the topology of the mesh. For example, several sweeps of a spatial Laplacian smoothing operator relaxes each adjustable vertex to the arithmetic average of adjacent vertices [78]. Alternatively, the smoothing could be incorporated into an optimization algorithm to allow adjustment of either individual or independent sets of vertices in parallel [79]. The amount of smoothing a vertex is subjected to could be controlled by hierarchical order of classification. Vertices are categorized by increasing rank levels, and those within the highest class are most affected by the smoothing operations.

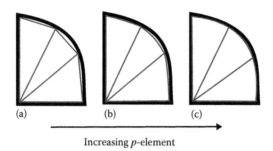

Increasing *p*-element

FIGURE 17.8
Observation of increasing *p*-elements in triangular/tetrahedral mesh. First-order linear elements do not capture the curved boundaries of the model (a). The mesh improves its adaption to the curvature of the model when the order of the *p*-element is increased to quadratic (b). Higher-order cubic element allows even better optimization as the mesh more accurately adapts to the curved regions of the model (c).

In mesh quality analysis, there are two types of element classifications that are applicable to both hexahedral and tetrahedral shapes. The low-order linear or quadratic *h-element* corresponds to the step size needed to converge the biomechanical behavior solutions or minimize the error obtained for the actual analysis. A smaller mesh size *h* represents a finer mesh consisting of a larger number of elements in the model. This is how a finer mesh in areas of high interest (e.g., areas of stress concentration) can be constructed. The *p-element* is a metric for the optimization of the mesh at a higher, polynomial, order: in *p*-element refinement, edges are no longer straight lines, but polynomial curves. The increased polynomial order *p* of the element allows the element edges to adapt to curved boundaries more accurately and thereby leads to minimization of discretization error and solution convergence during the analysis of the model. In contrast to *h*-elements, fewer elements are required to obtain convergence, and the surface discretization error can be reduced without increasing the number of elements within the mesh. Figure 17.6 demonstrates how a mesh can be refined by *h*-elements, while optimization using *p*-elements is illustrated in Figure 17.8.

17.3.4 Tetrahedral versus Hexahedral Elements in Biomechanics

The preference of tetrahedral or hexahedral elements in FEM continues to be an unsolved topic of debate. Each has advantages and disadvantages. Tetrahedral elements are widely selected because of their geometrical flexibility, and they produce acceptable displacement behavior [80]. Hexahedral elements are well suited to model stresses and strains in tissues, and hexahedral elements are assumed to lead to more accurate simulation results. On the other hand, inaccurate approximation of the actual shape can be observed at jagged edge areas [81]. In addition, hexahedral meshes are more challenging to generate than tetrahedral meshes.

Meshes with tetrahedral elements can match simulation accuracy of hexahedral meshes when more and smaller elements are used (i.e., increased *h*-element). Four to 10 times the amount of elements are needed in tetrahedral meshes in order to achieve comparable levels of accuracy provided by hexahedral elements [82–84]. Tetrahedral elements of lower order are unduly stiff and lock in instances of modeling extensive stress deformations or materials that are nearly incompressible. They are also more prone to a failure of the inversion problem during analysis [85]. Many of these differences can be observed and justified when the examples in Figures 17.6 and 17.8 are considered. One possible solution to this dilemma is to create hybrid meshes that are constructed with an outer surface of all-tetrahedral elements and an inner volume of all-hexahedral elements [6,86].

17.4 Simulation

Once the mesh is generated, the actual analysis can be performed. The analysis consists of the assignment of material properties and boundary conditions, followed by numerically solving the constituent partial differential equations. Overall, this step represents a numerical *simulation* of the material behavior under the given boundary conditions.

It is debatable whether the assignment of material properties and boundary conditions is part of the meshing process or part of the simulation process. In meshes obtained from medical images, material properties are often extracted from the image. However, because material properties and boundary conditions can easily be changed for simulation purposes, they are covered in this section.

17.4.1 Boundary and Loading Constraints

Some of the nodes and elements of the mesh must be supplemented with additional information that is strongly dependent on the analysis application. Accurate simulation may require certain regions of the model to be loaded with prescribed displacements, nodal forces, pressure forces, body forces, or surface tractions, velocity, or flux. Such conditions occurring on the boundary are referred to as nonessential or *Neumann boundary conditions.* Specifications also need to be made in reference to how the model interacts with its surroundings. These are the essential or *Dirichlet boundary conditions* and refer to the rotation, support, or fixation of the region.

17.4.2 Material Properties

Material characteristic values (e.g., elastic modulus) are then assigned to the model in order to numerically distinguish it as bone, soft tissue, muscle, fluids, or a combination of materials from an engineering aspect in terms of strength, elasticity, durability, conductivity, and porosity. Material properties can be

- *Homogeneous*: Same at all locations
- *Nonhomogeneous*: Location dependent
- *Isotropic*: Same in any direction
- *Anisotropic*: Direction dependent
- *Orthotropic*: Symmetric with respect to x–y, y–z, or x–z planes

Examples for isotropic tissues are those in the cardiovascular system and neurological tissues. Typical anisotropic tissues are ligaments, tendons, and cartilage. Both cortical and trabecular bone exhibit orthotropic behavior. Soft tissue also exhibits *creep*, that is, its stress–strain behavior is time dependent. FEM solvers need to be capable of incorporating these different types of material descriptions for the simulation of biological tissues.

17.4.3 Governing Principle

In the basic theory of FEM, each subdivision or element is associated with a finite number of degrees of freedom, which are the unknown function values at the nodal points that the element is composed of. The constraints, mechanical properties, and loads applied at the nodes are condensed into discrete differential equations corresponding to the element's response. A node can be shared by several elements; therefore, the deflection at the shared node is representative of deflection of the sharing elements at the node location. Shape functions use interpolation to approximate deflection values occurring at all nonnodal points within an element. The assembly of these individual element equations leads to the generation of the global equations representing the entire meshed region. Both the individual and global equations are always expressed in the form

$$\{F\} = [K]\{u\}, \tag{17.1}$$

where

{F} is the column matrix of the applied external force or nodal loads.

[K] is a stiffness matrix containing the geometric and material information that determines the element's (or the mesh's) resistance to deformation when subjected to loading. Specifically, this matrix is

Symmetric, as a result of equal and opposite forces to ensure equilibrium.

Singular, since the equation has not been solved. Boundary conditions must be included at this point to alleviate this.

{u} is the column matrix of nodal displacements (i.e., the degrees of freedom) resulting from the application of load {F}. These values are interdependent since the body is continuous and elastic.

Equation 17.1 is solved for the nodal displacements {u}. Once this information is obtained, the stresses (σ) can be determined from kinematic relationships, and the strain (ε) is calculated through material or constitutive relationships in solid mechanics analysis. The general form of Equation 17.1 governs many physical phenomena in which the parameters {u} and {F} have different physical significance. It should also be noted in applications in which there is no measure of deformation that the matrix [K] is still referred to as the *stiffness matrix* to maintain uniformity in nomenclature and definition. Table 17.1 lists these physical phenomena and the interpretation of {u} and {F} for some applications.

TABLE 17.1

Interpretation of the Displacement Matrix {u} and Load Matrix {F} in Different Physical Problems That Obey the General Form of Equation 17.1

Analysis/Application	{u}	{F}
Acoustic fluid	Displacement potential	Particle velocity
Electrostatics	Electric potential	Charge density
General flow	Velocity	Flux
Heat conduction	Temperature	Heat flux
Potential flow	Pressure gradient	Velocity potential
Magnetostatics	Magnetic potential	Magnetic intensity
Structures and solid mechanics	Displacement	Mechanical load

It is possible to combine physical phenomena and subject them to a joint simulation. One example is blood flow in the vasculature. Fluid flow exerts shear stress on the tissue at the interface and can cause viscoelastic deformation. Deformation can also be caused by fluid pressure, such as blood pressure. Such models are referred to as *biphasic models*. The generation of biphasic models, especially those with nonlinear properties, can lead to models of appreciable complexity; however, these models still follow the general outline presented in Section 17.4.4.

17.4.4 Approximate Solution Determination

FEA solvers commonly obtain the approximate solution to Equation 17.1 via an indirect formulation method based on the minimum total potential energy (TPE). The TPE (Π) for a model composed of n elements and m nodes is the difference between the total strain energy (Λ) and the work done by the external forces ($F \cdot u$) and is given by

$$\Pi = \sum_{e=1}^{n} \Lambda^{(e)} - \sum_{i=1}^{m} F_i u_i, \tag{17.2}$$

where the strain energy per unit volume for linear elastic materials is

$$\Lambda^{(e)} = \frac{1}{2} \int \sigma \in dV. \tag{17.3}$$

This is ideal for models with solid materials where the strain energy of the system can be calculated. During deformation, the work done by the applied load F is stored as elastic or strain energy. The model is considered to be at equilibrium when the TPE is minimal with respect to displacement u. Therefore the solution is found by

$$\frac{\partial \Pi}{\partial u_i} = \frac{\partial}{\partial u_i} \sum_{e=1}^{n} \Lambda^{(e)} - \frac{\partial}{\partial u_i} \sum_{i=1}^{m} F_i u_i = 0 \tag{17.4}$$

in accordance to the law of conservation of energy. Each finite element will have its own TPE.

For simplicity, we will use the discrete connected system of springs in Figure 17.9 to illustrate the FEA procedure. There are four springs, three nodes, and two external loads present in the system. The TPE is given by

$$\Pi = \frac{1}{2} k_1 \delta_1^2 + \frac{1}{2} k_2 \delta_2^2 + \frac{1}{2} k_3 \delta_3^2 + \frac{1}{2} k_4 \delta_4^2 - F_1 u_1 - F_3 u_3, \tag{17.5}$$

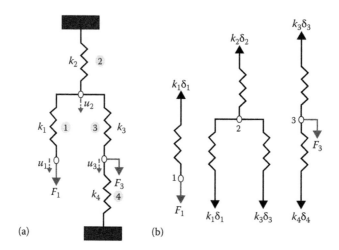

(a)   (b)

FIGURE 17.9
Discrete spring system used to derive FEA theory (a). The system is composed of four springs and is subjected to two external loads F_1 and F_3 as well as three displacements u_1, u_2, and u_3. Free-body diagram representing each spring component of the system's mechanical behavior (b).

where δ_1, δ_2, δ_3, and δ_4 correspond to the amount each spring stretches. These can be rewritten as

$$\begin{aligned}
\delta_1 &= u_1 - u_2 \\
\delta_2 &= u_2 \\
\delta_3 &= u_3 - u_2 \\
\delta_4 &= -u_3.
\end{aligned} \tag{17.6}$$

Now, substitution into Equation 17.5 yields

$$\Pi = \frac{1}{2}k_1(u_1 - u_2)^2 + \frac{1}{2}k_2u_2^2 + \frac{1}{2}k_3(u_3 - u_2)^2 + \frac{1}{2}k_4u_3^2 - F_1u_1 - F_3u_3 \tag{17.7}$$

such that u_1, u_2, and u_3 are the displacements of each node.

In order for equilibrium to be reached, the TPE needs to be minimized with respect to the three displacements as explained in Equation 17.4. Therefore, each spring's mechanical behavior can be defined by a set of differential equations:

$$\frac{\partial \Pi}{\partial u_1} = k_1(u_1 - u_2) - F_1 = 0$$

$$\frac{\partial \Pi}{\partial u_2} = -k_1(u_1 - u_2) + k_2u_2 - k_3(u_3 - u_2) = 0 \tag{17.8}$$

$$\frac{\partial \Pi}{\partial u_3} = k_3(u_3 - u_2) + k_4u_3 - F_3 = 0$$

These differential equations are converted into algebraic equations, followed by each k value being arranged into a stiffness matrix using the general form:

$$K^{(e)} = \begin{bmatrix} k_e & -k_e \\ -k_e & k_e \end{bmatrix},$$ (17.9)

where e represents the four spring systems (k_1, k_2, k_3, and k_4). Each of these system matrices can be combined such that a global stiffness matrix for the overall system is obtained and expressed as

$$K(G) = \begin{bmatrix} k_1 & -k_1 & 0 & 0 \\ -k_1 & k_1 + k_2 + k_3 & -k_2 - k_3 & 0 \\ 0 & -k_2 - k_3 & k_2 + k_3 + k_4 & -k_4 \\ 0 & 0 & -k_4 & k_4 \end{bmatrix}.$$ (17.10)

Based on the algebraic equation from each node,

$$\begin{aligned} k_1\delta_1 &= F_1 \\ k_2\delta_2 - k_1\delta_1 - k_3\delta_3 &= 0 \\ k_3\delta_3 - k_4\delta_4 &= F_3, \end{aligned}$$ (17.11)

and the boundary conditions of our system, the k_2 components in the third column as well as the fourth row and column of the matrix can be deleted owing to the spatial fixation of the nodes at those locations. Now, the algebraic form can be rewritten in the general form as presented in Equation 17.1

$$\begin{Bmatrix} F_1 \\ 0 \\ F_3 \end{Bmatrix} = \begin{bmatrix} k_1 & -k_1 & 0 \\ -k_1 & k_1 + k_2 + k_3 & -k_3 \\ 0 & -k_3 & k_3 + k_4 \end{bmatrix} \begin{Bmatrix} u_1 \\ u_2 \\ u_3 \end{Bmatrix}$$ (17.12)

and solved by inversion of the matrix $[K]$.

In order to observe the mechanical behavior of the spring system, let us assume that each spring has a uniform cross-section area A and length l when subjected to a force F. The average stress (σ) in a spring is given by

$$\sigma = \frac{F}{A}$$ (17.13)

and the average normal strain (ε) is the change in length Δl per unit original length of the spring

$$\varepsilon = \frac{\Delta l}{l}. \tag{17.14}$$

Hooke's law relates stress and strain in elastic regions through the equation

$$\sigma = E\varepsilon, \tag{17.15}$$

where E is the modulus of elasticity of the spring's material. Rearranging and substituting Equations 17.14, 17.13, and 17.15 to isolate F results in

$$F = \left(\frac{AE}{l}\right)\Delta l, \tag{17.16}$$

which bears resemblance to the equation of a linear spring. Therefore, we can conclude in this case that each spring has a stiffness k of

$$k_e = \frac{AE}{l}. \tag{17.17}$$

As described above, solving for the displacement values $\{u\}$ allows the stresses and strains to be determined. The stress for each spring is calculated by

$$\sigma = \frac{F}{A} = \frac{k_e(u_{i+1} - u_i)}{A} = \frac{\frac{AE}{l}(u_{i+1} - u_i)}{A} = E\left(\frac{u_{i+1} - u_i}{l}\right) \tag{17.18}$$

and the strain can be determined from Equation 17.15 or from the displacement of each spring at the nodes,

$$\varepsilon = \left(\frac{u_{i+1} - u_i}{l}\right). \tag{17.19}$$

Although we presented a simplified example, the FEM simulation obeys the exact same principle, because each node of the volumetric mesh is examined in the same fashion as the nodes in Figure 17.9, with the spring constants determined by the neighboring nodes and the material properties in the respective element. It should be noted that in more complex two-dimensional (2D) and 3D models, the directional components of stress and strain are considered (stress and strain tensors) and that the stiffness k is dependent on the area of the model and the analysis application (i.e., solid mechanics, heat transfer, etc.).

17.4.5 Nonlinear Analysis

Biomaterials often exhibit nonlinear behavior. A deviation from linear behavior (i.e., Hooke's law) not only occurs for large geometry changes that lead to fracture but also includes plastic deformation and creep. These situations result in nonlinear and even time-dependent σ–ε and ε–u relationships, where occurrences of stiffening, hardening, softening, or buckling are possible. In such cases, the stiffness matrix $[K]$ becomes time dependent. The solution is usually obtained by incremental or iterative methods, such as the implicit Newton–Raphson approach. In this approach, a load is applied in discrete time steps that advance the simulation from t to $t + \Delta t$. This technique addresses material nonlinearity by solving for the state at time $t + \Delta t$ when displacements at u^t are known. The load increment is applied such that the state is updated to $t + \Delta t$, and $u^{t+\Delta t}$ is the main variable. The principles of the Newton–Raphson approach can be integrated into the TPE method and represented as

$$\Phi(u^{t+\Delta t}) = \int \sigma \in (u^{t+\Delta t}) dV - F = 0, \tag{17.20}$$

where Φ represents the sum of internal and external residual forces and $\Phi = 0$ is a set of nonlinear equations in $\{u\}$. Given that $\Phi(u^{t+\Delta t}) = 0$, for an ith iteration:

$$u_{i+1}^{t+\Delta t} = u_i^{t+\Delta t} - \left[\frac{\partial}{\partial u} \Phi\left(u_i^{t+\Delta t}\right) \right]^{-1} \Phi\left(u_i^{t+\Delta t}\right) \tag{17.21}$$

can be rearranged such that

$$\delta u_{i+1} = u_{i+1}^{t+\Delta t} - u_i^{t+\Delta t} = -\left[\frac{\partial}{\partial u} \Phi\left(u_i^{t+\Delta t}\right) \right]^{-1} \Phi\left(u_i^{t+\Delta t}\right), \tag{17.22}$$

where

$$[K_{\mathrm{T}}] = \left[\frac{\partial}{\partial u} \Phi\left(u_i^{t+\Delta t}\right) \right]^{-1} \tag{17.23}$$

is the total tangential stiffness matrix for which holds

$$\left[K_{\mathrm{T}}\left(u_i^{t+\Delta t}\right) \right] = \left[K^a\left(u_i^{t+\Delta t}\right) + K^b\left(u_i^{t+\Delta t}\right) + K^c\left(u_i^{t+\Delta t}\right) \right], \tag{17.24}$$

where
   $[K]^a$ is a linear matrix that includes small strain and displacement model components.
   $[K]^b$ houses linear and quadratic strain terms and is considered the large displacement or stiffness matrix.
   $[K]^c$ is a nonlinear matrix composed of quadratic strains and nonlinearities associated with the material.

Substitution yields

$$\delta u_{i+1} = -K_T\left(u_i^{t+\Delta t}\right)^{-1}\Phi\left(u_i^{t+\Delta t}\right) \qquad (17.25)$$

and therefore

$$-\left\{\Phi\left(u_i^{t+\Delta t}\right)\right\} = \left[K_T\left(u_i^{t+\Delta t}\right)\right]\left\{\delta u_{i+1}\right\} \qquad (17.26)$$

is in the general form presented in Equation 17.1. This must be solved for each iteration *i* to advance the simulation by Δt and obtain the change in incremental displacements

$$u_i^{t+\Delta t} - u_i^t = \Delta u_i = \sum_{k=1}^{i}\delta u_k, \qquad (17.27)$$

whereby K_T and Φ are different for each iteration. A quadratic convergence rate toward a tolerance threshold ε_T is achieved when

$$\left|\left\{\Phi\left(u_{i+1}^{t+\Delta t}\right)\right\}\right| < \varepsilon_T. \qquad (17.28)$$

Because Φ needs an accurate stress value (σ) to obtain a current approximation of $u^{t+\Delta t}$, the updated Lagrangian approach is implemented as the solution process moves from $t \rightarrow \Delta t$ to iteratively follow elements of the model along their configuration. All derivatives and integrals are determined with respect to spatial coordinates.

17.5 Postprocessing: Output and Visualization

The solutions to equations evaluated in the analysis are stored as raw data. These solutions represent behavioral effects, such as stress, strain, pressure, or geometrical distortion attributed to the simulated forces. The postprocessing step can be either quantitative or qualitative, where the latter most often involves some form of *visualization* of the simulation results. The postprocessing step is the most application-specific step in the entire analysis chain, and only a general overview can be given.

Quantitative analysis would involve the examination of forces, stresses, or deformation in an automated fashion: computer software could, for example, provide a histogram of the stress magnitude for the examined volume. The histogram then displays the probability or absolute number of elements that experience a certain stress. Similarly, a threshold function would provide the simplest means to obtain a yes/no decision if material failure can occur.

Qualitative analysis usually involves the examination of the simulation results by a trained observer. For this purpose, simulation results are usually presented in graphical, visual form. Most frequently, the simulation results (e.g., the stress magnitude) is superimposed over the original geometry. For 2D simulations, visualization is fairly straightforward, but in three dimensions, some form of projection is required, where the object of interest is displayed from a camera perspective. The visualization software allows the user to position the object in its virtual space: rotate it, move it, or zoom in or out. In this fashion, the observer can focus on critical parts of the geometry.

There is an almost limitless number of visualizations, and in many ways, a good visual representation of the result contains a considerable artistic element. In fact, it is recommended that a *visualization strategy* [87] is developed beforehand, which is determined by the key conclusions of the simulation. However, there are a number of commonly used tools in the visualization process. These include the following:

- *False-coloring*: Magnitude can be displayed in grayscale, but more frequently, the magnitude is mapped to colors, because the human eye is more sensitive to differences in hues than to differences in gray shades.

- *Contours*: Similar to contour lines in topographical maps, contour lines that connect locations of equal value can be introduced. Contour lines facilitate the assessment of gradients as well as the shape of regions of interest.

- *Glyphs*: Vector fields (e.g., forces) can be visualized with glyphs. Glyphs are small 3D objects, such as arrows, that are placed along a vector field. Their size and direction indicate magnitude and direction of the vector field.

- *Partial transparency*: Most often, only the outer surface of a 3D object is visible. Scalar fields can be represented by an isosurface. However, some software programs make it possible to introduce transparency to a solid volume, and the amount of transparency can be made magnitude dependent. In this fashion, parts of a volume can be made *see-through*, allowing the visualization of different elements inside the volume.

- *Clip planes*: A clip plane allows cutting away parts of a 3D object, and the interior becomes visible at the cut surface.

- *Animation*: The time-dependent evolution of the simulation was introduced in Section 17.4. Visualizations can include animations to illustrate the time-dependent behavior of, for example, forces, stresses, and deformation.

In one specific case (GiD visualization software, CIMNE, Barcelona, Spain), deformation can be exaggerated. A likely approach is to take the spatial coordinates of each node at two time points t and $t + \Delta t$ and to compute the displacement vector. In the visualization, each node is then again displaced by a multiple of its displacement vector. Since material deformation often occurs on a small scale, this exaggeration can make deformation behavior particularly well visible.

Some of the visualization techniques are demonstrated in Figure 17.10 with the help of Paraview software. A more complex visualization, created with OpenDX, is shown in Figure 17.11, where the stress magnitude is represented by glyphs and the pressure is imprinted in false colors on an oblique clip plane. The geometry is superimposed in a transparent gray shade.

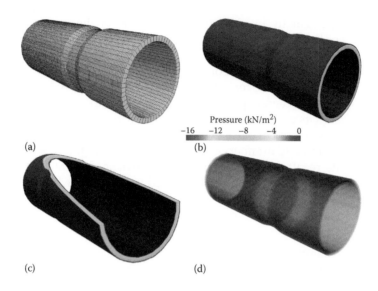

Pressure (kN/m²)

−16   −12   −8   −4   0

(a)   (b)

(c)   (d)

FIGURE 17.10
Visualization examples of a blood vessel phantom model. (a) The meshed model of the tubular phantom.
(b) View of the phantom after FE simulation with color-coded pressure values superimposed (surface view).
(c) View of the phantom with color-coded pressure, but after application of an oblique clip plane. This view better reveals the pressure distribution along the phantom and highlights a thinner section. (d) Rendering of the
phantom with partial transparency.

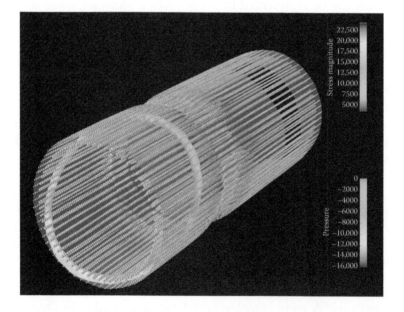

FIGURE 17.11
More complex visualization example of the phantom in Figure 17.10, created with OpenDX. The stress magnitude is represented by glyphs, and it can be seen that the thinner section of the phantom experiences larger
stress. The pressure is superimposed in false colors over an oblique ring. The geometry of the object is made
visible by overlaying a partly transparent gray surface.

17.6 Software

17.6.1 Commercial Software Packages

There are a large number of software options available for use in image segmentation, mesh generation, FEA, and visualization applications. Specifically, review of biomechanical FEA literature reveals the following frequently used commercial options:

Image Segmentation/Meshing:
- MIMICS (Materialise, Leuven, Belgium)
- ScanIP+FE (Simpleware Ltd., Exeter, UK)
- 3D-DOCTOR (Able Software Corp., Lexington, Massachusetts)

FEA/Visualization:
- Abaqus (Simulia [Dassault Systèmes], Vélizy-Villacoublay Cedex, France)
- Algor (Autodesk)
- ANSYS (ANSYS, Inc., Canonsburg, Pennsylvania)
- COMSOL (COMSOL, Inc.)

Software companies usually try to offer monolithic solutions. For example, many combined FEM and visualization packages also come with a model builder tool, which allows the assembly of models from relatively simple geometrical elements. In addition, these packages come with several import options to read either surface models or solid models that have been created with other packages. This collection of features makes these packages ideal for the analysis of classical load and stress problems in mechanical engineering. One advantage of the all-in-one approach of monolithic software is the ability of the individual steps to seamlessly interface with each other. Unlike solutions where multiple software modules need to use a common file format for data interchange, a monolithic package handles its data transfer internally and usually invisible to the user.

The creation of finite-element models from biomedical images is more challenging for the monolithic packages. Segmentation and surface parametrization is usually not included, and an external program, such as MIMICS, is needed to perform the first steps in the analysis chain. Although the segmentation and meshing software is aimed at a broad range of applications, it may fail in some special cases, in part because no universal segmentation and meshing approach exists. This shortcoming has led many research groups to develop application-specific modules (e.g., Refs. [69,88–90]). Meshing-related studies often do not address the issue of segmentation. In fact, segmentation is usually considered to be a separate step, although one preprocessing toolkit [21] specializes in combining segmentation and meshing of 3D models.

Analysis of the pertinent literature reveals that a focus of the software development lies on the meshing algorithm, because the transition from a voxel-based image to an analytical description of the object (i.e., the mesh) remains the most critical step in the entire FEM chain.

17.6.2 Image-Based Modeling with Open-Source Software

Frequently, research groups not only describe their methods but also release the actual software source code for use by other interested parties. In fact, a strong community-driven effort to develop and make available free, open-source software has evolved over the last several years, from which interested researchers can benefit immensely. The philosophy of the open-source community not only places an emphasis on free-of-charge availability of such software but more importantly encourages users to share software source code. As a consequence of this openness—and the associated freedoms to inspect and modify the software code—an Internet-connected community continuously works on improving the software and adding new features. Furthermore, the same community is generally available through Internet forums to respond to user questions. Free software, therefore, can be seen as a parallel model to the commercial software model, which is peer based, and which has analogous characteristics of software distribution and user support through the Internet. Since the software is free of license fees, a researcher can download and install software to try without further risk whether the software is suitable for the specific application.

In many cases, wide distribution and continuous improvement have led to the evolution of high-value software. Popular free, open-source software is available not only as program code. Rather, some members of the community create installation-ready software packages that can be conveniently installed without programming experience.* Specifically for medical image processing, segmentation and feature extraction, meshing, FEA, and visualization, there exist several options that make a fully open-source FEM toolchain feasible. Since this field of development currently exhibits a strong momentum, it is covered in detail in Sections 17.6.3 and 17.6.4.

Some examples for free open-source software packages that fulfill some of the functionality laid out in Figure 17.1 are as follows:

Image Processing and Segmentation:
- ImageJ (US National Institutes of Health, Bethesda, Maryland)
- OsiriX [91]
- Crystal Image [27]
- Seg3D (Scientific Computing and Imaging Institute, University of Utah)

Combined Segmentation/Meshing Applications:
- BiMECH [21]
- IA-MESH [92]
- Works presented in Refs. [71,72,93,94]

Meshing:
- BioMesh3D (Scientific Computing and Imaging Institute, University of Utah)
- Cleaver [95]
- Gmsh (http://www.geuz.org/gmsh/)
- MeshLab (http://meshlab.sourceforge.net/)
- Works presented in Refs. [6,69,85,88,96,97]

FEA:
- FeBio [98]
- FreeFEM (http://www.freefem.org/)

---

* One example is the repositories of the popular *ubuntu* operating system, which contain more than 20,000 installation-ready software packages ranging from office suites to scientific applications, including mesh handling and FEM. The repositories are linked to the operating system in such a fashion that the installation of new software is no more effort than a few mouse clicks.

- Elmer (CSC, Espoo, Finland)
- Tochnog (http://tochnog.sourceforge.net/)

Visualization:

- Paraview (Kitware, Inc., Clifton Park, New York)
- OpenDX (http://www.opendx.org/)

Open-source software for image-based FEM has not yet reached the mainstream of the FEM community, and a careful discussion of the advantages and limitations of a free-software approach is needed. Software modules that find their way into the open-source community are often incorporated to bridge a gap or overcome challenges encountered within the execution of the flow process outlined in Figure 17.1. As such, some open-source packages are limited to special cases. However, frequently those packages are *absorbed* by the wider community and integrated into a larger system of software modules.

Before integrating open-source software into the research process, the following actions can help determine the best overall approach:

- Identify what role(s) the needed software should address.
- Assess capabilities of the software options currently accessible within the research facility. First, site licenses reduce per-user fees for commercial software. Second, available software can be evaluated for suitability for a specific purpose.
- Assess capabilities of commercially available software. If the license fees of a commercial software package are not an obstacle, monolithic software can offer a streamlined solution that promises the least investment of time by the user.
- If an open-source package is being considered, a literature search is helpful to determine if similar solutions have been reported and whether a method is applicable to desired research objectives.

The most frequent contributions to open-source software related to biomechanical FEM analysis are in the form of meshing modules or toolkits that discretize the geometries obtained from segmentation of medical imaging data.* Suitable representations of biomedical objects often lead to excessive numbers of nodes, elements, vertices, and faces that tend to overwhelm the computational specifications of commercial meshing and FE software, which are usually designed to handle CAD-based analytical geometries. As previously mentioned, commercial meshing software is also often somewhat limited in mesh functionalities and capabilities. The other major factor contributing to the recent surge in published mesh generation methods and algorithms can be attributed to the diverse field of biomedical applications, including bone, soft tissue (muscles, organs, blood vessels, implants), the medical image source, and the properties of the mesh (e.g., allowable discretization error, mesh complexity, and the inclusion of material properties). Moreover, reproducibility is a key factor: since open-source software allows the user to examine the actual *inner workings* of the program, a very high level of transparency is inherent in the open-source model. For scientific applications, transparency (and, by association, reproducibility) is of prime concern. Commercial *black-box* software does not provide this advantage: it is well possible that slightly different numerical implementations can lead to

---

* A comprehensive list can be found at http://www.robertschneiders.de/meshgeneration/software.html, accessed August 24, 2013.

divergent results between different closed-source software packages, and even between different versions of the same package.

17.6.3 Completely Open Source–Based FEA

Some meshing modules have been developed with the sole aim of being interfaced or used in conjunction with a specific commercial FE software. To our knowledge, there are only two reported instances in which the entire analysis toolchain has been implemented exclusively with open-source software. The first instance examines patient-specific data in order to identify optimal locations for placement of implantable cardiac defibrillators [99,100] and the second study proposes a process to evaluate the biomechanical behavior of autologous tissue-engineered blood vessels [97]. The work presented by Jolley et al. [99,100] features customization through the addition and modification of visualization, mesh refinement, and finite-element calculation parameters within currently available open-source software (notably the software offered by the Scientific Computing and Imaging Institute, University of Utah). Our toolchain [97] revolves around the development of a hexagonal mesh-extraction module capable of adaptive mesh refinement; assignment of material properties, loading, and boundary conditions; and automatic generation of input file data needed to conduct the actual analysis performed with stand-alone FE and visualization software. Both studies compare the results obtained to those provided by commercial counterparts for proof-of-principle validation.

17.6.4 Limitations of Open-Source Software

The vast assortment of currently available open-source software options for image processing, meshing, analysis, and visualization may give rise to the misconception that construction of a FEM toolchain can be done with ease. Fortunately, the continuing adoption of open-source software into scientific computing in general leads to significant streamlining of the data analysis process. Through the organization of community-based libraries, such as the Insight Segmentation and Registration (ITK), Finite Element (FETK), and Visualization (VTK) toolkits, there exists often a central *hub* or headquarters in which developers share, debug, update, modify, and provide cross-platform support for related open-source software. To provide one example, the Scientific Computing and Imaging Institute at the University of Utah (http://www.sci.utah.edu) has provided a comprehensive package of interrelated modules for image-based FEA. Notable elements of this package are Seg3D for volumetric image segmentation, BioMesh3D as a mesh generator for segmented biomedical images, and SciRUN, termed *problem solving environment*, which allows operations with significant manual interaction, such as manual delineation and segmentation. The same research group provides FEBio for solving nonlinear FEA problems specifically in biomedical applications [98], PreView and PostView for pre- and postprocessing, ImageVis3D for volume rendering and visualization, and AtlasWerks for medical image atlas generation.

Not all software is as streamlined as this suite of packages. Frequently, use of open-source software requires some familiarity with computer programming. In some cases, the software is provided in source-code form *only*, and the user has to compile the software (i.e., convert it into an executable application). The compilation process requires that development tools are installed and available. Furthermore, such software often depends on libraries (such as the ITK and VTK libraries mentioned above) that have to be installed separately.

The main challenge that the creation of a completely open-source FEM toolchain poses is the interfacing between different software applications. Since the need to interface different software programs is a known problem, some file formats are likely to emerge as universal mesh data exchange formats. For example, the STL format (STL stands for *stereo lithography*) is widely used to describe arbitrarily complex surfaces, and it is probably best known as the input format for rapid prototyping. A file format known as STEP (Standard for the Exchange of Product Data) has become an ISO standard exchange format for representing 3D data. IGES (Initial Graphics Exchange Specification) is a NIST (National Institute of Standards and Technology)-supported file format that allows the exchange of information among CAD software. DXF (Drawing Exchange Format) is an alternative file format, created by AutoDesk, to exchange drawing information between CAD programs. STL and DXF files contain geometry, but not material properties or boundary conditions. STEP, which can serve as input for FreeFEM, is a format under development, but the flexible format definition would allow a STEP file to carry all information needed for FEM analysis.

In some instances, special files are needed. For example, Tochnog is a versatile solver for a large number of PDE-based physical problems, including stress/strain, heat transfer, and fluid dynamics (cf. Table 17.1). Tochnog also contains mechanical models for time-dependent, nonlinear materials, which makes it very attractive for modeling of biological tissue. Tochnog uses a nonstandard plaintext input file that contains the spatial coordinates of all mesh vertices, the list of elements and their associated vertices, material groups and the assignment of elements to material groups, boundary conditions, and control instructions. Although Tochnog output is directly readable by Paraview and OpenDX, special software is needed to generate the input file from an existing mesh. It is therefore almost inevitable that Tochnog users need to write a small translation program that reads a mesh in its existing format (e.g., the widely used STL file format) and writes a Tochnog input file.

At this point of software availability, however, the creating of small filter programs to link individual applications is a small price to be paid for the advantage of source code availability. Commercial software is distributed in black-box form, and user support only reaches the extent of the existing software as provided. Given the complexity of biological geometry, the software often becomes overwhelmed and freezes or stops processing. The authors have experienced this effect with two different commercial packages that attempt to create their own volumetric mesh from a given surface mesh, yet fail with complex geometries, such as the volumetric CT image of dentures, or even an inhomogeneous tubular phantom [97]. Because of the black-box nature of commercial software, the failure reason cannot be determined beyond the help available from customer support. Conversely, an open-source package would allow the identification of the point of failure and either remedy the problem (e.g., by increasing the memory limits) or adjust the input file to create a workaround that avoids the point of failure.

17.7 The Open-Source Toolchain—A Case Study

17.7.1 Problem Statement and Underlying Volumetric Image

The skeleton of a rhinoceros (*Diceros bicornis*) was donated to the School of Veterinary Medicine at the University of Georgia. A photo of the skeleton as it is currently on display is shown in Figure 17.12. In the process of preparation, the left hind foot was damaged, and

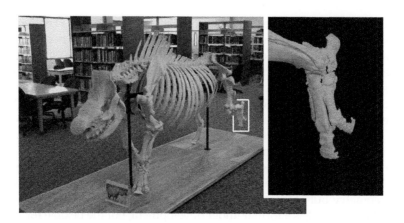

FIGURE 17.12
Photo of the rhinoceros skeleton on display at the University of Georgia School of Veterinary Medicine. The inset shows a close-up photo of the left hind foot.

a repair was attempted by means of inserting metal rods to fixate the bone fragments. A CT scan was performed to verify the placement of these rods. The volumetric CT image was provided to the authors courtesy of Dr. Steven D. Holladay. In this section, we demonstrate the application of the individual steps described in Sections 17.2 through 17.5 to obtain the stress and strain distribution under a defined load.

17.7.2 Segmentation

The CT image (one slice is shown in Figure 17.13a) allows segmentation with purely first-order methods because of the large contrast between bone and the surrounding air and the similarly large contrast between metal and bone. A region-growing process yields the

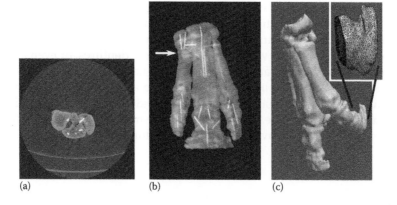

(a)   (b)   (c)

FIGURE 17.13
CT imaging results of the rhinoceros foot. (a) Raw cross-sectional CT image; one slice is shown at about the height indicated by a white arrow in (b). Bright white areas indicate metal. Below the bone, the slightly curved patient tray can be seen. The image shows dark streak artifacts that are partly attributed to beam hardening. (b) Projection view of the segmented foot where the metal regions are shown in white and the bone has been assigned a transparent color to make the embedded metal rods visible. (c) Projection view of the meshed volume, rotated to match the observer position of the inset in Figure 17.12. The inset shows a magnified section with the mesh edges highlighted.

bone area and eliminates the patient tray and the foam cushion on which the foot rested during imaging. Morphological operations were used to fill small discontinuities caused by the streak artifacts. In a second step, purely intensity-based thresholding was used to separate bone and metal. We used Crystal Image to perform these steps. A rendered view of the segmented foot, created with OpenDX, is shown in Figure 17.13b.

17.7.3 Meshing

Meshing was performed with Biomesh3D and Cleaver. A rendered image of the mesh, visualized with Paraview, can be seen in Figure 17.13c. In preparation for meshing, the volumetric image was rescaled to one-third of its original size, because Cleaver does not offer any mesh scaling option: the number of voxels in the image directly determines the number of nodes in the mesh. The bone region in the unscaled image (voxel size, 0.5 × 0.5 × 1 mm) occupies 3.5 million voxels. The number of bone voxels in the scaled image was approximately 132,000. The volume mesh produced by Cleaver was composed of 1,045,415 tetrahedral elements and 216,627 vertices. With this number of elements, a simulation run with Tochnog requires almost 16 GB of memory, and the available memory is the main limiting factor for initial mesh refinement. For example, scaling the image by 1/2 instead of 1/3 increases the number of nodes by a factor of 3.5, and memory requirement increases from 16 to 64 GB. These numbers again highlight the key role of the meshing software in image-based FEM. Objects with known analytical geometry can be meshed with much fewer elements, because the optimum model, notably with p-refinement, is known. Conversely, in image-based FEM, the optimum model is unknown, and the meshing software needs to decide to what extent p- and h-refinement can be used. In the simplest case (i.e., Cleaver), no refinement takes place. Biomesh3D allows some control over the level of detail in the mesh, but a Biomesh3D run can take several days to complete.

17.7.4 Simulation

Consistent with the limitations discussed in Section 17.6.4, we wrote a simple script that translated the Cleaver output file into a Tochnog input file. The script was also responsible for scaling the vertex coordinates by the voxel size and supplementing the loading and boundary conditions. In this example, we simulated a situation where the isolated foot rested on a surface (simulated by fixation of the nodes in space), and where a force was applied to the middle toe.

Given its skeletal form, the rhino foot was modeled as an elastic, isotropic, nonlinear solid composed of cortical bone and the titanium rods used to join and fixate the bone fragments. The strain energy (TPE) method for material deformation containing both distortional (deviatoric) and volumetric components of the deformation gradient is defined in Tochnog by

$$\rho v_i = \frac{\partial \sigma_{ij}}{\partial x_{ij}} + (1 - \beta T)\rho g_i - d\frac{\partial v_i}{\partial x_i} + f_i, \tag{17.29}$$

where
    ρ is the density of the material,
    v_i is the material velocity in the i direction,
    σ_{ij} is the material stress matrix,
    x is the space coordinate,

β is the material expansion volume, or measurement of the volume change of a solid in response to a change in pressure or stress,

T is the temperature of the material (assumed to be constant in our case),

g_i is gravity,

d is the damping coefficient of material (negligible in our case), and

f_i is the pressure tensor source (in our case, a force is applied to the middle toe).

17.7.4.1 Boundary and Loading Conditions

The following conditions were assigned to the meshed model (Figure 17.14a):

Boundary:

- Nodes corresponding to lower portions of each outer toe were fixed in the x, y, and z directions to mimic their attachment to a surface.

Loading:

- A constant load of 9.8 N ($\approx$1 kg or 2.2 lb) was applied to the nodes near the lower portion of the middle toe. In order for the force to be evenly distributed, each of the 19,777 nodes in the region was assigned a force of -4.9×10^{-4} N. This force was applied in the y direction and assigned a negative value to simulate a load directed downward onto the toe based on the rhino foot's orientation.

17.7.4.2 Material Properties

The material property input parameters and units for both materials are provided in Table 17.2.

17.7.5 Visualization

The results of the FE simulation are presented in Figure 17.14. The behavior exhibited in the rhino foot subjected to an applied load in Figure 17.14a is similar to a diver on a diving board. The board is fixated at the edge of a pool in the manner the foot is secured to the tray. The middle toe and the free edge of the diving board are comparable. As the diver walks to the end of the platform, the board is likely under minimal amounts of stress. However, once the diver jumps and lands back on the diving board in preparation for the dive, the largest stresses are observed at the point of impact, resulting in deformation of the board (strain) to accommodate the intensity of the stress (Figure 17.14b and c). This partially explains why the observed changes in stress and strain behavior are restricted to the boundary between areas of the middle toe subjected to the load and areas that are not.

In the case of the rhino foot, the bone fragment's fixation by the titanium rods near the edge of the middle toe also contributes to the stress and strain behavior observed. Additionally, the stress and strain values reported correlate with the known mechanical properties of bone and metal. Such materials exhibit high strength as reflected by their large elastic modulus values and are able to withstand large amounts of stress (in this case, 10^9 Pa) with only minimal deformation or strain (10^{-4}). Movement throughout the middle toe in response to the boundary conditions, applied load, and mechanical properties of the materials can be seen in Figure 17.14d. Although the values are relatively small $\left(10^{-4} \dfrac{\text{m}}{\text{s}} \right)$,

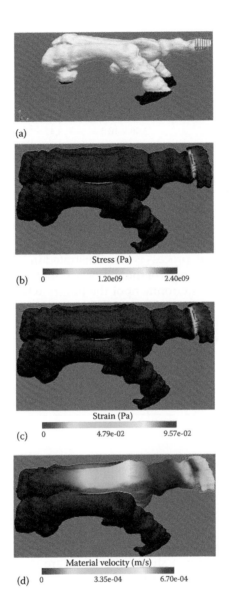

FIGURE 17.14
Visualization results of the rhino foot simulation. Boundary and loading conditions applied to the rhino foot mesh (a). All nodes of each outer toe's lower portion (black) are fixed in the x, y, and z directions. The intermediate colors represent the boundary between fixated and nonfixated nodes. A load of 9.8 N was evenly distributed over the 19,777 nodes near the end of the lower toe (orange arrows). Stress and stain distribution behavior are nearly identical and higher levels are restricted to a thin region where the bone fragment near the end of the middle toe is held in place by a titanium rod (b and c). Although the model is subjected to large amounts of stress, the strain or deformation values observed are very small in comparison. The material velocity is representative of the movement of the center toe in response to the applied load and boundary conditions (d).

TABLE 17.2

Material Property Parameters Used in FE Simulation

Property (Units)	Cortical Bone	Titanium Rods	Reference
Density, $\rho\left(\dfrac{kg}{m^3}\right)$	3.315×10^5	4.430×10^3	[101,102]
Poisson ratio	3.00×10^{-1}	3.42×10^{-1}	[102,103]
Elastic modulus, E (GPa)	18.6	113.8	[102,104]

the most movement is observed in the areas of applied force and where there is a connection of bone fragments via the titanium rods. In Figure 17.14, the effect is most prominent in the material deformation, which is represented as velocity (Figure 17.14d), that is, the spatial change of the nodes over one simulated time step Δt. Once again, the deformation is consistent with the diving-board analogy.

A side benefit of the meshing process is also illustrated in Figure 17.12. At some point, it was decided that the damaged bones of the rhinoceros foot were beyond repair and at risk of coming apart in the lively environment of the library where the skeleton is exhibited. We decided to use the meshed model (Figure 17.13c) to extract the surface and used a 3D printer to create an exact representation of the foot. The left hind foot shown in Figure 17.12 is actually the 3D-printed construct, and only very astute observers actually recognize the difference.

17.8 Future Perspective

The need for robust, completely automatic methods for image segmentation and mesh generation of geometric models obtained from medical imaging data continues to drive the research within this realm. As the capabilities of medical imaging coupled with FEA continue to expand past engineering and computational mathematics-based laboratories into hospitals and research groups composed of medical professionals, engineers, and statisticians, techniques that are accurate and reproducible, require minimal user intervention, and can generate models within a short time frame are in high demand. The evolving focus areas of computer-aided diagnosis and computer-aided visualization and analysis (CAVA) have catalyzed biomedical FEA applications and thereby are largely responsible for the formulation of such multidisciplinary teams. Computer-aided diagnosis is applied in the detection and diagnosis of disease, lesions, and abnormalities while CAVA involves the study and development of computerized methods, such as the ones discussed in this chapter, to catalyze new strategies, education, and training [29,105–107]. To provide one example, the biomechanical response behavior obtained from FEA could assist in clinical research trials to measure changes in condition attributed to drug and radiation therapies.

The creation of registration, template, and atlas-based databases; rapid prototyping; and computational fluid dynamics are a few CAVA-related developments that can further facilitate the growth of computer-aided diagnosis. Integration of a novel meshing algorithm that *morphs* itself around a presegmented medical image based on a template or atlas of the desired geometry provides a convenient way to evaluate clinical data for multiple patients at varying stages of disease and treatment [108–113]. Rapid prototyping allows the creation of physical models manufactured from 3D data obtained from medical images and is ideal for anatomical instruction/education, presurgical planning, and the design, verification, and manufacturing of medical implants and prosthetics [114–116]. Lastly, the adaptation of computational fluid dynamics, a numerical simulation technique designed for the analysis of fluids and of biphasic solid and fluidic models, to accommodate nonlinear and complex flow patterns provides real-time simulations of blood flow and cerebrospinal fluid through ventricles in the vascular and neurological cavities [117,118].

References

1. R. Courant, Variational methods for the solution of problems of equilibrium and vibrations, *Bulletin of the American Mathematical Society* 49 (1) (1943) 1–23.
2. D. J. Hawkes, D. Barratt, J. M. Blackall, C. Chan, P. J. Edwards, K. Rhode, G. P. Penney, J. McClelland, D. L. G. Hill, Tissue deformation and shape models in image-guided interventions: A discussion paper, *Medical Image Analysis* 9 (2) (2005) 163–175.
3. T. Hopp, M. Dietzel, P. Baltzer, P. Kreisel, W. Kaiser, H. Gemmeke, N. Ruiter, Automatic multi-modal 2D/3D breast image registration using biomechanical FEM models and intensity-based optimization, *Medical Image Analysis* 17 (2) (2013) 209–218.
4. K. Miller, A. Wittek, G. Joldes, A. Horton, T. Dutta-Roy, J. Berger, L. Morriss, Modelling brain deformations for computer-integrated neurosurgery, *International Journal for Numerical Methods in Biomedical Engineering* 26 (1) (2010) 117–138.
5. T. A. Sundaram, J. C. Gee, Towards a model of lung biomechanics: Pulmonary kinematics via registration of serial lung images, *Medical Image Analysis* 9 (6) (2005) 524–537.
6. J. Teo, C. Chui, Z. Wang, S. Ong, C. Yan, S. Wang, H. Wong, S. Teoh, Heterogeneous meshing and biomechanical modeling of human spine, *Medical Engineering & Physics* 29 (2) (2007) 277–290.
7. W. Parr, U. Chamoli, A. Jones, W. Walsh, S. Wroe, Finite element micro-modelling of a human ankle bone reveals the importance of the trabecular network to mechanical performance: New methods for the generation and comparison of 3D models, *Journal of Biomechanics* 46 (1) (2013) 200–205.
8. M. Mononen, M. Mikkola, P. Julkunen, R. Ojala, M. Nieminen, J. Jurvelin, R. Korhonen, Effect of superficial collagen patterns and fibrillation of femoral articular cartilage on knee joint mechanics—A 3d finite element analysis, *Journal of Biomechanics* 45 (3) (2012) 579–587.
9. M. Bajuri, M. R. A. Kadir, M. M. Raman, T. Kamarul, Mechanical and functional assessment of the wrist affected by rheumatoid arthritis: A finite element analysis, *Medical Engineering & Physics* 34 (9) (2012) 1294–1302.
10. C. Lally, F. Dolan, P. J. Prendergast, Cardiovascular stent design and vessel stresses: A finite element analysis, *Journal of Biomechanics* 38 (8) (2005) 1574–1581.
11. P. J. Prendergast, C. Lally, S. Daly, A. J. Reid, T. C. Lee, D. Quinn, F. Dolan, Analysis of prolapse in cardiovascular stents: A constitutive equation for vascular tissue and finite-element modelling, *Journal of Biomechanical Engineering* 125 (5) (2003) 692–699.
12. P. Mortier, G. Holzapfel, M. De Beule, D. Van Loo, Y. Taeymans, P. Segers, P. Verdonck, B. Verhegghe, A novel simulation strategy for stent insertion and deployment in curved coronary bifurcations: Comparison of three drug-eluting stents, *Annals of Biomedical Engineering* 38 (1) (2010) 88–99.
13. H. Huang, J. Hsu, L. Fuh, M. Tu, C. Ko, Y. Shen, Bone stress and interfacial sliding analysis of implant designs on an immediately loaded maxillary implant: A non-linear finite element study, *Journal of Dentistry* 36 (6) (2008) 409–417.
14. M. Ghajari, S. Peldschus, U. Galvanetto, L. Iannucci, Effects of the presence of the body in helmet oblique impacts, *Accident Analysis and Prevention* 50 (2013) 263–271.

15. A. Erdemir, T. M. Guess, J. Halloran, S. C. Tadepalli, T. M. Morrison, Considerations for reporting finite element analysis studies in biomechanics, *Journal of Biomechanics* 45 (4) (2012) 625–633.

16. M. A. Haidekker, *Medical Imaging Technology, SpringerBriefs Series in Physics*, Springer, New York, 2013.

17. L. Allard, G. Cloutier, L. Durand, 3D power Doppler ultrasound imaging of an in vitro arterial stenosis, *Acoustical Imaging* 23 (1997) 267–272.

18. Z. Guo, A. Fenster, Three-dimensional power doppler imaging: A phantom study to quantify vessel stenosis, *Ultrasound in Medicine and Biology* 22 (8) (1996) 1059–1069.

19. Z. Guo, L.-G. Durand, L. Allard, G. Cloutier, A. Fenster, In vitro evaluation of multiple arterial stenoses using three-dimensional power doppler angiography, *Journal of Vascular Surgery* 27 (4) (1998) 681–688.

20. G. Cloutier, Z. Qin, D. Garcia, G. Soulez, V. Oliva, L.-G. Durand, Assessment of arterial stenosis in a flow model with power Doppler angiography: Accuracy and observations on blood echogenicity, *Ultrasound in Medicine and Biology* 26 (9) (2000) 1489–1501.

21. C.-K. Chui, Z. Wang, J. Zhang, J. S.-K. Ong, L. Bian, J. C.-M. Teo, C.-H. Yan, S.-H. Ong, S.-C. Wang, H.-K. Wong, S.-H. Teoh, A component-oriented software toolkit for patient-specific finite element model generation, *Advances in Engineering Software* 40 (3) (2009) 184–192.

22. R. Andresen, H. J. Werner, H. C. Schober, Contribution of the cortical shell of vertebrae to mechanical behaviour of the lumbar vertebrae with implications for predicting fracture risk, *British Journal of Radiology* 71 (847) (1998) 759–765.

23. C.-S. Kuo, H.-T. Hu, R.-M. Lin, K.-Y. Huang, P.-C. Lin, Z.-C. Zhong, M.-L. Hseih, Biomechanical analysis of the lumbar spine on facet joint force and intradiscal pressure—A finite element study, *BMC Musculoskeletal Disorders* 11 (1) (2010) 1–13.

24. D. Withey, Z. Koles, Medical image segmentation: Methods and software, in: *Noninvasive Functional Source Imaging of the Brain and Heart and the International Conference on Functional Biomedical Imaging, 2007. NFSI-ICFBI 2007. Joint Meeting of the 6th International Symposium on*, IEEE, 2007, pp. 140–143.

25. M. Gao, J. Huang, X. Huang, S. Zhang, D. Metaxas, Simplified labeling process for medical image segmentation, in: *Medical Image Computing and Computer-Assisted Intervention–MICCAI 2012*, 2012, pp. 387–394.

26. G. Dougherty, *Digital Image Processing for Medical Applications*, Vol. 1, Cambridge University Press, Cambridge, United Kingdom, 2009.

27. M. Haidekker, *Advanced Biomedical Image Analysis*, John Wiley & Sons, Hoboken, NJ, 2011.

28. K. Ciesielski, J. Udupa, A framework for comparing different image segmentation methods and its use in studying equivalences between level set and fuzzy connectedness frameworks, *Computer Vision and Image Understanding* 115 (6) (2011) 721–734.

29. X. Chen, J. K. Udupa, A. Alavi, D. A. Torigian, GC-ASM: Synergistic integration of graph-cut and active shape model strategies for medical image segmentation, *Computer Vision and Image Understanding* 117 (5) (2013) 513–524.

30. M. Kass, A. Witkin, D. Terzopoulos, Snakes: Active contour models, *International Journal of Computer Vision* 1 (4) (1988) 321–331.

31. R. Malladi, J. Sethian, B. Vemuri, Shape modeling with front propagation: A level set approach, *Pattern Analysis and Machine Intelligence, IEEE Transactions on* 17 (2) (1995) 158–175.

32. S. Osher, R. P. Fedkiw, Level set methods: An overview and some recent results, *Journal of Computational Physics* 169 (2) (2001) 463–502.

33. A. X. Falcão, J. K. Udupa, S. Samarasekera, S. Sharma, B. E. Hirsch, R. D. A. Lotufo, User-steered image segmentation paradigms: Live wire and live lane, *Graphical Models and Image Processing* 60 (4) (1998) 233–260.

34. S. Lloyd, Least squares quantization in PCM, *Information Theory, IEEE Transactions on* 28 (2) (1982) 129–137.

35. J. C. Bezdek, *Pattern Recognition with Fuzzy Objective Function Algorithms*, Kluwer Academic Publishers, Norwell, MA, 1981.

36. Y. Boykov, G. Funka-Lea, Graph cuts and efficient ND image segmentation, *International Journal of Computer Vision* 70 (2) (2006) 109–131.
37. L. Vincent, P. Soille, Watersheds in digital spaces: An efficient algorithm based on immersion simulations, *IEEE Transactions on Pattern Analysis and Machine Intelligence* 13 (6) (1991) 583–598.
38. J. K. Udupa, S. Samarasekera, Fuzzy connectedness and object definition: Theory, algorithms, and applications in image segmentation, *Graphical Models and Image Processing* 58 (3) (1996) 246–261.
39. A. K. Jain, R. P. W. Duin, J. Mao, Statistical pattern recognition: A review, *Pattern Analysis and Machine Intelligence, IEEE Transactions on* 22 (1) (2000) 4–37.
40. K. I. Laws, Texture energy measures, in: *Proc. DARPA Image Understanding Workshop*, 1979, pp. 47–51.
41. R. K. Yip, P. K. Tam, D. N. Leung, Modification of Hough transform for circles and ellipses detection using a 2-dimensional array, *Pattern Recognition* 25 (9) (1992) 1007–1022.
42. T. Cootes, C. Taylor, D. Cooper, J. Graham, Active shape models—Their training and application, *Computer Vision and Image Understanding* 61 (1) (1995) 38–59.
43. T. Cootes, G. Edwards, C. Taylor, Active appearance models, in: *Computer VisionECCV98*, 1998, pp. 484–498.
44. T. Heimann, H.-P. Meinzer, Statistical shape models for 3D medical image segmentation: A review, *Medical Image Analysis* 13 (4) (2009) 543–563.
45. D. Lesage, E. D. Angelini, I. Bloch, G. Funka-Lea, A review of 3D vessel lumen segmentation techniques: Models, features and extraction schemes, *Medical Image Analysis* 13 (6) (2009) 819–845.
46. S. Ghose, A. Oliver, R. Martí, X. Lladó, J. C. Vilanova, J. Freixenet, J. Mitra, D. Sidibé, F. Meriaudeau, A survey of prostate segmentation methodologies in ultrasound, magnetic resonance and computed tomography images, *Computer Methods and Programs in Biomedicine* 108 (1) (2012) 262–287.
47. Z. Dokur, T. Ölmez, Segmentation of ultrasound images by using a hybrid neural network, *Pattern Recognition Letters* 23 (14) (2002) 1825–1836.
48. C. Petitjean, J.-N. Dacher, A review of segmentation methods in short axis cardiac MR images, *Medical Image Analysis* 15 (2) (2011) 169–184.
49. M. M. Fraz, P. Remagnino, A. Hoppe, B. Uyyanonvara, A. R. Rudnicka, C. G. Owen, S. A. Barman, Blood vessel segmentation methodologies in retinal images—A survey, *Computer Methods and Programs in Biomedicine* 108 (1) (2012) 407–433.
50. L. Szilágyi, S. M. Szilágyi, B. Benyó, Z. Benyó, Intensity inhomogeneity compensation and segmentation of mr brain images using hybrid c-means clustering models, *Biomedical Signal Processing and Control* 6 (1) (2011) 3–12.
51. A. P. Dhawan, S. Juvvadi, Knowledge-based analysis and understanding of medical images, *Computer Methods and Programs in Biomedicine* 33 (4) (1990) 221–239.
52. F. Masulli, A. Schenone, A fuzzy clustering based segmentation system as support to diagnosis in medical imaging, *Artificial Intelligence in Medicine* 16 (2) (1999) 129–147.
53. M. Clark, L. Hall, D. Goldgof, R. Velthuizen, F. Murtagh, M. Silbiger, Automatic tumor segmentation using knowledge-based techniques, *Medical Imaging, IEEE Transactions on* 17 (2) (1998) 187–201.
54. D. Zhang, S. Chen, A novel kernelized fuzzy c-means algorithm with application in medical image segmentation, *Artificial Intelligence in Medicine* 32 (1) (2004) 37–50.
55. A. Papadopoulos, D. Fotiadis, A. Likas, An automatic microcalcification detection system based on a hybrid neural network classifier, *Artificial Intelligence in Medicine* 25 (2) (2002) 149–167.
56. F. Xie, A. C. Bovik, Automatic segmentation of dermoscopy images using self-generating neural networks seeded by genetic algorithm, *Pattern Recognition* 46 (3) (2013) 1012–1019.
57. S. Gibson, Constrained elastic surface nets: Generating smooth surfaces from binary segmented data, in: *Medical Image Computing and Computer-Assisted Intervention MICCAI98*, 1998, pp. 888–898.
58. W. Lorensen, H. Cline, Marching cubes: A high resolution 3D surface construction algorithm, *Computer Graphics* 21 (4) (1987) 163–169.

59. I. Takanashi, S. Muraki, A. Doi, A. Kaufman, 3D active net for volume extraction, in: *Proc. SPIE*, Vol. 3298, 1998, pp. 184–193.

60. M. A. Yerry, M. S. Shephard, Automatic three-dimensional mesh generation by the modified-octree technique, *International Journal for Numerical Methods in Engineering* 20 (11) (1984) 1965–1990.

61. M. S. Shephard, M. K. Georges, Automatic three-dimensional mesh generation by the finite octree technique, *International Journal for Numerical Methods in Engineering* 32 (4) (1991) 709–749.

62. S. Lo, Volume discretization into tetrahedra—I. Verification and orientation of boundary surfaces, *Computers & Structures* 39 (5) (1991) 493–500.

63. S. Lo, Volume discretization into tetrahedra—II. 3d triangulation by advancing front approach, *Computers & Structures* 39 (5) (1991) 501–511.

64. B. Delaunay, Sur la sphère vide, *Izvestia Akademii Nauk SSSR: Otdelenie Matematicheskikh i Estestvennykh Nauk* 7 (1934) 793–800.

65. T. D. Blacker, R. J. Meyers, Seams and wedges in plastering: A 3-d hexahedral mesh generation algorithm, *Engineering with Computers* 9 (2) (1993) 83–93.

66. T. Li, R. McKeag, C. Armstrong, Hexahedral meshing using midpoint subdivision and integer programming, *Computer Methods in Applied Mechanics and Engineering* 124 (1) (1995) 171–193.

67. R. Schneiders, A grid-based algorithm for the generation of hexahedral element meshes, *Engineering with Computers* 12 (3) (1996) 168–177.

68. T. J. Tautges, T. Blacker, S. A. Mitchell, The whisker weaving algorithm: A connectivity-based method for constructing all-hexahedral finite element meshes, *International Journal for Numerical Methods in Engineering* 39 (19) (1996) 3327–3349.

69. Z. Yu, M. J. Holst, J. Andrew McCammon, High-fidelity geometric modeling for biomedical applications, *Finite Elements in Analysis and Design* 44 (11) (2008) 715–723.

70. S. Azernikov, A. Miropolsky, A. Fischer, Surface reconstruction of freeform objects based on multiresolution volumetric method, in: *Proceedings of the Eighth ACM Symposium on Solid Modeling and Applications*, ACM, 2003, pp. 115–126.

71. Y. Zhang, C. Bajaj, B.-S. Sohn, 3d finite element meshing from imaging data, *Computer Methods in Applied Mechanics and Engineering* 194 (48) (2005) 5083–5106.

72. N. Ribeiro, P. Fernandes, D. Lopes, J. Folgado, P. Fernandes, 3-d solid and finite element modeling of biomechanical structures-a software pipeline, in: J. Ambròsio (Ed.), *Proceedings of the 7th EUROMECH Solid Mechanics Conference*, Lisbon, Portugal, 2009.

73. G. B. Dantzig, L. R. Ford, D. R. Fulkerson, A primal-dual algorithm for linear programs, *Linear Inequalities and Related Systems* (38) (1956) 171–181.

74. L. A. Freitag, C. Ollivier-Gooch, Tetrahedral mesh improvement using swapping and smoothing, *International Journal for Numerical Methods in Engineering* 40 (21) (1997) 3979–4002.

75. T. Ju, F. Losasso, S. Schaefer, J. Warren, Dual contouring of hermite data, *ACM Transactions on Graphics (TOG)* 21 (3) (2002) 339–346.

76. S. Schaefer, J. Warren, Dual marching cubes: Primal contouring of dual grids, *Computer Graphics Forum* 24 (2005) 195–201.

77. S. Schaefer, T. Ju, J. Warren, Manifold dual contouring, *Visualization and Computer Graphics, IEEE Transactions on* 13 (3) (2007) 610–619.

78. L. R. Herrmann, Laplacian-isoparametric grid generation scheme, *Journal of the Engineering Mechanics Division* 102 (5) (1976) 749–907.

79. L. Freitag, M. Jones, P. Plassmann, A parallel algorithm for mesh smoothing, *SIAM Journal on Scientific Computing* 20 (6) (1999) 2023–2040.

80. M. Puso, J. Solberg, A stabilized nodally integrated tetrahedral, *International Journal for Numerical Methods in Engineering* 67 (6) (2006) 841–867.

81. D. L. Camacho, R. H. Hopper, G. M. Lin, B. S. Myers, An improved method for finite element mesh generation of geometrically complex structures with application to the skullbase, *Journal of Biomechanics* 30 (10) (1997) 1067–1070.

82. A. Cifuentes, A. Kalbag, A performance study of tetrahedral and hexahedral elements in 3-D finite element structural analysis, *Finite Elements in Analysis and Design* 12 (3) (1992) 313–318.

83. V. I. Weingarten, The controversy over hex or tet meshing, *Machine Design* 66 (8) (1994) 74–76.
84. A. Ramos, J. Simoes, Tetrahedral versus hexahedral finite elements in numerical modelling of the proximal femur, *Medical Engineering & Physics* 28 (9) (2006) 916–924.
85. K. H. Shivanna, S. C. Tadepalli, N. M. Grosland, Feature-based multiblock finite element mesh generation, *Computer-Aided Design* 42 (12) (2010) 1108–1116.
86. Z. Wang, J. Teo, C. Chui, S. Ong, C. Yan, S. Wang, H. Wong, S. Teoh, Computational biomechanical modelling of the lumbar spine using marching-cubes surface smoothened finite element voxel meshing, *Computer Methods and Programs in Biomedicine* 80 (1) (2005) 25–35.
87. D. Thompson, J. Braun, R. Ford, *OpenDX—Paths to Visualization*, Visualization and Imagery Solutions, Inc., Missoula, MT, 2001.
88. G.-H. Kwon, S.-W. Chae, K.-J. Lee, Automatic generation of tetrahedral meshes from medical images, *Computers and Structures* 81 (2003) 765–775.
89. W. Lee, T.-S. Kim, M. Cho, Y. Ahn, S. Lee, Methods and evaluations of MRI content-adaptive finite element mesh generation for bioelectromagnetic problems, *Physics in Medicine and Biology* 51 (2006) 6173–6186.
90. P. Perré, Meshpore: A software able to apply image-based meshing techniques to anisotropic and heterogeneous porous media, *Drying Technology* 23 (2005) 1993–2006.
91. A. Rosset, L. Spadola, O. Ratib, Osirix: An open-source software for navigating in multidimensional dicom images, *Journal of Digital Imaging* 17 (3) (2004) 205–216.
92. N. M. Grosland, K. H. Shivanna, V. A. Magnotta, N. A. Kallemeyn, N. A. DeVries, S. C. Tadepalli, C. Lisle, IA-FEMesh: An open-source, interactive, multiblock approach to anatomic finite element model development, *Computer Methods and Programs in Biomedicine* 94 (1) (2009) 96–107.
93. L. Antiga, M. Piccinelli, L. Botti, B. Ene-Iordache, A. Remuzzi, D. A. Steinman, An image-based modeling framework for patient-specific computational hemodynamics, *Medical and Biological Engineering and Computing* 46 (11) (2008) 1097–1112.
94. Q. Fang, D. A. Boas, Tetrahedral mesh generation from volumetric binary and gray-scale images, in: *Proceedings of the Sixth IEEE International Conference on Symposium on Biomedical Imaging: From Nano to Macro*, IEEE Press, 2009, pp. 1142–1145.
95. J. R. Bronson, J. A. Levine, R. T. Whitaker, Lattice cleaving: Conforming tetrahedral meshes of multimaterial domains with bounded quality, in: *Proceedings of the 21st International Meshing Roundtable*, Springer, 2013, pp. 191–209.
96. S. K. Boyd, R. Müller, Smooth surface meshing for automated finite element model generation from 3D image data, *Journal of Biomechanics* 39 (7) (2006) 1287–1295.
97. A. Madison, M. A. Haidekker, A completely open-source finite element modeling chain for tubular tissue-engineered constructs, *International Journal of Computer Science and Application (IJCSA)* 1 (2) (2012) 44–55.
98. S. A. Maas, B. J. Ellis, G. A. Ateshian, J. A. Weiss, FEBio: Finite elements for biomechanics, *Journal of Biomechanical Engineering* 134 (1) (2012) 011005-01–011005–10.
99. M. Jolley et al. Open-source environment for interactive finite element modeling of optimal ICD electrode placement. in: *Functional Imaging and Modeling of the Heart*, Springer, Berlin, Heidelberg, 2007, pp. 373–382.
100. M. Jolley, J. Stinstra, S. Pieper, R. MacLeod, D. H. Brooks, F. Cecchin, J. K. Triedman, A computer modeling tool for comparing novel ICD electrode orientations in children and adults, *Heart Rhythm* 5 (4) (2008) 565–572.
101. R. Andresen, M. Haidekker, S. Radmer, D. Banzer, CT determination of bone mineral density and structural investigations on the axial skeleton for estimating the osteoporosis-related fracture risk by means of a risk score, *British Journal of Radiology* 72 (858) (1999) 569–578.
102. R. F. Boyer, E. Collings, *Materials Properties Handbook: Titanium Alloys*, ASM International, Materials Park, OH, 1994.
103. D. C. Wirtz, N. Schiffers, T. Pandorf, K. Radermacher, D. Weichert, R. Forst, Critical evaluation of known bone material properties to realize anisotropic FE-simulation of the proximal femur, *Journal of Biomechanics* 33 (10) (2000) 1325–1330.

104. M. Cuppone, B. Seedhom, E. Berry, A. Ostell, The longitudinal Youngs modulus of cortical bone in the midshaft of human femur and its correlation with CT scanning data, *Calcified Tissue International* 74 (3) (2004) 302–309.
105. J. K. Udupa, V. R. LeBlanc, Y. Zhuge, C. Imielinska, H. Schmidt, L. M. Currie, B. E. Hirsch, J. Woodburn, A framework for evaluating image segmentation algorithms, *Computerized Medical Imaging and Graphics* 30 (2) (2006) 75–87.
106. K. Doi, Computer-aided diagnosis in medical imaging: Historical review, current status and future potential, *Computerized Medical Imaging and Graphics* 31 (4–5) (2007) 198–211.
107. H. Kobatake, Future cad in multi-dimensional medical images: Project on multi-organ, multi-disease cad system, *Computerized Medical Imaging and Graphics* 31 (4) (2007) 258–266.
108. L. Baghdadi, D. A. Steinman, H. M. Ladak, Template-based finite-element mesh generation from medical images, *Computer Methods and Programs in Biomedicine* 77 (1) (2005) 11–21.
109. I. A. Sigal, M. R. Hardisty, C. M. Whyne, Mesh-morphing algorithms for specimen-specific finite element modeling, *Journal of Biomechanics* 41 (7) (2008) 1381–1389.
110. M. A. Baldwin, J. E. Langenderfer, P. J. Rullkoetter, P. J. Laz, Development of subject-specific and statistical shape models of the knee using an efficient segmentation and mesh-morphing approach, *Computer Methods and Programs in Biomedicine* 97 (3) (2010) 232–240.
111. M. Bucki, C. Lobos, Y. Payan, A fast and robust patient specific finite element mesh registration technique: Application to 60 clinical cases, *Medical Image Analysis* 14 (3) (2010) 303–317.
112. G. D. Santis, M. D. Beule, K. V. Canneyt, P. Segers, P. Verdonck, B. Verhegghe, Full-hexahedral structured meshing for image-based computational vascular modeling, *Medical Engineering & Physics* 33 (10) (2011) 1318–1325.
113. C. Lederman, A. Joshi, I. Dinov, L. Vese, A. Toga, J. D. V. Horn, The generation of tetrahedral mesh models for neuroanatomical MRI, *NeuroImage* 55 (1) (2011) 153–164.
114. R. Petzold, H.-F. Zeilhofer, W. Kalender, Rapid prototyping technology in medicinebasics and applications, *Computerized Medical Imaging and Graphics* 23 (5) (1999) 277–284.
115. R. Bibb, J. Winder, A review of the issues surrounding three-dimensional computed tomography for medical modelling using rapid prototyping techniques, *Radiography* 16 (1) (2010) 78–83.
116. T. Boehler, D. van Straaten, S. Wirtz, H.-O. Peitgen, A robust and extendible framework for medical image registration focused on rapid clinical application deployment, *Computers in Biology and Medicine* 41 (6) (2011) 340–349.
117. K. B. Chandran, S. C. Vigmostad, Patient-specific bicuspid valve dynamics: Overview of methods and challenges, *Journal of Biomechanics* 46 (2) (2013) 208–216.
118. V. Kurtcuoglu, D. Poulikakos, Y. Ventikos, Computational modeling of the mechanical behavior of the cerebrospinal fluid system, *Transactions of the ASME-K-Journal of Biomechanical Engineering* 127 (2) (2005) 264–269.

Index

Page numbers followed by f and t indicate figures and tables, respectively.